Cells,
Aging, and
Human Disease

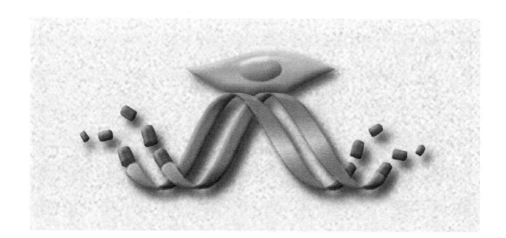

Cells, Aging, and Human Disease

MICHAEL B. FOSSEL, M.D., PH.D.

OXFORD
UNIVERSITY PRESS
2004

OXFORD
UNIVERSITY PRESS

Oxford   New York
Auckland   Bangkok   Buenos Aires   Cape Town   Chennai
Dar es Salaam   Delhi   Hong Kong   Istanbul   Karachi   Kolkata
Kuala Lumpur   Madrid   Melbourne   Mexico City   Mumbai   Nairobi
São Paulo   Shanghai   Taipei   Tokyo   Toronto

Published by Oxford University Press, Inc.,
198 Madison Avenue, New York, New York, 10016

www.oup.com

Oxford is a registered trademark of Oxford University Press

Library of Congress Cataloging-in-Publication Data
Fossel, Michael.
Cells, aging, and human disease /
Michael B. Fossel.
p. cm.   Includes bibliographical references and index.
ISBN 0-19-514035-4
1. Aging.
2. Cells—Aging.   I. Title.
QP86.F68 2004   612.6'7—dc22   2003060938

Cover and frontpiece figures adapted from
and courtesy of Geron Corporation.

9 8 7 6 5 4 3 2 1

Printed in the United States of America
on acid-free paper

To Len Hayflick

Good comes from those who care what others think; greatness, from those that don't.

To Louis Pasteur and Robert Koch

Great ideas pivot on the Janus'd cusp of history: looking forward they are obviously foolish, looking backwards they appear foolishly obvious. We are doubly blind.

Acknowledgments

My thanks to the following—friends mostly—who have my respect and who made this book a necessity and a possibility. If they hadn't done so much work, they could have saved me (and the reader) a lot of bother. My gray hair and presbyopia are their doing. This is (more or less) the book that they had wanted me to write the first time.

Bill Andrews (for working too hard and laughing)

Bob Arking (wine and cheese on Lake Tahoe)

Bob Butler (who still owes me a paper)

Judy Campisi (whose fairness won)

Vince Cristofalo (we never age anyway)

Rita Effros (and her laughter)

Richard Faragher (and Marrakech)

Tuck Finch (and his leather vest)

Walter Funk (and microbrews in Menlo Park)

George Martin (and his wife's seeds in Italy)

Barbara Gilchrest (who wanted something here)

Carol Greider (her letter to my RHA editor)

Cal Harley (for the candy jar and his TTAGGG stool)

Len Hayflick (Len and Ruth, laughing at dinner)

Tom Kirkwood (who arranged Italy)

Mark Lane (for making me executive director)

Owen McGettrick (for everything)

Graham Pawelec (for e-mail)

Olivia Pereira-Smith (for a Tuscany hilltown)

Suresh Rattan (and dinner in Aarhus)

Michael Rose (and the Roman Empire)

George Roth (why couldn't he be sole director?)

Jerry Shay (and his hot tub)

Hubert Warner (and the NIA)

Bob Weinberg (for speaking)

Rick Weindruch (jogging with me in San Antonio)

Mike West (who can never be found)

Woody Wright (his famous guitar)

Apologia

There are limitations—intrinsic and human, absolute and relative—in writing a book on cell senescence, aging, and disease. Four limitations played foremost in this text and circumscribed its outcome:

1. The entire field cannot be covered. Having to shortchange something, I neglect dozens of areas from telomere structure to cholesterol metabolism, methylation to tau proteins, free radical scavengers to presbyopia. The restriction here is one of focus; available pages and reader interest dictate a Procrustean approach to textbook writing.

2. Even a defined area cannot be covered flawlessly, and here the fault is a human one. None of us perhaps—not myself certainly—can perfectly comprehend and plainly convey a topic as large as this one, even shorn of its conceptual appendages.

3. Even with genius, the field is full of pitfalls and lacunae. Much is unknown, some of what we think is known is probably in error, and the result is uneven coverage and an inconsistency not due to human limitation but scientific limitation. Writing demands that we accept what we daily work to overcome in science.

4. Finally, health of a field is implied if a book is out of date before it is published. Literature progresses in all directions. Flux and evolution of a field are the delight of the researcher, the curse of the writer.

Request to the Careful Reader

Error-free textbooks are impossible for human authors. The copy editor (doubtless with *Fowler's Modern English Usage* encoded in her genes) corrected hundreds of stylistic errors and, by extrapolation and Bayesian statistics, thereby increased the already high probability that this text must contain undiscovered substantive errors. The author is grateful to readers who find such errors (whether of commission, omission, or intention), and email them to oxfordtext@earthlink.net, so that the second edition, already in progress, may prove more useful and accurate for future readers. Thank you.

Preface

The major danger of technology is not that we may play God, but that we may refuse to work at being fully human. Compassion is the highest of human motivations, allowing us first to understand, then to prevent, the suffering, fear, and tragedy of others. Our enemy is not death, which will forever be with us, but avoidable suffering, which need not be. The ubiquity of disease is no more ordained than is the rarity of individual compassion, but it is in our power to lessen the former through our dedication to the latter.

The aim is to understand how diseases of aging occur, that we may prevent human suffering. Helping those around us is not "playing God," but is, if it has a sacred meaning, God's *work*. To denigrate this dedication, to avoid our responsibility, to ignore the suffering of those around us is neither human nor forgivable. We cannot assume that if someone suffers, the creator of the universe must have wanted it that way. Our ignorance of divine intent is no justification for a lack of mercy.

Finally, the age of those who suffer does not mitigate nor alter our responsibility to them. Few are callous enough to ignore the suffering of children, some would ignore and trivialize suffering in the elderly. Having been children, perhaps we remember our own helplessness and fear, yet remain unable to predict or understand the suffering of those who walk ahead of us in time. Compassion for the young is common; an equal compassion for the old should be no less equally common. Its lack indicts our basest egoism and rests upon a willful ignorance of life.

Contents

Part I   The Aging Cell

1. The Context, 3

2. Cell Senescence, 16

    Telomeres, Telomerase, and Cell Senescence, 16
    The History of Cell Senescence, 24
    Telomerase and Its Function, 28
    Is Telomerase Good for Anything?, 33

3. Cell Senescence in Aging, 38

    What Is Cell Senescence?, 38
    The Limited Model: Cells Senesce, 45
    The General Model: Cell Senescence Results in Organismal Aging, 56
    FERTILIZATION RESETS TELOMERE EFFECTS, 59
    CRITICISM GONE AWRY, 61
    CELLS TO ORGANISMS, 63

4. The Aging Cascade, 66

    The Jigsaw Puzzle of Aging, 66
    Upstream from Cell Division, 71
    Cell Turnover and Gene Expression, 71
    Between Cells: Cells, Tissues, and Pathology, 73

5. Cancer, 75

    Cancer in Its Cellular Context, 75
    Cancer and Cell Senescence, 76

Diagnosis, 79
DERMAL CANCER, 82
HEMATOPOETIC CANCER, 83
PULMONARY CANCER, 85
BREAST CANCER, 87
MALE GENITAL CANCER, 90
FEMALE GENITAL CANCER, 92
RENAL AND URINARY TRACT CANCER, 97
GASTROINTESTINAL CANCER, 99
CENTRAL NERVOUS SYSTEM CANCER, 104
OTHER CANCER, 107
Prognosis, 108
Therapy, 110

6. Parasitic Disease, 122

    Pathology and Incidence, 122
    Cell Senescence and Intervention, 124

Part II   The Aging Organism

7. The Progerias, 129

    What They Are, 129
    Werner Syndrome, 130
    Hutchinson-Gilford Syndrome, 133

8. The Skin, 140

    Structure and Overview, 140
    Aging and Other Pathology, 143
    The Role of Cell Senescence, 147
    Intervention, 157

9. Cardiovascular System, 161

    Structure and Overview, 161
    Aging and Other Pathology, 162
    The Role of Cell Senescence, 168
    Intervention, 173

10. Orthopedic Systems, 179

    Structure and Overview, 179
    Aging and Other Pathology, 181
    The Role of Cell Senescence, 184
    Intervention, 187

11. Hematopoetic and Immune Systems, 191

    Structure and Overview, 191
    Aging and Other Pathology, 192
    The Role of Cell Senescence, 195
    REGULATION OF TELOMERASE EXPRESSION, 200

CELL SENESCENCE IN OTHER HEMATOLOGIC DISEASE STATES, 202
Intervention, 205

12. Endocrine Systems, 208

    Structure and Overview, 208
    Aging and Other Pathology, 211
    The Role of Cell Senescence, 217
    Intervention, 220

13. Nervous System, 224

    Structure and Overview, 224
    Aging and Other Pathology, 227
    The Role of Cell Senescence, 234
    Intervention, 238

14. Kidneys, 245

    Structure and Overview, 245
    Aging and Other Pathology, 248
    The Role of Cell Senescence, 249
    Intervention, 250

15. Muscle, 252

    Structure and Overview, 252
    Aging and Other Pathology, 253
    The Role of Cell Senescence, 256
    Intervention, 258

16. Gastrointestinal System, 261

    Structure and Overview, 261
    Aging and Other Pathology, 263
    The Role of Cell Senescence, 267
    Intervention, 270

17. The Eye, 271

    Structure and Overview, 271
    Aging and Other Pathology, 273
    The Role of Cell Senescence, 277
    Intervention, 280

18. Towards Therapy, 283

    Interventions, 283
    TECHNIQUES, 284
    CAVEATS, 288
    OBSTACLES, 288
    Implications, 289

    References, 291

    Index, 469

PART I

The Aging Cell

CHAPTER 1

The Context

*A*GING is cell aging.

This bald statement, shorn of caveats and qualifications, is a simplistic (and so inaccurate) statement of the cell senescence model of aging. While reflecting the central tenet of this book, the model as proposed is complex, misunderstood, and ardently disputed and has little direct, confirming data. Despite this, a growing body of experimental work and the powerful implications of the hypothesis (Fossel, 1996; Liu, 1999) make it imperative that the model be defined, allowing it to become understood, testable, and perhaps even disproved.

Although the central role of cells in human disease was first described by Rudolph Virchow one and a half centuries ago (Virchow, 1858), the invocation of cell senescence in this context is of more recent provenance. First described by Hayflick and Moorhead (1961), cell senescence has been a tempting model to explain aging and aging disease (Martin, 1977a).

Ironically, although the hypothesis has never been clearly formulated, it has received frequent criticism in absentia. It is tempting to cite Darwin's (1859) dismissal of such critics as "writers who have not taken the trouble to understand the subject," but the fault lies in necessarily understanding two abstruse and interrelated areas: cell biology and human pathology. Although cell biology is necessary to an accurate understanding of human pathology (Rubin, 2002b), it is the latter—human pathology—that is of primary concern here. The focus of this book is on the pathology, but fundamental therapy for age-related disease requires the language and facts of cell biology. Pathology (and, by implication, therapy) remains paramount, however, and is required if we are to understand what cell biology has to tell us.

Lacking this macaronic understanding of the pathology, some (e.g., Wallace, 2000) have stated that cell senescence cannot play a role in aging diseases because cells do not divide in relevant organs. Likewise, Clarke (1999) suggests that cell senescence cannot play a clinical role because "the majority of cells in our bodies" don't senesce. Others (Goyns and Lavery, 2000) have suggested that not only do most cells not senesce, but there is insufficient senescence among those that do to have a clinical impact. Human pathology contradicts assumptions that cells are identical or function independently, or that senescence is an all-or-nothing affair. The common mistake is confusing nondividing cells with cells central to the pathology (Martin, 1977b), resulting in a counterfeit certainty (Macieira-Coelho, 2000). Consider Kirkwood's (1999, p 157) conclusion that since brains and muscles "certainly age" and the cells of those organs don't divide (approximately true), then cell aging cannot play a role in aging disease (Kirkwood, 2001). Paraphrasing, since myocardial cells don't divide, cell division couldn't play a role in age-related heart disease such as myocardial infarction. Similar desultory reasoning suggests that since myocardial cells do not accumulate cholesterol, cholesterol couldn't possibly play a role in myocardial infarctions. Experience suggests otherwise.

A mutual understanding of cell biology and pathology is rare and ill-conceived conclusions are the result. The pathology of aging and many diseases are consistent with the cell senescence model, although there is only a modicum of data implying causation. A more seduous view is occasionally personified in de Grey (1999), who concludes that the model is consistent with human pathology. Aging and age-related pathology might be caused by senescing cells whose dysfunction might in turn "harm non-dividing cells." He merely faults the model as unproven, which summarizes its current status (Rudolph et al., 1999).

The aim is to understand how cell senescence affects human aging and disease, separating what is known from the speculative and elusive. This aim is not academic, but that we may intervene in diseases. Voltaire (1764), echoing Cicero's earlier dictum (Einhard, 1960), said that a book "must be new and useful, or at least have great charm." Lacking charm, the hope is that this book will provide something new and useful.

The urge to ameliorate aging was first recorded in the *Epic of Gilgamesh* 4700 years ago (Sandars, 1960). Gilgamesh obtains a plant that "restores his lost youth to a man," then loses it, in a conspicuously Biblical motif, to a snake. Fourteen hundred years later, Egypt gave us far grander examples of immortality, although none of age reversal. This difference—between a merely long or a healthy life—remains a quotidian ethical distinction, echoed in hospitals and nursing homes.

In classical Greece, Aurora, daughter of Zeus, loved Tithynos, a mortal. At her pleading, Tithynos obtained immortality, but not eternal youth. He became older and older, his body crippled, his mind gone until, "he babbled endlessly, words of no meaning" (Hamilton, 1940). At what price is immortality, if paid for in the coin of dementia?

In an ironic blessing, modern biology cannot offer immortality but instead offers a chance, through an understanding of disease, to treat and prevent human suffering. It is dementia we wish to prevent, not merely early death. Treating the diseases of aging is more desirable than a fictional immortality. Our fear, that like Tithynos we might simply extend dependence and disease, is groundless. Extending the human lifespan *cannot be done without preventing age-related disease*. Reasonably, we prefer the death of Tithynos's son Memnon at the gates of Troy: healthy and active to the end. Luckily, this preference encompasses the goal and spirit of modern biology. We may achieve the opposite of Tithynos, not the irony and pathos. His minatory myth is, thank God, inconsistent with human biology.

Until recently, not only had aging interventions eluded us but even a consensus understanding appeared suspect. Recently, however, cell biology has given us novel and accurate insight into aging, recasting apparent certainties (Rose and Nusbaum, 1994; Rose, 1999a). Historically, we have increased mean but not maximum lifespan. In early hominids, maximum lifespan may have been far less (Smith, 1993), but within historical times, the maximum has been stable at about 120 years.

The threefold increase in mean lifespan over two centuries contrasts markedly with an immutable maximum lifespan (Fig. 1–1). In developed nations, mean lifespan has gone from approximately 25 years (1800), to 50 years (1900), to the current 75 years (2000). Even these rough figures raise the hackles of academic demographers: historical data are sparse and unreliable; compared to the privileged, figures for most of the population are unreliable; and previous populations are inappropriate for modern comparisons. Nonetheless, due to several social and medical factors, mean lifespan has tripled while the maximum hasn't budged. Rectangularization of the survival curve implies that mean lifespan responds to behavioral, dietary, and medical interventions, but the maximum lifespan is "pinned" by fundamental, elusive biological constraints (Kirkwood, 1996; Holloszy, 2000; Kvitko, 2001). Retrospectively, there is nothing to suggest that maximum lifespan has been or ever will be extended. Contrary claims have been the result of insufficiently large samples (i.e., less than a billion, as in Wilmoth et al., 2000), exaggerations, outright fictions, or unsubstantiated data. Such exaggerations include Marco Polo's 150- to 200-year-old Indian Yogis who ate only rice, milk, sulphur, and, in spectacular disregard for their safety or lifespan, mercury (Latham, 1958). Yogis were pulling Polo's leg or he, ours. Dozens of other fictional candidates exist, such as Candide's 172-year-old man drinking liqueurs in El Dorado's diamond goblets (Voltaire, 1759) or Elie Wiesel's codification of the Wandering Jew legends (Wiesel, 1968). Claimants abound in the literature of each age and culture. Perhaps the most well-known, in the Judeo-Christian tradition, are the antediluvian biblical patriarchs living almost a thousand years, until God apparently changed his mind with Noah, and limited us to 120 years (Genesis 6:3). There is a time beyond which God no longer "strives" in a person (Hebrew: "Y'don"). Buddhist tradition (i.e., Abdhidamma) surpasses this limit, giving

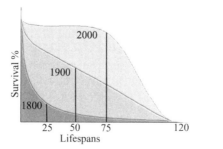

Figure 1–1 Survival curves. Over the past 200 years, the approximate mean lifespan in most developed nations has gone from 25 years (in 1800), to 50 years (in 1900), to 75 years (in 2000), but the maximum lifespan has been invariant at an estimated 120 years.

" no definite limit to the duration of life" (Narada, 1968, p 244), a remarkable thought. Despite such accounts, or perhaps in light of their provenance, and despite continual (Oeppen and Vaupel, 2002) increases in mean lifespan, there has been no reason to believe that the maximum lifespan or aging is mutable. Contrary claims were based on profit, not data.

A broad and careful look at the biology of aging, however, suggests that while maximum lifespan cannot be increased by the methods that have improved the mean— reliable access to calories and other nutrients, immunization and antibiotics, and access to a safe water supply—maximum lifespan is nevertheless alterable (Nusbaum et al., 1996). This statement is not theory but reflects current facts: aging is neither immutable nor biologically ubiquitous. The immutability and universality of aging belie reliance on limited interventions, narrow perspectives, and species provincialism. Aging is not ubiquitous among organisms, nor is it immutable among those that age.

Many unicellular organisms (e.g., most bacteria) do not age while most multicellular organisms (e.g., mammals) do. This suggests that aging is a side effect of multicellularity, an intrinsic limit to communal survival. Perhaps aging just "happens" because time passes and is an emergent phenomenon of multicellular gestalts; data contradict this. Aging is a necessary concomitant of neither chronology nor multicellularity. The rate of aging varies between and within species. Unicellular organisms such as *Saccharomyces cerevisiae* age (Lundblad and Szostak, 1989), while some multicellular organisms do not, although a clear understanding of aging remains elusive (Austad, 2001). In his encyclopedic work, *Longevity, Senescence, and the Genome*, Finch (1990) devotes an entire chapter to "negligible senescence" in lobsters, Quahog clams, tortoises, and bristlecone pines. If these organisms age, they take an extraordinarily long time doing so.

Similar inconsistencies occur within cells. As Weismann suggested a century ago, normal somatic cells senesce, whereas cancer cells and germ cells do not (Weismann, 1884). Aging occurs in some cells, but at different rates or not at all in others (Curtis, 1963; Austad, 2001). Were aging mere entropy, we could not explain such inconsistencies, key hints to fundamental mechanisms. Complex and subtle processes trigger, modulate, and direct entropy.

Were aging mere chronology, mere accumulated damage from free radicals and similar processes (Kowald and Kirkwood, 1996; Kirkwood and Kowald, 1997; Kirkwood, 1998, 2002), we would face the contradiction of the overwhelming "age" of every cell line. If the vox populi is correct—"free radicals are the engine of aging"—then the engine is controlled and modulated. Each cell derives from preceding cells, whose ancestry weaves (due to sexual and other recombination, including viral transfer) backward through earlier cell lines. This retrospective cell line—for *every* cell—is three and a half billion years old. In a basic and inescapable sense, every cell is three and a half billion years old. Eukaryotic cells themselves form an unbroken cell lineage of a billion and a half years of hosting symbiotic mitochondria, the major source of the free radicals (Loschen et al., 1974; Chance et al., 1979; Turrens, 1997). This unbroken three-and-a-half-billion-year cell lineage begs the question of why cell senescence has not accumulated retrospectively in the germ cell lines (Beach, 2000). Why has time and free radical damage not aged all cells, instead of only *somatic* cells? Germ cell lines maintain themselves over billions of years; somatic cell lines accumulate damage and age over a mere handful of years.

Cell senescence begins at defined times, occurs only in specific cells, and shows a clear temporal inflection in doing so. Furthermore, cell senescence correlates with cell divisions, not with time. Without division, cell aging stops, regardless of time duration, and restarts when the cell divides again. Cell "aging" is not the same thing as the duration of exposure to damage. Cellular aging occurs in somatic cells, but not in the germ cells from which they derive. In particular cell lines we can say that aging did not occur (back to the dawn of life) until fertilization occurred. But why then? Aging is continually reset in cancer and germ cell line. What interventions, until now impossible, allow us to reset aging in somatic cells? That aging is not universal or that cell aging can be reset does not imply that organism aging can be easily altered. Quite the contrary. Facile claims notwithstanding, aging is robust.

Caloric restriction delays aging and aging diseases (Masoro 1984; Weindruch and Walford, 1988; Yu, 1993), as obesity shortens life (Fontaine et al., 2003), but the mechanisms of the former are unclear (Masoro, 2001). There is limited evidence (Lin et al., 2000a) supporting the contention that caloric restriction works via changes in gene expression (Allison et al., 2001; Teillet et al., 2002) and may link caloric restriction and cell senescence (Campisi, 2000a). Gene expression changes (Lee et al., 1999a; Nusbaum and Rose, 1999; Imai et al., 2000), specifically, transcriptional silencing occurs (Lin et al., 2000a; Rogina et al., 2002), and correlates with delayed cell senescence (Pignolo et al., 1992; Wolf and Pendergrass, 1999), but this may be a response to rather than a necessary mechanism of caloric restriction. There is initial evidence that while transcriptional silencing may be important, at least in yeast (Jazwinski, 2000d), it is not required in caloric restriction (Jazwinski, 2000c).

Hormonal explanations (Sonntag et al., 1999b; Mobbs et al., 2001) and potential links between corticosteroids and stress in the aging brain (Lee et al., 2000c) notwithstanding, there is no evidence that these mechanisms explain caloric restriction. Despite potential benefits (Smith, 2000), there is no evidence that growth hormone, melatonin, dehydroepiandrosterone (DHEA), or oral supplements have any effect on aging nor on the *maximal* lifespan of any species. To the extent that there are data on hormonal interactions with aging, clinical benefits may be restricted to or mediated by specific tissues (e.g., estrogens on vaginal epithelium). Claims that hormonal interventions affect aging, like most other claims for aging interventions, are false. Nonetheless, aging *is* mutable and contrary claims are equally false.

Accelerating aging (with appropriate disputes as to whether this is aging) is trivial. Environmental stresses such as UV radiation (e.g., dermal photoaging), recurrent trauma, infections, hyperoxia, toxins, and dietary inadequacies or alterations (Arking, 1998; Kapahi et al., 1999) accelerate aging, although these processes may simply increase mortality without affecting aging. As George Roth once observed, if you hit a young organism with a hammer, you increase early mortality, but not aging. Are "photoaging and intrinsic aging two distinct entities" (as per Kaminer and Gilchrest, 1994) or do both processes use the common pathologic pathways and thereby deserve common discussion (Li et al., 2003)? Photoaging may be a distinct entity, as progeria is distinct from normal aging, yet may aid in understanding aging. Incomplete but useful models for accelerated aging include human progerias (Fossel, 1996, 2000c) and animals bred for rapid aging (Arking, 1998), such as *Mus* (Takeda et al., 1981) and *Drosophila* (Rose and Charlesworth, 1981). The questions of whether progerias are true aging and whether animals demonstrate rapid aging or merely rapid pathology remain arguable (Harrison, 1994), yet provide insights.

Decreasing the aging rate is more difficult but more interesting and has profound clinical implications. Three current interventions delay aging: (*1*) selective breeding, (*2*) caloric restriction, and (*3*) genetic alteration.

Selective breeding can increase the lifespan and slow the rate of aging in domestically bred and experimental laboratory animals (Rose and Nusbaum, 1994; Banks and Fossel, 1997), including the nematode *Caenorhabditis elegans* (Johnson, 1987; Larsen et al., 1995; Hekimi et al., 2001), the fruit fly *Drosophila melanogaster* (Luckinbill et al., 1984; Rose, 1984; Arking, 1987b; Arking and Dudas, 1989; Jazwinski, 1996), and mice (Atchley et al., 1997; Miller, 2001). In humans, this approach is scientifically impractical, ethically unacceptable, and clinically pointless. The same caveats are accepted in fiction (Heinlein, 1958). Human selective breeding would be paradoxical: experimenters have equivalent lifespans, requiring a multigenerational experiment and undercutting the self-interest of the experimenters. Nor is there clear benefit: the eugenic implications are strikingly distasteful and would undercut financial or political support. The ethics devolve into the same concerns as intentional and enforced selection of humans for any trait. Selection occurs haphazardly and naturally (Perls et al., 2000) as each of us chooses a mate, but this process reflects personal, not social enforced choices and rarely achieves the same level of opprobrium. The haphazard nature assures a more varied species gene pool than a single criterion, such as extended lifespan. Our clinical goal is not solely to prevent future suffering by selecting for healthier humans but to prevent or cure the diseases we now suffer from. Aside from practical and ethical objections, selection offers no benefit to patients. Despite this, an understanding of how selection delays aging remains practically, ethically, and clinically relevant. By consensus, such breeding selects for genes involved in basic energy metabolism, antioxidant efficacy (Dudas and Arking, 1995), metabolic efficiency, and free radical metabolism in the broadest sense (Arking, 1998). Curiously, epidemiologic analysis suggests that these experiments may not be selecting for lower mortality with aging, but for much lower mortality overall (Curtsinger et al., 1995; Pletcher et al., 2000).

Caloric restriction, by about 30%–40% of ad libitum intake with careful maintenance of nutrient balance (Pugh et al., 1999a), works through restricting *total* caloric intake, rather than any specific nutrient or calorie source (Weindruch and Walford, 1988; Sohal and Weindruch, 1996). A minor exception, lifespan extension of *Caenorhabditis elegans* through specific restriction of coenzyme Q, has been attributed to reduced generation and enhanced scavenging of intracellular reactive oxygen species (Larsen and Clarke, 2002).

First described in rats (McCay et al., 1935), caloric restriction appears to work in a fair number of nonmammalian species (Kirk, 2001), in all tested mammalian species (Lane et al., 1998a; Roth et al., 1999), including primates (Lane et al., 1992, 1997b; Ingram et al., 1993), and likely in humans (Roth et al., 2003). Caloric restriction may have an analog in yeast (Imai et al., 2000; Jazwinski, 2000b; Jiang et al., 2000). *Saccharomyces* starvation, however, accelerates cell senescence, though only for one generation (Ashrafi et al., 1999). Philosophically, we might ask whether caloric restriction extends lifespan or the normal ad libitum diet shortens it. In the natural environment, caloric restriction might be the control group while ad libitum diet constitutes an increased, but suboptimal and unnatural, caloric intake. However we view caloric restriction, the optimal diet is not what most organisms choose in the wild, in captivity, or, in modern humans and their lucullan diet, in the supermarket.

Caloric restriction affects many (Lane et al., 1997a; Wolf and Pendergrass, 1999; Roth et al., 2003), but not all biomarkers of aging (Nakamura et al., 1998). Exceptions include age-related changes in healing rates (Roth et al., 1997), serum lipid ratios, and lipid oxidation (Cefalu et al., 2000), although it does decrease protein oxidation (Youngman et al., 1992). Epidemiologic analysis suggests that caloric restriction affects aging per se, rather than simply mortality (Pletcher et al., 2000). Correlated with its other benefits, in some circumstances caloric restriction "is accompanied by more youthful rates of cell replication" (Pendergrass et al., 1999b; Wolf and Pendergrass, 1999). Caloric restriction delays the onset of age-related diseases, including cancer (Weindruch et al., 1991; Weindruch, 1992; Volk et al., 1994), which may be linked to an increased cell sensitivity to apoptotic death (Muskhelishvili et al., 1995).

Human (leaving aside Marco Polo) and primate data are limited. During the early 1940s, the incidence of most age-related diseases fell in The Netherlands (Hoogendoorn, 1990) and has been attributed to the limited caloric intake (near starvation in some cases) resulting from the Nazi occupation. Initial results (Lane et al., 1998a) in rhesus macaques (Ingram et al., 1990) support but do not confirm (Roth et al., 1999) the suggestion that caloric restriction may be effective in humans (Roberts et al., 2001). Circumstantially, the limited current data imply potential human clinical benefits (Hadley et al., 2001; Lee et al., 2001a; Roth et al., 2003). Caloric restriction probably lowers the incidence of atherosclerosis (Verdery et al., 1997) and risk factors known to play a role in its pathology (Edwards et al., 1998; Cefalu et al., 1999; Lane et al., 1999). The same is likely true of other age-related diseases and their respective risk factors (Lane et al., 2000).

Given human nature, however, caloric restriction has limited direct practical value. Human patients are notoriously resistant to permanent dietary change, let alone a 30% reduction in caloric intake (Hass et al., 1996). Nonetheless, when it can be enforced, stringent dietary changes have been shown to lower the incidence of heart disease (Ornish et al., 1998). As with selective breeding, caloric restriction may achieve clinical application through increased understanding of mechanisms rather than through use of its methods. Caloric restriction is likely to involve fundamental energy metabolism (Lane et al., 1995; Roth et al., 1995a; Luckinbill and Foley, 2000), perhaps paralleling those implicated in selective breeding. Drugs that affect energy expenditure (Ramsey et al., 1998), especially glucose mimetics (such as 2-deoxyglucose), result in some benefits of caloric restriction without caloric restriction (Lane et al., 1998b, 2002; Poehlman et al., 2001; Weindruch et al., 2001). Initial work shows that glucose mimetics have neuroprotective effects against oxidative damage (Guo and Mattson, 2000b). Alternatively, such a basic change in the cellular energy budget may increase protein (Gafni, 2001; Gottesman and Maurizi, 2001) and lipid membrane turnover, with effects on respective function (see mathematical analysis in Chapter 3). Mechanisms aside, caloric restriction remains the most reliable method of postponing aging in mammals (Arking, 1998).

Among invertebrates, a parallel example is found in the nematode, *Caenorhabditis elegans*, which enters the dauer phase (with conceptual but no etymological justification, this may be thought of as hibernation) if food is scarce. Caloric restriction or not (Lane, 2000), it extends lifespan by restricting metabolism approximately 12-fold (O'Riordan and Burnell, 1989). The *daf-2* and *age-1* genes play a role and are homologous to the human insulin receptor tyrosine kinase gene (Kimura et al., 1997). *Drosophila* lifespan is extended by mutation of *daf-2* homologs, the insulin-like receptor gene *InR* (Tatar et al., 2001), or an insulin receptor substrate, *chico* (Clancy et al., 2001). Multiple mutations, directly affecting intermediate metabolism, double the *Drosophila* lifespan (albeit in a line starting with a shorter than average lifespan) without apparent costs to fertility or activity (Rogina et al., 2000). In *Caenorhabditis elegans*, mutations of *daf-2* (Larsen et al., 1995) or *age-1* (Larsen, 1993) may result in extended dauer phases and extended lifespans (Gems et al., 1998), with the central nervous system gene expression being paramount in these effects (Wolkow et al., 2000), although telomere-like sequence may play a significant but unknown role (Jones et al., 2001). Mutations of the "Clock genes," especially *clk-1* coupled with *daf-2*, result in a fivefold lifespan extension in these worms (Lakowski and Hekimi, 1996). The Clock genes act as metabolic regulators (Ewbank et al., 1997; Felkai et al., 1999; Branicky et al., 2000) and may act to increase telomere length. *Clk-2*, whose overexpression shortens telomeres in *C. elegans*, is homologous with *TEL2*, which regulates telomere length in yeast (Benard et al., 2001; Lim et al., 2001; Rothman, 2002). By whatever mechanism, these mutations mimic caloric restriction (Strauss, 2001) and, with caveats (Lane, 2000), might employ the same underlying mechanisms (Lakowski and Hekimi, 1998) or perhaps employ an independent third mechanism different from those of loss-of-function mutations in the insulin-like signaling pathways or the Clock genes (Braeckman et al., 2000). Curiously, though perhaps predictably, several of the genes that extend lifespan in *Caenorhabditis elegans*, specifically *age-1*, *clk-1*, and *spe-26*, may have segmental and independent effects upon the lifespan curve. *Age-1*, for example, selectively lowers late mortality, whereas *spe-26* lowers early mortality (Johnson et al., 2001b). Lifespan-extending genes may work by radically different mechanisms.

The effect of the *daf-2* mutation upon lifespan is not mediated by autonomous cells that in turn control the organism's lifespan through their effect on the other cells of the body (harking back to hormonal and similar theories of human aging), but is a simultaneous effect in multiple, if not all, cell lineages within the organism (Apfeld and Kenyon, 1998). Ablation of the germ cells, however, does cause such a generic effect on the remaining cells of the organism, apparently through the same *daf-2* mechanism and insulin signaling (Hsin and Kenyon, 1999), although hormonal effects have been suggested (Arantes-Oliveira et al., 2002). A similar effect pertains to mutations of the sensory cilia cells; once again, mutations of a few cells can affect the lifespan of the entire organism (Apfeld and Kenyon, 1999). The *daf-2* gene effect on lifespan requires the activity of the *daf-16* gene, which encodes a member of the hepatocyte nuclear factor 3/forkhead family of transcriptional regulators, antagonized by insulin (Lin et al., 1997). Mutations of the *DAF-16* transcription factor (a homologue of the mammalian insulin receptor) can bypass these effects of the *daf-2* mutation (Ogg et al., 1997). In these and other studies (Guarente et al., 1998; Paradis and Ruvkun, 1998; Tissenbaum and Ruvkun, 1998), there is a recurrent and tantalizing implication that basic energy metabolism plays a role in lifespan determination. While mutants have normal metabolic rates, lifespan is increased by altering glucose sensing, glucose transport, or glycolysis (Lin et al., 1997). Lifespan determination in mutants and that in calorically restricted mammals share common metabolic mechanisms but retain differences (Lane, 2000).

The paradoxical observation in nematodes—energy metabolism changes without apparent effect on the gross metabolic rate—is echoed in mammalian caloric restriction work, in which metabolic rate remains unaltered (McCarter and Palmer, 1992). While unadjusted total body energy expenditure is decreased (Lane et al., 1996) in restricted rhesus macaques, which have a smaller body mass than ad libitum macaques (Ramsey et al., 1997; Colman et al., 1998, 1999c; Black et al., 2001), energy expenditure per lean or total body mass is unchanged. Differences in physical activity do not explain caloric restriction (McCarter et al., 1997), but the mechanisms remain arguable.

Glucose metabolism (Masoro et al., 1992; Lane et al., 1998b), glycation (Cefalu et al., 1995; Teillet et al., 2002), free radical production (McCarter, 1995; Kim et al., 1996; Wachsman, 1996), oxidative damage (Weindruch, 1996; Kim et al., 1997a; Wanagat et al., 1999; Hall et al., 2000), antioxidant production (Luhtala et al., 1994; Suzuki et al., 1997), individual cell or mitochondrial energy expenditure (Lass et al., 1998), mito-chondrial damage (Aspnes et al., 1997; Harper et al., 1998; Lee et al., 1998b), immune changes (Roecker et al., 1996; Weindruch et al., 1997), or hormonal changes in insulin (Wang et al., 1997), somatostatin (Sonntag et al., 1995), growth hormone (GH; Xu and Sonntag, 1996a, 1996b), or IGF-1 (Sonntag et al., 1999b) have been used to explain caloric restriction. More likely, however, caloric restriction involves basic changes in gene expression, perhaps via transcriptional silencing (Campisi, 2000a; Lin et al., 2000a), that underlie, contribute to, and tie together these plethora of other, perhaps more facile and superficial, explanations. Perhaps an explanation lies in the forest—altered *patterns* of gene expression—and not the trees.

Experimental genetic interventions extend the lifespans of relatively simple multi-cellular species (Guarente and Kenyon, 2000), such as *Caenorhabditis elegans* (Kenyon et al., 1993; Larsen, 1993; Dorman et al., 1995; Lin et al., 1997; Hekimi et al., 1998; Murakami and Johnson, 1998; Yang and Wilson, 1999). Such intervention in *C. elegans* amounts to a "fountain of youth" for nematodes (Kenyon, 1996; Guarente and Kenyon, 2000). A parallel finding in *Saccharomyces cerevisiae* is the *FOB1* mutation that slows the generation and accumulation of extrachromosomal ribosomal DNA circles (see below), an apparent counting mechanism for yeast senescence (Defossez et al., 1998). This finding links chromosomal structure, gene expression, metabolism, and aging (Guarente, 1996, 1997a; Defossez et al., 1999). Increasing the gene dosage of Sir 2p extends lifespan, probably by related mechanisms (Kaeberlein et al., 1999) or via tran-scriptional silencing or recombination suppression (Imai et al., 2000). Similar extended-lifespan mutations are found in mice, with again the implication that insulin metabolism is central to the effect (Dozmorov et al., 2001).

Lifespan determination is complex, but is alterable by simple mutation as well as selection. Though not determined solely by genetics (Arking, 1988; Finch and Tanzi, 1997), lifespan is extraordinarily responsive to selective breeding. In *Drosophila*, breed-ing is enormously effective in extending or shortening lifespan (Rose and Charlesworth, 1981; Arking, 1987c; Arking and Dudas, 1989; Rose, 1989), despite technical barriers and theoretical criticisms (Arking and Buck, 1995). The mechanisms are complex and difficult to characterize (Rose, 1989; Arking et al., 1993) even in this simple, termi-nally differentiated organism (Kowald and Kirkwood, 1993a). Although the effect has been localized to *Drosophila*'s third chromosome (Arking et al., 1991; Buck et al., 1993b), the genes and mechanisms remain unclear (Hutchinson et al., 1991; Dudas and Arking, 1994; Nusbaum and Rose, 1994; Force et al., 1995; Arking et al., 1996). Per-haps coincidentally, a gene that lengthens *Drosophila* telomeres is on the same chro-mosome (Siriaco et al., 2002). With considerably less funding, Aristotle observed, "it is not clear whether . . . it is a single or a diverse cause that makes some to be long-lived, others short lived" (from Ross, 1908, p 464b).

Flies bred for longevity are probably more efficient in combating oxidative damage (Hari et al., 1998). The family of small heat shock proteins, which play a role in oxidative stress, has been implicated (Kurapati et al., 2000; Verbeke et al., 2001; Walker et al., 2001) and has raised the issue of hormesis (beneficial effects of low level physiological stressors) in extending lifespan (LeBourg, 2001; Rattan, 2001). Mild stress, like caloric restriction, may be the natural condition (Hayflick, 2001), but repeated stresses shorten lifespan (Jazwinski, 2001). Hormesis may trade short-term survival for long lifespan (Cypser and Johnson, 2001), but practical implications await an understanding of the genetic mechanisms (Lithgow, 2001).

Lifespan is inversely correlated with body temperature within strains, but there is no correlation with lifespan between strains bred for long or short lifespans (Arking et al., 1988). Longer lifespan is not a matter of living (and using energy) more slowly, but something more subtle, echoing the mutations of *C. elegans*. The cost of a nematode's longer lifespan is a prolonged dauer phase; the cost of a fly's longer lifespan is delayed development (Buck et al., 1993a). Just as age is delayed in the longer-lived strain, so too is the entire pattern of events (e.g., the rate of amino acid uptake, protein synthesis) in adult life (Pretzlaff and Arking, 1989; Arking and Wells, 1990). There is an interaction between lifespan and fecundity (Hutchinson and Rose, 1991; Kirkwood and Rose, 1991). Fecundity alone will select for longer-lived organisms (Rose et al., 1992b). How these are related remains unclear.

Does this apply to humans? The genetics (Rose, 1999b) and most basic metabolic functions are identical or closely analogous (Rose et al., 1992a). Similarities tempt us to believe that invertebrate data offer generic insight into mechanisms of mortality (Nusbaum et al., 1993) and into mechanisms of vertebrate, specifically human, aging (Schachter et al., 1993). Temptations notwithstanding, there are no corresponding data from mammalian experiments. Invertebrate lifespan extension genes modulate oxygen consumption, free radical metabolism, cellular respiration, or basal metabolism (Ogg et al., 1997; Paradis and Ruvkun, 1998; Tissenbaum and Ruvkun, 1998; Gems, 1999; Honda and Honda, 1999; Paradis et al., 1999; Van Voorhies and Ward, 1999), echoing the caloric restriction data (Kimura et al., 1997). Within vertebrates, few models bear upon these genetic findings; those that do reflect changes in resistance to oxidative stress (Kapahi et al., 1999; Migliaccio et al., 1999).

That a few genes modulate aging (in invertebrates or otherwise) is startling. That random mutation apparently improves biological function, which is complex and far from random, is so improbable as to strenuously imply unappreciated survival costs. There is evidence of such costs (Kuether and Arking, 1999), although their significance and extent is unclear. Mutation may remove metabolic restrictions having only occasional benefits and having reproductive or survival costs in the wild (Kirkwood, 1997; Westendorp and Kirkwood, 1998) though not easily demonstrable in the laboratory (Hsin and Kenyon, 1999). Such costs probably accrue to developmental viability and are selected against in the wild (Buck et al., 2000).

In humans, only circumstantial evidence suggests that aging or maximum lifespan can be altered. Segmental progerias, such as Hutchinson-Gilford syndrome, Werner syndrome, and trisomy 21, have isolated features that resemble normal aging. They may result from single mutations, single chromosome duplications (Brown, 1992), or epigenetic abnormalities. While not equivalent to normal aging at the gross or cellular levels (Brown et al., 1985; Oshima et al., 1995; Kipling and Faragher, 1997), cells do show senescent changes that may underlie these syndromes, such as fibroblasts in Hutchinson-Gilford progerics and lymphocytes in trisomy 21 patients. In Werner syndrome, a single mutation underlies the clinical and cell senescence abnormalities (Yu et al., 1996). Surprisingly, telomerase circumvents the accelerated senescence, resetting telomere length (Ouellette, 2000b; Wyllie et al., 2000) and gene expression and partially normalizing cell function (Choi et al., 2001).

Whatever the species, there are two overarching themes: interventions that extend the lifespan or that delay aging alter energy metabolism or chromosomal function. Not only are free radical metabolism (Harman, 1956, 1999) and mitochondrial dysfunction (de Grey, 1997, 1999; Richter, 1999) central to aging (Finkel and Holbrook, 2000), they are probably necessary to explaining caloric restriction (Feuers et al., 1993) and genetic alteration of lifespan (Larsen, 1993).

Purely metabolic explanations are insufficient. The evidence of germ and cancer cell lines, helicase abnormalities in Werner syndrome (Yu et al., 1996), and growing literature on telomeres (Moyzis, 1991; Losi and Dal Cin, 1999) and telomerase (Yegorov, 1999) suggest that chromosomal function modulates not only cellular (Kipling, 1995b) but perhaps also organismal aging (Fossel, 2001b). The thesis of this book is that chromosomal function, and specifically alterations in gene expression, plays a key role in human (and mammalian) aging by modulating the changes in energy metabolism and mitochondria that drive aging in all organisms (not merely those that, like humans, demonstrate cell senescence). The role of energy metabolism in aging is biologically universal; the roles of chromosomal function and gene expression in aging are more restricted. The driving forces underlying aging are ubiquitous; the genetic *control* of such forces differs between species. Adult insects (Finch, 1990; Arking, 1998) are terminally differentiated (their cells no longer divide). They age by running out of cells, with cell losses set by free radical damage and mitochondrial dysfunction (Yan and Sohal, 1998). Cell senescence plays little role in the aging of terminally differentiated organisms. Not surprisingly, these organisms have different ("non-canonical"; Hawley, 1997) telomere mechanisms (Pardue et al., 1996; Martinez et al., 2001a, 2001b). Insects actively maintain telomeres (Kipling, 1995b) and recognize them as nondamaged chromosomal terminations (Ahmad and Golic, 1999; Ahmed and Hodgkin, 2000), even if the telomere and maintenance mechanisms are strikingly different (Biessmann et al., 1997; Kamnert et al., 1997). That telomeres are "similar in structure" (Pryde et al., 1997) may apply to yeast and vertebrate organisms (Dubrana et al., 2001), but is less true in multitudes of other organisms such as *Drosophila* (Pardue et al., 1996; Savitsky et al., 2002), *Borrelia* (Hinnebusch and Barbour, 1991; Kobryn and Chaconas, 2002), certain other bacteria (Goshi et al., 2002), and viruses (DeMasi et al., 2001; Kobryn and Chaconas, 2001).

In some single-celled organisms that, although intuitively surprising, demonstrate aging, telomeres play a role (Sinclair et al., 1998b). Yeasts lose telomere length with age (although see D'Mello and Jazwinski, 1991) and simultaneously accumulate curious extrachromosomal ribosomal DNA circles (ERCs) within the nucleolus (Defossez et al., 1998; Johnson et al., 1998; Sinclair et al., 1998a), which may result from DNA repair (Park et al., 1999). Blocking ERC creation extends yeast lifespan (Defossez et al., 1999). The relationship, if any, between these circles and "supertwisted" DNA minicircles found in the mitochondria of some candidal yeast species (Tomaska et al., 2000) is unclear. Whether these circles have human parallels (Shore, 1998a) is unknown and even their role in yeast remains uncertain (Jazwinski, 2000d). Circle location matches hTR and hTERT location within the human nucleolus (Etheridge et al., 2002; Yang et al., 2002b), a location that varies with malignancy and cell cycle (Wong et al., 2002).

Telomeres at chromosome terminations are probably necessary for cells with linear chromosomes (Sandell and Zakian, 1993; Ishikawa and Naito, 1999) as well as de novo chromosomes, e.g., in *Ascaris* (Muller et al., 1991) and *Euplotes* (Mollenbeck and Klobutcher, 2002). Exceptions (Levis, 1989; Biessmann et al., 1990a) or interesting complications (Biessmann et al., 1990b; Ravin et al., 2001) occur, but telomeres are universal on linear chromosomes, even on linear mitochondrial chromosomes (Morin and Cech, 1988). This necessity was confirmed experimentally in new telomeres, formed experimentally (Anglana and Bacchetti, 1999) or normally (Jentsch et al., 2002), and artificial chromosomes (Grimes et al., 2002) in which telomeres are required for normal function (Runge and Zakian, 1993; Ascenzioni et al., 1997; Grimes and Cooke, 1998; Mills et al., 1999b).

Curiously, telomere-like sequences are found throughout the chromosomes of many organisms, e.g., horses (Lear, 2001) and primates (Hirai, 2001). In *Tetrahymena*, these sequences (Yu and Blackburn, 1991) probably result from telomerase-induced chromosomal repair or "healing" (Greider, 1991a; Harrington and Greider, 1991; Collins and Greider, 1993).

Unlike invertebrates, vertebrates have many cell lines that divide throughout the lifespan, replacing typical and constant cell loss, providing a peculiar twist to the cell dynamics of aging. Within vertebrates, and within mammals, aging differs, not so much in the basics of intermediate metabolism but in changing *control* of metabolism and hence aging. If all mammals were to start with the same intermediate metabolism and mitochondria, differences in rates of energy use (and hence free radical accumulation) and patterns of gene expression would drastically alter the outcome and pathology (e.g., Goldstein and Moerman, 1984; von Zglinicki et al., 2000a). Compared to humans, mice have higher metabolic rates, fewer body cells, longer telomeres (at least in some strains; Hande et al., 1999b), different patterns of gene expression (or marginally different genes), and, as a result, faster overall aging. Aging is not simply telomere length, nor any other single factor. These differences reflect the evolutionary pressures on mice, in which aging is seldom the weakest link in survival (Wright and Shay, 2000).

The intent is not to explain universal patterns of metabolism, nor interspecies differences in the genetic control and expression of aging (Kirkwood, 1992), but to illuminate *human* aging. Specifically, the intent is to explore a practical model of human age-related pathology. Rather than an ivory-tower, conceptual bagatelle, aging is the concrete and daily accrual of personal dysfunction and discomfort. Aging is arthritis, angina, strokes, dementias, incontinence, and infections. Aging is, etymologically and experientially, emphatically a dis-ease. It is distinctly tangible, fundamentally human, and unavoidably real.

Finally, cell senescence is consistent with our current understanding of age-related clinical disease and myriad hypotheses regarding aging. It explains how hypertension and tobacco may cause pathology. It explains exceptions, such as atherogenesis in progeric children who lack other risk factors. That aging now occurs on the stage of cell senescence does not change our usual actors, but it does introduce new and important characters to our play. Free radicals may be villains in this drama, but the script is that of cell senescence and it is here we can intervene most effectively. The importance of cell senescence lies in how it defines human pathology and then only if we can alter the script and prevent age-related disease.

CHAPTER 2

Cell Senescence

Cell senescence appears carefully arranged as cells divide; aging appears to be a more haphazard affair. For cells, this has prompted a semantic distinction between aging and senescence, but organisms may age or senesce without fear of scholarly argument.

Until 40 years ago, cells were not believed to age or senesce. Cells simply divided and survived indefinitely. By implication, aging was an emergent property of multicellularity with unavoidable repercussions the cells. Cells were immortal; organisms (collections of cells) were not. Aging was failure of the gestalt between rather than any mechanism within cells. Cells might be immortal, but the anarchy of aging was the body's unavoidable destiny.

Data were meager, causes elusive, theories rampant. Was aging due to hormonal imbalance, metaphysical failure of cellular social contracts, or trade-off of procreative for survival energy (although energy remained ill-defined)? Lacking evidence of cell aging until past the middle of the twentieth century, aging remained the product of multicellular interaction by default. Though false, the belief that cells did not age was vigorously defended. The crucial breakthrough occurred serendipitously and despite dogged attempts at disproof. That cell senescence occurred was revolutionary; that it might have clinical implications for aging remains so. To understand the revolution in our concept of aging, we must first explore telomeres (the terminal portion of linear chromosomes), telomerase (the enzyme that extends telomeres), and our concept of cell senescence.

Telomeres, Telomerase, and Cell Senescence

In 1888, Waldeyer described dark nuclear clumps, naming them *chromosomes*. Half a century later, investigators described terminal portions of chromosomes and, in 1938,

Hermann Muller named them *telomeres* (Muller, 1938). Barbara McClintock, who won a Nobel prize for her work on maize, did the initial work on telomeres and found them essential to chromosomal integrity. Succinctly, "nature does not like DNA with free ends" (Brenner, 1997). Lacking telomeres (Shore, 1998b), chromosomes become unstable, "sticky," and prone to mutation (McClintock, 1941; Lundblad, 2001). The poetic and common—although, strictly speaking, inaccurate—metaphor is that telomeres "keep our chromosomes from unraveling."

Although research has been done in plants (Richards and Ausubel, 1988; McKnight et al., 1997; Zentgraf et al., 2000; Riha et al., 2001), most work was done on animal telomeres. Telomeric organization is similar in plants (Kilian et al., 1995; Ohmido et al., 2001), although with differences (Armstrong et al., 2001). Telomeric structure and sequence suggest distinct clades (Adams et al., 2001) although some species have lost the normal telomere mechanism (Cunado et al., 2001). Readers are referred elsewhere for details (Gall, 1995) and early reviews (Biessmann and Mason, 1992; Blackburn and Greider, 1995) of those who established a preliminary understanding of telomeres (see Greider, 1991c).

Sometimes referred to as a "chromosomal cap" (Cervantes and Lundblad, 2002), the telomere has been compared to the terminal plastic sleeve or "aglet" on the chromosomal "shoelace" (Gottschling and Stoddard, 1999). Correctly stressing their importance, this comparison incorrectly suggests a passive role and disregards the active nature of telomere maintenance (Bryan and Cech, 1999; Dandjinou et al., 1999; Dubrana et al., 2001). Telomere loss has widespread consequences throughout cells—the "telomere deletion response"—including up-regulation of energy production, mitochondrial proliferation, and wholesale alterations in gene expression (Nautiyal et al., 2002). Far from mere DNA ferrules on chromosomal handles, telomeres actively and assiduously modulate cell function (Kim et al., 2002f). Far more importantly, as the telomere shortens (Levy et al., 1992), the cell cycle slows (Morin, 1997a), as does cell division (Maigne et al., 1998), leading to growth arrest (Harley et al., 1990) long prior to apocryphal unraveling.

Linear chromosomes, and hence telomeres, create problems (Hawley, 1997), foremost among them, replication (see Fig. 2–1). Telomere function cannot be divorced from mechanisms maintaining them and permitting duplication (Zakian, 1995; Lingner and Cech, 1998; Blackburn, 2000b), especially telomerase (Harley, 1994; Lundblad and Wright, 1996; Evans et al., 1999). Predicted in 1971 (Olovnikov, 1971; Watson, 1972), telomerase was identified in *Tetrahymena* (Greider and Blackburn, 1985), the preeminent organism in early telomere research (Turkewitz et al., 2002). Before considering them together in cell senescence (Greider, 1990), we will consider first the telomere, then telomerase.

The telomere comprises DNA and proteins (Kipling, 1995b; Campisi et al., 2001), forming a complex (Cong et al., 2002) sufficient to permit DNA replication and protect chromosomal stability (Blackburn and Szostak, 1984; Gottschling and Cech, 1984; Gottschling and Zakian, 1986). Telomeric DNA is rigorously (de Lange et al., 1990) repetitive (Blackburn and Gall, 1978); the protein structure is specific to and defines the action of the telomere (Henderson, 1995). The complex allows the cell to distinguish telomeres unambiguously from other chromosomal breaks (Wynford-Thomas and Kipling, 1997). In some species, the telomere is the site of attachment for a "tether" between partner chromatids during anaphase separation (LaFountain et al., 2002).

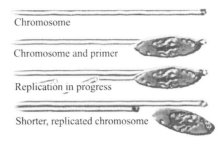

Chromosome

Chromosome and primer

Replication in progress

Shorter, replicated chromosome

Figure 2–1 Telomere shortening. Telomere shortening occurs because the DNA primer, though initiating replication, "hides" and thus prevents replication of the distal telomere of the replicated strand.

The DNA portion, repetitive hexameric nucleotides, is typically several kilobase pairs long. In humans, the sequence is TTAGGG: thymine, thymine, adenine, guanine, guanine, guanine (Moyzis et al., 1988). Some organisms display variation in the G-rich sequence (Blackburn and Szostak, 1984; Blackburn, 1990b), even with only a single telomerase RNA gene (Forstemann and Lingner, 2001). The boundaries of telomere variation may reflect unknown but required functions (Shoeman et al., 1988; Guo et al., 1992; Villanueva et al., 1999). The TTAGGG sequence is shared by vertebrates, slime molds, trypanosomes, and many other organisms (Zakian, 1989; Greider, 1990; Blackburn, 1991). Some yeasts have a hexameric portion, but the repeats may range up to 25 bases (McEachern and Blackburn, 1994). Distal bases are turned over more frequently than innermost bases (McEachern et al., 2002). Similar sequences are found elsewhere in chromosomes ("interstitial sequences") and may be more labile—prone to breaks and faulty repair—than telomere sequences (Balajee et al., 1994) and may represent erroneous insertion during double-strand break repair (Faravelli et al., 2002), end-fusions, and segmental duplications (Uchida et al., 2002).

The telomere is not a simple structure but forms a terminal loop (Greider, 1999b), at least in mammals (de Lange, 2001). To an extent, this loop forms a protective cap (de Lange, 2002) and disruption is interpreted as DNA damage (Eller et al., 2002). This "lariat" or telomere duplex loop (t-loop) structure probably forms immediately after duplication (Wright et al., 1999) when the longer, guanosine-rich, 3' end (Wright et al., 1997) of the overhang (the tail) bends backward and attaches slightly proximally from the termination ("invades the duplex telomeric repeat"), displacing the normally complementary 3' strand and taking its place on the complementary, more proximal, cytosine-rich 5' strand of the telomere (Griffith et al., 1999a). The normally complementary displaced portion of the 3' strand becomes the d-loop (for displacement loop) (Fig. 2–2).

An analogous circular arrangement occurs in yeast (Wellinger et al., 1992, 1993b; Wright et al., 1992), although other mechanism may predominate (de Lange, 2001). A critically short telomere (triggering cell cycle arrest) is probably one too short to form t-loops (Yegorov et al., 1997) and this length may determine p53 binding (Stansel et al., 2002). Overhang length is variable and directly proportional to the rate of telomere base loss, perhaps explaining variation in shortening rates between different cells (Huffman et al., 2000) and rapid shortening in certain mutations (Bucholc et al., 2001). Longer overhangs may be more prone to damage, access by DNA repair proteins (von Zglinicki,

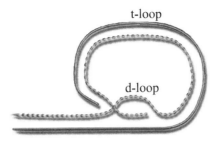

Figure 2–2 Telomere structure. Telomeres routinely form complex, looped structures: the larger loop is the telomere duplex loop (t-loop), the displaced portion of the 3' strand forms a smaller displacement loop (d-loop).

2000), and accelerated loss. Overhang length (Jacob et al., 2001) is apparently independent of telomerase (Hemann and Greider, 1999; Nikaido et al., 1999), at least in murine mTERT null cells, but there is disagreement (Stewart et al., 2003), and models suggest that length variation may be due to template abnormalities (Hao and Tan, 2002). Finally, telomeres can form four-stranded structures, G-quartets (see Kipling, 1995b; Henderson, 1995; Moine and Mandel, 2002), or even larger structures (Sen and Gilbert, 1992; Scherthan, 2001), with functional (Ferguson et al., 1991; Phan and Mergny, 2002) and perhaps clinical (Brown et al., 1998b) implications.

Human telomeres comprise at least two specific binding proteins, telomere-repeat binding factors 1 and 2: TRF1 and TRF2 (Chong et al., 1995; Bilaud et al., 1997; van Steensel and de Lange, 1997). These and a growing number of other proteins (Fang and Cech, 1995; Shore, 1997b; d'Adda di Fagagna et al., 1999; Classen et al., 2001; Kamma et al., 2001) regulate telomere length (Ishikawa, 1997; Griffith et al., 1998; Shay, 1999a). Proteins, such as Cdc13p (Grandin et al., 2001; Mitton-Fry et al., 2002), open the G-quartet structure, permitting replication (Izbicka et al., 2001; Lin et al, 2001). Proteins in the MRX complex such as MRE11, Rad50p, and Xrs2p (Diede and Gottschling, 2001; Tsukamoto et al., 2001), fulfill maintenance functions including checkpoint signaling and DNA replication (D'Amours and Jackson, 2002), and preserve chromosomal integrity in animals (Booth et al., 2001; Goytisolo and Blasco, 2002) and plants (Daoudal-Cotterell et al., 2002), if not necessarily, yeast. Amounts and ratios of these proteins (e.g., MRX proteins) may change significantly in cancer cells (Matsutani et al., 2001b). Heterogenous nuclear ribonucleoproteins (hnRNPs) may regulate length (Ford et al., 2002). Telomere associated proteins may be linked to oxidative damage or single-strand fragment production (Saretzki et al., 1999; von Zglinicki et al., 2000a). Whatever the mechanism, telomerase and longer telomeres are protective against apoptosis (Ozen et al., 1998; Holt et al., 1999b; Ren et al., 2001; Gorbunova et al., 2002).

TRF1 and TRF2 regulate telomere length and maintain homeostasis (Shore, 1997a; de Lange, 2000; Watanabe, 2001; Ancelin et al., 2002), preventing indefinite lengthening and unlimited cell proliferation. Judging from the function of similar proteins (such as Rap1p) in *Saccharomyces* (Conrad et al., 1990; Wright and Zakian, 1995; Marcand et al., 1997a; Li et al., 2000a) and in *Kluyveromyces lactis* (Blackburn, 1997; Blackburn et al., 1997; Maddar et al., 2001), and overexpression causing telomere loss in telomerase-positive tumors that normally display stable telomeres (van Steensel and de Lange, 1997),

TRF1 and perhaps TRF2 provide feedback regarding telomere length (Smogorzewska et al., 2000; Karlseder et al., 2002). A frequent, concise observation is that TRF1 negatively regulates elongation whereas TRF2 protects chromosome ends and inhibits end-to-end fusions (Matsutani et al., 2001a; de Lange, 2002; Karlseder et al., 2002).

Both TRFs bind duplex telomeres in vivo, especially long telomeres. Neither affects telomerase expression or activity in vitro, but blocks telomere elongation in vivo, probably by sequestering the 3' terminus in loops, preventing telomerase access and therefore activity (Smogorzewska et al., 2000). Both TRFs contain a C-terminal Myb domain that binds telomeres (Hanaoka et al., 2001); both have equivalent α-helical architectures that resemble twisted horseshoes, permitting homodimerization and almost identical binding (Fairall et al., 2001; Nishikawa et al., 2001). They are found in vertebrates, but not necessarily in budding yeasts (Wellinger et al., 1993c; Lin and Zakian, 1994; Li et al., 2000a). A TRF2 analog, Taz1p, is found in fission yeasts such as *Saccharomyces pombe* (Cooper et al., 1997; Matsutani et al., 2001b). Telomere maintenance mechanisms are more similar in fission yeasts and humans than fission and budding yeasts (Park et al., 2002b). With exceptions, e.g., *Caenorhabditis elegans* (Yi et al., 2001), most plants and animals have analogous (if not equivalent) binding proteins (Hwang et al., 2001b). Pot1 protein, binding single-stranded DNA, may bind the terminus of the protein in ciliates, fission yeast, and mammals, and perhaps most eukaryotes (Baumann and Cech, 2001).

TRF1 (aka Pin2) and other proteins probably maintain stability (Yajima et al., 2001) by signaling normal, undamaged chromosomal terminations (Ancelin et al., 1998; Karlseder et al., 1999), blocking inappropriate elongation (Shore, 1997a; van Steensel and de Lange, 1997), and inhibiting telomerase (Ancelin et al., 2002). TRF1 binds a potent telomerase inhibitor, PinX1 (Zhou and Lu, 2001). TRF1 is regulated cell cycle–specifically; it binds to, and regulates microtubules and mitotic spindles (Nakamura et al., 2001b, 2002b). Meiotic spindle function, by contrast, requires functional telomeres and perhaps telomerase (Liu et al., 2002d). TRF1 molecules dimerize (Bianchi et al., 1999; Fairall et al., 2001), bind to duplex TTAGGG, induce a shallow bend in the DNA, and lead to loop formation. The sequence of TRF1 varies between species. Although certain (presumably key) regions of the proteins are conserved at the N-terminus and in the middle, overall there is only a 67% homology between mTRF1 and hTRF1. TRF genes are not syntenic, lying on different chromosomes in mice compared to those of humans (Broccoli et al., 1997).

TRF2 probably caps newly formed telomeres (Bailey et al., 2001), remodeling (Stansel et al., 2001) and stabilizing (Shay, 1999a) t-loops. It prevents end-to-end fusions (Hiyama et al., 1998b; van Steensel et al., 1998; Karlseder et al., 2002), probably by favoring d-loop formation or stability (Griffith et al., 1999a). TRF2 inhibition removes this protection, causing loss of the 3' tail, activation of p53, end-to-end fusions, apoptosis, DNA damage checkpoint activation, and even senescence, including senescent morphology and β-galactosidase expression (de Lange, 2000). Telomeric genes for proteins inhibiting apoptosis may be implicated (Li and Altieri, 1999). Absent TRF2, exposure of telomere ends, rather than short telomeres, may trigger the senescent phenotype (Karlseder et al., 2002). TRF2 binds telomeric repeats, even interstitially along the chromosome (Mignon-Ravix et al., 2002), but preferentially at the loop–tail junction (Griffith et al., 1999a), where it may stabilize t-loops at the binding of the 5' strand, displacing the corresponding d-loop from duplex telomere. In doing so, it may "hide" the single-strand 3' tail, which would otherwise be mistaken for single-strand, damaged DNA and initiate an inappropriate (e.g., apoptotic or senescent) response (Karlseder et al., 1999, 2002). Mutant TRF2 overexpression induces end-to-end fusions and growth arrest, which suggests that normal senescence may be triggered by TRF2 loss (van Steensel et al., 1998; Karlseder et al., 2002). Overexpression of normal TRF2 delays senescence and reduces the senescent "checkpoint" by several kilobases, but also accelerates telomere shortening (Ancelin et al., 2002; Karlseder et al., 2002), similar to TRF1 overexpression (Smogorzewska et al., 2000).

Tankyrase (Smith et al., 1998; Zhu et al., 1999c; Rippmann et al., 2002) is a poly(ADP-ribose) polymerase (PARP) that inhibits TRF1 binding and whose sub-cellular location correlates with TRF1 (Seimiya and Smith, 2002). Tankyrase is cell cycle–dependent (Smith and de Lange, 1999) and probably has two forms; functional differences, if any, are unknown (Cook et al., 2002). PARPs protect protein stability against oxidative damage and correlate with species longevity (Burkle, 2000). That DNA polymerases may play a role in telomere maintenance (Ohya et al., 2002) is neither surprising nor enlightening.

Ku, a heterodimeric protein with a high binding affinity for double-stranded DNA ends, nicks, and gaps, functions in DNA repair and telomere maintenance in some viruses (Jeanson and Mouscadet, 2002), yeasts (Peterson et al., 2001; Cosgrove et al., 2002; Gravel and Wellinger, 2002), plants (Riha et al., 2002), eukaryotes (Conway et al., 2002), and mammals (Bailey et al., 1999; d'Adda di Fagagna et al., 2001; Espejel and Blasco, 2002; Espejel et al., 2002a), including humans (Hsu et al., 1999; Gasser, 2000). Mammalian Ku may prevent telomeric fusions (Samper et al., 2000). Recent work finds that Ku binds specifically to hTERT (Chai et al., 2002). Homologs (Chen et al., 2001c), binds to undamaged telomeres, "G-quartet conformation" or not (Bianchi and de Lange, 1999), and may identify intact telomeric structures as undamaged DNA (Teo and Jackson, 2001).

Two ATM kinases, Tel1p and Mec1p, maintain telomeres, acting directly rather than through telomerase, in *Saccharomyces cerevisiae* (Chan et al., 2001) and perhaps humans (D'Amours and Jackson, 2001). La, a component of ribonucleoprotein complexes, interacts with hTR; overexpression results in telomere shortening (Ford et al., 2001). DNA-dependent protein kinase catalytic subunits (DNA-PKCs) are implicated in telomere maintenance and telomere capping (Espejel et al., 2002b), particularly in mice with severe combined immune deficiency (SCID; Gilley et al., 2001). DNA primases may regulate telomerase activity, at least in yeast (Diede and Gottschling, 1999) and ciliates (Ray et al., 2002), ensuring simultaneous activity on both chromosomal strands, obviating long, unmatched strands. Additional candidate proteins, including p80 and p95 in *Tetrahymena*, associate with telomerase, but have no proven role in telomere maintenance (Mason et al., 2001).

TIN2 (Kim et al., 1999; Simonsson, 2001), E-Cbs (Klobutcher et al., 1998), replication factor C (Uchiumi et al., 1996, 1998, 1999; Mossi and Hubscher, 1998), Nijmegen breakage syndrome (NMS) protein (Ranganathan et al., 2001), and others (e.g., Grunsteing, 1997; Fanti et al., 1998) could play a role, as may chromatin structure (Slijepcevic et al., 1997; Lowell and Pillus, 1998). Some species may have idiosyncratic approaches to telomere stability, for example, the repetitive inclusion of β-D-glucosyl-hydroxymethyluracil, in trypanomome telomeres (van Leeuwen et al., 2000). Telomerase activity, hence length and stability, may be controlled through access to the telomere (Shay, 1999a). Telomerase may even regulate its own activity, through splice variants (Krams et al., 2001). One of six variants, hTERT-α, lacks catalytic core residues, inhibiting activity and causing shortening (Colgin et al., 2000).

That genes regulate telomere length is likely, but that there are supportive data (Blackburn et al., 1997) is fascinating, for it clarifies their dominance (Wright et al., 1996a), inheritance (Manning et al., 2002), and location (Hinkley et al., 1998), even if their regulation remains unclear (Kipling, 1995b, pp 111–113; Greider, 1996; Shore, 1997a). Whatever mechanisms are involved, they are largely shared throughout eukaryotes (Greider, 1993; Dokudovskaya et al., 1997), with the lessons of one species likely relevant to another.

Crossbreeding *Mus musculus* (telomeres >25 kb) and *M. spretus* (5–15 kb) clarifies factors controlling telomere length. Longer length is dominant; controlling genes localize to a 5 cM region on distal chromosome 2 (Zhu et al., 1999c). Whether these mechanisms correspond to those discussed above remains unknown, but they are, to a degree, cell phenotype–specific (Coviello-McLaughlin and Prowse, 1997) and likely responsive to selection pressure (Weinstein and Ciszek, 2002).

Even within species, lengths vary between telomeres, but specific chromosomes may have specific telomere lengths (Zijlmans et al., 1997; Slijepcevic and Hande, 1999) and those lengths correlate directly with length of their chromosome (Suda et al., 2002), although lengths may vary among a minority of sister chromatids (Bekaert et al., 2002). Murine telomere lengths correlate with length of their respective arms; telomeres are shorter when closer to centromeres and p-telomeres are shorter than q-arm telomeres. Mice have acrocentric centromeres (Kipling et al., 1991, 1994), but the correlation remains in humans and Chinese hamsters, with more central centromeres (Slijepcevic, 1998b). Whether active mechanism or accidental correlation, there are suggestions of a functional link between centromeric and telomeric heterochromatin in mammals, *Drosophila*, and yeast (Netzer et al., 2001). Curiously, 600 telomere sequences added to yeast chromosomes had no obvious effect, while a dozen centromere sequences were rapidly destabilizing (Runge et al., 1991). Telomere maintenance (Moreau et al., 2001; Romney et al., 2001; Schwartz et al., 2001) may be critical to radiation resistance (Bouffler et al., 2001; Finnon et al., 2001), but surviving radiation-induced dicentrics rarely display intermediate telomere sequences (Cornforth et al., 1989).

The pivotal function of telomeres, cell survival (Muniyappa and Kironmai, 1998), is deceptively clear in outline but unsettled in detail. The necessity for specific base sequences, for example, and their influence on cell survival has received little attention and is largely unexplained (Marusic et al., 1997; Ware et al., 2000).

Telomeres "match" meiotic chromosomes (Hiraoka, 1998) and localize them during transcription (Blackburn, 1991; Gray and Celander, 1991), but these roles are passive. Telomeres are not static structures (Blackburn, 1995; Cooke, 1995; Kipling, 1995b). First the Russian (Olovnikov, 1971), then the English (Watson, 1972) literature pointed out that linear replication implied loss of part of the telomere during every division. Replication begins not at the terminus (Wellinger et al., 1993a) but at the DNA replication "primer." Telomere replication may occur late in S phase (McCarroll and Fangman, 1988) and vary even within an organism (Hultdin et al., 2001). The "lagging" strand underlying the primer would usually go unreplicated (Nozawa et al., 2000). The "leading" strand may have its own problems (Lingner et al., 1995). This model, supported experimentally (Ohki et al., 2001), implies incomplete replication of the lagging end of each strand, hence incomplete chromosome copying. Chromosomes shorten with each division. This "end replication problem" implies progressive telomeric erosion (Greider, 1995) and, ultimately, loss of chromosomal integrity.

In increasing probability, this implies that

1. immediately upon evolving, telomeres eroded and life with linear chromosomes became extinct,
2. chromosomes replicate in another fashion and telomere shortening does not occur, or
3. an unknown mechanism relengthens telomeres (at least in germ cells) and maintains species survival.

Readers may dismiss the first mechanism, while the second has a modicum of truth. We do not fully understand replication nor the gamut of mechanisms responsible for telomere maintenance. The third mechanism proved accurate. Early theory (Blackburn and Szostak, 1984; Zakian, 1989) has yielded to data on telomere-extending mechanisms (Greider and Blackburn, 1985; Greider, 1995), especially telomerase.

Telomerase, or telomere terminal transferase (Greider and Blackburn, 1985; Greider, 1991b, 1995), binds (Price et al., 1992) and relengthens eukaryotic telomeres (Kipling, 1995b; Campisi et al., 1996; Counter et al., 1997). It is a reverse transcriptase (Cech et al., 1997) that reextends telomeres by adding terminal TTAGGG repeats.

Telomerase comprises two primary components (Morin, 1989): a dimeric RNA template (hTR) configured for the correct (e.g., TTAGGG) telomere sequence (see Blackburn, 1999) and a catalytic component (hTERT) that does the enzymatic work (Blackburn, 1990a; Barinaga, 1997; Lingner et al., 1997) (Fig. 2–3). The catalytic component is commonly called *hTERT* (human telomerase reverse transcriptase); *TE* stands for telomerase, *RT* for reverse transcriptase. The RNA component should then be *hTER* (human telomerase RNA), *TE* standing for telomerase, *R* for RNA. However, the literature prefers *hTR*, and we bow to this more common usage.

There is considerable (Greider, 1995; Kipling, 1995b) and growing (Cong et al., 1999) evidence that other proteins modulate telomerase in humans and yeast (e.g., Lin and Zakian, 1995; Hughes et al., 1997), but the primary components reextend telomeres in vitro (Autexier and Greider, 1994; Wen et al., 1998). Telomerase is largely responsible for telomere maintenance and ultimately for cell viability (Dandjinou et al., 1999) and continued replication (Shay and Bacchetti, 1997). Without telomerase, linear chromosome replication is a finite, biologically unrewarding affair.

The importance of telomere loss in cell senescence was first pointed out by Alexey Olovnikov (1971). Going beyond theoretical necessity, Olovnikov compared telomeres

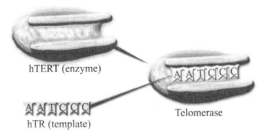

Figure 2–3 Telomerase structure. Human telomerase comprises both a template component (hTR) and an active enzymatic component (hTERT).

to a clock, counting cell divisions and timing cell senescence, connecting telomeres and cell aging.

The History of Cell Senescence

As microbes 300 years previously, cell senescence was initially heresy. This is surprising and ironic, in light of Weisman's early distinction between "immortal germ cell lines" and mortal somatic cells (Weismann, 1884). Even Freud commented in 1920 that the somatic cell "alone is subject to mortal death" (Freud, 1961). Unfortunately, Weismann suggested that aging was an active genetic process. Some have resurrected this notion (Skulachev, 1997), but portraying aging as having a selective advantage remains unconvincing (Kirkwood and Austad, 2000). For whatever reason—faulty theory or technical flaws in cell culture—dogma favored cell immortality. Weismann's quondam distinction was prescient, but thoroughly and promptly ignored.

Early work indicated that all cells were biologically immortal (Kirkwood and Cremer, 1982). Two dominant scientists, Alexis Carrel and Albert Ebeling, asserted that *all* cells grew indefinitely (Carrel and Ebeling, 1921). Had their cells divided until their work was refuted in 1961, "the mass of chicken cells . . . would have been greater than the sun" (Hayflick, 1994). Ironically, cells can be immortal, given telomerase, but absent this, Carrel and Ebeling were simply wrong (Shay and Wright, 2000a).

Against this faith and error, it took courage for Leonard Hayflick and Paul Moorhead, at the Wistar Institute in Philadelphia, to suggest (Hayflick and Moorhead, 1961) that earlier researchers were wrong and that cells have "lifespans." Then a mere parvenu, the "Hayflick limit" is now a pillar of biology. Germ, stem, somatic, and cancer cells have individual replicative limits (Hayflick, 1968, 1992, 1998a, 1998b).

Germ cell lines are biologically immortal if properly cultured in vitro, and by definition in vivo (hence, the reader's existence). Although not immortal in a strict sense (keeping them alive is technically daunting), they are immortal in the biological sense: they do not senesce. Theoretically, all cells derive from ancestral cell lines with a common origin three and a half billion years ago, eukaryotes branching off perhaps one and a half (Margulis, 1970) to two billion years ago, hominids perhaps seven and a half million years ago (Leakey, 1992, p 80), and *Homo sapiens* perhaps half of that, although dating is technically difficult (Shay, 1997a) and conceptually moot.

In contrast, somatic cells divide a limited number of times in vitro or (with considerable circumstantial evidence) in vivo (Schneider and Mitsui, 1976). Stem cells—not by definition (Potten and Loeffler, 1990), but not surprisingly—have replicative limits, greater (Ramirez et al., 1997) than those of somatic cells that derive from them (van der Kooy and Weiss, 2000). Embryonic stem cells, which give rise to all cell types and show profound medical promise (Lanza et al., 1999b; Okarma, 1999), have the least restriction in their replicative limits, particularly when including the organism's future germ cells (ova and sperm).

With fates largely controlled by surrounding cells (Kiger et al., 2000; Tran et al., 2000), early stem cells differentiate into fetal endothelium, mesothelium, and ectothelium, with differentiation varying within specific tissues. Hematopoetic stem cells include less (from which all blood elements derive) and more differentiated (from which only particular cells, e.g., leukocytes derive) cells. On the basis of theoretical reasoning and data (e.g.,

Yashima et al., 1998b), each stem cell type has characteristic replicative limits, while their derivative somatic cells have shorter limits. At birth, there is little telomere variability among different somatic cells within (but not between) organisms and no significant variation between males and females (Okuda et al., 2002).

A distinction is drawn between true stem cells (dividing, but not differentiating), transit cells (dividing and differentiating slightly), and functionally competent somatic cells (fully differentiated, dividing only into equally differentiated cells). True stem cells reside in a "microenvironment that regulates the self-renewal and output of a stem cell population" (Wasserman and DiNardo, 2002), whose regulatory mechanisms are gradually becoming clearer (Kiger et al., 2002; Tulina and Matunis, 2002). Transit cells, intermediate between stem and differentiated cells, occasionally confuse discussions of stem cell capabilities (Potten and Loeffler, 1990). The fully differentiated somatic cell—hepatocyte, leukocyte, neuron, myocyte, etc.–has a replicative limit particular to each species and cell phenotype.

Distinction between mortal somatic and immortal germ cells prompted a search for the switch controlling cell senescence. Early reports showed senescence dominating in fused senescent and nonsenescent somatic cells (Pereira-Smith and Smith, 1982) and with few exceptions mortality dominates (Pereira-Smith et al., 1990b) when mortal human fibroblasts (Pereira-Smith and Smith, 1983) or T lymphocytes (Pereira-Smith et al., 1990a) fuse with immortal cells. Similarly, in heterokaryons of mortal human fibroblasts (young versus senescent), senescence dominates (Norwood et al., 1974), although senescent human fibroblasts could be rescued by fusing hamster cells (Goldstein and Lin, 1972).

Factors (Lumpkin et al., 1986b; Spiering et al., 1988) enforcing such senescence in fused cells were labile and could be isolated in cytoplasts (Pereira-Smith et al., 1985). Four complementation groups (Pereira-Smith and Smith, 1988; Smith and Pereira-Smith, 1989b; Smith et al., 1992) were found in T and B lymphocytes, fibroblasts, and endothelial cells (Goletz et al., 1994a). The genetics of cell senescence were thought crucial (Berube et al., 1998; Smith and Pereira-Smith, 1990) and there was success at assigning complementation factors to chromosomal locations (Ning et al., 1991a; Goletz et al., 1993; Tominaga et al., 2002), such as chromosome 1 (Hensler et al., 1994; Vojta et al., 1996), chromosome 4 (Ning and Pereira-Smith, 1991; Ning et al., 1991b; Pereira-Smith and Ning, 1992; Pershouse et al., 1997), and chromosome 7 (Ran and Pereira-Smith, 2000).

The mechanisms by which complement groups caused senescence were investigated (Pereira-Smith, 1992), especially inhibition of DNA synthesis (Spiering et al., 1991). Factors included mortalin (Kaul et al., 1995; Wadhwa et al., 1995), mortality factor 4 (Bertram et al., 1999), and SDI1 (Noda et al., 1994), although the roles of the latter two are more complex (Smith et al., 1996a; Bryce et al., 1999). Mortality factor 4 (MORF4) appears to be located on chromosome 4 and has motifs suggesting transcriptional regulation (Ran and Pereira-Smith, 2000; Leung and Pereira-Smith, 2001) that may play a role in the changes in gene expression (e.g., Irving et al., 1992) that define cell senescence (Tominaga et al., 2002).

Other factors (p53, CIP1, WAF1, p21) led into the cell cycle (Johnson et al., 1994; Nakanishi et al., 1995b; Tahara et al., 1995c). Antisense p21 (a cell cycle factor) reinstates DNA synthesis and mitosis in senescent fibroblasts (Nakanishi et al., 1995a), complementing wild p21, which inhibits telomerase expression (Kallassy et al., 1998).

This research elucidated the function of cell cycles in senescence (Kill and Shall, 1990), particularly via cyclic-dependent kinases (Stein et al., 1991; Nakanishi et al., 1995c; Gerland et al., 2001) and other mechanisms of cell cycle braking (Rubelj and Pereira-Smith, 1994). Although there were hints that chromosomal mechanisms, such as methylation, might be involved (Henderson et al., 1990; Ferguson et al., 1991; Vertino et al., 1994; Mitchell et al., 1996), much remained unclear and without a unifying theoretical framework.

Absent knowledge of telomere dynamics, some investigators suggested that cells have a stochastic risk of becoming mortal at each division, of "committing" to senescence (Kirkwood and Holliday, 1975; Holliday et al., 1977). This resembled modern stochastic views of senescence (Rawes et al., 1997) and was not contradicted by available data, although a nonstochastic limit—the Hayflick limit—remained immutably present (Harley and Goldstein, 1980; Shmookler Reis et al., 1980). In the 1980s, cell senescence theories (Kirkwood, 1984, 1987) attempted to incorporate earlier aging theories, including error catastrophe (Gallant and Prothero, 1980) and free radical theory (Harman, 1956). In the early 1990s, attempts were made to revive these theories (Kowald and Kirkwood, 1994). Despite such efforts, cell senescence remained a mystery (Goletz et al., 1994b).

For two decades, the insights of Olovnikov and Watson lay fallow, with little credence paid to telomere mechanisms. The focus remained on somatic cells and the distinction between somatic and germ cell mortality, largely ignoring cancer cell immortality (Crocker, 2001), despite clinical implications. Cancer cells typically have no limitation on their divisions, do not senesce (Shay and Wright, 1996a, 1996b), and maintain stable telomere lengths (Shay and Wright, 2001a, 2001b). By implication, such cells must not only express (Morin 1989; Counter et al., 1992; Kim et al., 1994; Harley and Villeponteau, 1995) and perhaps regulate (Gorbunova et al., 2003) telomerase but regulate excess telomere extension (Blackburn et al., 1997; Shay, 1999a).

Roughly, germ cells and cancer cells are immortal, somatic cells have defined replicative lifespans (Linskens et al., 1995b), and stem cells are intermediate cells. Stem cells have prolonged, though restricted, lifespans compared to their somatic daughter cells. Transformation is a two-way street: immortal germ cells produce cells with limited lifespans, mortal somatic cells can give rise to immortal cancer cells. Cancer overcomes dominant mortality; cellular mortality is reversible.

Early work suggested that there were two independent but necessary mortality stages to cell immortality: M1 and M2. M1 is executed via p53, perhaps through binding to the t-loop of the telomere (Stansel et al., 2002) or via proteins in the p16/Rb pathway (Shay, 1998a), though this latter pathway may not function in mice (Smogorzewska and de Lange, 2002). This stage may have subdivisions and backup mechanisms to ensure senescence (Morris et al., 2002a). M1 is not senescence but (e.g., induced by photoactivated psoralen) may mimic it (Ma et al., 2002b). At M1, cells lose responsiveness to normal mitogens (except SV40 T antigen), arresting near G1/S. Many tumor viral proteins bind p53 and p16, block their inhibition, and allow cells to bypass M1. Cell replication then continues until M2. M2 coincides with telomere shortening; bypassing M2 requires telomerase (Park et al., 2002a). Cells undergo crisis (Wright et al., 1989), distinct from normal senescence in that cells "detach from culture dishes en masse and undergo apoptosis" (Hubbard and Ozer 2000; Macera-Bloch et al., 2002). Bypassing both stages, cells achieve immortalization and indefinite lifespans (Wright and Shay, 1996; Duncan and Reddel, 1997).

Cellular "lifespan" is the number of divisions cells undergo before division slows (Maigne et al., 1998) or stops (Hayflick, 1970). Retrospectively, all cells have *been* immortal (i.e., derive from immortal germ cells), but prospectively, few cells remain so. Rare cells retain immortality, having unrestricted replicative potential. Cancer cells reattain, and abuse, this potential (Hayflick, 1967; Kipling, 1995a; Greider and Blackburn, 1996). Somatic cells have defined replicative lifespans characteristic of their species, phenotype, and donor age (Hayflick, 1989; Cristofalo and Pignolo, 1993). Embryonic human somatic cells average 50 successive doublings (Hayflick, 1985, 1994), although some phenotypes may double this (Duthu et al., 1982). Reproducible differences in replicative lifespans between species, between cell types, and between age of cell donors raise two questions: (*1*) what is the clock governing replicative limits (Hayflick, 1965), and (*2*) is there a relationship between replicative limit and aging within the organism?

Olovnikov (1971) answered the first question and was proven correct a decade ago. In 1990, Calvin Harley, Carol Greider, and Bruce Futcher (Harley et al., 1990) showed that fibroblast telomere lengths correlate with replicative limits in culture. Other correlative studies followed, as did a suggestive and confirmatory, but circumstantial study (Wright et al., 1996a), showing that telomeric oligonucleotides extend telomeres and cell lifespans in hybridized senescing cells. This argument culminated in the publication of a study (Bodnar et al., 1998) proving causation and "ending the debate" (de Lange, 1998). The crucial work was done by Harley's group (at Geron Corporation) and colleagues at the University of Texas Southwestern Medical Center (Jerry Shay and Woody Wright) and was confirmed repeatedly (Counter et al., 1998a; Vaziri, 1998; Vaziri and Benchimol, 1998). Transfecting hTERT into human somatic cells (lung fibroblasts, skin fibroblasts, and pigmented retinal epithelial cells) resulted in cells lacking a measurable replicative limit or senescent pattern of gene expression but that were otherwise normal. In four decades, telomerase has changed from Watson's theoretical "loose end" to a method of immortalizing human somatic cells with enormous clinical potential. In answer to our first question: telomeres and telomerase control cell senescence.

The second question, the potential relevance of cell senescence for aging (Cristofalo et al., 1994; Hayflick, 1998a), has occupied many researchers over four decades (Hayflick, 1989, 1991) and is the foundation for this book. The potential relevance for aging provided a strong impetus for research (Cristofalo, 1996), but little was initially known (Hayflick, 1984a). Attempts to fill this void included defining the characteristics of senescence (Cristofalo et al., 1967; Cristofalo, 1988; Pignolo et al., 1994; Cristofalo and Pignolo, 1996) and conditions under which normal cells immortalize (Gorman et al., 1984). SV40, for example, immortalizes murine cells (Hubbard and Ozer, 2000) but only 1 in 10^{-8} human fibroblasts (Shay and Wright, 1989; Cheng et al., 1997). Equally studied were factors inducing cell senescence (Wright and Hayflick, 1975; Pignolo et al., 1998a; Tresini et al., 1998) and altered responses of senescent cells (Balin et al., 1977; Cristofalo et al., 1989; Phillips et al., 1990). Research naturally segued from growth factor response (Cianciarulo et al., 1993) to cell protein expression (Ferber et al., 1993; DiPaolo et al., 1995; Keogh et al., 1996a) and then into the basic molecular (Carlin et al., 1994; Allen et al., 1995; Keogh et al., 1996b), signaling (Cristofalo and Tresini, 1998), and genetic (Choi et al., 1995; Wang et al., 1996; Tresini et al., 1999) mechanisms. As techniques improved, research became increasingly molecular (Cristofalo et al., 1992b; Allen et al., 1997; Pignolo et al., 1998b) and focused on senescent patterns of gene expression (Smith and Pereira-Smith, 1989a; Cristofalo et al., 1992a; Doggett et al., 1992; Medcalf et al., 1996), giving us an expanded and detailed understanding of senescence (Cristofalo et al., 1998a, 1998b; Teng et al., 2002). Senescent human fibroblasts, for example, display impairment in Cdk2and Cdk4 activation in response to mitogens, secondary to increased binding of p16 to Cdk4 and increased association of Cdk2 with cyclin D1 and p21 (Morisaki et al., 1999). The past decade, marked by accelerating interest and citations, has been succinctly, albeit informally, reviewed elsewhere (Marx, 2002). While the second half of this text will address the clinical relevance of cell senescence, the remainder of the first half explores our growing knowledge of cell senescence at the molecular and genetic levels.

Telomerase and Its Function

Knowledge of telomerase function (Blackburn, 2001) has grown, but appreciation of our ignorance has grown faster. Telomerase is a reverse transcriptase that adds DNA bases to human telomeric DNA using an RNA template (Greider and Blackburn, 1985; Yu et al., 1990; Singer and Gottschling, 1994). Human telomerase conserves many generic characteristics of reverse transcriptases (Bosoy and Lue, 2001), but, unique from most reverse transcriptases (such as HIV reverse transcriptase), retrotransposons (Moore and Haber, 1996; Teng et al., 1996; Arkhipova and Morrison, 2001), and the extensive family of DNA retroelements, telomerase does not cleave the DNA strand prior to inserting new bases (Eickbush, 1997) and has regions outside the reverse transcriptase domain critical to telomerase and DNA primer activity (Beattie et al., 2000; Armbruster et al., 2001). Molecules may inhibit HIV reverse transcriptase without effect on hTERT (Mizushina et al., 2000). Instead of infecting the host or increasing DNA burden, as do other reverse transcriptases (Boeke, 1996), telomerase (excepting carcinogenesis) benefits the cell and organism. In some species, retroposons may serve a similar end, as maintaining telomeres in *Drosophila melanogaster* (Sheen and Levis, 1994; Pardue et al., 1996). Human telomerase comprises the RNA template (hTR) and the catalytic component (hTERT). There is also an uncertain number of telomerase associated proteins (TEP) (Nugent and Lundblad, 1998; Le et al., 2000; Scheffer et al., 2000).

The RNA template is specific for the telomere sequence that varies slightly among vertebrates, yeast, and other organisms (Chen et al., 2000c). The dimeric template is functional only as a homodimer; heterodimers consisting of a wild-type hTR and a mutant hTR unit are almost inactive (Wenz et al., 2001). hTR has additional non-template bases with functions, such as alignment (Gavory et al., 2002), in humans and other vertebrates (Autexier et al., 1996; Hinkley et al., 1998; Lukowiak et al., 2001; Chen et al., 2002c), as well as in nonvertebrates, such as tetrahymena (Autexier and Greider, 1995; Gilley and Blackburn, 1999; Blackburn et al., 2000; Ware et al., 2000), and yeast (Roy et al., 1998; Tzfati et al., 2000). Functionally, the non-template portion of this phylogenetically diverse enzyme is more important. A single, short "template-recognition" element defines adjacent residues as a template for telomere synthesis (Miller and Collins, 2002). Folded into a long hairpin structure, the 5'-terminal template domain remains accessible; the 3'-terminal domain folds into a hairpin-hinge-hairpin-tail structure (Antal et al., 2002).

Although other regions vary among vertebrates, 10 helical regions of the RNA remain almost invariant. The global architecture is likewise almost universal even in many nonvertebrates (Chen et al., 2000c; Rhodes et al., 2002). Disruption of non-template regions reduces or abolishes DNA synthesis (Autexier and Greider, 1998; Chen et al., 2002c), or causes replication beyond normal template boundaries, with consequent abnormal telomere maintenance and cellular growth defects (Tzfati et al., 2000). Some telomerases accept RNA primers, suggesting an evolutionary origin as an RNA-dependent RNA polymerase (Collins and Greider, 1995). The hTR gene maps to chromosome 3q26.3 (Soder et al., 1997), correlating with local telomerase repression (Newbold, 1997). Control of expression, however, is more complicated and dependent on many interacting sites (see below).

hTR is by no means the passive player to hTERT's active role as an enzyme (Blackburn, 1999; Smith and Blackburn, 1999). Specific domains determine binding of hTERT and TEPs (Bachand et al., 2001). Approximately 270 bases downstream of the template is a sequence required for in vitro assembly of the active telomerase. Either of two fragments of hTR (nucleotides +33–147 or +164–325) combined with hTERT cannot produce telomerase activity separately but do so together (Tesmer et al., 1999). In humans, other vertebrates, and many invertebrates, the telomere sequence is a series of tandem repeats of TTAGGG (thymine, thymine, adenine, guanine, guanine, guanine), usually for several thousand base pairs. The corresponding hTR template is complementary, but overlaps and is capable of "climbing" telomeres as bases are added (Greider, 1996).

Most normal human somatic cells have a low but stable hTR concentration; stem, cancer, and hTERT-transfected cells often have higher or more variable hTR concentrations. hTR activity is increased (often with increased gene copy numbers) in some carcinoma cells (Soder et al., 1997; McCaul et al., 2002). Since it is constitutively expressed in most normal human somatic cells (Blasco et al., 1995, 1997a; Feng et al., 1995; Avilion, 1996), hTR is probably not rate limiting for telomerase activity. Nonetheless, in some human and other species (Avilion et al., 1992) cells, the RNA component may be actively regulated.

hTR and hTERT expression may be independent (Avilion et al., 1992) or reciprocal (Stanta et al., 1999), but theory suggests a positive correlation and most data support this. The hTR half-life (approximately 5 days in hTERT-negative human cells) increases markedly (as do hTR levels) if cells express hTERT. In extreme cases (H1299 tumor cells), the half-life is 4 weeks, longer than other cellular RNA. Surprisingly, whether hTERT is endogenous (as in stem or cancer cells) or exogenous (as in transgenic cells) profoundly effects hTR transcription rates. Exogenous hTERT does not alter hTR transcription, but endogenous hTERT markedly increases transcription. This origin has no effect on hTR half-life, however, which increases 1.6-fold regardless of hTERT source (Yi et al., 1999). hTERT affects hTR synthesis and degradation; the hTERT source somehow modulates hTR transcription. If telomerase transcription, degradation, and activity vary with cell phenotype, cell state, and a variety of intracellular factors, small wonder that differences in hTERT source and expression should affect hTR expression.

The catalytic component of telomerase, human telomerase reverse transcriptase, or hTERT (previously hEST2; Meyerson et al., 1997), is a catalytic protein and the active half of telomerase. The number of molecules present in cells demonstrating hTERT activity may be surprisingly small. Using assays sensitive to 0.004 molecules per cell, hTERT molecules are estimated at between 0.2 and 6 per cell (Ducrest et al., 2001). Combining hTR and hTERT in vitro (Weinrich et al., 1997) or in vivo (Counter et al.,

1998b) reconstitutes telomerase activity with normal enzymatic properties. The amino acid and gene sequences of hTERT are known (Collins et al., 1995; Nakamura et al., 1997; Nakayama et al., 1998). The specific effect of protecting (as opposed to lengthening) the telomere (see discussion below) localizes at the COOH terminus of hTERT (Huang et al., 2002), but specific functional locations may vary between yeast and higher organisms and are still being teased apart (Banik et al., 2002).

hTERT is probably the most distal gene (5p15.33) on chromosome 5p (Bryce et al., 2000; Shay and Wright, 2000b). Most human somatic cells do not express hTERT constitutively; it is therefore the controlling element for telomerase activity in most such cells (Harrington et al., 1997b; Kilian et al., 1997; Lingner et al., 1997; Nakamura et al., 1997; Nakayama et al., 1998). Exceptions include germ and stem cells, and likely a few potentially proliferative cells in otherwise telomerase-negative tissues. These include mitotically inactive cells, such as breast lobular epithelium, and mitotically active, regenerating cells, such as proliferating basal cells underlying human epidermis (Harle-Bachor and Boukamp, 1996; Kolquist et al., 1998).

Most mouse somatic cells constitutively express the catalytic component of telomerase (mTERT), although expression probably remains carefully regulated (Greenberg et al., 1998; Martin-Rivera et al., 1998; Blasco, 2002b) and overexpression may increase malignancy risk (Artandi et al., 2002). mTERT may be constitutively expressed, but its activity may be more restricted than that of hTERT (Prowse et al., 1993). The regulation of hTERT expression may be the norm for human cells, but with exceptions. Human lymphocytes may express hTR and hTERT, while telomerase activity remains undetectable. While hTERT levels may be regulated by transcription (Ducrest et al., 2001), activity can be independently regulated by unknown post-transcriptional mechanisms (Liu et al., 1999), perhaps proteolysis (Holt and Shay, 1999) or inhibition by hTERT variants (Colgin et al., 2000). Synthesis may often be rate limiting for activity, and other processes may also play a role: hTERT transport into the nucleus, assembly of the holoenzyme, recruitment to the telomere, and post-translational modifications (Aisner et al., 2002). Increases in hTERT gene numbers occur in some tumor cell lines (Bryce et al., 2000) and might conceivably regulate hTERT in normal cells.

The holoenzyme (Shay et al., 2001) comprises hTR, hTERT, and TEPs (Le et al., 2000), including TEP1 (Harrington et al., 1997a), hStau, and L22. These apparently independent proteins may play roles in hTR processing, telomerase assembly, or localization within the cell. Their function and necessity (Liu et al., 2000b) remain ambiguous. Other proteins may modulate telomerase activity. These include molecular chaperones such as p23 and Hsp90 (Masutomi et al., 2000; Akalin et al., 2001; Forsythe et al., 2001) that bind to the catalytic subunit of telomerase (Holt et al., 1999a) and (in yeasts) DNA primases (Diede and Gottschling, 1999), an F-box protein (Katayama et al., 2002), and inhibitory hTERT variants (Colgin et al., 2000).

Telomerase may have other roles than extending telomeres, such as telomere repair (Collins and Greider, 1993) or preventing senescence by "capping" telomeres (Blackburn, 2000c), the latter being mediated by the hTERT COOH terminus (Huang et al., 2002). Not only can the mere presence of telomerase (absent net telomere lengthening or activity) increase replicative potential (Cao et al., 2002a), provide a selective growth advantage (Forsythe et al., 2002; Xiang et al., 2002), and perhaps limit DNA damage–protein binding, but subtelomeric DNA can cause capping (Chan and Blackburn, 2002). The extent and significance of these roles remain uncertain. Just as telomerase may do more than merely lengthen telomeres, the obverse occurs: telomeres can lengthen without telomerase. Alternate lengthening of telomeres [ALT] is discussed below (Chapter 5).

Typically, normal somatic cells constitutively express the RNA but not the catalytic component (Greenberg et al., 1998). Thus there may be three ways to test the effect of telomere length on cell senescence and gene expression:

1. *transfect* the catalytic gene into a somatic cell that normally lacks it (as in Bodnar et al., 1998),
2. *knock out* the catalytic gene from a cell or organism (as in murine cells that constitutively express telomerase; see below), or
3. *reversibly* control expression of the catalytic component in cells that lack constitutive expression.

Roughly speaking, we can add the gene to a cell that lacks it, subtract the gene from a cell that has it, or produce a cell in which we can turn it on and off at will. We are capable of transfection in vitro, ex vivo, and, potentially (with limited "take"), in vivo. Gene knockouts are standard in genetic laboratories as in, for example, the telomerase knockout mouse. Reversible induction occurs routinely in hematopoetic and perhaps other stem cell lines (Hiyama et al., 1995d; Soares et al., 1998; Holt and Shay, 1999). The same appears to occur in rats (and probably other species) during hepatic regeneration when telomerase is transiently turned on and then back off when regenerative proliferation terminates (Tsujiuchi et al., 1996, 1998; Golubovskaya et al., 1997). We are experimentally capable of reversibly controlling gene expression in vitro (Steinert et al., 2000) and there is increasing focus on mechanisms controlling hTERT expression (Poole et al., 2001). This effort has clear implications for treating cancer and (at a more distant resolve) age-related diseases (Gonzalez-Suarez et al., 2001).

hTERT levels may be predominantly controlled (not by degradation but) by gene expression, specifically transcription (Horikawa et al., 1999; Gunes et al., 2000; Ducrest et al., 2001). In many cell lines, perhaps in general, telomerase activity declines with differentiation (Fukutomi et al., 2001). After cell cycle exit, terminal differentiation, and loss of detectable telomerase activity (Holt et al., 1997a), proteolysis may play a greater role in telomerase regulation (Holt and Shay, 1999). Major control is, however, vested in transcription and is tightly restrained by promoter (Takakura et al., 1999; Koga et al., 2000; Kyo et al., 2000b; Poole et al., 2001) and repressor mechanisms (Fujimoto et al., 2000; Kanaya et al., 2000). Beyond expression, synthesis, and mere presence of hTERT, however, lie complex controls on activity (Aisner et al., 2002).

The hTERT gene lies within a 37 kb region and consists of 16 exons, with an identifiable promoter region flanking it on the GC-rich 5' end. This regulatory region contains a TATA-less promoter located in a CpG island (Horikawa et al., 1999) and the proximal 181 bp core promoter of hTERT has five binding sites for Sp1 and two for c-Myc (Wick et al., 1999; Takakura et al., 2001). Maximal promoter activity can be assigned to a 59 bp region (-208 to -150) that appears to contain the Myc binding site. Insertion of c-Myc plasmids (Horikawa et al., 1999) or retroviral infection (Falchetti et al., 1999) results in rapid telomerase transcription and activation. Transcriptional switching has been accomplished using a conditional v-Myc-estrogen receptor protein (Falchetti et al., 1999) with resultant estrogen-dependent telomerase activity.

Regarding hTERT promoters, current interest focuses on c-myc as a preeminent promoter of transcription (Cerni, 2000; Biroccio et al., 2002). c-*myc*, a ubiquitous transcription factor and protooncogene, directly induces of hTERT transcription. hTERT and c-*myc* are expressed in actively dividing cells, but down-regulated in nondividing cells. Constitutive expression induces immortalization, but c-*myc* rapidly induces hTERT expression regardless of the proliferation status (Wu et al., 1999c). The hTERT promoter region contains numerous c-myc binding sites and is active in cancer, but not in normal cells. Myc directly interacts with these sites, activating hTERT transcription in vivo and in vitro and may be required for telomerase activation in cancer cells (Oh et al., 1999a). The effects of c-myc on hTERT transcription can be overcome. Suppression by herbimycin A blocks transcription independent of direct effects on exogenous telomerase activity (Akiyama et al., 2000b), a finding indicating that suppression can (and does) occur effectively at transcription, rather than by inhibition of activity.

Although our knowledge of the promoter mechanisms for hTERT is increasing rapidly, little is known of the repressor mechanisms (Liu, 1999; Oh et al., 1999b). These are probably complex (Reddel, 1998b; Liu, 1999; Shay, 1999b), although much has become clear in the past few years (e.g., Takakura et al., 1999; Kyo et al., 2000b). Some inhibitory elements may lie within the larger promoter sequence (Braunstein et al., 2001). E2F-1 may have two putative binding sites proximal to the transcriptional start site of the promoter and function as a key regulator of the gene in human cells (Crowe et al., 2001; Crowe and Nguyen, 2001). Methylation alone is not responsible for telomerase repression (Guilleret et al., 2002b), although it may play a role (Dessain et al., 2000; Hoare et al., 2001; Bechter et al., 2002; Guilleret et al., 2002a; Neumeister et al., 2002). The issue of the Polycomb-group proteins in immortalization and telomerase regulation has been raised but not clarified (Jacobs et al., 1999; Itahana et al., 2003).

Effects from other regions have been examined. In keratinocytes, telomerase expression is normally repressed by at least one gene that has been tentatively mapped to the short arm of chromosome 3p (Loughran et al., 1997; Newbold, 1997; Parkinson et al., 1997; Tanaka et al., 1998a). This nicely matches data from renal cell carcinomas, in which restoration of normal chromosome 3 function restores cell senescence (and reciprocally abolishes telomerase activity) within this otherwise immortal tumor cell line (Ohmura et al., 1995). In immortalized breast epithelial cells, insertion of a normal chromosome 17 inhibits telomerase activity (Yang et al., 1999b). Other work has implicated chromosome 5 (Kugoh et al., 2003) as well as chromosomal regions 1q and 17p as having inhibitory effects and 3q and 8q as having promoter effects on telomerase expression. The c-*myc* gene is located on 8q and the *p53* gene on 17p, perhaps explaining part of this correlation (Loveday et al., 1999). In cervical cancer, hTERT expression appears to be controlled by a repressor on chromosomes 6 (Steenbergen et al., 2001) and in HeLa cells, by repressors on chromosomes 3 and 4 (Backsch et al., 2001). While it is likely that telomerase control is a complex and interactive phenomenon, it is equally likely that much remains to be learned that will simplify and give order to the current data.

One possible candidate is the transcription factor Mad1, a second member of the myc/marx/mad network. Initial work suggests that mutation of Mad binding sites causes de-repression of hTERT, which can be counteracted by Myc. The relative amounts of Mad and Myc proteins may be negatively correlated and these levels are appropriate for the hTERT expression found in normal versus malignant cells (Oh et al., 2000). Mad1 repression is dependent on the NH2 terminal domain in association with a corepressor, mSin3 (Gunes et al., 2000). Additional candidates for hTERT suppression include human interleukin-4 (IL-4; Fu et al., 2000a) and interferon-alpha (IFN-α), which represses telomerase transcription (but not hTR or TP1) and telomerase activity in Burkitt's lymphoma cells, apparently by a c-myc–dependent mechanism (Akiyama et al., 1999).

Suppression may vary among cell phenotypes, as occurs with the Wilms' tumor 1 suppressor gene (*WT1*) in renal cells. Alteration of the binding site markedly derepresses hTERT transcription in renal cells, although not in HeLa cells, probably because they lack WT1 expression. At least in some cell lines, *WT1* represses the hTERT promoter and therefore telomerase transcription (Oh et al., 1999b). A growth hormone releasing factor antagonist (MZ-5-156) down-regulates hTERT gene expression (and thereby telomerase activity) but had no effect on hTR or TP1 levels in a glioblastoma cell line (Kiaris et al., 1999). Information on other possible suppressors (e.g., Mendoza et al., 2000) remains scant.

Is Telomerase Good for Anything?

Absent telomerase, cellular renewal of organs in vivo or the serial passage of somatic cells in vitro leads to telomere shortening and changes in gene expression (Hayflick, 1984a; Linskens et al., 1995a; Jansen-Durr, 1998), cell morphology (Matsumura et al., 1979b; Pignolo et al., 1994) and the rate of cell cycling (Matsumura et al., 1979a; Faragher and Kipling, 1998). As the telomeres shorten, the expression of multiple, dominant genes halt DNA synthesis. Virally transformed senescent cells reactivate DNA synthesis and divide even with critically short telomeres. This end run of cell cycle braking can result from viral oncogenes that encode proteins, especially the SV40 T antigen (Pereira-Smith and Smith, 1981, 1987; Counter et al., 1994a; Hayflick, 1997b). Not all oncogenes are as effective (Lumpkin et al., 1986a). The SV40 T antigen binds and inactivates p53 and retinoblastoma (pRb) tumor suppressor proteins (Shay et al., 1991a), which, along with basic helix-loop-helix (HLH) transcription factors (Desprez et al., 1995), otherwise suppress proliferation (Hara et al., 1996). Destabilization of the genome ensues, encouraging further mutations that permit cell immortalization (Stewart and Bacchetti, 1991). SV40 and hTERT can induce immortalization in human mammary epithelial cells (with telomere elongation), but the former causes aberrant differentiation, loss of DNA damage response, karyotypic instability, and occasional tumorigenicity, while the latter results in intact DNA damage responses and more normal differentiation (Toouli et al., 2002). SV40 can induce telomerase activity, at least in mesothelioma cells (Foddis et al., 2002). Factors such as phosphorylation (Yan et al., 1997; Venable and Obeid, 1999; Kharbanda et al., 2000) and methylation (Sonoda et al., 2000) changes may play a role in SV40 immortalization. Overexpression of the Id family of HLH proteins inhibits cell differentiation while activating telomerase and inactivating retinoblastoma protein in human keratinocytes. Such immortalized cells have an impaired p53-mediated response to DNA-damage response (Alani et al., 1999). The story remains complex and incompletely understood.

The notion that cell senescence is timed by a mechanism that measures telomere shortening is probably "the best explanation" (Campisi, 1997b), though perhaps not the only one (Spitkovsky, 1997). Although it remains supported by literally hundreds of studies over the past decade, some studies question the necessity (and at times the utility) of telomerase. Mouse embryonic fibroblasts (MEFs), nullizygous for telomerase RNA, spontaneously immortalize without telomerase activity (Blasco et al., 1997a; Hande et al., 1999a), although normal telomere structure and function may be required (Espejel and Blasco, 2002). Mouse embryonic fibroblasts become immortal given optimal in vitro conditions (Mathon et al., 2001; Shay and Wright, 2001c; Tang et al., 2001). Although inhibition of mTERT activity appears to interrupt proliferation, some subclones escape inhibition and continue dividing (Boklan et al., 2002). Spontaneous immortalization is 10 million–fold more likely in murine than in human cells (Wright and Shay, 2000). Occasional reports (Romanov et al., 2001) notwithstanding, spontaneous immortalization is extraordinarily rare in human cells. Although the majority (perhaps 90%) of human malignancies express telomerase, there are immortal human cell lines with long telomeres but lacking detectable telomerase activity (Bryan et al., 1995; Gollahon et al., 1998). These may be attributable to technical limits, suggesting greater reliability (and telomerase expression) as methods improve (Wright et al., 1995; Shay et al., 1997; Norton et al., 1998). The general rule suggests there is an all-but-consistent repression of telomerase in normal somatic cells (Hastie et al., 1990) and overwhelming expression in malignant ones (Harley and Kim, 1996). Overall, telomerase is required for immortalization (Dessain et al., 2000).

Mice are useful for aging research because they are cheap, well understood, and have short lifespans. Initially negative results (Blasco et al., 1997a) from a telomerase RNA (mTR) knockout, or telomerase null, mouse (mTR–/–) were greeted with surprise and uncertainty (Sedivy, 1998). Unlike humans, mice have baseline telomerase activity in most (Chadeneau et al., 1995b; Prowse and Greider, 1995; Greenberg et al., 1998) although not all (Bednarek et al., 1995) somatic cells, making telomerase a poorer marker for murine than human malignancy (Kipling, 1997a, 1997b; King et al., 1999). Nonetheless, telomerase activity does increase during murine carcinogenesis (Bednarek et al., 1995; Miura et al., 1998).

Rats show similar constitutive activity (Yoshimi et al., 1996; Nozawa et al., 1999), at least in many somatic cells (Borges and Liew, 1997; Golubovskaya et al., 1997, 1999). In rats, telomerase activity declines with age (Kang et al., 1999), but (as in humans) there is wide variation depending on cell phenotype and stimulatory conditions (Yamaguchi et al., 1998). The same is true of many other small mammals, including some primates, such as tamarins (Tobi et al., 2001). Constitutive telomerase expression occurs in Syrian hamsters (Russo et al., 1998) and chickens (Venkatesan and Price, 1998), although immortalized chicken cell telomeres remain stable without telomerase activity (Kim et al., 2001a). In most birds (penguins, finches, and swallows), telomere length declines with age, although in storm petrels, a longlived species, telomere lengths may increase (Haussmann et al., 2002). Whether this correlates with telomerase expression remains unknown. Telomeres may control nonhuman cell senescence and carcinogenesis, but there may be striking differences in how telomerase activity (as opposed to expression) is controlled (Forsyth et al., 2002) and how telomere length is regulated (Serakinci et al., 1999) in these organisms compared to in primates (Steinert et al., 2002) and especially humans (Blasco et al., 1999).

Murine constitutive telomerase activity and its associated high incidence of cancer (Prowse and Greider, 1995; Holliday, 1996; Greenberg et al., 1998) made the telomerase knockout mouse a research priority. Despite what are now known to be significant intracellular abnormalities (Liu et al., 2000b), mTR knockout (Blasco et al., 1997a) and mTERT knockout (Nikaido et al., 1999) mice initially appeared to suffer no ill effects.

Consider the implications. While most normal human somatic cells lack telomerase and do well for decades, some embryonic cell lines (Mantell and Greider, 1994; Wright et al., 1996b; Yashima et al., 1998b), the germ cell line, and some stem cell lines (see below) depend on telomeres maintenance to continue dividing. In the long run, telo-mere maintenance is necessary to species survival and perhaps (in the short run) for normal fetal development (Kojima et al., 2001). The initial results of the knockout mice therefore startled many. Lifespans (more or less), motor activity, weight gains, hematopoetic histology, peripheral blood counts, immune response, and in vitro cell growth remained unaffected (Blasco et al., 1997a; Lee et al., 1998c). Bluntly, telomerase activity was unnecessary for murine "organogenesis or postnatal organ function or maintenance" (Lee et al., 1998c).

Subsequent results put the initial data in a different light (Lee et al., 1998c; Rudolph et al., 1999; Blasco, 2002a). Early-generation mice were subtly abnormal and abnor-malities increased with age (Herrera et al., 1999b). Some first-generation mice had ero-sive dermatitis. Fertility problems became apparent by the fifth generation and there were no sixth-generation offspring. This was partially attributable to cell losses and organ changes in reproductive systems, but other organs with highly proliferative cells were similarly affected (Blasco, 2002a). Hematopoetic stem cell renewal diminished in vitro, although not demonstrably in peripheral or marrow histology. Responses to blood loss (Samper et al., 2002), wound healing (Rudolph et al., 1999), immune function (Blasco, 2002a), angiogenesis, and vascularization (Franco et al., 2002b) were impaired. Lympho-cytes showed a marked increase in late apoptotic cells, suggesting that telomerase and long telomeres were (in certain cases) protective against apoptosis (Ozen et al., 1998; Holt et al., 1999b; Seimiya et al., 1999; Ren et al., 2001). Abnormal chromosomal fusions and other evidence of genomic instability (Chang et al., 2001) increased over generation times (Slijepcevic, 1998a), perhaps in a chromosome-specific manner (Hande et al., 1999a). Curiously, mice null for telomerase RNA and INK4a tumor suppressor genes (part of the DNA damage response) have fewer tumors in vivo and less malignant transformation in vitro. This partially resolves with reintroduction of mTER (Greenberg et al., 1999a). Short telomere mTR knockout mice are less prone to epithelial tumors (Gonzalez-Suarez et al., 2000) and melanomas (Franco et al., 2002b) than normals.

The long delay in these defects has been attributed to the long telomeres found in this murine strain (and in hamsters; Slijepcevic and Hande, 1999). With a longer telomeric buffer, they began to suffer only when the telomere had all but completely eroded (Lee et al., 1998c). This vague explanation accords with later data comparing mTR knock-outs in mice with longer or shorter telomeres. Original mice with longer telomeres sur-vived for six generations; those with shorter telomeres only survived for four generations (Herrera et al., 1999b). The telomere plays a role in timing *something*, if not within, then between generations.

The primary importance of this work is that t*elomerase expression and telomere length per se are often not critical in individual organisms*. This cannot be overly stressed: absolute (as opposed to relative) telomere lengths do not determine aging or aging pa-thology within an organism. Failure to appreciate this difference has led to the unwar-ranted conclusion that telomere shortening may determine cell senescence in humans but not in mice, because their cells arrest without "significant telomere shortening" (Hornsby, 2001). Shortening may be minimal in proportion to total telomere length, but discounting its effect on gene expression is premature. The fundamental issue is neither telomerase expression nor absolute (or initial) telomere length (Golubev, 2001; Serra and von Zglinicki, 2002), but the alteration of patterns of gene expression (West et al., 1996; Shelton et al., 1999; Ly et al., 2000), only indirectly attributable to relative changes in telomere lengths and even more distantly to telomerase expression (Li and Liu, 2002). In cell senescence, the critical issue is gene expression, modulated by a (poorly understood) linkage that depends not on absolute initial telomere length but on the relative change in telomere length as cells divide. This change in length may be minor as a percentage of total length, yet have major effects upon gene expression. The mechanism linking changes in telomere length to distant effects on gene expression (and therefore any measure of senescence within the cell) is, of necessity, reset upon germ cell fertilization (see below).

Comparing telomere lengths between specific murine chromosomes, there is predictable consistency of specific chromosomes and rate of telomere loss within individual cells, but (also predictably) no consistency of telomere lengths between different chromosomes (Zijlmans et al., 1997) nor between individual mice, even within fully inbred populations (Kipling and Cooke, 1990). This agrees with the model suggested here: telomere length is irrelevant; telomere loss is critical. The controlling variable is not absolute length (Rubio et al., 2002; Serra and von Zglinicki, 2002), but relative loss of length since fertilization. Consider falling from a building: the 50th percentile for survival (LD_{50})in humans is approximately 2.5 stories. On the other hand, jumping from 5000 feet (200 x LD_{50}) is safe if it goes only 4 inches (e.g., from the sidewalk to the street in Denver). Survival is determined, not by absolute altitude, but by relative loss of altitude. Changes in gene expression are determined, not by absolute length, but relative loss of length. Lack of correlation between telomere length or knockout status and lifespan is irrelevant.

Gene expression must be separated conceptually from which genes the organism possesses (Goyns et al., 1998). Specific genes have been implicated in aging and used to extend lifespan in some species (Jazwinski, 2000a). Despite understandable interest in "longevity genes" (Hodes et al., 1996b; Pedersen, 2000; Yashin et al., 2000; Perls et al., 2002) or "vitagenes" (Rattan, 1998a, 1998b), the concern is gene expression (Linskens et al., 1995a; Shelton et al., 1999). *All* genes affect lifespan, but not necessarily aging. Critical genes deserve attention for their clinical and biological implications (Martin, 2000) and affect aging's "pace" (Guarente, 1997a), but cell immortality is determined by gene expression. Within cells, aging is not a matter of longevity genes, but longevity pattern of gene expression. Germ cells have the same genes as somatic cells, but express them differently. Cell immortality and senescence are determined by gene expression, not a change in genes. Resistance to oxidative damage, characteristic of long-lived avian species, is determined not by the presence of specific genes but by their pattern of expression (Ogburn et al., 2001).

While the genes the organism possesses (its genome) determine the "universe" of possible expression, this set includes a subset enabling cell immortality, i.e., indefinite survival, as occurs in germ cells. An organism lacking such a pattern precludes germ cell and hence species survival. It is the *control* of this subset of gene expression that concerns us. When will a cell express a senescent pattern and when an immortal pattern?

Fertilization is a major determinant of gene expression. Normal fetal development occurs only if nonfetal patterns are repressed, then proceeds with progressive differentiation and decreasing cellular immortality: germ cells become somatic cells. Telomerase gene transfection ("telomerization") is an experimental determinant, switching somatic cells from mortal to immortal without disruption of the remainder of the pattern of gene expression (Bodnar et al., 1998; Funk et al., 2000). This process of gene control is central to cell aging and experimental intervention. Resetting gene expression occurs in knockout mice, cloning, and other interventions, permitting us to make sense of how cell senescence causes aging in organisms.

CHAPTER 3

Cell Senescence in Aging

What Is Cell Senescence?

Defining cell senescence is surprisingly difficult. Current discussions often confuse telomere length, population doublings, and cell morphology, prompting misunderstanding and contradiction. Degree of senescence is frequently ignored, with similar outcomes. One person's senescence is another's normal cell. As Voltaire (1764, p 225) said, "Define your terms . . . or we shall never understand one another."

Cell senescence is not simply the cessation of division. Adult human neurons and myocytes have long been considered incapable of division although exceptions occur. Nor is cell quiescence equivalent to senescence (Pignolo et al., 1993; Faragher et al., 1997b; Holt and Shay, 1999). Many cells are "normally quiescent," not dividing without external stimulation, including hepatocytes (Aikata et al., 2000), lymphocytes (Lansdorp, 1998), ocular stromal keratocytes (Tuft et al., 1993), and corneal endothelial cells (Mishima, 1982; Treffers, 1982; Schultz et al., 1992). Not dividing, they remain capable of doing so and are not senescent. The distinction between quiescent and senescent may be based on the cell cycle: quiescent cells are in G0Q and senescent cells, in G0S (Norwood et al., 1990a).

Cell senescence generally refers to changes in cells as they divide repeatedly. These include not only morphology but G1 DNA content (Gorman and Cristofalo, 1981), changes in gene expression (Sheshadri and Campisi, 1990; Wistrom and Villeponteau, 1992; Shelton et al., 1999), unique antigenic determinants (Porter et al., 1990), and, perhaps most importantly, changes in cell function (Faragher et al., 1997b; Obeid and Venable, 1997).

Cell senescence was originally considered to occur in somatic cells after many (typically 60 or more) divisions. Cells slow and finally cease dividing. Cell cycle deceleration is accompanied by morphological changes that are consistent within cell pheno-type (Hayflick, 1979). Such changes are extensive; a review by Hayflick (1980) required six pages to list known alterations two decades ago. The sheer volume and the ease of a numerical approach to those limits, however, prompted oversimplification. A single number—population doublings—came to define senescence. Cells were senescent when reaching a cell phenotype–specific number of population doublings that was thought to represent the equivalent number of divisions. Although a cell culture might have doubled 10 times, specific cells were unlikely to have undergone exactly 10 divisions, except as a population mean. Some cells might be "senescent" early, others might be "young" well after the usual "senescent" number of doublings. Errors were intrinsic; watching each cell divide was impractical, counting doubled volumes was simple. The literature—appropriately, honestly, but misleadingly—gave data in PDs (population doublings); this came to be equivalent to cell divisions. Cell senescence was occurring as a mean, and senescent variance rose nearly as fast as the population doublings, i.e., exponentially.

Some authors (e.g., Faragher et al., 1997b) suggested that senescence was an en-tirely quantal, stochastic process (Rawes et al., 1997) in that a cell has a small but equal chance of achieving senescence at each division. Some data (Smith and Whitney, 1980) and theory (Shall and Stein, 1979) support the suggestion. In Russian-roulette view, cells were senescent or not: there was no spectrum of senescence. Cell senescence was all-or-nothing and each cell division "pulled the trigger" (Faragher et al., 1997b) until the odds of senescence became overwhelming (Shall, 1997). The number of population doublings offered no insight into the mechanics of senescence. A more moderate ver-sion suggests that perhaps seven cell divisions remain once the cell commits to senes-cence (Gallant and Prothero, 1980; Prothero and Gallant, 1981).

Observation of individual cell morphology, by contrast, suggests that senescence is gradual, not binary, but morphology is subjective. Observers have differed in whether cells look young or like senescent fried eggs. Cell cycle deceleration gave a more reli-able (perhaps more valid) measure, but was demanding. Observers needed to watch large numbers of individual cells without interruption for days to be accurate.

In 1990, cell senescence was found to correlate with telomere length (Harley et al., 1990). This useful observation made telomere lengths a marker for cell senescence. Technically demanding (Baerlocher et al., 2002; Pommier and Sabatier, 2002; Scherthan, 2002), it was relatively objective and permitted ready comparison based on kilobase pairs (kbps). Young cells might have 15 kbps, senescent cells a mere 3. A specific (Hao and Tan, 2001) critically short telomere might induce senescence (Dimri et al., 2000; Lundblad, 2001), but single telomeres are rarely sufficient (Lansdorp, 2000). In a popu-lation of cells, however, *mean telomere lengths* might mean no more than *mean divi-sions*. Was a mean telomere length of 2 kbps more accurate in describing individual cells or population variance than 50 population doublings? Neither measure accounted for the considerable variance (Allsopp and Harley, 1995; Lauzon et al., 2000). While making progress in quantifying cell aging (Grant et al., 2001; Poon and Lansdorp, 2001; Cawthorn, 2002; Fordyce et al., 2002; Meeker et al., 2002a), individual telo-meres are difficult to measure, prompting some investigators to simply weigh the entire telomeric DNA and call it even (Bryant et al., 1997). Even worse, the telomere length at which the human fibroblast senesce may vary with age (Figueroa et al., 2000) or other factors.

DNA damage (Ahmed and Hodgkin, 2000) such as hypoxia, hyperoxia (von Zglinicki et al., 1995; Honda et al., 2001; Saretzki and von Zglinicki, 2002), oxidative damage by hydrogen peroxide (Chen et al., 1998; Beach, 2000; von Zglinicki et al., 2000a), chromatin remodeling, and oncogenic forms of Ras (Serrano et al., 1997; but see Hutter et al., 2002) or Raf, E2F1 (Dimri et al., 2000), as well as other interventions (Shibanuma et al., 1997; Toussaint et al., 2002) can apparently induce cell senescence (Proctor and Kirkwood, 2002), although this effect may be due to cell divisions (Dumont et al., 2001), loss of effective telomere capping (Peitl et al., 2002), and DNA damage (Gorbunova et al., 2002) rather than senescence, and proteomic effects differ from telomeric senescence (Dierick et al., 2002). Telomerase may protect chromosome by capping the telomere or limiting DNA damage responses, independent of the canonic effect of telomere lengthening (Chan and Blackburn, 2002), perhaps by protecting single-strand overhangs (Stewart et al., 2003). In the case of E2F1, cell senescence might result from repression of hTERT (Crowe et al., 2001). Whether these interventions induce senescence or mimic it is unknown. Confluent cultures occasionally undergo cell senescence without sufficient divisions, although this apparently requires p16(INK4A) and perhaps p27(KIP1) expression and may be reversible (Munro et al., 2001; Sviderskaya et al., 2002). This effect may vary among human, mouse, and chicken fibroblasts (Kim et al., 2002b).

Telomerase works directly as well as having enzymatic effects on telomere length (Blackburn, 1999, 2000a, 2000c). In mTERT heterozygous mice, telomerase activity insufficient to maintain length protects against fusions and genome instability (Liu et al., 2002e), perhaps capping the telomere, as it does in yeast (Blackburn, 1999) or via other mechanisms (Gollahon et al., 1998). Ectopic expression of hTERT in human fibroblasts with short telomeres can effectively avert crisis and prevent chromosomal instability even without extending the telomere. Such cells can continue to proliferate despite progressively eroding telomeres shorter than those of control cells that have already entered crisis (Zhu et al., 1999b). Apparently, hTERT permits cell proliferation without telomere lengthening.

Perhaps we need a more universal marker of cell senescence, such as changes in cell function. Changes in morphology and cell cycle timing, and altered response to environmental stimuli reflect altered cell function and result from current patterns of gene expression. Patterns of gene expression define the difference between fibroblasts and leukocytes; perhaps they can define the difference between senescent and non-senescent cells (Linskens et al., 1995a; Shelton et al., 1999). This is not arbitrary or circular. We require a useful definition, not merely a descriptive one. Context and intent determine utility of definition and consequent risk of denotative confusion. We intend to discuss changes occurring in senescing cells; changes in gene expression applies nicely in the context. Senescent cells express their genes in a senescent pattern rather than a nonsenescent pattern, just as fibroblasts are cells that express their genes in a fibroblast pattern rather than a leukocyte pattern.

Senescence is not simply cumulative cell damage causing changes in gene expression, but senescence and accumulating damage result from changes in gene expression. This allows us to discuss senescence in practical, operational terms: by measuring gene expression we not only define a cell as senescent but gain insight into how and why it is senescent. Does the altered patterns of gene expression affect cell growth (Irving et al., 1992)? Is inflammatory gene expression altered (Shelton et al., 1999)? What about the genes responsible for energy metabolism? Has expression changed in genes for cell cycle factors and what precedes this change (Obeid and Venable, 1997)? From a scientific standpoint, basing our definition of cell senescence on gene expression not only provides a complex, measurable, and objective definition but immediately provides information as to potential mechanism and, better, avenues to further experimentation and intervention (Shelton et al., 1999). Unfortunately, this definition presents an overabundance of data. Senescence becomes a state-of-the-art technical measurement of differential expression in tens of thousands of genes (Shelton et al., 1999). This is more difficult than counting population doublings, though also more rewarding experimentally, theoretically, and clinically.

Orthogonally to the problem of measuring senescence is the problem of agreeing to a cutoff: how senescent is "senescent"? Backtracking to a definition base on cell divisions, if a young cell has zero divisions and the cell can undergo a maximum of 50 divisions, then what is our cutoff for senescence? Does a cell become senescent at 25, 40, or 49 divisions? Must a cell have stopped dividing to be senescent? Despite proclamations that "there is no such thing as a half senescent cell"(Faragher et al., 1997b), some authors refer to "near senescent" cells, capable of rescue via telomerization (Steinert et al., 2000). Others (Cristofalo and Pignolo, 1993) refer to "conditionally senescent states," citing cells in an "obligatory arrested state" that, under proper conditions, can still undergo DNA, if not cell replication.

We unconsciously employ different assumptions, different definitions, and inconsistent criteria. Parameters, cutoffs, and whether senescence is all-or-nothing or a more gradual process vary randomly throughout the literature. Honest researchers find contradictory results: one finds 1% of cells are senescent in centenarians, another that 99% of cells are senescent, even in a single biopsy from a single centenarian. To achieve useful insights into cell senescence and aging (Hayflick, 1976), we need to identify changes in cell function, measure the degree of each change, and specify assumptions.

In the entire picture of cellular change, senescence is not all-or-nothing, but a matter of degree. Deceleration of cell cycling begins gradually, morphologic change is a continuum. Confusion reigns when we lose sight of what actually occurs in senescing cells, which undergo wholesale but gradual changes in patterns of gene expression and, secondarily, cell function. With the advent of telomerization, i.e., hTERT transfection (Bodnar et al., 1998), cell senescence can be prevented. This is no longer merely an academic but now a practical question: can we reset senescence in senescent or "near senescent" cells (Steinert et al., 2000)? The answer depends on our definition. Assume we agree on a measuring stick for senescence running from zero to 100 (e.g., telomere length). Maximally "young" cells (longest telomere), without any senescence, are at 100; maximally senescent cells are at zero (a scale corresponding to percentage of telomere loss?). Cells with low numbers are senescent and cannot be rescued by telomerization or other intervention, but at how low a number and how completely "rescued"? Are cells irrevocably senescent at 20? Fifty? No longer arbitrary, senescence becomes a matter of measurable effect based on a defined intervention.

While no one suggests we can reset cells at zero (are such cells dead?), there is disagreement as to what degree of cell senescence can be reversed (Faragher et al., 1997b). As St. Augustine once observed, "It is not so much a question of what men's opinions are, but what the truth is" (Schopenhauer, 1965). There is little disagreement that certain cells, senescent or nonsenescent, can be immortalized (Bodnar et al., 1998).

There is a publicly unstated, but general assumption that there is a point of no return for senescing cells, but this point is ambiguous, partly through inconsistent definition, partly through our lack of complete data.

In defining cell senescence, Bodnar et al. (1998) employed telomere length and population doublings. These and other markers for senescence, such as colony size, which correlates with in vitro and in vivo aging in several species (Smith et al., 1978, 1980), are historically sanctioned, but measure populations, not cells. Evaluation of cell senescence requires a valid and reliable parameter reflecting intracellular events, one that allows us to compare different cell phenotypes, different species, and different organism ages. It is misleading and pointless to discuss whether two cells are equally senescent while relying on population doublings or even cell divisions. We require a marker that accounts for changes in cellular state, i.e., gene expression. By default and without overt intent, gene expression may become standard in discussions of cell senescence.

β-galactosidase (β-gal) has become a common marker of senescence in skin fibroblasts (Dimri and Campisi, 1994a; Dimri et al., 1995; Katakura et al., 1997; Watanabe et al., 1997), retinal pigmented epithelial cells (Matsunaga et al., 1999a), and mesothelial cells (Thomas et al., 1997), yet this method has been criticized (Yegorov et al., 1998; Severino et al., 2000). Single gene–based definitions are neither appropriate nor well supported. Patterns of gene expression (Linskens et al., 1995a) vary with cell phenotype and senescence (Funk, 1998; Shelton et al., 1999; Ly et al., 2000) and permit operational and useful distinctions. Moreover, patterns of gene expression determine cell function, organ function, and clinical disease.

As cells senesce and gene expression alters, they become increasingly dysfunctional and accrue damage. Damage is ubiquitous and, at least historically, has been attributed primarily to free radicals. This is not a simple, passive accumulation of damage (Kirkwood and Franceschi, 1993). Even restricting consideration to free radicals still results in four independent processes:

1. *Production:* the number of free radicals produced per mole of ATP increases.
2. *Sequestration:* the mitochondrial lipid membranes become less effective.
3. *Scavenging:* free radical scavenging mechanisms become less effective.
4. *Repair and replacement:* the effective response to such damage diminishes.

Changes in gene expression underlying any of these will increase cell damage. Free radical damage accumulates when the cell increases free radical production (Allen et al., 1999; Chen et al., 2001a) or fails to sequester or trap them (Hall et al., 2001), and then only when damage exceeds the cell's ability to repair (Moriwaki et al., 1996; Gilchrest and Bohr, 1997) or replace (Finch, 1990; Arking, 1998; Donati et al., 2001) cell components.

Somatic cell mitochondria differ from those of immortal cells (Duncan et al., 2000). Although constant in number, there are subtle changes in mitochondrial morphology in normal and progeric aging (Goldstein and Korczack, 1981; Goldstein and Moerman, 1984). Mitochondrial protein synthesis falls with age (Beaufrere and Boirie, 1998; Proctor et al., 1998; Short and Nair, 1999), as do binding affinities (Liu et al., 2002b) and other functions. More importantly, aging mitochondria produce an increasing percentage (normally 1%–4%) of reactive oxygen species (ROS) for every mole of ATP (Richter, 1988; Joenje 1989). As production increases, so does membrane leakage. Proton escape increases (Porter et al., 1999) as lipid membrane turnover decreases (Harper et al., 1998; Donati et al., 2001).

The outcome is an increasing probability of damage to intracellular molecules, damage which the aging cell is less able to replace or repair (Lamb, 1977; Kowald and Kirkwood, 1994). Granted the increasing production and leakage of free radicals, it is the deceleration of turnover, rather than faulty synthesis, that underlies much of the cell's accumulating damage. Age-related synthesis of faulty proteins (Stadtman, 1992) or the archaic notion of aging as a vicious cycle of errors in protein synthesis—error catastrophe (Kirkwood, 1977)—is tempting, but unlikely (Rattan and Clark, 1999). There is no evidence that errors in protein synthesis cause cellular senescence; there is considerable evidence that transcription fidelity is maintained (Harley et al., 1980; Wojtyk and Goldstein, 1980; Goldstein et al., 1985), although subtle effects may occur (Rattan and Clark, 1999).

Oxidative DNA damage alone occurs perhaps 10,000 times per day per cell (Ames et al., 1993), requiring at least 130 known DNA repair genes (Wood et al., 2001b). Even if this damage were constant (Lindahl and Wood, 1999), repair is not (Goldstein, 1971b). A number of studies over the past decade (Higami et al., 1994; Moriwaki et al., 1996; Gilchrest and Bohr, 1997) support the consensus that DNA repair declines with age (Hadshiew et al., 1999), although not uniformly in all cells (Liu et al., 1982, 1985; Christiansen et al., 2000b), nor equally in all types of DNA repair (Hadshiew et al., 1999). The resulting damage accumulation is neither predictable nor uniform among cells (Singh et al., 1990) or individuals (Singh et al., 1991). Theories attributing aging solely to accumulated DNA damage (e.g., Szilard, 1959) have been discounted (Kirkwood, 1988a, 1989; Arking, 1998), although DNA damage does occur (Ramsey et al., 1995; Tucker et al., 1999; Spruill et al., 2000) and accumulates in aging organisms (Bohr and Anson, 1995; Kaneko et al., 1996; Vijg, 2000), in aging organs (Higami et al., 1994), and in senescent cells (Brown et al., 1978; Weirach-Schwaiger et al., 1994; Gilchrest and Bohr, 1997).

Senescing human fibroblasts and osteoblasts may show a parallel decrease in DNA repair (Goldstein, 1971b) although repair of UV damage is unaffected (Christiansen et al., 2000b). Whether decreasing DNA repair causes senescence or vice versa would remain unsettled (Sen et al., 1987; Bohr and Anson, 1995) were it not for data showing that cell senescence can be indefinitely deferred (e.g., Bodnar et al., 1998) or even reversed (Vaziri 1998; Vaziri and Benchimol, 1998), apparently without directly increasing DNA repair (Roques et al., 2001). Moreover, hTERT immortalization of human fibroblasts indefinitely prevents any decline in DNA repair (Roques et al., 2001). Experimental abrogation of DNA repair or other components of genomic maintenance (Hasty and Vijg, 2002), including double-strand break repair (Vogel et al., 1999) and helicase function (de Boer et al., 2002), can induce premature clinical aging. Telomerase knockout mice, though as sensitive to radiation damage, show a striking problem with DNA repair, with delayed DNA break repair kinetics, persistent chromosomal breaks, chromosomal aberrations, and fragmentation (Wong et al., 2000), as well as complex nonreciprocal translocations (Artandi et al., 2000), chromosomal aberrations that may also induce telomere shortening (Modino and Slijepcevic, 2002).

Many proteins play a dual role in telomere maintenance and DNA repair, especially double-strand break repair (Weaver, 1998; Lewis et al., 2002). Cells from patients with ataxia telangiectasia (ATM), whose chromosomes are prone to fusions, end associations, and breaks (as well as more sensitive to radiation), have shorter than normal telomeres (Hande et al., 2001). There is an inverse correlation between telomere length and chromosomal end associations (Pandita et al., 1995). This has been attributed to problems of telomere maintenance (Greenwell et al., 1985; Pandita, 2001) and specifically to defective telomeric chromatin (Pandita and Dhar, 2000; Scherthan et al., 2000). Some problems, specifically premature cell senescence, disappear when ATM cells are immortalized (Sprung et al., 1997), although other abnormalities, such as radiosensitivity, telomere fusions, and cell cycle defects, remain (Wood et al., 2001a). The latter can be related to defective TRF1 function (Kishi and Lu, 2002) and a failure of double-strand DNA repair (Pandita, 2002). Nijmegen breakage syndrome, likewise having characteristic genomic instability and cancer susceptibility, has defective telomere maintenance (Lombard and Guarente, 2000). In these diseases, it is telomere lengthening and the prevention of cell senescence that improves chromosome stability (Counter et al., 1992; Amit et al., 2000), not the reverse, which suggests that longer telomeres may be essential to chromosomal stability (Golubovskaya et al., 1999).

With the sole exception of DNA (Singer and Berg, 1991), cellular molecules are not repaired but replaced. The rate of turnover is surprisingly critical (Rattan and Clark, 1999), even absent any change in rate of damage with age. If the rate of damage (here arbitrarily 1% of molecules per day) and the total number of molecules in the pool (here 100%) remain constant, but the turnover rate varies (r = % molecules replaced per day), then the percentage of damaged molecules (X) on day (N) will be X_N. At equilibrium, $X_N = X_{N-1}$. This can be calculated as the number damaged on a particular day, plus the number of damaged molecules remaining from the previous day ($X_{N-1} \times M$), minus the number of previously damaged molecules replaced during the past day ($X_{N-1} \times r$), divided by the total number of molecules (M) in the cell. At equilibrium:

$$\text{Equilibrium protein damage:} \quad X = 1 + [X(100 - r)/100]$$

If the molecular turnover rate (r) is 50%, then:

$$X = 1 + 0.5X$$
$$X = 2$$

Given a damage rate of 1%, if the turnover rate were 50%, then at equilibrium, 2% of the molecules are damaged on any given day.

If the molecular turnover rate (r) is 2%, then

$$X = 1 + 0.98X$$
$$X = 50$$

Given a damage rate of 1%, if the turnover rate were only 2%, then at equilibrium, 50% of available molecules would have been damaged (see Fossel, 1996, p 260).

Turnover rates—whether protein, lipid, or other molecules—have a profound effect on the burden of damaged molecules within a cell, i.e., on cell dysfunction. This process might conceivably contribute to caloric restriction, since relative starvation increases protein turnover (Gottesman and Maurizi, 2001). The cell, hungry for specific amino acids, increases protein turnover, resulting in a decreasing percentage of damaged proteins and prolonged cell function.

Lipid membranes are known to change with age (Zs-Nagy, 1997), but the importance of this change is unproven. Increased lipid peroxidation is found in atherogenesis (Morel et al., 1984; Steinberg and Gotto, 1999), but whether this is the fault of turnover is unknown. In rats, lipid membrane turnover probably decreases (Rothstein, 1995; Donati et al., 2001), accounting for greater free radical permeability (Tsai et al., 2001) and a failure of membranes to sequester free radicals within the mitochondria (Kim et al., 1996).

Protein synthesis falls in senescing cells (Cristofalo and Sharf, 1973) and protein turnover probably slows with age (Rattan and Clark, 1999; Donati et al., 2001), although little is known in detail (Gafni, 2001). Protein turnover is a balance between synthesis and the "recycling" of ubiquinated proteins destroyed in proteosomes (Goldberg et al., 2000). Although difficult to assess accurately for individual protein fractions, protein turnover shows an overall decrease with age and protein half-life increases (Rothstein and Evans, 1995), in accord with predictions (Grune et al., 2001). Given the complexity of changes occurring in aging cells, some proteins might display increased turnover, even if net turnover decreases.

Increasing data suggest that cell senescence is not merely an accumulation of damage but an accumulation of damage secondary to changes in gene expression (Ahmed and Hodgkin, 2000). These may alter free radical production and sequestration, DNA repair, and molecular turnover, but they also encompass altered responses to extrinsic cell signals, altered cell secretion, and altered patterns of gene expression (Shelton et al., 1999; Ly et al., 2000). Until recently, however, it has been difficult to distinguish cell damage from underlying changes in gene expression. Older aging studies often looked at the entire organism, averaging all somatic cells. We can scarcely expect to distinguish between cells that divide and senesce (e.g., endothelial cells and microglia) from those that do not (e.g., muscle cells and neurons) on the basis of whole-organism data. Even studies of specific organs or tissues may reflect similar confounding, as when coronary endothelial cells are assayed with myocardial cells or glial cells with neurons. Within specific tissue types—bone marrow or epidermis—stem cells senesce slowly while other cells differentiate and senesce rapidly. Recently, gene array data allow specific, often quantitative answers to questions regarding changes within specific cell phenotypes as they senescence. Cells change in specific, predictable, and measurable ways as they senesce and these changes have profound effects on neighboring cells.

The Limited Model: Cells Senesce

Cell senescence may change cell function, but what causes cells to senesce? The limited model of the cell senescence theory of aging (Harley et al., 1992; Allsopp, 1996; Harley, 1998b) addresses this issue, at least within the cell. The general model addresses the implications of cell senescence for the organism in the following section.

Until 1990, explanations of cell senescence—for example, soluble factors (Wistrom et al., 1989)—went largely untested. Since then, despite occasional eccentric fusillades (Rubin, 1998), there has been increasing consensus for the limited model (Faragher et al., 1998; Kipling et al., 1999). Although much remains unclear (Reddel, 1998a; Perrem and Reddel, 2000; Marcotte and Wang, 2002), the overall outline (Engelhardt and Martens, 1998; Ishikawa, 2000b) is well supported by data and has gained wide acceptance (Boukamp, 2001). Simply put, cell senescence occurs because telomere shortening results in a change in the linkage (see below), which results in significant and cell phenotype-specific changes in the expression of critical genes, such as those regulating growth (Campisi, 1997b) and cell division (Ly et al., 2000). The segue from telomere erosion to gene expression (Campisi, 2000a) is probably the result of telomeric chromatin changes: alterations in the histone proteins that play a central role gene expression (Jenuwein and Allis, 2001). Gene expression, not genes, distinguish myocyte from fibroblast and young cells from senescent ones; telomeres are the controlling variables in altering gene expression during cell senescence.

This summary is inaccurate and unfair. Cell senescence is not a simple domino mechanism progressing from telomeres to linkage to genes. Not only is the mechanism from telomere to gene expression much more complex than this catenation suggests, but this portrayal ignores preceding (why did the telomere shorten?) and succeeding events (so what if gene expression changes?) that place cell senescence in a broader cellular and biological context.

Many of us assume that the passage of time causes cell senescence. This reflects an unjustified, though common assumption: things falls apart as time passes. Unfortunately, vague allusions to wear-and-tear explanations of cell senescence and are contradicted by a passing knowledge of biology. All living cells are three and a half billion years old. The keratinocyte on the back of my left hand is doing fairly well considering its provenance. But total time living is not age. All cells may be three and a half billion years old, but they are certainly not equivalent. Some cells senesce and some don't, no matter how many eons have passed since life began.

A second option might be to measure a cell's age from its last cell division. The keratinocyte on the back of my left hand is now merely a few days old. But defining cell age as the time since last division would suggest that cell senescence cannot occur over a number of divisions, which it does. Measuring age from last division suggests that every time a cell divides, it is renewed and biologically "born again." Yet cells are known to senesce over dozens of divisions, reliably and predictably for each cell phenotype.

Cell senescence is neither total age (since life began), nor age since division. We might compromise on the colloquial definition, "chronological age," measuring cell age as time since fertilization. In this sense, cell age is equivalent to the age of the organism. Keratinocytes on the back of my left hand are neither three and a half billion years old nor a few days old, but somewhat more than five decades old. Our age since fertilization seems like common sense, because it is in keeping with what most of us (even biologists who should be a bit more broad-minded and canny) assume we mean by age, cells or otherwise. Unfortunately, different cells senesce at markedly different rates independent of chronological age. Frequently dividing cells such as arterial endothelial cells and basal keratinocytes rapidly show senescent changes, whereas non- (or rarely) dividing cells such as myocytes and neurons undergo considerable damage and pathology, but not senescence. Furthermore, frequently dividing cells (exposed keratinocytes on my hand) senesce more rapidly than phenotypically identical cells that divide more slowly (protected keratinocytes on the buttock). Finally, phenotypically different cells dividing at about the same rate can "senesce" at different rates. If we measure senescence as the percentage rate of decline in the cycling fraction of cells per population doubling, human dermal fibroblasts and human peritoneal mesothelial cells show differential rates (0.89% vs. 2.2% per population doubling, respectively) of cell senescence (Thomas et al., 1997).

Cell senescence is clearly not the simple passage of time, whether we use age since life began, age since division, age since fertilization, or any other measure of time. Aging is not a matter of time (Hayflick, 1984b), but a matter of intracellular events. In some complex fashion, time is *correlated* with aging and cell senescence, but doesn't *cause* them. Leaving time in abeyance for a moment, let's move on to the more recent but almost equally problematic model of telomere length. The simple (and invalid) version of this model would be that telomere length defines cell senescence in all cells. If this is so, then why do some cells with long telomeres (such as some murine strains; Zhu et al., 1999b) senesce faster than other cells with shorter telomeres? Among primates, humans have the longest lifespans but the shortest telomeres (Kakuo et al., 1999). In his *Almagest* almost 2000 years ago, Ptolemy tried to fix his geocentric model of the universe by adding epicycle upon epicycle to the orbits of the planets until it became clumsy and a useless mere list of positions, different for each planet, and ad hoc throughout. Yet despite exceptions, much of the telomere data, just as in the Ptolemaic model of the solar system, are in accordance with the simple model. There *is* a rough (negative) correlation between relative telomere length and cell senescence. Copernicus solved the problem by assuming heliocentricity. Can we do something analogous?

The assumption is frequently made that telomere length translates directly into gene expression, but the assumption is misleading and, in specific cases, wrong (Mathon and Lloyd, 2001). Gene expression is neither a direct, unmediated outcome of telomere length nor of the rapidity of base pair loss from the telomere. Abundant cellular examples falsify this simple but inaccurate relationship. In the (mTR–/–) telomerase knockout mouse (Blasco et al., 1997a), for example, there is no evidence that cells of matched phenotype are (at least initially) more senescent in the telomerase knockout animal than in the normal mouse, despite the cumulative loss of telomere lengths in each succeeding generation of the knockout animals. Equally, *Mus musculus* has telomere lengths of > 25 kb, while *Mus spretus* has telomere lengths of 5–15 kb (Zhu et al., 1998). Cells of different telomere lengths can exist in equivalent cell phenotypes (from different strains) without necessary differences in cell senescence. Nonetheless, there is a correlation between telomere maintenance and generational viability within the knockout mice (Herrera et al., 1999b).

An equally effective example is found in nature's experiments. Even in inbred populations of mice, there is significant variation ("hypervariable" telomere lengths) in the otherwise Mendelian inheritance of banding patterns as the length of telomeres varies within individuals (Kipling and Cooke, 1990). Within individuals, however, the somatic cells show predictable, cumulative loss of telomere lengths. If cell senescence is the dependent variable, then the operative independent variable is not telomere length, but the change in telomere length post-fertilization. While one might assert that telomere length is irrelevant to cell senescence, this recommends itself more for shock than veracity, particularly at short telomere lengths where additional considerations apply.

Despite varying telomere lengths among different knockout generations, among different species, among different strains, and among different individuals, normal somatic cells show telomere erosion and it correlates with cell senescence within that cell line. The telomere may act effectively as a timer, but we must remember that it does not operate in isolation (Reddel, 1998a). Despite the metaphorical appeal and value of sobriquets (Counter, 1996; Chiu and Harley, 1997), telomeres are neither clocks (Stewart and Weinberg, 2002), nor "hourglasses" (Rensing et al., 2001), nor the "watchmaker's masterpiece" (Ishikawa, 2000a). Although the term is awkward, Hayflick is correct to call telomeres "replicometers" (Hayflick, 1997a, 2000a). Even if human and murine telomeres had equivalent lengths, we cannot expect them to erode at equivalent rates (even per cell division) or cause identical changes in gene expression.

Consider cells as time bombs, a useful analogy in discussing telomeres (Harley, 1991). Extending the trope, suppose the telomere is a fuse and the altered pattern of gene expression (that ensues as the telomere shortens) the explosive. Fuse length alone cannot predict what happens: we need to know where we have applied the match, the rate of burn, and the amount of explosive. Telomere length alone doesn't predict senescence: we need to know the length at fertilization, the rate of telomere loss, and the likely changes in gene expression. Cats have longer telomeres than humans, but feline telomere loss, due to cell kinetics, is also higher (Brummendorf et al., 2002). Some strains of mice have longer telomeric "fuses" than humans, but how fast do each of their cells divide, at what length does gene expression start to change, and what changes occur? There is extensive variance in the rate of cell division among species; extensive variance within a species and among individuals (e.g., dependent on environmental factors); and extensive variance within individuals, among cell phenotypes. Some cells (stem keratinocytes in the basal epidermis) divide frequently, some nearly not at all (adult mammalian neurons and myocytes). Some smaller organisms (mice and rats) have high metabolic rates (McCarter and Palmer, 1992), while some larger organisms (humans) have relatively slow rates. Even holding metabolic rates and number of divisions constant, the "burn rate" of telomeric fuses per division is still important. The number of DNA bases lost per cell division may not only vary among species but among cell phenotypes. Single-strand breaks, repaired elsewhere, may not be repaired within the telomere (von Zglinicki, 1998; von Zglinicki et al., 2000a), offering another variable affecting the rate of telomere erosion. Variance in number of telomeric base pairs lost per division (or even in the absence of division) is attributable to oxidative damage (Saretzki et al., 1999; von Zglinicki et al., 2000a; Goyns, 2002; von Zglinicki, 2002), environmental variables (e.g., differential ultraviolet exposure; Kruk et al., 1995; Hande et al., 1997), metabolic differences such as differential rates of free radical production (Chen et al., 2001a) or the presence of ascorbate (Furumoto et al., 1998), mutation (e.g., the activation of the H-*ras* oncogene; Serrano et al., 1997), and perhaps other variables. Even knowing the length of the telomeric fuse, the rate of base loss per division, and the burn rate of cell divisions per unit time is insufficient to adequately predict senescence. Senescence depends on the amount and type of the genetic explosive. If gene expression changes dramatically (perhaps even with the earliest, most minimal loss of telomere length), the outcome may be catastrophic. In the converse case, we might posit a cell phenotype with minimum gene expression occurring only when the telomere has all but disappeared.

Cell senescence is not a change in telomere length (the fuse), but a change in function (the explosion). As we are now capable of measuring such expression and changes in gene expression that underlie cell senescence (e.g., Shelton et al., 1999; Ly et al., 2000), gene expression is, appropriately, the basis for denoting senescence. To accurately understand the reality of cell senescence and its role in aging, we need to understand what genes change expression and how a loss of telomeric length relative to initial length (no matter how small a proportion of total length) induces these changes. A unilateral understanding of absolute initial telomere length (Rubio et al., 2002; Serra and von Zglinicki, 2002) and rate of telomere base loss does not speak to the issue.

In cell senescence, the issue remains neither telomerase, nor telomeres, nor cell division, but their practical outcome and variables, such as changes in gene expression. If cell senescence directly alters the expression of genes controlling extracellular matrix maintenance, inflammation, and mitosis (Dandjinou et al., 1999; Ly et al., 2000), then these changes in gene expression, rather than telomere lengths, would become critical to subsequent pathology. In some species, changes may include recombination, as occurs in subtelomeric regions of *Plasmodium falciparum* (Freitas-Junior et al., 2001; Figueiredo et al., 2002), but differential gene silencing is a common mechanism (Stavenhagen and Zakian, 1994; Shore, 1995) occurring via a "telomere position effect" in *Saccharomyces* (Gottschling et al., 1990; Aparicio et al., 1991; Renauld et al., 1993; Stavenhagen and Zakian, 1998), other species (Tham and Zakian, 2002), and probably in humans (Baur et al., 2001; Koering et al., 2002). In *Saccharomyces cerevisiae*, for example, telomere elongation is capable of silencing reporter genes (Denisenko and Bomsztyk, 2002). Differential gene silencing is a biologically ubiquitous process and is required to "stably maintain distinct patterns of gene expression during eukaryotic development" (Laible et al., 1997), but similar changes in transcriptional silencing may define cell senescence. If cell senescence has implications for age-related pathology, it will be understood most directly through our increasing knowledge of changes in gene expression that occur during cell senescence, not through a simpleminded measure of kilobase pairs.

None of this is intended to undermine the causal or conceptual importance of telomeres in cell senescence (Greider, 1998b). Absolute telomere length and erosion rates may not be primary variables, but they are by no means inconsequential. Telomeres don't cause aging, but they do provide an effective point of intervention. Gene expression may be the orchestra of cell senescence, but telomeres are conductors. To obtain a clinical benefit, we must focus on the conductor. The conductor, not the first violinist, chooses the score. By maintaining the telomere, gene expression may be reset and maintained indefinitely (Bodnar et al., 1998; Jiang et al., 1999).

The linkage between the telomere and gene expression has been looked at in detail, predominantly in yeast (*Saccharomyces*), a eukaryote that may bear little resemblance to human cells in this regard (Price, 1999), yet offers insights into mammalian telomere function and gene expression (Kipling and Cooke, 1992). The leading assumption is that changes in heterochromatin are involved (Gottschling, 1992; Shay et al., 1994; Jazwinski et al., 1995) and several models have been developed (Wright and Shay, 1992a; Howard, 1996; Grunstein, 1997; Villeponteau, 1997; Imai and Kitano, 1998). Most investigators assume that heterochromatin alters with telomere shortening and that heterochromatin changes cause transcriptional silencing (Venetsanakos et al., 2002) or permit expression of genes previously trapped beneath the heterochromatin (Wright and Shay, 1996). The latter would permit gene expression by genes now located within a euchromatin domain and might signal the M1 mechanism, the first stage of cell crisis. The former, transcriptional silencing or the telomere position effect (Stavenhagen and Zakian, 1998), may occur at least in the subtelomere region (Stavenhagen and Zakian, 1994; Shore, 1995; Stevenson and Gottschling, 1999; Krogan et al., 2002; Venditti et al., 2002) and be independent of the telomere's role in chromosomal stability (Sandell et al., 1994; Wiley and Zakian, 1995; Lin and Zakian, 1996), though it is perhaps still linked to telomere length regulation (Morin, 1996b) in *Saccharomyces* (Runge and Zakian, 1996) and perhaps humans (Baur et al., 2001). The subtelomere may have additional functions in yeast (Pryde and Louis, 1997) and perhaps in mammalian chromosomes. Human subtelomeric sequences, or "telomere associated DNA" (Blackburn and Szostak, 1984), are partially repetitive, but variable (Brown et al., 1990; Cooke and Smith, 1996) and their function, if any (Allshire et al., 1989), remains unknown.

Among other possibilities, gene amplification may occur more frequently in these regions (Brannan et al., 2001; Corsini et al., 2001) and variation has served to define hybrid relationships in yeasts (Casaregola et al., 2001). Although the mechanisms of heterochromatin modulation of gene expression, especially transcriptional silencing, are being elucidated (Monson et al., 1997; Bi, 2002), it is probably operating in *Saccharomyces* (Hecht et al., 1996; Lustig, 1998; Wright et al., 1999) and perhaps other eukaryotes (Kurenova et al., 1998; Cryderman et al., 1999), if not necessarily in mammals. Initial data on silencing protein homologs (Perrod et al., 2001) and on telomere position effects are consistent with this proposition (Baur et al., 2001). The functional association between telomeres, heterochromatin, and gene expression is probably common among eukaryotic cells (Kurenova and Mason, 1997), although with variation in detail.

One model of telomere–gene expression linkage is an altered chromosomal structure (Ferguson et al., 1991), such as a heterochromatin "hood" that covers the telomere and a variable length of the subtelomeric chromosome (Fossel, 1996; Villeponteau, 1997; Wright et al., 1999). As the telomere shortens, the hood slides further down the chromosome (the heterochromatin hood remains invariant in size and simply moves with the shortening terminus) or the hood shortens (as the telomere is less capable of retaining heterochromatin). In either case, the result is an alteration of transcription from portions of the chromosome immediately adjacent to the telomeric complex, usually causing transcriptional silencing, although the control is doubtless more complex than merely telomere effect through propinquity (Aparicio and Gottschling, 1994; Singer et al., 1998; Stevenson and Gottschling, 1999). These silenced genes may in turn modulate other, more distant genes (or sets of genes). There is some direct evidence for such modulation in the subtelomere (see below), but overall, while experimental data imply the existence of some undefined (Campisi, 2000a) but direct and causal linkage between telomere shortening and changes in gene expression, the mechanisms of the linkage remain unclear and arguable (Ouellette et al., 2000a).

Much of what we know of telomeric heterochromatin and its function has come from the study of yeasts, the most common being *Saccharomyces cerevisiae*, the common bread yeast (Runge and Zakian, 1990; Wang and Zakian, 1990a, 1990b; Zakian, 1996). Yeast and human beings are strikingly different at the macroscopic level and may differ in the details of gene transcription and gene expression (Francon et al., 1999) as well as telomeric heterochromatin, its function, and replicative timing (Wellinger et al., 1996; Wright et al., 1999; Taggart et al., 2002). The last few decades have made it clear, however, that yeast and human cells share striking similarities (Allshire, 1995; De Rubertis et al., 1996; Gotta and Cockell, 1997; Laible et al., 1997) and may offer useful clinical and genetic insights for human organisms (Bridger and Bickmore, 1998; Brown et al., 1998a; Perfect et al., 1998), including mechanisms of telomere–gene interaction (Aparicio, 1991). Most species differ, not so much in telomere organization as in telomere regulation (Pardue and DeBaryshe, 1999), allowing us to identify general mechanisms by which telomeres modulate gene expression.

In eukaryotic cells, including human cells, gene expression is modulated by overall heterochromatin arrangement and "wrapping" of chromosomes around nucleosomes (with a 50-fold condensing of the duplex DNA), which generally represses local gene expression. One hundred and sixty-eight base pairs of helical DNA wind around a single nucleosome, composed of an octomer of histone proteins (two each of H2A, H2B, H3, and H4). Although this set of histones completes the nucleosome body in yeast and other small eukaryotes, more complex eukaryotes have an additional histone, H1, the largest of the histone group, which ties together the double helix as it enters and leaves the nucleosomal loop (Singer and Berg, 1991). Histones in the telomeric heterochromatin can have local (Lenfant et al., 1996) and more distant (Marcand et al., 1996) effects on gene expression, including changes concomitant with senescence (Parseghian et al., 2001). Even relatively distant (20 kb) genes, beyond the reach of non-histone effects such as those of the Sir complex (see below), are influenced by telomeric histones (Wyrick et al., 1999), perhaps through telomere loop effects (Zaman et al., 2002). On a theoretical note, simplistic models have even tried to ascribe all of aging to "progressive heterochromatinization" (Lezhava, 2001a, 2001b).

In yeast, genes integrated near the telomeres have their expression regulated by the silent information regulatory proteins Sir2p, Sir3p, and Sir4p. These proteins bind to heterochromatin in the nucleosome and repress gene expression cell cycle dependently (Laroche et al., 2000). Within the peritelomeric region, RAP1 (repressor/activator protein 1) and Sir complex may have more predictably local effects on gene expression and particularly transcriptional silencing (Bourns et al., 1998; Cockell et al., 1998, 2000; Roy and Runge, 2000; Moretti and Shore, 2001) than do the histones and nucleosomes. RAP1 and its homologs regulate transcriptional activation, silencing, and telomere function in several yeasts (Grossi et al., 2001; Haw et al., 2001; Wahlin and Cohn, 2002). Sir3p may affect transcriptional silencing through its effects upon the nucleosome and heterochromatin structure (Vega-Palas et al., 1998). Not only may it play a prominent role in the basic changes in gene expression that underlie caloric restriction (Lin et al., 2000a), but it may explain the effects of helicase mutations on aging, at least in yeast (Sinclair et al., 1997).

The mapping of peritelomeric genes is progressing rapidly (Kipling et al., 1995) and specific genes (e.g., the α-globin locus on human chromosome 6p13.3) have been mapped to this region (Smith and Higgs, 1999). Curiously, although these regions are prone to recombination (Mefford and Trask, 2002) and many genetic syndromes demonstrate subtelomeric abnormalities (Cotter et al., 2001; Tsien et al., 2001; Veltman et al., 2002), subtelomeric translocations are more frequently associated with mental retardation (Bonifacio et al., 2001; Joyce et al., 2001; Baker et al., 2002; Clarkson et al., 2002) or autism (Wolff et al., 2002) than with other congenital anomalies (Rosenberg et al., 2001). Telomeric probes may have a role in prenatal counseling (Benzacken et al., 2002), and subtelomeric defects improve diagnosis in idiopathic mental retardation (Rio et al., 2002; Martin et al., 2002a, 2002b). These regions are comparatively similar but unstable within the primates (van Geel et al., 2002), prompting consideration of a putative relationship to rapid neurologic evolution within this clade.

A number of transcription factors (Skammelsrud et al., 1999) are found associated with the human telomere, as well as the telomeres of other species (Strahl-Bolsinger et al., 1997). The most well-studied is probably the general DNA-binding protein RAP1 from yeast (Wright and Zakian, 1995; Krauskopf and Blackburn, 1998; Prescott and Blackburn, 2000), which binds to telomeric DNA repeats (Krauskopf and Blackburn, 1996), contributes to telomere length control and to telomeric silencing (Lustig et al., 1990), and is a major component of telomeric chromatin (Enomoto et al., 1997). It is also involved in gene activation and repression. Recent studies suggest additional roles for RAP1 in heterochromatin boundary-element formation and chromatin opening, allowing this abundant DNA-binding protein to participate in a diverse array of chromatin-related functions (Morse, 2000) and be a central mechanism in telomere homeostasis (Blackburn et al., 1997; Lundblad, 2000). These effects on telomere length regulation may be shared by and interact with other factors such as the Sir complex (Guarente, 1999; Mills et al., 1999a; Venditti et al., 1999b), particularly Sir3p (Venditti et al., 1999a) and Rif1p and Rif2p (Marcand et al., 1997b; Gasser et al., 1998).

It is worth mentioning other possible linkage mechanisms. Olovnikov, author of the original proposal of telomere shortening as a mechanism for cell senescence (Olovnikov, 1971) and a good record of theoretical prediction, has posited ionic "fountains" (Olovnikov, 1999). Telomeres distribute peripherally (Pfeifer et al., 2001) and specific regions of the telomere (Carlton and Cande, 2002) bind to the inner nuclear membrane in a "telomeric bouquet" during meiotic prophase (Seimiya et al., 2000; Wai-Hong and Zakian, 2000; Chikashige and Hiraoka, 2001), perhaps modulated by specific membrane telomere binding proteins (Dol'nik et al., 2001), although the telomere is probably dispensable (Franco et al., 2002a). In the ionic fountain model, membrane binding modulates local ion concentrations and their availability to chromosomes, thereby modulating transcription. The model may not be inconsistent with known data, for example, the effects of gene proximity to the nuclear membrane (Blackburn and Szostak, 1984; Cockell and Gasser, 1999) and relationships between gene silencing and the nuclear periphery (Tham et al., 2001), but lacks supporting data.

While we do not understand the linkage, it is critical to recognize its existence and importance. An intermediate variable, it cannot be neglected in an attempt to adequately understand or discuss senescence. We must distinguish three separate but interacting aspects of cell senescence: the telomere, the linkage, and gene expression. The shortening (not the length) of the telomere may control the movement of the linkage (potentially and probably a heterochromatin sheath), but the two are not equivalent and may be manipulated independently in experimental settings. Likewise, the linkage may modulate gene expression, but is emphatically not the only operative variable. Put simplistically, but not inaccurately, everything affects gene expression in a cell; a shift in the linkage is only one input (and in the overall genetic scheme, a fairly minor one) among many inputs over the cell's lifetime. The hypothesis that the telomere linkage causes wholesale patterns of change in gene expression in no way gives licence to take such effects out of context. Senescence-associated changes in gene expression, although central to age-related pathology, are a minor part of a cell's world. The importance of this point comes when considering what must logically occur to the linkage during cell fertilization in organisms with varying telomere lengths, such as clones (Miyashita et al., 2002), and varying abilities to express telomerase, such as (mTR–/–) knockout mice or (mTR+/–) heterozygous interspecies mice (Hathcock et al., 2002). Absolute telomere length is not an operative variable in cell senescence, nor is its linkage the major determinant of gene expression.

Finally, the linkage is not alone in translating telomere changes to changes in cell behavior (Shay et al., 1992b). An additional mechanism, and one almost certain to play a role in human cell senescence, is the p53–dependent checkpoint (Shay et al., 1992a; Gollahon and Shay, 1996; Filatov et al., 1998), i.e., the cell cycle braking system (Harley and Sherwood, 1997b; von Zglinicki, 1998; Carr, 2000; Webley et al., 2000). The cell employs a battery of DNA damage–signaling proteins, which detect DNA damage and trigger a common pathway (Ahmed and Hodgkin, 2000; Rouse and Jackson, 2002) involving a minimum of several dozen factors, including p53 (Shay et al., 1992a; Chin et al., 1999), p21 (Brown et al., 1997b), D cyclins, and cdks (Watanabe et al., 1998), among others (Lundberg and Weinberg, 1999; Wynford-Thomas, 1999). This mechanism stops the cell cycle and up-regulates DNA repair. As a result, normal cells either repair chromosomal errors or remain fully braked, unable to divide further (Carr, 2002). The mechanism need not be all-or-nothing: short telomeres may be interpreted as damaged (Buchkovich, 1996; Ahmed and Hodgkin, 2000), accounting for cell cycle slowing during senescence (Morin, 1997a; Maigne et al., 1998). This may be independent of other changes in gene expression modulated by other linkage mechanisms. Cell senescence shares several common pathways with apoptosis (Seimiya et al., 1999; Joaquin and Gollapudi, 2001; Wang et al., 2001a) and intracellular defenses against malignant transformation.

Considering genes as a cellular orchestra, genes do not go out of tune so much as they play an alternate score. The instruments are neither missing, nor out of tune: they are merely playing discordantly because the conductor has chosen a discordant score. The difference between Amadeus Mozart and John Cage is not the quality of the instruments but the pattern of notes played; the difference between a young and a senescent cell is not the quality of the genes but the pattern of genes expressed. Cells do not senesce because of wear and tear, but because they permit wear and tear to occur because of an altered pattern of gene expression. Telomerization effectively replaces the score, allowing the genes to express their previous pattern. While telomerization can abort cell senescence, there is probably a point beyond which this rescue is unlikely or even impossible. To define the interventional limit of telomerization in senescing cells, we need to more clearly define senescence.

The simplification that there are only two types of cells—somatic cells, which lack telomerase and senesce in lock step, and germ cells, which express telomerase and are immortal—is inaccurate. For one thing, this ignores exceptions and intermediate cell types. Though typically immortal (Sela, 2000), cancer cells often have short telomeres (de Lange, 1995) and altered telomere maintenance (Greider, 1994). Moreover, some cancer cells have long telomeres and some even senesce. Some cells—dermal fibroblasts from Hutchinson-Gilford syndrome patients—apparently begin life already senescent, but then continue to senesce in a more or less normal fashion (Allsopp et al., 1992). Others, from Werner syndrome (Thweatt and Goldstein, 1993; Oshima et al., 1995) or Fanconi's anemia (Adelfalk et al., 2001; Hanson et al., 2001; Callen et al., 2002a, 2002b) patients, start out normally (Schulz et al., 1996) but senesce quicker than normal cells. During normal human fetal development, most 16- to 20-week somatic cells (excepting brain tissue) express telomerase (Wright et al., 1996b), as do trophoblasts within the early chorion, though later placental (Kyo et al., 1997d) or amniotic fluid cells do not (Mosquera et al., 1999). In bovine fetal tissue, telomerase activity decreases during oocyte maturation and subsequent development to the eight-cell stage but then increases again in the morula and blastocyst stages (Betts and King, 1999). There are data suggesting at least two regulatory mechanisms control hTERT activity in human fetal cells: (*1*) transcriptional regulation of the hTERT genes, and (*2*) alternate splicing of hTERT transcripts (Ulaner and Giudice, 1997; Ulaner et al., 1998; Colgin et al., 2000). Even in cells expressing telomerase, not every telomere is necessarily extending during every cell division (Forstemann et al., 2000). Although the variance in telomerase expression may have implications for human pathology (Kojima et al., 2001), its regulation is only marginally understood.

Although most somatic cells never express telomerase, a restricted set of somatic stem cells can do so upon appropriate stimulation. Such cells include hematopoetic, basal skin, gastrointestinal crypt, hepatic, hair follicles, and potentially several other stem cell lines (see below). In these cells, telomerase expression and activity is carefully controlled within the cell and may be modulated via cell–cell interactions, e.g., through interleukins (Soares et al., 1998) and lymphokines in lymphocyte precursors. Typically, such stem cells transiently express telomerase, reextending their telomeres, and divide. One daughter cell differentiates and becomes unable to reexpress telomerase even in the face of further cytokine stimulation, its telomeres shortening progressively with further divisions. The other daughter cell remains in the stem cell line with a marginally shorter telomere and is capable of reexpressing telomerase to appropriate cytokine stimulation and of dividing. Stem cell telomeres therefore shorten more slowly than other cells with similar rates and numbers of divisions (Fig. 3–1). Teleologically, this allows stem cells to divide over the life of an organism, such as a human who may require an astronomically high number of cells over a century or more. Other dividing somatic cells show a predictable erosion of telomere lengths (Butler et al., 1998; Tsuji et al., 2002). In nondividing somatic cells the telomere lengths remain intact.

In cells that show telomere loss, the intracellular effects are ubiquitous and variable, but probably share common features. Senescent cells have slower protein elongation and protein turnover (Finch, 1990; Arking, 1998), resulting in a gradual accretion of dysfunctional enzymatic and structural proteins. DNA repair becomes slower and less effective (Bohr and Anson, 1995), resulting in genomic instability in senescent cells, an effect magnified in cells lacking telomerase (Wong et al., 2000; Chang et al., 2001). Mitochondria produce a higher frequency of ROS per mole of ATP produced (Harper et al., 1998), resulting in diminished cell energy economy and an increased risk of oxi-

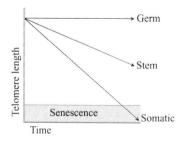

Figure 3–1 Naive model: germ, stem, somatic cells. Naive models suggest that germ cells maintain telomere length, while somatic cells and stem cells both lose telomere length linearly—the former rapidly, the latter slowly (due to intermittent telomerase activity).

dative damage. As discussed, mitochondrial sequestration in increasingly faulty, while free radical trapping decreases as trapping compounds of intracellular origin are less available. These several problems result in a marked increase in cell dysfunction as senescence ensues. The cell becomes increasingly resistant to apoptotic signals (Holt et al., 1999b; Lundberg and Weinberg, 1999; Wang et al., 2001a) as well as messengers such as ceramide (Miller and Stein, 2001), the cell cycle slows, and cell becomes less capable of dividing and replacing local tissue losses.

Cell senescence also has extracellular effects and these are paramount in explaining disease and age-related tissue and organ changes. Not only do senescent cells change their pattern of gene expression but the result is a change in the production of secretory products, such as trophic (Cristofalo et al., 1998b; Shelton et al., 1999) and replication factors (Pendergrass et al., 1999a). The same is true of structural or enzymatic secretory products, such as collagen (Furth et al., 1997), elastin, collagenase, elastase, or β-galactosidase (Burke et al., 1994; Dimri and Campisi, 1994a; Matsunaga et al., 1999a). Inflammatory factors and cytokines change as the cell senesces. Some cells (e.g., skin fibroblasts) show a decreased pattern of inflammatory cytokines (Shelton et al., 1999). Other cells (e.g., endothelial cells) show an increasingly inflammatory pattern.

Senescence in one cell accelerates senescence in surrounding cells. If one set of cells is stressed and prone to cell loss, remaining cells divide, senescing more rapidly. Senescing cells drag down other cells. Extracellular effects may start locally as a subtle change in the function of a neighboring cell or a subtle change in the extracellular matrix (West et al., 1996), but the effects progress to neighboring tissues planes, to entire organs, to downstream parts of the vascular bed in which they lie, and, ultimately, throughout the organism. What begins as cell senescence ends as age-related disease.

The limited model of cell senescence—shortening telomeres induce changes in gene expression that cause gradual accrual of secondary cellular damage—stands in contrast to wear-and-tear views of aging in which DNA and mitochondrial damage cause cell senescence. If we reset telomeres, resetting gene expression (replacing the score in our metaphorical orchestra), cell function is largely or completely restored (Bodnar et al., 1998). Immortalized, but otherwise normal, somatic cells (Franco et al., 2001; MacKenzie et al., 2002) have reset cell senescence as reflected not only in replicative capability and telomere length but in gene expression pattern (Shelton et al., 1999). This implies that cells do not senesce because they are damaged, but permit damage because they senesce. Homeostatic processes suffice indefinitely in germ cell lines; they suffice in somatic cells if senescence is abrogated.

Interventions that rescue a cell from senescence should vary in efficacy depending on the degree of senescence; some cells may be sufficiently senescent to preclude rescue. Against this, however, in vivo tissue may show a tendency toward clustering of almost but not irremediably senescent cells. Cell division may slow in more senescent cells, placing the divisional burden on neighboring but less senescent cells. The degree to which a tissue is senescent, however, is not a matter of the degree to which a cell has an altered pattern of gene expression but the degree to which individually altered cell behavior has an impact on cell–cell interactions and tissue function. We might imagine a markedly senescent cell with marginal impact on surrounding tissue cells or a marginally senescent cell with marked impact on surrounding tissue cells. The degree of impact depends on the tissue and on specific cell function within that tissue. Moving from cell senescence to tissue senescence introduces complications. Cell senescence is more than telomere length; tissue senescence is more than percentages of senescent cells and degrees of senescence.

The General Model: Cell Senescence Results in Organismal Aging

Cell senescence underlies human aging. This describes the general model, but simplicity stops there. The verb reflects the subtle nature of the causal process at work in aging. Consider the parallel issue in atherosclerosis: does cholesterol cause, contribute to, or underlie the pathology? It doesn't strictly cause atherosclerosis, yet does more than contribute. Cells may senesce, but cell senescence is surely not equivalent to organismal aging (Norwood et al., 1991b; Cristofalo et al., 1998a; Smith et al., 2002). Free radicals might be said to cause aging, yet they don't cause cumulative damage in germ cells. Senescence plays a permissive role that, at the level of the organism, is reflected in dysfunctional tissues and organs, clinical pathology, and aging changes.

With qualification, some (McCormick and Campisi, 1991; Peacocke and Campisi, 1991; Campisi, 1996, 1997b; Imai and Kitano, 1998; Klapper et al., 2001; Mikhelson, 2001) have speculated that cell senescence might play such a role, perhaps minor or ill defined, in organismal aging, at least in tissues with dividing cells. There has also been speculation that cell senescence plays some role in age-related disease generally (Hayflick, 1979; Chang and Harley, 1995; Rawes et al., 1997; Faragher and Kipling, 1998) or in specific age-related diseases (Harley, 1997; Morin, 1997b), including essential hypertension, non-insulin–dependent diabetes mellitus (Goldstein and Harley, 1979), atherosclerosis, and cancer (Aviv and Aviv, 1998).

In addition to the model suggested here, that changes is gene expression underlie aging, other telomere-related mechanisms have been suggested. For example, telomere loss might lead to genomic instability and a loss of heterozygosity, with the consequent expression of latent disease-causing genes (Aviv and Aviv, 1998, 1999). Alternatively, cell senescence might cause pathology by interfering with apoptosis (or the apoptotic response; Pritchard et al., 2001), resulting in the accumulation of apoptosis-resistant "junk" cells that interfere with normal young cell function (Wang and Warner, 1989; Warner et al., 1992; Joaquin and Gollapudi, 2001). Apoptosis eliminates both "damaged and presumably dysfunctional cells (e.g., fibroblasts, hepatocytes), which can then be replaced by cell proliferation, thereby maintaining homeostasis," and "essential postmitotic cells (e.g., neurons, cardiac myocytes), which cannot be replaced, thereby leading to pathology" (Warner, 1997; Warner et al., 1997). Proponents suggest that we might effectively intervene in this process (Joaquin and Gollapudi, 2001).

The notion that cell senescence might play a more generic role in age-related diseases has been downplayed (Le Bourg, 2000; Ahmed and Tollefsbol, 2001), often because of a difficulty in appreciating how cell senescence in dividing cells could possibly cause clinical pathology in nondividing (and therefore presumptively nonsenescent) cells. Privately, some have resorted to what might flippantly be termed "infectious" senescence (compare Faragher, et al., 1997b), in which senescent cells trigger a reactive senescence in adjacent cells. However, the position that cell senescence cannot logically be responsible for major age-related diseases is flawed: dividing arterial wall cells certainly have enormous impact on nondividing brain and heart cells. The notion that pathology in nondividing cells (e.g., myocardial infarction or cerebrovascular stroke) cannot be attributed to dividing cells (e.g., arterial endothelium) belies ignorance of pathology.

The position that human aging and age-related disease are products of cell senescence has been stated and fleshed out (Fossel, 1996, 1998a and b, 2000a, 2001b; Banks and Fossel, 1997). Gradual accumulation of data over the past few years and a sophisticated view of the complex pathology involved in age-related diseases have made this view more supportable. More to the point (and more practically), to the extent that we can prevent or reverse cell senescence, we may be able to alter age-related diseases (Faragher, 2000). We might consider the model to a question rather than a theory. Altering cell aging, what happens to age-related human pathology? Is cell senescence consistent as a fundamental variable in age-related human pathology? This is a question raised not only within this chapter but throughout the book.

To say that aging is cell aging is imprecise, inaccurate, and often inapplicable (in insects, for example). Moreover, it does not imply that cell senescence "causes" human aging or that either can be reversed, prevented, or slowed. Besides aphoristic clarity, the advantage of the simple statement, aging is cell aging, is in provoking argument and therefore exploration of the pathology and current data. The statement that human aging is cell aging is not a radical dictum. Shorn of the causal direction implied, it is not even particularly novel (compare Gilchrest and Yaar, 1992).

The intent of this section is to set the stage by making it clear what the theory is — and to make equally clear what it is not. Difficulties consistently arise from a blithe and thoughtless attribution of causation. Causation is not simple. Biological "causes" are multiple and notoriously interactive. Even with a well-defined and complete sequence of intracellular events, we can be misled by the apparent simplicity. In apoptosis, for example, where causation may depend on cell state and extracellular events, "the role of a given protein may be entirely contextual" (Lockshin et al., 2000). Causation in apoptosis, particularly regarding mitochondrial involvement (Finkel, 2001; Wei et al., 2001a) is still argued. The simplicity of linear causation is meretricious, luring us away from a complex reality. Telomeres do not cause aging nor does cell senescence cause organismal aging. To argue that telomeres don't cause aging is disingenuous. Telomeres are a rough cellular "clock" (Aviv and Harley, 2001) that indirectly modulate gene expression and are a useful (if limited) marker for cell senescence in the laboratory.

The important issue is not causation but a realistic understanding of the complexity of aging, which we can efficiently intervene for clinical benefit. Aging is caused by time, free radicals, protein turnover rates, telomeres, cell senescence, gene expression, cell divisions, methylation, heterochromatin changes, DNA damage, lipid peroxidation, environmental insults, the entire cell genome, cell–cell effects, and manifold other variables. Do we need to intervene in all of these causes? And as with proteins in apoptosis, causes of aging are contextual, depending on species, cell phenotype, and cell history, and have an interactive effect on one another. Telomere length determines cell senescence only in specified contexts. Telomeres do not cause aging any more (or any less) than a key causes a car to go down the highway. The context — available gas, whether the brakes are set, the state of the tires, the road, etc. — remains critical to the behavior of the car. Like a key, telomeres are an available and effective point of intervention.

Cholesterol is often considered to cause atherosclerosis, yet some atherosclerotic patients have low cholesterol (Mehta et al., 1998; Jee et al., 1999; Lee et al., 1999b), and others with normal vessels have high cholesterol. This does not imply that cholesterol plays no role in atherosclerosis. Cholesterol may not "cause" atherosclerosis, but the interventional implications remain: lowering cholesterol "causes" a lower risk of atherosclerotic morbidity and death (Stamler et al., 2000). The practical intent—intervention—is more amenable to both logical discussion and practical solution than are theoretical discussions of causation. Cholesterol doesn't cause atherosclerosis, but it is a major factor, a convenient marker, and an effective point of intervention. Lack of strict causation is scarcely a recommendation for ignoring one's serum or dietary cholesterol.

The appropriate focus is intervention (Rattan, 2000b): what happens when we alter a complex system, under what conditions, with what limitations? In atherosclerosis, the pertinent question is the *effect* (if any) of lowering serum cholesterol (Grundy, 2000). In regards to free radicals in aging, the appropriate question is the effect of decreasing UV exposure or increasing dietary tocopherols or other dietary components, such as carnitine (Hagen et al., 2002; Liu et al., 2002a, 2002b). If enzymatic activity or the expression of superoxide dismutase (SOD) (Tyler et al., 1993; Allen et al., 1995; Mockett et al., 1999; Serra et al., 2003) or other enzymes (Fleming et al., 1993; Lorenz et al., 2001; Muller, 2001) play a role in aging, what are the effects of more active genes? Very little, at least in mice (Huang et al., 2000). What of other points of experimental intervention?

Mitochondria change markedly in senescent cells. They may decrease in volume (Chen et al., 2001a). They leak, their protein synthesis rates fall (Beaufrere and Boirie, 1998; Proctor et al., 1998; Schwarze et al., 1998a; Short and Nair, 1999), and they produce more free radicals, including hydrogen peroxide (Allen et al., 1999) and superoxide (Chen et al., 2001a), per unit of ATP (Harper et al., 1998; Schwarze et al., 1998b). Changes occur in vitro and in vivo (Michikawa et al., 1999). Everything within mitochondria turns over except mitochondrial DNA (mtDNA; de Grey, 1999), but turnover rates slow and defect rates climb with age (de Grey, 1997; Lee and Wei, 1997; Lee et al., 1997), probably for many reasons (Lee et al., 1994a; Wanagat et al., 2001). Although the damage rate is variable among species, cell phenotypes, and mitotic states, it may be constant until well into adulthood, then undergo a sudden inflection (Herrero and Barja, 2001), suggesting a separate, more fundamental triggering process.

Mitochondrial DNA is circular in most but not all organisms (Nosek et al., 1998; Duby et al., 2001). In organisms (such as *Tetrahymena*) with linear mitochondrial chromosomes, telomeres have tandem repeats, similar to nuclear DNA, but with surprising diversity (Morin and Cech, 1988), sufficient to identify yeast species diagnostically or taxonomically (Nosek et al., 2002). The evolutionary conversion between ring and linear was relatively simple and telomere binding proteins show homology (Tomaska et al., 2001). Circular human mtDNA codes for only 13 proteins (Anderson et al., 1981), each crucial to oxidative metabolism. Damage occurs in nuclear and mtDNA, sometimes involving transfer from one to the other (Shay and Werbin, 1992), but mtDNA damage (Denver et al., 2000) is many-fold higher (Herrero and Barja, 2001; Wanagat et al., 2001), ranging from 3- (Richter, 1999) to 20- (Kadenbach et al., 1999) fold that of nuclear DNA damage. This is largely due to proximity to reactive oxygen species, lack of protective histones (Caron et al., 1979), and lack of introns (Anderson et al., 1981). Worse, mtDNA repair (Croteau et al., 1999) is relatively less effective (Street et al., 1999; Dobson et al., 2000; Kolesnikova et al., 2000). Balancing this, however, each mitochondria may have 5–10 DNA copies and each cell may have 100–1000 mitochondria (Kadenbach et al.,

1999). Overall, it is unclear how a relatively small (< 5%) amount of age-associated mtDNA damage can be responsible for aging (Lee and Wei, 1997; Anson and Bohr, 2001). In some cells, e.g., human T lymphocytes, there is no evidence for age-related increase in mtDNA damage (Ross et al., 2002).

Though endocrine systems change with age—Pacific salmon undergo an endocrinological catastrophe—this begs the question of what in turn times endocrine aging. Why should hormone secreting cells wear out? If another cell (e.g., in the hypothalamus or pituitary gland) regulates the secreting cell, why does the regulating cell age? The naive notion that the endocrine system controls aging conflicts with what we know of pathology, aging, and endocrine function.

Some investigators assume that aging and age-related diseases are merely "wear and tear," like a car that "rusts out" (Hayflick, 1999, 2000a) or a "Mars space probe" not designed to maintain itself (Comfort, 1970; Goldstein, 1971a). Similar views (Olshansky et al., 2002a, 2002b) rely on misunderstanding and dogmatism rather than a wide perspective on biology and often fail to survive editorial review. Mechanical analogies are poor analogies for biological systems, in which energy input gives theoretical license for indefinite maintenance (Hasty and Vijg, 2002). Germ cell lines maintain themselves for several billion years despite free radical damage, mitochondrial damage, and allegorical rust to the cellular undercarriage—some car.

The cell senescence model suggests that when cells divide in response to cell loss, these cell senesce with consequent dysfunction within the cell, between cells (the intracellular matrix), in neighboring nonsenescent cells (e.g., subendothelial cells respond to senescing endothelial cells), and in distant cells dependent on dividing cells (e.g., myocardial cells depending on arterial endothelial cells). The overall process (within cells and tissues) constitutes aging. Cell senescence doesn't cause aging so much as it is aging.

Fertilization Resets Telomere Effects

A major conceptual solecism can occur in the interpretation of the telomerase knockout, knock-in, and cloning data: confusing telomere length with a more crucial variable, altered gene expression. The linkage (or linkages) between these two variables remains a black box.

Certain outcomes of the linkage are clear. In successful fertilization, "the donor nucleus must be reprogrammed . . . so that it can direct the development of the embryo" (Prather, 2000). Equally, in viable knockout, knock-in, or cloned animals gene expression must be reset to an undifferentiated (normal fetal) state. Production of a healthy (Lanza et al., 2001) young clone from an older animal argues that proliferative capacity (Wilmut et al., 2000) and epigenetic programming (Rideout et al., 2001) must be appropriately reset (Betts et al., 2001). This need not, in a naive sense, "reset the telomere clock" (Miyashita et al., 2002), but fertilization does imply that the linkage (whatever its mechanism) must be reset to permit normal fetal gene expression. If gene expression were not reset, the organism would display abnormalities in gene expression. Clones derived from embryonic stem (rather than somatic) cells are less likely to have such abnormalities and more likely to survive (Wakayama et al., 1999; Rideout et al., 2000; Eggan et al., 2001). This has been attributed to epigenetic factors in the reprogramming of such cells (Vastag, 2001b) and there is evidence supporting this (Humphreys et al., 2001). Though a tempting analogy, an embryonic cell is not a tabula rasa but has a specific pattern of gene expression appropriate to early fetal development and continued tissue differentiation (Rideout et al., 2001). The resetting of such epigenetic effects, including the linkage between (relative) telomere length and (nonsenescent) gene expression, can be central to understanding the effects of cloning and telomerase knockouts on cell senescence.

The lifespans of knockout mice, clones, and animals with exceptional telomere lengths, such as some wild murine strains and hamsters (Slijepcevic and Hande, 1999), should be unaffected as long as the linkage is appropriate for normal gene expression during fetal development (Fossel, 2000b). Initial telomere length should be largely irrelevant. Consider three supportive examples.

For the first example, posit two *Mus* strains, one with long (20 kb) telomeres (*Mus* strain A) and one with short (10 kb) telomeres (*Mus* strain B), but otherwise equivalent genomes (except genes enforcing differential telomere length maintenance). Should they have different lifespans? If viable, zygotic gene expression should be reset and appropriate for a cell that will soon divide and differentiate into multiple phenotypes. Imprinting (Tilhgman, 1999) of perhaps 100 human genes (Tilghman, 2000) on this genetic palimpsest probably occurs via methylation (Forejt et al., 1999), adding to the complexity of the soi disant tabula rasa (Hark et al., 2000; O'Neill et al., 2000; Schmidt et al., 2000). Faulty imprinting causes epigenetic disease, such as Beckwith-Wiedemann syndrome (Zhang et al., 1997; Caspary et al., 1999; Tilghman, 2000). In our two *Mus* strains, telomere lengths may be different, but the pattern of gene expression must be normal: we have viable murine zygotes. If telomere lengths differ and gene expression is remains equivalent, then the linkage must differ correspondingly. Strain A has 20 kb telomeres with a matching 20 kb linkage. Strain B has only 10 kb long telomeres, but gene expression is the same because B's linkage is 10 kb long, thus matching its telomere. *Mus* strain A (with 20 kb telomeres) should have the same lifespan as *Mus* strain B (with 10 kb telomeres). Regardless of initial telomere length, the rates of telomere base loss, linkage movement, changes in gene expression, and cell senescence will occur at the same rate in both experimental strains. Senescence is determined (indirectly) by change in telomere length, not by prefertilization telomere length. More directly, the linkage determines cell senescence. Given otherwise matched genomes, and even granting the necessity for telomeres in fertilization (Liu et al., 2002c), prefertilization telomere length may have no significant impact on lifespan.

As a second example, consider clones. Posit a donor animal which normally has 20 kb telomeres. An adult somatic cell, used for the clone, might have 10 kb telomeres. In this respect the clone may be older than its donor (Hornsby, 2000; Vogel, 2000), but an abnormal zygotic patterns of gene expression may not be viable (a common outcome). Clonal viability implies a reset linkage, telomere length notwithstanding. Indeed, the initial result with Dolly, the cloned sheep, was shorter than normal telomeres (Shiels et al., 1999). Except in limiting cases (discussed below) and barring genetic damage, many cloned animals appear healthy and normal (Kubota et al., 2000a; Lanza et al., 2001) with lifespans typical of uncloned animals. Telomere length prior to cloning does not determine the subsequent telomere length (Betts et al., 2001), lifespan, or development in the cloned animal. Unexpectedly, some clones have longer telomeres than their donors and cells may undergo 50% more population doublings (Lanza et al., 2000b). Various explanations have been offered (Wilmut et al., 2000), but the finding requires duplication and explanation.

For a third example, consider telomerase knockout (mTR–/–) mice. Telomeres show progressive loss with each generation (Hande et al., 1999a) and we might naively expect progressively shorter lifespans. To some extent this occurs (Herrera et al., 1999b; Rudolph et al., 1999), but a gross shortening of lifespan would be inconsistent with either the theory espoused here or our knowledge of embryology. The viability F1 telomerase knockouts suggests normal gene expression, implying that the linkage has been reset appropriately. With two exceptions, shorter telomeres in a telomerase knockout mouse should have no necessary effect on lifespan. First, after sufficient generations, regardless of linkage position, zygotes will lack sufficient telomeres for viability. Predictably, knockouts are infertile by the sixth generation (Blasco et al., 1997a) or by the fourth in strains with shorter baseline telomeres (Herrera et al., 1999b). Second, rapidly dividing cells might have initially normal gene expression but completely run out of telomeres. Even early knockout generations show dysfunction in organs with highly proliferative cells, including abnormal spermatogenesis and hematopoesis (Lee et al., 1998c; Herrera et al., 1999b). We might further expect decreased fertility or an increased number of developmental defects: each succeeding generation demonstrates more frequent neural tube defects (Herrera et al., 1999a). In a parallel plant example, *Arabidopsis* mutants lacking telomerase activity may survive for up to 10 generations, displaying unstable genomes, increasingly shorter telomeres, and cytogenetic abnormalities (McKnight et al., 2002).

Do extremely long or critically short telomeres have no effect on lifespan or pathology? As above, critically short telomeres (Lustig, 1999) cause dysfunction in organs with highly proliferative cells, ensuring mortality via the weakest link, rather than wholesale aging acceleration. Extremely long telomeres are also probably detrimental (McEachern and Blackburn, 1995; Blackburn et al., 1997), subtly impeding quotidian chromosomal mechanics and cell replication. Though they have a higher incidence of malignancy (Artandi et al., 2002) and better wound healing (Gonzalez-Suarez et al., 2001), telomerase knock-in animals do not address this issue, as these animals still maintain normal telomere lengths. The outcome (pathology, aging, and lifespan) may depend on the length at which telomeres stabilize and how firmly they are maintained at this length.

Critically short or extremely long telomeres may cause dysfunction and demonstrable pathology; merely longer (some murine strains) or shorter (knockout mice) prefertilization telomeres should not cause gross changes in aging. Cell senescence is not determined by telomere length but by the change in telomere length during the life of the organism. The cell senescence model of aging explains much about human disease that was otherwise puzzling (e.g., Hutchinson-Gilford atherosclerosis) and is supported by current data but remains equally unproven, requiring that we falsify the model or validate it in clinical testing.

Criticism Gone Awry

Too often, criticism founders on the rocks of misconstrued data or faulty logic. For example, the importance of nondividing cells in age-related disease (e.g., myocytes in myocardial infarction) is frequently raised, but ignores the dependence of nondividing cells on dividing cells. Furthermore, senescence may not be restricted to dividing cells alone. "Reactive" as opposed to "constitutive" senescence (Faragher et al., 1997b) may be triggered by mutation (Serrano et al., 1997), ultraviolet or other high-energy photon exposure (Kruk et al., 1995), free radical (von Zglinicki et al., 2000a) or oxidative damage (Kagawa et al., 1999; Saretzki et al., 1999; Seidman et al., 2000; de Magalhaes et al., 2002), or oncotherapeutic agents (Brenneisen et al., 1993; Khaw et al., 1993). Ultraviolet photons and dimethylsulfoxide (DMSO) exposure may also trigger transient telomerase expression (Alfonso-De Matte et al., 2001). Nondividing myocardial cells might undergo reactive senescence from the hypoxia of coronary stenosis (in turn induced by endothelial cell senescence).

Invalid arguments often use strawman reasoning. The initial example is clearly false: myocardial cells don't accumulate cholesterol (valid, but irrelevant), therefore, cholesterol can't contribute to myocardial infarction (invalid conclusion). Nevertheless, a parallel is occasionally used to attack the putative role of cell senescence: myocardial cells don't senesce (valid, but irrelevant), therefore, cell senescence can't contribute to myocardial infarction (invalid conclusion). Strawmen reveal more about the logical disabilities of the disputant than about human pathology. Yet the same strategy has been used repeatedly in criticizing cell senescence as a overall factor in aging: some cells in the body don't become senescent (valid, but irrelevant), therefore cell senescence can't cause aging (invalid conclusion). The fact that some cells never senesce while others could but have not yet done so is neither a surprise nor an issue. Compare arguments that might have been made against microbial theory: bacteria can't always be cultured from every sample, therefore bacteria can't cause infections. In cellulitis, 20% of cultures (at best) yield positive growth and patients die of infections without infectious organisms in every tissue, but proof of bacterial etiology lies in clinical response to appropriate antibiotic intervention.

Consider an even more glaring illustration in the arena of malignancy: some noncancerous cells exist in dying cancer patients, therefore, cancer can't be the cause of their death. The diagnosis of cancer does not require the entire body to be malignant. A sufficient number of cancer cells will cause dysfunction and mortality, though most body cells are normal and nonmalignant at death. Cancer cells, like senescent cells, do not kill by being nonfunctional but by being dysfunctional. The impressive cachexia and asthenia of advanced malignancy, as well as of sepsis, severe trauma, and other catabolic conditions (Hasselgren et al., 2002), is due to systemic intercellular effects (Bruera and Sweeney, 2000; Kurzrock, 2001; Inui, 2002), not to the wholesale conversion of normal cells into malignant ones. Cancer cells and senescent cells impose their dysfunction on cells around them, systemically as well as locally, aggressively undermining overall tissue and organ function.

It is not necessary for all cells to senesce, but some do and are sufficient. This is a far cry from the strawman argument that cell senescence cannot play a role in aging because not all cells are senescent in old patients. Even the oldest animals (Kohn, 1975) or humans (Cristofalo et al., 1998a) have nonsenescent, functional cells still capable of division. The question is not whether all cells are senescent (or even dead?) but whether enough sufficiently senescent cells are present in some tissues to undermine organ function and cause clinical pathology. Moreover, the preeminent issue is not mere presence but active interference with function. Lipomas (benign fatty tumors) do little to interfere with other tissues and body function generally; malignant tumors aggressively interfere with other cells and organ function. Senescent cells do not simply drop out of collective tissue function but interfere with such function. Whether in malignancy or senescence, a small minority of cells may cause major morbidity or mortality.

Criticisms misconstruing the model (e.g., telomeres cause aging) hit the wrong target. Criticism based on deficient understanding of clinical pathology (neurons don't divide, so cell senescence can't cause Alzheimer disease), tissue function (not all cells are senescent, so cell senescence can't cause aging), or the events of fertilization (telomerase knockout mice have normal lifespans, so telomeres don't cause aging) are neither apropos nor telling. The severest test lies in the need for direct confirmatory data.

Cells to Organisms

Telomere lengths vary among species and do not correlate well with comparative species lifespan in knockout mice (Blasco et al., 1997a), *Mus musculus* versus *spretus* (Zhu et al., 1998), rats (Yoshimi et al., 1996), or other species—nor should they. When comparing animal species, lifespan depends not merely on mean fetal telomere length but on innumerable other factors. Within cells these include metabolic rate, ultraviolet exposure, free radical trapping efficiency, DNA repair, and cell cycle differences (e.g., von Zglinicki et al., 2000a). Age-related pathology depends on species-specific changes in gene expression as well as on species-specific cell–cell interactions and organ differences. Species differ significantly at all levels: their cells, the interactions between cells, and their organs. Murine cells have higher metabolic rates than do corresponding human cells and murine SOD is less efficient as well (Cutler, 1985); additional changes occur at every level. Telomere lengths do not determine the marked disparity in mean murine and human lifespans.

In tissues comprising dividing cells (as in skin), a minority of relatively senescent cells may suffice to produce aging changes. As senescing cells divide more slowly, younger cells may increase their division rate reciprocally. Near-senescent human fibroblasts have variable telomere lengths (Steinert et al., 2000); each tissue will equilibrate somewhat, yet have variable percentages of not-yet senescent cells. It is probably unlikely that senescent cells ever become a majority within in vivo tissue.

In tissues comprising nondividing cells (as in myocardium), a small minority of relatively senescent cells elsewhere (as in coronary arteries) may suffice to produce pathologic changes. Of approximately two-thirds of a million myocardial infarction patients dying in the United States annually, almost all have otherwise normal (but infarcted) cardiac myocytes (Lakata, 1994). Endothelial cells lining arterial walls divide, their telomeres shorten, and they senesce (Chang and Harley, 1995), likely triggering atherogenesis (Kumazaki, 1993; Cooper et al., 1994; Bodnar et al., 1998; Yang and Wilson 1999). Myocytes do not have to senesce; they die nonetheless.

Whether the tissue's cells divide or not is irrelevant when the tissue (like all human tissues) depends on other tissues whose cells divide. In the epidermis, senescence of epidermal cells affects only neighboring epidermal cells. In the brain, microglia senescence also affects intermingled neuronal cells. In the arteries, endothelial cell senescence affects both neighboring subendothelial and distant myocardial cells. Senescence also results in the altered expression of genes responsible for extracellular matrix and its maintenance. Dermal overexpression of plasminogen activator activity, for example, may progressively disrupt the extracellular matrix, leading to degenerative changes (West et al., 1996), though only a modicum of cells senesce.

In any tissue, interdependence increases the potential outcome of senescent cells. Myocardial infarction begins in endothelial cell dysfunction. Equally, Alzheimer dementia might begin in microglia dysfunction. Oligodendrocytes and most glia may not divide, but microglia do (Sturrock, 1976). Neurons depend on glial maintenance of ionic milieu, guidance during arborization, insulation from excitatory transmitters, metabolic support, and, perhaps most critically, trophic factors (Nishi, 1994). In the glial–neural interaction, this may be the crucial factor in the etiology of neural apoptosis. Until recently, neurons and myocytes were considered postreplicative. While neurons may not divide, neuronal stem cells do and may even play a role in learning and memory. Satellite cells may likewise replace adult myocyte loss. This occurs in rat myocardium with consequent myocyte telomere shortening (Kajstura et al., 2000). Such exceptions, though fascinating, are academic and orthogonal to the point: even if none of these cells divide, nondividing cells depend on dividing cells. Dependence translates into age-related pathology.

Occasionally, there have been attempts to measure telomere length to assess biological age (Tsuji et al., 2002; Cawthon et al., 2003). While there might be a narrow value in length, it does not express the effects of changes in gene expression, local effects of cell dysfunction, or the frequently significant (even fatal) effects on distant tissues. Moreover, cells do not divide in lock-step, even within an apparently homogenous tissue. The classic graph of telomere lengths versus time suggests that germ cell lengths are constant, while somatic cell lengths fall linearly. In reality, somatic cell telomeres do not show a linear or uniform decrease but vary substantially over time (Fig. 3–2) (Butler et al., 1998). Every cell pursues a separate vector. No two daughter cells are likely to maintain the same vector, as they are unlikely to receive the same integration of signals favoring and restraining cell division, bear the same environmental stresses, or have the same direct cell–cell interactions. At every cell division, daughter cell lines diverge, curve, overlap, tangle, and all but knot themselves as the daughter cells continue their gradual, discontinuous, and unsteady course into a complex and interactive senescence.

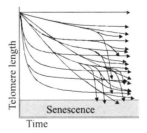

Figure 3–2 Reality of telomere shortening. Realistic appraisal of cell dynamics suggests that telomere loss is far from linear in any cell line. The differing fates of daughter cells during stem cell division (as one differentiates and one remains in the stem cell compartment), disparate oxidative stress, and widely varying (over time and between cell types) demands for cell division enforce complex trajectories in plotting telomere lengths over time.

Cells not only vary in their rates of telomere loss but, far more importantly and interestingly, in the onset and effects of their senescence. Aging tissues show a broadening range of senescence as displayed not by telomere lengths but by gene expression, morphology, function, and implication. That senescing cells (as a population average) should be equivalently senescent by any measure verges on inconceivably improbable. That aging tissues should display a majority of senescent cells, equivalent or otherwise, is almost equally improbable.

CHAPTER 4

The Aging Cascade

The Jigsaw Puzzle of Aging

By providing a broader, more inclusive framework for understanding aging, cell senescence resolves many apparent conflicts among aging theories, as well as adding to our understanding of age-related clinical pathology. How does this fit within the framework of other, previous aging models (Balcombe and Sinclair, 2001)? Although this is not the appropriate venue to explore the historical background and prior theories in detail, it is appropriate to examine the consistency of cell senescence with previous models and with current biology and pathology.

The belief that free radicals (reactive oxygen species [ROS]) cause damage in aging organisms (Grune and Davies, 2001) has a firm theoretical foundation and, despite a surprising lack of proof, has achieved widespread acceptance in their role. Recent work has attempted to move this model into intervention clinically (Yu, 1999) and scientifically (Chen et al., 1995; Yuan et al., 1995; Saretzki et al., 1998). Synthetic superoxide dismutase/catalase, more active than the wild enzyme, extends lifespan by half in *Caenorhabditis elegans*, although mouse data are less compelling (Melov, 2000; Melov et al., 2000).

Free radicals are not a complete explanation of aging. The eukaryotic germ cell line, for example, has been subject to ROS damage from symbiotic mitochondria for more than a billion years without senescing. Yet damage rapidly accumulates in somatic cell lines. Free radical researchers should not be asking how free radicals cause aging but why they don't usually cause aging. Free radicals may underlie aging and may even play some role in telomere erosion (von Zglinicki et al., 2000a), but there is something fundamental controlling the occurrence or accumulation of cellular free radical damage, something controlling the balance between damage and homeostasis. Free radical damage accumulates in somatic cells, but homeostasis is a sufficient match in germ cell lines. Alteration in gene expression, modulated by telomere length, is a likely candidate for such control. Without this or a similar explanation, wear-and-tear theories are not so much wrong as inadequate.

One exception is a novel and thoughtful explanation (Kowald and Kirkwood, 2000) suggesting defective mitochondria as the cause of aging: damaged mitochondria are preferentially selected in postmitotic somatic cells compared to rapidly dividing cells. This theory, first sketched out by de Grey (1997) and subsequently refined and extended (de Grey, 1999), is more consistent than previous mitochondrial (e.g., Linnane et al., 1992; Richter, 1992; Kowald and Kirkwood, 1993b) or most nonmitochondrial models: it explains the biological immortality of the germ cell line. Germ cells outdivide their damaged mitochondria, and somatic cells unavoidably accumulate damaged mitochondria. Other wear-and-tear or mitochondrial theories (Kalous and Drahota, 1996; Finkel and Holbrook, 2000) remain incomplete without additional theorization to explain this difference; mitochondrial theory (as we shall see) requires only stochastic selection.

The incidence of defective mitochondria is higher in older organisms (Linnane et al., 1990; Hattori et al., 1991; Yen et al., 1991; Michikawa et al., 1999), but is this a primary effect (as de Grey suggests) or (as most data suggest) secondary to the lack of appropriate support from the nucleus as gene expression alters with senescence? In yeast, for example, a "retrograde response" from the nucleus ameliorates mtDNA damage (Jazwinski, 2000d, 2000e). Such interactions between nuclear and mtDNA may be crucial to eukaryotic cell longevity (De Benedictis et al., 2000). Cumulative mitochondrial dysfunction is predicted from cell senescence theory, attributing the increasing mitochondrial defects to altered nuclear DNA expression and hence altered function not only within the cell in general but in the mitochondria in particular. Indeed, at least in tumor cells, immortalization is accompanied by characteristic changes (the immortalization-associated d-loop) in the mitochondria (Duncan et al., 2000) that may explain the failure of mitochondria to induce damage in such immortal cells.

In normal cells, however, cell senescence causes progressive changes in cell function. Consequences include slowed mitochondrial turnover (Lee and Wei, 1997; Korr et al., 1998), greater oxidative damage (due to damaged mitochondrial lipid membranes and those mitochondrial proteins synthesized from nuclear DNA), ineffective phagocytic degradation of the damaged mitochondria (Donati et al., 2001), and decreased mitochondrial volume (Chen et al., 2001a). Furthermore, there is an age-related increase in mitochondrial proton leakage in vivo, but not necessarily in vitro (Porter et al., 1999): mitochondrial aging may be secondary. In contrast, mitochondrial theory attributes increasing mitochondrial defects to ineffective phagocytic degradation as a result of ineffective oxidative "tagging" of the inner mitochondrial membranes (see below); mitochondrial aging is primary, not secondary. Mitochondrial theory raises two questions: (1) why should defective mitochondria accumulate preferentially, and (2) how do we deal with the growing data on cell senescence, particularly the work showing that cell senescence can be prevented (or reversed) via telomerase?

Mitochondrial theory, as initially outlined (de Grey, 1997), dealt with the issue of mitochondrial selection. More recent mathematical models (Kowald, 1999; Kowald and Kirkwood, 1999) provide further detail. Free radicals cause progressive damage to mitochondrial DNA (Korr et al., 1998; Kovalenko et al., 1998), in turn interfering with ATP production, resulting in cell dysfunction and (ultimately) aging. We might expect the cell to destroy defective mitochondria or stimulate mitochondrial replication as it senses decreasing ATP availability and it is not clear that mitochondrial damage is sufficient to explain aging (Gadaleta et al., 1992). Defective mitochondria are normally degraded by lysosomal phagocytosis, with consequent mitochondrial turnover (Korr et al., 1998) and renewal (Kadenbach et al., 1999), although the rate of turnover may decline with age (Donati et al., 2001).

Mitochondrial theory suggests that turnover fails and defective mitochondria preferentially accumulate. While some explanations do not stand up to data (Kowald and Kirkwood, 1999), de Grey (1997) suggests that defective mitochondria might not degrade as readily. Mitochondria typically turn over every 1 to 4 weeks (Huemer et al., 1971; Menzies and Gold, 1971; Korr et al., 1998) depending on species and cell phenotype. If damaged mitochondria are tagged for degradation by their level of oxidative damage to the inner mitochondrial membrane, but if defective mitochondria have a slow enough rate of respiration, they may have less rather than more oxidative tagging and hence a slower rate of turnover. Defective mitochondria would accumulate in older, nondividing cells.

Defective mitochondria have an increased ratio of free radical production (Bandy and Davidson, 1990; Lee and Wei, 1997, 2001), but their proton pumps are even more defective, lowering the overall rate of perhydroxyl formation (as fewer protons are available). Since perhydroxyl radicals oxidize lipids, membrane damage is lower and there is less oxidative tagging of the defective mitochondria (Kowald and Kirkwood, 1999).

Since human mitochondria turn over after a mean of 14 days, are there reserve mitochondria from which other mitochondria derive (as there are erythrocyte stem cells)? If damaged mitochondria turn over, is damage reset in the stem mitochondria by the process of division (as it is in erythrocyte stem cells)? The alternative is (reductio ad absurdum) that *all* mitochondria degrade approximately 14 days after last division. Unless there are stem mitochondria, all eukaryotic cells quickly die of mitochondrial loss. Alternatively, mitochondrial turnover is asymmetric: degradation must be completely reset in one of the two dividing mitochondria. Eukaryote survival apparently implies that mitochondrial division can reset mitochondrial degradation even in nondividing cells.

Regarding cell senescence, initial mitochondrial data appear to contradict the model. Cell senescence theory predicts a higher percentage of damaged mitochondria in dividing (more nearly senescent) cells, but data suggest that defective mitochondria are found preferentially in nondividing, postmitotic (hence nonsenescing) cells (Cortopassi et al., 1992; Sugiyama et al., 1993; Lee et al., 1994b). But are these postmitotic cells already senescent? While some of these studies were done on nondividing myocytes (striated and cardiac), suggesting that mitochondrial aging operates independent of senescence (Kwong and Sohal, 2000), other cells (hepatocytes) may have been postmitotic due to cell senescence, muddying the theoretical waters. Even the myocytes (see Chapter 15) could have been functionally senescent due to satellite cell replacement. Curiously, mitochondrial changes were not found in testes, which might represent nonsenescing germ or other cell phenotypes (Yashima et al., 1998b).

That cell senescence and defective mitochondria might independently play roles has experimental implications (Kowald and Kirkwood, 1999; Sozou and Kirkwood, 2001). The rapid divisions of in vitro studies might show significant senescence effects but little mitochondrial effect as multiple divisions dilute out defective mitochondria. In vivo studies might balance the two processes or favor mitochondrial failure as the primary cause of cell dysfunction. In pheochromocytoma cells, high telomerase levels correlate with less mitochondrial dysfunction (Fu et al., 1999). Senescent cells do show defects in free radical metabolism, including increased superoxide (Chen et al., 2001a), elevations in cytochrome-c oxidase and NADH dehydrogenase activity, hydrogen peroxide generation, and catalase activity (but not its mRNA) as well as a decrease in GSH peroxidase (GPx) mRNA abundance (Allen et al., 1999). Work on telomerase-negative mice (Rudolph et al., 1999) show only minimal effects on cell dysfunction and longevity (see above) until the sixth generation, but misunderstanding (Kowald and Kirkwood, 1999) such data does not rule out the importance of cell senescence for in vivo aging. The issue, as discussed above, is not telomere length (and the loss of the telomerase gene) but the effects of telomere shortening (Tsuji et al., 2002) on gene expression in critical cells over the organism's lifespan. Telomere length prior to fertilization does not alter cell viability, except when it is so critically short that it precludes telomere maintenance and cell survival, as occurs by the sixth generation.

Mitochondrial damage is central to aging, but whether this is primary (caused by the failure to degrade defective mitochondria) or secondary (to changes in gene expression within the nucleus) remains unsettled. Permissive accumulation of defective mitochondria may be the outcome of cell senescence. Just as protein turnover slows in senescent cells, so too does mitochondrial turnover. As slower protein turnover results in the preferential accumulation of defective proteins (Grune et al., 2001), slower mitochondrial turnover results in preferential accumulation of defective mitochondria. This may occur independently of changes in oxidative tagging, recognition of defective mitochondria, or rate of damage.

Cell senescence may explain slower mitochondrial turnover and mtDNA changes (Chung et al., 1994) even in nondividing cells. In a cardiac myocyte, for example, the vascular supply becomes inadequate (due to endothelial cell senescence). Even as postmitotic cells with stable telomere lengths (Takubo et al., 2002), myocardial cells are dependent on dividing, senescing endothelial cells in the coronary arteries. As atherosclerosis progresses, relative anoxia ensues. Anoxia, like hyperoxia (Carvalho et al., 1998), causes increased free radical (Serebrovs'ka et al., 1999; Grune et al., 2000; Seidman et al., 2000) and mitochondrial damage (Johnston et al., 2000b). Lipid peroxidation as well as protein and DNA damage (Taylor et al., 1999) are due to the oxygen dependence of our free radical defenses and to a shift toward anaerobic metabolism (Nordstrom and Arulkumaran, 1998). The lipid damage further interferes with free radical sequestration. Moreover, hypoxia may result in altered patterns of gene transcription, including some pathways of apoptosis (Mishra and Delivoria-Papadopoulos, 1999). This may cause further mitochondrial damage and invocation of apoptosis pathways (Pollack and Leeuwenburgh, 2001) more characteristic of senescent than of nonsenescent cells. Free radical and mitochondrial damage occur preferentially in hypoxic conditions, whether caused by low environmental oxygen, anemia, or low flow. The pathology of ischemia is prominent in myocardial, neuronal, and sensory tissues (Seidman et al., 2000). Mitochondrial damage occurs within nondividing cells as a result of senescence in dividing cells. Although both mitochondrial theory and cell senescence are consistent with mitochondrial damages, mitochondrial theory cannot explain the indefinite deferral or reversal of cell senescence occurring in telomerized cells.

Other popular but less scientific theories attribute aging to hormonal or organ-level clocks, e.g., DHEA, growth hormone, or melatonin. Mass attribution, however, is irrelevant (Fossel, 2001a): science is not subject to majority vote. Not only are there no data showing that aging can be altered by such approaches (Kala et al., 1998; Wolfe, 1998), but each begs a basic question: if hormonal decline causes aging, then what causes the hormonal decline in the first place? If we run out of hormones, why do cells stop producing hormones at different times in different species? What genetic clock sets the hormonal one? Hormones may have beneficial, even lifespan-increasing effects, but there is no evidence that their lack causes aging. Adequate diet, good hygiene, immunizations, seatbelts, regular exercise, and screening exams may all increase lifespan, without any effect on aging. Only three interventions (caloric restriction, breeding, and genetic alteration) validly affect aging.

Caloric restriction causes a substantial increase in the mean and maximum lifespan and a substantial postponement of age-related disease processes including (in relevant species) atherosclerosis and cancer. Although there are growing data on the effects of caloric restriction on specific organs, e.g., microvascular density and blood flow in the nervous system (Lynch et al., 1999), we still lack a clear understanding of the process. Most explanations focus on insulin and glucose metabolism (Kemnitz et al., 1994), metabolic efficiency, and free radical generation, though without consensus (Roth et al., 1999). Cell senescence is consistent with caloric restriction (Wolf and Pendergrass, 1999) and offers a broader explanation for aging and aging diseases. Comparisons of ad libitum and restricted animals demonstrate striking and intriguing differences in patterns of gene expression (Lee et al., 1999a). The altered pattern of expression in genes regulating energy production, protein synthesis, and DNA repair suggests that any explanation of the effects of caloric restriction on aging might best be understood in terms of gene expression (Marx, 2000). Caloric restriction may slow cell senescence (and perhaps replication), rendering cells more efficient and less likely to produce free radicals, or the cells of smaller, calorically restricted animals (Black et al., 2001) might have undergone fewer divisions, but there is little evidence for this. A single study did find a lower percentage of senescent cells in calorically restricted animals (Li et al., 1997), but a link remains vague and poorly substantiated.

Work on selective breeding (reviewed in Rose and Charlesworth, 1980; Arking, 1987a; Arking and Dudas, 1989; Jazwinski, 1996; Rose, 1998) and genetic alteration, especially in *C. elegans* (Larsen, 1993; Larsen et al., 1995; Guarente and Kenyon, 2000), generally emphasizes genes relevant to energy and free radical metabolism (Lin et al., 1997). Aging can be slowed by either removing inefficient genes (e.g., in *Caenorhabditis*), selecting for more efficient genes (e.g, in *Mus* or *Drosophila*), or altering the pattern of gene expression of existing genes (e.g., through the telomerization of somatic cells). The outcomes are similar whether accomplished by telomerase (resetting or postponing senescence associated gene expression), breeding (selecting for specific genes involved in senescence or its postponement), or gene replacement (affecting energy and free radical metabolism and thereby delaying the damage cascade). Genetics is crucial to any attempt to understand aging (Johnson, 1997; Miller 1999): genes play the major role (Rattan, 2000a) and are the stage on which cell senescence occurs (Pereira-Smith, 1997). Purely genetic theories of aging are, however, insufficient. Our genes play the major roles, but chromosomes (Guarente, 1996) direct the entire tragedy. Aging and age-related disease are not a matter of which genes we have, but of how gene expression changes as critical cells senesce.

Upstream from Cell Division

Cell division occurs not because we age but because we live. Living, we lose cells and replace them by replication of those remaining. This can be continuous as in the skin and hematopoetic system or a response to injury as in the liver, or almost nonexistent as in the brain and heart. Cell replacement is not so much a response to time as to environmental events. We continuously replace keratinocytes in our skin, but only because we lose so many from dermal trauma. We continuously replace erythrocytes, but more rapidly in infection or trauma. This response to events is more obvious in tissues with lower turnover, such as endothelial cells in the arterial wall. Here, cell turnover is affected by dozens of factors, some obvious and well known, others subtle, suspected, or unproven. Suggesting that cell senescence is central to aging is like suggesting that the commentator is central to the evening news. It appears true only by neglecting unseen, unappreciated, and essential events occurring offstage. In atherosclerosis, to argue that cell senescence is central to the pathology makes us prone to two misleading errors. First, it erroneously suggests that all we know of atherosclerosis is wrong. Second, it erroneously suggests that cell senescence stands alone, deus ex machina, causing aging independently.

Cell senescence is merely a common denominator between upstream risk factors and downstream pathology. In atherosclerosis, hypertension increases tension upon the aorta, stressing the endothelial cells. This is more evident (and atherosclerosis more common) at bifurcations. Tobacco products, circulating in the blood vessels, act as cell toxins and they do so first and in their greatest concentrations on the endothelial cells that line those vessels. Each of the circulating factors that have been implicated in atherosclerosis—lipids, glucose, dietary toxins, bacteria, viruses—reach the endothelial cells preferentially in their circulation. Cells are damaged, missing cells are replaced, and cell senescence advances.

Central to pathology, cell senescence is nevertheless the effect of upstream causes and the cause of downstream effects. In atherosclerosis, such upstream causes include complex genetic variables (including predilections for exercise, hypertension, tobacco addiction, diabetes, hyperlipidemia) and environment variables (social impetus for exercise, available diet, stress, infections, access to tobacco). Cell senescence offers an opportunity to understand the link between causes and effects. Cell senescence does not stand alone from nor in contradiction to previous theories of aging and disease but offers an integral framework to explain how age-related pathology occurs and suggests unique promise as a therapeutic target.

Cell Turnover and Gene Expression

Taking atherosclerosis as our perennial example, cholesterol does not cause coronary artery disease simply because there is a lot of it circulating in our arteries. The web of effects that results in cholesterol plaques is difficult to summarize in one accurate sentence; the notion that cholesterol causes heart disease is an inaccurate summary. Nonetheless, cholesterol does play a role and clinical recommendations to prevent heart disease include lowering cholesterol levels through diet, medication, exercise, or a combination. Why, then, is it unreasonable to say that cholesterol causes heart disease?

The simple response cites exceptions. Some patients with abnormally high cholesterol have no atherosclerosis; some patients with abnormally low cholesterol have severe atherosclerosis. Progeric children (with normal cholesterol) die of severe atherosclerosis before puberty.

The more accurate response notes high serum cholesterol is but one of many risk factors. High cholesterol can be mitigated by other factors or other risks may be sufficient to overwhelm normal defenses.

The thorough response would be difficult, involving a consistent and detailed explanation of how independent and interacting variables go into the equation for atherosclerosis so that the dependent variables (heart attack, death) can be calculated. Readers may be relieved if I do not attempt such an equation.

What we require is a response that provides an overview of how complex variables interact and identifies efficient interventions in age-related disease. While we can intervene in environmental variables, cell senescence may be more effective. It is in cell turnover where complex variables come together to cause pathology.

Changing patterns of cell division (Warner et al., 1992) and gene expression are the result of transcriptional changes (Dimri et al., 1996). How gene expression alters as cells become senescent has been investigated for years (Campisi, 1992a), permitting the identification of cell phenotype–specific patterns of change (Jazwinski et al., 1995; Shelton et al., 1999). The details constitute a list of genes that alter their expression as senescence progresses and, collectively, tell us about altering cell functions.

Some of the changes in gene expression are predictable. The cell cycle (and hence cell turnover and replacement) slows down; changes in gene expression reflect shifts in the cell cycle and in modulators of growth regulatory genes. For example, there is repression of the c-fos component of the AP1 transcription factor, the Id1 and Id2 helix-loop-helix (HLH) proteins that negatively regulate basic HLH transcription factors, and the E2F-1 component of the E2F transcription factor. All three modulators may be required for normal cell cycling and their loss might help to explain many of the changes characterizing senescence. Curiously, E2F-1 has two binding sites proximal to the transcriptional start site of the hTERT promoter and functions as a transcriptional repressor of hTERT (Crowe et al., 2001). Loss of c-fos alters the balance between cell cycle promoting factors (such as AP-1 components with its effect on c-jun) and inhibiting factors (such as QM), culminating in growth arrest and senescent gene expression (Dimri et al., 1996).

Senescent cells (and progeric cells) become less responsive to some stimuli (Chen et al., 1986), including serum induction of Id-1H and Id-2H mRNAs (Hara et al., 1994). Although senescent cells demonstrate many genes responsive to mitogens, several E2R regulated genes that operate in late G1 stage are no longer inducible (Dimri et al., 1994). Other cell cycle–related components show what might be considered predictable changes (Dimri et al., 1994; Good et al., 1996). Senescent human, but not necessarily rodent (Wei et al., 2001b), fibroblasts show increased p14(ARF) expression (Dimri et al., 2000) and decreased expression of cyclins A and B (as well as dihydrofolate reductase, E2F-1, E2F-4, and E2F-5, though not p107, E2F-3, DP-1, or DP-2). Furthermore, cells deficient in the ARF transcriptional activator DMP1 are readily immortalized and those lacking it do not senesce (Inoue et al., 2000). Expression vectors for E2F-1 and DP-1 were only weakly active in senescent human cells, suggesting that such cells fail to express late G1 genes at least partly because E2F-1 is repressed and its activity lacking. Other independent factors play a role, at least in some cells, such as human fibroblasts (Dimri et al., 1994). The mRNA expression of several growth regulatory genes (c-*fos*, c-*jun*, *Id-1*, *Id-2*, *E2F-1*, and *cdc2*) are repressed in senescent cells (Dimri et al., 1994; Hara et al., 1996), and one or more basic helix-loop-helix (bHLH) factors that cooperate with pRb, or pRb-related proteins, are probably expressed, suppressing proliferation (Hara et al., 1996). Similarly, there is a general change in the expression of growth- and differentiation-specific genes as well as transcription factors that parallel the induction of senescence. These include increased expression of one of three TFIID complexes and OctBP, while there was a reduction in the expression of AP1, CREBP, and CTF complexes in senescent cells, and no change in GREBP, NF-κ B, and SP1 complexes. The alteration in the single TFIID complex was dependent on the presence of a functional retinoblastoma protein (Dimri and Campisi, 1994b). Telomerase itself is down-regulated in most somatic cells, apparently in parallel with differentiation (Fukutomi et al., 2001). Stem cells express telomerase but show transcriptional repression upon exiting the cell cycle, probably with proteolysis in terminal differentiation (Holt and Shay, 1999).

Other changes in gene expression are less predictable from the change in cell cycle mechanics. The constitutive expression of a ribosomal subunit (the mRNA for L7, a structural human protein with close homologs in the mouse and rat), for example, declines several-fold in senescent fibroblasts from human lung or foreskin, even though it is not a cell cycle–related protein. The mRNAs for five other ribosomal proteins (L5, P1, S3, S6, and S10) showed a similar decline, unrelated to the cell's growth state or its rate of overall protein synthesis (Seshadri et al., 1993).

Like the changes in gene expression themselves, the effects may be categorized as either (*1*) effects on slowing cell replacement, usually shared by dividing cells, or (*2*) effects on cellular function, usually peculiar to a cell phenotype. Predictably, the former results in fewer cells available within a given tissue, such as the epidermis, the circulating erythrocyte population, the endothelial lining of an artery, or the recruiting response of leukocytes during infectious challenge. The latter, more idiosyncratic effects, however, have been less well investigated. These changes differ between dermal fibroblasts, vascular endothelial, or retinal pigment epithelial cells. Such patterns are not only characteristic of a cell phenotype but correlate with the age-related diseases characteristic of tissue type for that cell (Shelton et al., 1999). Inflammatory genes are strongly expressed in dermal fibroblasts, for example, paralleling the clinical characteristics of senescent skin. Data correlating tissue- and cell-specific patterns of senescent gene expression are limited; the human diseases they cause are not.

Between Cells: Cells, Tissues, and Pathology

Multicellularity requires interdependence. In pathology, disease is never due to the lack of function within a single cell, and even disease due to the lack of function of a single cell phenotype (the loss of the islet of Langerhans cells in type I, insulin-dependent diabetes) is less common than disease due to aberrant cell function. Pathology is more commonly a sin of commission than omission. Pathological cells seldom passively fail to perform so much as they actively interfere with other nonpathological cells. The "innocent bystander effect" (Fossel, 1996) is typical of age-related diseases, as in myocardial infarction from aberrant endothelial function. Vascular endothelial cells do not simply fail, but fail in a spectacularly active and novel way. Subendothelial tissues shows marked inflammatory change and active lipid accumulation, not merely an unassuming necrosis. Aging and age-related pathology only become evident as pathology between cells. Some pathological interactions are purely local cell–cell interactions, involving cell–cell contact or trophic factor transmission. Some are distant cell–cell interactions, involving gross vascular dysfunction (as in coronary artery disease) or hormonal interactions (as in alterations in serum estrogen, insulin, or erythropoietin levels).

Local cell interactions often result from alterations in secreted products, such as cytokines, which act over short distances as autocrine or paracrine hormones (Bissell, 1998). These secreted products can cause changes in surrounding cells by their presence (e.g., secretion of inflammatory factors) and absence (e.g., dependence on trophic factors). These changes allow senescent cells to compromise function and integrity at the tissue level (Faragher et al., 1997b) and trigger pathology. While the origin of pathology is an old question, the suggestion that cell senescence plays a role (Campisi, 1996) is novel. Cell senescence occurs; pathology occurs. At issue is the link between the two—the effects of cell dysfunction on tissue dysfunction—for this is the level at which pathology becomes evident.

The link between aging and disease is clear demographically (Mueller et al., 1995) as epitomized by the Gompertz equation. While genes determine the onset and susceptibility (Johnson, 1997) of age-related disease (Rose and Archer, 1996), intervention requires that we understand the nature of the link (Kipling and Faragher, 1997). Cell turnover clearly occurs and has effects in aging and disease (Hodes, 1999). Replicative senescence also occurs, with changes in the rate of division and patterns of gene expression likely contributing to age-related pathology (Smith and Pereira-Smith, 1996; Campisi, 1997b). There has been extensive discussion of mechanisms by which cell senescence might cause organ pathology (Fossel, 1996; Faragher and Kipling, 1998) and there is firm correlational evidence that cell senescence occurs in age-related diseases.

To what extent, however, is there evidence that cell senescence results in pathology? Before moving on to an organ-by-organ exploration of this question, we need to explore a disease in which cells do not senesce.

CHAPTER 5

Cancer

Cancer in Its Cellular Context

Cancer is a disease in which cells do not senesce. Our natural defenses against cancer can be grouped into intra- and extracellular defenses: cell senescence plays a role in both. Intracellularly, there are passive lines of defense (sequestration of DNA in the nucleus and production of free radicals in the mitochondria) as well as three active, sequential lines of defense: DNA repair, the cell cycle braking system, and cell senescence. Extracellularly, there is a passive requirement for angiogenesis in solid tumors (Barinaga, 2000), inflammation (Hudson et al., 1999), and active immunosurveillance (Allison et al., 1998). The failure of these mechanisms (Benson et al., 1996) together contribute to the exponential rise in cancer with age.

Free radical sequestration in the mitochondria is insufficient to prevent DNA damage. Throughout the cell, thermal damage disrupts purine-deoxyribose-*N*-glycosyl linkages five to ten thousand times daily in each cell (Singer and Berg, 1991). Granted the ubiquity of damage, DNA repair is stunningly effective but imperfect (Grossman and Wei, 1995; Lindahl and Wood, 1999). Damage is often to silenced tumor suppressor genes (Raza, 2000) or to genes that inhibit growth or ensure apoptosis (Chin et al., 1999; Lundberg and Weinberg, 1999; McCormick, 1999b; Akiyama et al., 2002). Cancers derive from the genetic errors (if not necessarily generic instability; Zimonjic et al., 2001) of such single clonal cells (Raza, 2000), although polyclonal cancers (Schwartz et al., 2002) may occur.

Failing repair, the cell limits its DNA replication. The cell cycle breaking system distinguishes normal from malignant cells (Hartwell and Kastan, 1994; Jacks and Weinberg, 1996). Cells normally recognize and repair DNA damage (Hoeijmakers, 2001), but failing recognition or pending repair, the cell cycle remains blocked (Carr, 2000). Checkpoints occur at several points, each necessary to ensure chromosomal stability (Dhar et al., 2000). If braked, for example, by a checkpoint kinase (Hirao et al., 2000), the cell (*1*) up-regulates DNA damage repair and (*2*) blocks the cycle and DNA replication.

Damaged DNA binding proteins, by binding, release p53 and up-regulate cell-cycle inhibitor p21^{WAF1} as well as invoking changes in p16 (Parkinson et al., 2000), p19 (Carnero et al., 2000b), p73 (Ichimiya et al., 2000), PARP (Tong et al., 2001), D cyclins, cdks, and ARF (Li et al., 1994; Wynford-Thomas, 1999; Sherr, 2000b). A rapid, alternate Cdc25A-mediated pathway, independent of p53 and p21, results in G1 cell cycle arrest (Mailand et al., 2000). However accomplished, DNA damage up-regulates braking and repair functions (Sherr, 2000a). Cells bypassing these inhibiting mechanisms (Shay et al., 1991b) are biologically, if not yet clinically, malignant.

Until 1989, there was no fundamental cellular distinction in which to drive a therapeutic wedge. Aberrant cell cycling (Artandi and DePinho, 2000b), by distinguishing cancer from normal cells (Yang et al., 2000), might permit oncologists to find a therapeutic "magic bullet" (Soria et al., 1998). The most frequently mutated human cancer gene (Levrero et al., 2000) is a mutant *p53* (Shay et al., 1992a; Chen et al., 1993; Zhang et al., 1994; Gollahon and Shay, 1996). Sixty percent (Rao, 1996; Sherr, 1996) of human cancers share defective *p53* (McCormick, 1999a), whose abnormal binding (Chen et al., 1993; Zhang et al., 1993a) renders it ineffective (Zhang et al., 1993b). Similar allelic variation of *p53* is found in spontaneously immortalized cells from a high-dose atomic bomb survivor (Honda et al., 1996).

Patients with germ-line *p53* mutations show an increased incidence of all cancer types; in patients with Li-Fraumeni syndrome (see Rogan et al., 1995), this is especially evident in their increased incidence of breast cancer (Shay et al., 1995a). Normal *p53* is essential to limiting cell division, as demonstrated when it is switched on and off (Carnero et al., 2000a). Mutant *p53* renders cancer cells more resistant to hypoxia and to angiogenesis inhibition (Yu et al., 2002). Conversely, mice with an overactive *p53* have a lower tumor incidence (Ferbeyre and Lowe, 2002; Tyner et al., 2002). When *p53* is missing in H1299 human non–small cell lung cancer cells, transfection of a wild-type (i.e., normal) *p53* gene causes loss of telomere signal and apoptosis (Mukhopadhyay et al., 1998). Activation of *p53* leads to growth arrest or apoptosis, but its deletion effectively prevents this only if done early in oncogenesis, prior to the cascade of "genetic catastrophe" (Chin et al., 1999). Liposomal delivery of wild-type *p53* to radiation-resistant squamous cell carcinomas results in increased radiation-induced apoptosis and tumor regression in mice (Xu et al., 1999). An adenovirus, tailored to divide only in cells with absent or abnormal p53, could infect and kill tumor cells and has shown good initial results against prostate tumors, hepatic tumors, head and neck tumors, and gastrointestinal (GI) tumors, although adjuvant chemotherapy appears to improve the results (Kirn et al., 1998; McCormick, 2000). The concept of a magic bullet remains quixotic, but only to a degree.

Cancer and Cell Senescence

Cell senescence is the last intracellular defense against cancer (Campisi, 1992b; Shay, 1997b, 1998a; Weinberg, 1998; Serrano and Blasco, 2001). A "dead man switch," senescence slows and ultimately prevents cell division and hence malignant growth

(Counter et al., 1994a). A common analogy has an accelerator, brake, and gas tank (de Lange and DePinho, 1999). Absent external signals (accelerator), normal cells (cars) are quiescent (stopped). Damaged DNA (accelerator stuck down) causes division, but cells detect the problem and invoke cell cycle braking (apply the brake). If cell braking fails, then telomere shortening enforces senescence (the car runs out of gas). Cancer cells express telomerase (Sugihara et al., 1996) and divide (refill the tank) indefinitely.

Mechanisms of cell cycle braking overlap senescence (Vaziri, 1997; Sherr and DePinho, 2000; Wynford-Thomas, 2000; Ahmed et al., 2001). Despite differences in regulation (Harrington and Robinson, 2002; Kim et al., 2002b), *p53* may inhibit activity through TEP1 binding (Li et al., 1999a), while telomere shortening appears to activate *p53* and, conversely, telomere repeats specifically stabilize the p53 protein (Milyavsky et al., 2001). Cells losing *p53* function proliferate a limited number of times beyond the replicative limit for phenotype. Similarly, lack of functional retinoblastoma (Rb) protein (or loss of p16INK4 function, abrogating regulation by retinoblastoma protein) permits only transient extension of proliferation (Duan et al., 2001), despite contrary claims (Duncan et al., 2000). The transient effect may be epigenetic (Yaswen and Stampfer, 2001). These two effects are additive, independently controlling division, and while sharing mechanisms, they are largely independent of telomere shortening, which continues in cells lacking p53 or Rb (Reddel, 1998b), though with exceptions (Garcia-Cao et al., 2002). Absent telomere maintenance, cells lacking p53 or Rb cannot replicate indefinitely (Cerni, 2000). Likewise, DNA repair flaws are more common in telomerase-deficient cells (Artandi et al., 2000; Wong et al., 2000), perhaps explaining the higher risk of malignant transformation in senescent cells. While senescence limits replication in individual cells, it increases risk of malignant growth in surrounding cells (Krtolica et al., 2001).

Evading these defenses risks genetic catastrophe and, in extremis, terminates both divisions and cell survival (Chin et al., 1999; Sohn et al., 2002). McClintock (1941) pointed out that chromosomes are unstable without telomeres but, curiously, damage and aberrations are more frequent in telomeres than elsewhere (Bouffler, 1998). This "delicacy" (Cottliar and Slavutsky, 2001; Lee and Huang, 2001) may be due to their critical role or the complexity of telomere maintenance.

The risk of such delicacy balances the risk of malignancy. Since cell senescence and its secondary pathology occur post-reproductively, the evolutionary costs of replicative limits are acceptable (Lithgow and Kirkwood, 1996; Westendorp and Kirkwood, 1998; Kirkwood and Austad, 2000) to the species if not the individual. The general concept—antagonistic pleiotropy—describes genes that benefit the young but incur less important post-reproductive costs (Harley, 1988; Rose and Graves, 1989; Rose and Finch, 1993; Weinstein and Ciszek, 2002). The aging body is "disposable" (Kirkwood and Holliday, 1979; Kirkwood, 1988b): aging is the serotinous cost of reproductive safety (Kirkwood and Rose, 1991; Wick et al., 2000) and results from necessary evolutionary choices (Kirkwood, 1992, 2000) that assure species survival (Rose, 1991). Teleologically, aging is a side effect of mechanisms that are meant to protect against cancer (Wang et al., 2000c) and consequent reproductive failure (Shay, 1997a). Cell senescence prevents malignant growth by limiting cell division (Campisi, 1997b; Reddel, 2000). Poetically, this "double-edged sword of cell senescence" (Campisi, 1997a, 1998a) is the evolutionary trade-off between aging and cancer (Zakian, 1997; Campisi, 2000b; Dimri et al., 2000).

The role of telomerase in cancer is neither simple (Shay, 1995; Holt et al., 1996a; Shay and Gazdar, 1997) nor uncomplicated (Tsao et al., 1998). Rather, it plays multiple (Blasco, 2002c; Stewart et al., 2003), complex (Autexier and Greider, 1996; Lubbe et al., 1997; Greider, 1998a) roles, even independent of telomere length (Stewart et al., 2002). While cell senescence limits division (Mera, 1998; Klingelhutz, 1999), it paradoxically facilitates carcinogenesis by compromising genomic stability (Artandi, 2002). Senescence increases instability (Golubovskaya et al., 1999; Holt and Shay, 1999; Artandi and DePinho, 2000a) and decreases immune surveillance (Pawelec, 1999b), favoring malignancy. The role of the telomere in chromosomal stability (Blagosklonny, 2001; Campisi et al., 2001; Hackett et al., 2001) argues that telomerase protects against carcinogenesis (Chang et al., 2001; Gisselsson et al., 2001), especially early in carcinogenesis when genetic stability is critical (Elmore and Holt, 2000; Kim and Hruszkewycz, 2001; Rudolph et al., 2001), as well as protecting against aneuploidy and secondary speciation (Pathak et al., 2002). The role of telomerase depends on the stage of malignancy as well as cofactors (Ohmura et al., 2000); expression is late and permissive, not causal (Seger et al., 2002).

Telomerase expression and especially telomere length may protect against malignant transformation in the rapid cell turnover of myelodysplastic syndrome, for example, by maintaining genomic stability (Ohyashiki et al., 1999). Transgenic insertion of exogenous hTERT is likewise protective against malignant transformation (Morales et al., 1999) and genetic instability (Amit et al., 2000 Elmore et al., 2002b; Zou et al., 2002). In combination with oncogenes (SV-40 large-T oncoprotein or an allele of H-*ras*), however, ectopic hTERT expression can transform human fibroblasts and epithelial cells (Hahn et al., 1999b). As elsewhere, hTERT is necessary but not sufficient (O'Hare et al., 2001).

Neither hTR (Avilion et al., 1996; Cerni, 2000) nor hTERT expression defines cancer absolutely, though hTERT is present in most human tumors (Shay and Bacchetti, 1997; Holt and Shay, 1999; Dessain et al., 2000) and effectively creates immortal human cell lines (Hahn et al., 1999). There are exceptions to the rule that tumors and immortalized cells (Mayne et al., 1986; Wright et al., 1989; Wright and Shay, 1992b; Bryan et al., 1995) demonstrate hTERT activity. Some immortalized human cells lack activity yet have stable telomeres (Bryan et al., 1997b); some cancer cells with telomerase activity still demonstrate telomere (TRF) loss down to 5 kb, while other cells lengthen, shorten, and plateau at initial lengths (Jones et al., 1998). In colon cancer cells (Bolzan et al., 2000), sarcomas (Yan et al., 2002), and rat bladder cancers (Shimazui et al., 2002) activity correlates minimally with length. Some maintain long telomeres (Henderson et al., 1996a; Xia et al., 1996; Gollahon et al., 1998) and even in telomerase-positive cells, length does not correlate well with malignancy (Kim et al., 1994; Hiyama et al., 1995b; Broccoli and Godwin, 2002) or clinical staging (Schneider-Stock et al., 1998a). While long telomeres or high activity may suffice (Matsutani et al., 2001a), exceptionally long telomeres may be detrimental in rapidly dividing cells (Savre-Train et al., 2000). Selection pressure may favor stable telomeres, regardless of length (Shay et al., 1995b; Bryan et al., 1998).

Expression is not activity. There are control points after expression, including nuclear transport, holoenzyme assembly, recruitment to the telomere, and post-translational modifications (Aisner et al., 2002; Collins and Mitchell, 2002). Fifty percent of oligodendroglial tumors express hTERT, but lack activity (Chong et al., 2000). Genistein

(4,5,7-trihydroxyisoflavone) prevents nuclear translocation: activity is normal, but telomeres shorten nonetheless (Alhasan et al., 2001). Splice variants inhibit activity in humans (Colgin et al., 2000; Yi et al., 2000; Krams et al., 2001; Villa et al., 2001) and other species (Guo et al., 2001). Some helicases (e.g., Pif1p) catalytically inhibit activity (Schulz and Zakian, 1994; Zhou et al., 2000; Mangahas et al., 2001) and fork replication (Ivessa et al., 2000), although without clear relationship to the Werner's helicase. SGS1 helicase mutation causes premature yeast aging, apparently via Sir3 silencing (Sinclair et al., 1997). Alteration of hTERT carboxyl terminus maintains activity but not telomere length (Ouellette et al., 1999). Differentiated cells may inhibit telomerase via proteolysis (Holt and Shay, 1999; Nozawa et al., 2001). Radiating murine leukemic cells (but not human fibroblasts or murine marrow cells) increases activity without demonstrated effects on c-myc, tankyrase, mTERT, or mTR levels (Finnon et al., 2000). Murine oncogenesis begins with rising mTR, increasing further with tumorigenesis; activity occurs later, not paralleling levels. Early tumors may express telomerase RNA, yet lack activity (Blasco et al., 1996). Despite these exceptions, hTERT expression generally implies activity (Wu et al., 1999a).

Given several decades of interest in genetic mechanisms of malignancy, it is not surprising that tumor suppressor genes and oncogenes (e.g., Steenbergen et al., 1996; Westerman and Leboulch, 1996; Hwang, 2002) are linked to telomerase expression, although the relationship is poorly understood (Bacchetti, 1996). Recent evidence shows that Myc up-regulates hTERT, which interacts closely with HPV E7, a viral product linked to cell immortalization (Greider, 1999a). But while HPV gene products increase mutation frequency and permit bypassing the senescence checkpoint, senescence continues unabated without active hTERT (Kang and Park, 2001). The number of hTERT gene copies (typically >3, but as high as 11) increases in some cancer cell lines, suggesting one road to up-regulation (Bryce et al., 2000). Some human squamous cell carcinomas, though not cholesteatomas (Watabe-Rudolph et al., 2002), show not only up-regulation but also "overrepresented or amplified" expression, in keeping with the frequent presence of isochromosome 3q (Parkinson et al., 1997). Rearrangement of hTERT repressors, e.g., the polymorphic minisatellite in introns 6 or 2 (containing binding sites for c-Myc, a known hTERT promoter), probably have no role in human carcinogenesis (Szutorisz et al., 2001). Neither simple nor linear, the link between c-myc overexpression (a hallmark of human cancer) and hTERT up-regulation depends on cell type, senescence, and other factors (Drissi et al., 2001; Tollefsbol and Andrews, 2001). Finally, certain tumor characteristics (e.g., hypoxia at the core of solid tumors) may affect telomerase activity (as well as mitogen-activated protein kinase activity, c-fos expression, and resistance to apoptosis). Increased hTERT activity may ameliorate the cell's response to hypoxia, which would otherwise increase genetic damage (Seimiya et al., 1999). These issues have profound clinical implications, offering diagnostic and therapeutic leverage (Meeker and Coffey, 1997; Zippursky, 2000).

Diagnosis

Several aspects of senescence may distinguish normal from cancer cells (Ide and Tahara, 1996; Kim, 1998; Shay, 1998b). Well over a thousand studies document the correlation between malignancy and telomerase (Matthews and Jones, 2001). While the importance of telomere (Gan et al., 2001a; Slijepcevic, 2001) and subtelomere (Sismani et al., 2001) lengths have been touted, most studies focus on telomerase (Blechner and Mandavilli, 2001). The diagnostic sensitivity of a polymerase chain reaction (PCR)-based assay— perhaps 1 cancer cell in 104 normal cells (Haber 1995)—entices the clinician. While PCR inhibitors may interfere, this can be overcome (Gollahon and Holt, 2000). The therapeutic potential is equally enticing (Buys, 2000; Larsen, 2000). Magic bullet or not, the data nonetheless endorse optimism (McKenzie et al., 1999; Urquidi et al., 2000).

Telomerase expression has excellent specificity (excepting stem and germ cell tissues) and approximately 90% sensitivity (Kim et al., 1994; Dhaene et al., 2000b). Dogs show similar sensitivities (Yazawa et al., 1999); their telomeres shorten with age (McKevitt et al., 2002) and they have similar overlap between normal and cancer cell expression (Carioto et al., 2001; Nasir et al., 2001). Figures vary for the percentage of human clinical cancer cells expressing telomerase, but the range is narrow (Blasco et al., 1996; Shay and Gazdar, 1997; Urquidi et al., 1998). Clinical sensitivities (assay errors, inaccurate biopsies, insufficient body fluid samples, and other exigencies of oncology) are probably worse.

Cancer is not equivalent to telomerase expression. Consider four possible states of cell type and expression: (*1*) cancer with telomerase, (*2*) cancer without telomerase, (*3*) normal with telomerase, and (*4*) normal without telomerase. The first and last are unremarkable; the second and third offer more insight.

Cancers without telomerase usually exhaust their telomeres and undergo senescence. For example, telomerase status predicts malignant versus benign outcome in neuroblastomas (Hiyama et al., 1995a, 1997a; Maitra et al., 1999). Although this is the general rule, some tumors survive indefinitely without telomerase (Bryan et al., 1995, 1997b; Blasco et al., 1997a), implying an alternative mechanism to maintain telomeres. Without such maintenance (or if insufficient), crisis (Multani et al., 1999a; Maser and DePinho, 2002), chromosomal fusions (Murnane et al., 1994), genetic instability (Morin, 1996a; Bryan et al., 1998; Dandjinou et al., 1999; Lo et al., 2002), and cell death (Lee et al., 1998c) occur. Even with oncogene activation (e.g., Myc), loss of the T-cell antigen gene (Rubelj et al., 1997), or loss of tumor suppressor function (e.g., Rb/p53), telomere maintenance remains critical (de Lange and DePinho, 1999; Vaziri and Benchimol, 1999; Neidle and Parkinson, 2002). Telomerase is, like Myc (Greenberg et al., 1998; Wang et al., 1998a), nearly universal in human cancers; inhibition arrests and ultimately kills malignant cells (Counter et al., 1992; de Lange and DePinho, 1999; Zhang et al., 1999b).

Cancer cells maintain stable telomeres (Shay, 1999a) using telomerase (Kim et al., 1994) or alternative lengthening of telomeres (ALT; Bryan et al., 1995; McEachern and Blackburn, 1996; Blasco et al., 1997a, 1997b; Bryan et al., 1997b; Colgin and Reddel, 1999). There are at least two (Sugimoto, 1998; Le et al., 1999b) and probably several (Bryan et al., 1997a; Reddel et al., 1997) independent ALT pathways (Huschtscha and Reddel, 1999; Reddel et al., 2001). Recombination (via proteins Rad52p and Rad50p) may be more common in yeasts (Lundblad, 2002), while sequence copying from donor to recipient is more common in humans (Varley et al., 2002). A "rolling circle mechanism" has also been described (Lindstrom et al., 2002; Natarajan and McEachern, 2002).

Prospective components have been identified, including Dna2 helicase-nuclease, a component of telomeric chromatin (Choe et al., 2002). One possible mechanism (Shammas and Shmookler Reis, 1999), consistent with detectable extrachromosomal telomeric DNA in telomerase-negative but not in telomerase-positive immortal or normal somatic human cells (Ogino et al., 1998), is gene conversion (Wang and Zakian, 1990b). Nuclear ring structures containing promyelocytic leukemia protein, telomeric DNA, and telomere binding proteins are associated with (Yeager et al., 1999) and may play a role in ALT (Aragona et al., 2000c; Grobelny et al., 2000). ALT is apparently repressed in normal cells, perhaps by binding proteins, including TRF1 and TRF2 (Lindahl et al., 1997; Perrem et al., 2001), that form part of the promyelocytic leukemia nuclear body, becoming unavailable to the telomerase complex. Chromosome 6 has been implicated in repression (Kumata et al., 2002). Length is less actively and stringently controlled in cells using ALT (Perrem et al., 1999; Varley et al., 2002), occasionally resulting in longer than normal telomeres (Henderson et al., 1996a). Complementation group data (Ishii et al., 1999) suggest that ALT may inhibit a dominant mechanism that (normally) rapidly deletes excess telomere bases. This mechanism may explain inactivated X-chromosome and X-chromosome aneuploidy, in which telomere shortening accelerates markedly (Surralles et al., 1999). Despite ALT (Scheel and Poremba, 2002), most human malignancies express telomerase (Holt et al., 1997b; Shay and Gazdar, 1997) and even more metastases do so (Multani et al., 1999b; Chang et al., 2003).

The second exception to equating telomerase and cancer is telomerase expression in normal somatic cells (Holt et al., 1997b; Hiyama et al., 2001). These include germ (or supporting) cells and stem cells. The latter include basilar skin cells (Harle-Bachor and Boukamp, 1996), hematopoetic cells (Hiyama et al., 1995d), GI crypt cells (Bach et al., 2000), hair follicle cells (Ramirez et al., 1997; Ogoshi et al., 1998), and perhaps others (Ramirez et al., 1997; Shay and Bacchetti, 1997). Noncancerous but diseased cells may also express telomerase—e.g., telomerase correlates with aggressiveness in immune-associated lung diseases (Hiyama et al., 1998f). The same occurs in hepatic cirrhosis (Rudolph et al., 2000), viral hepatitis (Tahara et al., 1995b), hyperplasia (Miura et al., 1997), normal hepatic regeneration (Leevy, 1998), and perhaps hepatic stem cells (Burger et al., 1997). Here (Takaishi et al., 2000) as in other tissues, quantitative telomerase expression might distinguish cancerous from merely abnormal cells.

As a promising cancer marker, telomerase is one among many (Gazdar et al., 1998; Mori et al., 1999), but has already proven useful (Breslow et al., 1997). There remain two practical caveats: (1) assays are in flux, and (2) results depend on the target of the assay.

Current assays are neither completely sensitive nor specific, though accuracy increases incrementally (Hirose et al., 1997, 1998; Schmidt et al., 2002). Real-time hTERT assays are now practical in human tissues (Buchler et al., 2001) and blood (Dasi et al., 2001), as is flow cytometry in mixed-cell samples (Ali et al., 2000). Cell-level hTERT activity measurement, first demonstrated in an in situ telomeric repeat amplification protocol (TRAP) assay (Wright et al., 1995; Ohyashiki et al., 1996, 1997c), is likely to achieve clinical use (Hirose, 1998; Dalla Torre et al., 2002).

Assay parameters vary: hTERT versus hTR (not well correlated with malignancy; Avilion et al., 1996), expression versus activity, or telomere length versus TRF. Despite concerns for reliability and validity (Dahse and Mey, 2001), telomerase activity is the most clinically intriguing parameter and measurement is improving (Gan et al., 2001b). To the extent that cell biologists use globally accepted oncologic cladistics (conventional tumor definitions and staging) and accurate laboratory assays, data will be comparable.

Dermal Cancer

The most feared dermal cancer is melanoma. Melanomas have been called a "modern black plague and genetic black box" (Chin et al., 1998). Although this might apply to every cancer, growing incidence and characteristic resistance make melanoma a cancer among cancers. Melanomas show a propensity for genetic abnormalities correlated with high metastatic potential. Among the chromosomal aberrations and gene mutations (Slominski et al., 2001), deletions are common, particularly near the D1Z2 locus in the subtelomeric region of 1p36 (Poetsch et al., 1999). The transition from normal to malignant melanocyte is characterized by the loss of cell senescence (Haddad et al., 1999; Bandyopadhyay et al., 2001; Bennett and Medrano, 2002) and correlates with telomerase activity (Yang and Becker, 2000). Spontaneous regression of Sinclair swine cutaneous melanoma is associated with absence of activity as well as loss of telomere length, abnormal telomeric configurations, and abnormal associations. Contrarily, in the nonregressing fetal variant, activity remains and telomeres are maintained (Pathak et al., 2000). Human melanomas parallel these findings (Miracco et al., 2002).

hTR levels are moderate to high in melanomas and basal cell carcinomas, but variable in the peripheral cells of squamous cell carcinomas (Avilion et al., 1996). hTR is not predictive of hTERT activity in most human skin tumors; while present in tumors with hTERT activity, it is also present in those lacking activity. hTERT levels are more reliable, as they do not correlate with age, sex, clinical history, proliferative state, or histologic subtype (Ogoshi et al., 1998). Proliferating melanocytes show evidence of neither activity nor hTERT mRNA (Bandyopadhyay et al., 2001), arguing against hTERT as characteristic of normal cell proliferation. Expression is not merely up-regulated in telomerase competent precursor cells, but reactivated during the transition to melanoma (Dhaene et al., 2000a).

Melanomas are generally hTERT positive and hTERT activity shows some correlation with malignant transition. Of eight malignant melanoma cell lines, all were hTERT positive (Glaessl et al., 1999). In comparison, hTERT activity was found in 9/10 (90%) of uveal melanomas but in no control samples (Rohrbach et al., 2000). Likewise, hTERT activity was found in 28/31 (90%) of primary melanomas, 12/13 (92%) of metastatic melanomas, and 4/5 (80%) of atypical nevi. Although weak, hTERT activity was found in 10/36 (28%) common melanocytic nevi and 4/34 (12%) normal human skin samples, but none of the normal fibroblasts (Glaessl et al., 1999). This suggests that activity correlates with transition from benign through atypical nevi, to malignant melanoma and metastasis. More importantly, hTERT activity (TRAP assay) and hTR correlate with clinical staging (Ramirez et al., 1999). Metastases, whether subcutaneous or lymphatic, have high activity; melanoma in situ has lower levels that increase with tumor penetration. hTR expression was all but exclusively found in tumor cells rather than in infiltrating lymphocytes.

hTERT activity is similar in many dermal cancers (Taylor et al., 1996), including basal cell carcinomas (73/77 or 95% of samples) and nonmetastatic cutaneous squamous cell carcinomas (15/18 or 83% of samples), as well as melanomas (6/7 or 86% of samples). Merkel's tumors, a rare tumor type found predominantly in elderly patients and probably deriving from basal keratinocytes, likewise express telomerase (Stoppler et al., 2001). Newborn epidermis, sun-damaged skin, psoriatic lesions, and skin from poison ivy dermatitis show increased activity (although less than tumors) compared to sun-protected normal adult skin.

Normal skin demonstrates limited telomerase activity (Yasumoto et al., 1996). Activity was found in 2/16 (12.5%) of normal samples, 1/16 (6%) of benign proliferative lesions (including viral and seborrhoeic warts), and 11/26 (42%) of premalignant actinic keratoses and Bowen's disease (Parris et al., 1999). The same study found activity in dermal malignancies, including 10/13 (77%) of basal carcinomas and 22/32 (69%) of melanomas, but only 3/12 (25%) of squamous carcinomas. Normal dermal telomerase expression is probably limited to the basal (stem cell) layer of the epidermis (Harle-Bachor and Boukamp, 1996; Dellambra et al., 2000), whereas other cell types, including differentiated epidermal cells, lack expression (Lee et al., 2000a).

One might suppose that telomeres shorten progressively until hTERT activity causes relengthening, implying little correlation between activity and length. No simple relationship is found (Parris et al., 1999). Predictably, given faster cell turnover, telomeres are (mean 2.5 kb) shorter in epidermal than dermal cells, whether from normal or tumor samples (Wainwright et al., 1995), but telomere lengths of tumor cells within the two skin layers are less predictable. Basal cell carcinomas had (mean 3.1 kb) longer telomeres than did matched epidermal cells in 13/20 (65%) of cases but shorter telomeres in the other 7/20 (35%). Curiously, facial wrinkling with age appears to correlate inversely with the risk of basal cell carcinoma (Brooke et al., 2001).

Kaposi's sarcoma is usually found in patients with acquired immune deficiency syndrome (AIDS), whose malignant nature has been disputed. In one study, 100% (22/22) of Kaposi's sarcoma samples were positive for telomerase and had relatively long telomeres, perhaps consistent with malignancy (Chen et al., 2001d). In other sarcomas, telomerase activity and level of expression both correlated with clinical aggressiveness (Tomoda et al., 2002).

Cutaneous lymphomas, dermal in location if not derivation, show telomerase activity in peripheral blood mononucleocytes (8/10 or 80%) and skin-homing T cells (16/18 or 89%), whereas normal samples have weak levels. These skin-homing T cells and peripheral blood mononucleocytes have high activity and short telomere lengths. Activity may correlate with transition from "early stages of cutaneous T-cell lymphoma such as parapsoriasis" (Wu et al., 1999b; Wu and Hansen, 2001).

Hematopoetic Cancer

Most hematopoetic cells circulate; phlebotomy permits easy access and diagnosis in hematopoetic cancer. Unfortunately, while malignant cells may express telomerase, normal leukocytes (whether in peripheral circulation, cord blood, or bone marrow) express baseline telomerase (Counter et al., 1995), at least in stem cells. Hematopoetic stem cells routinely respond to proliferative signals by expressing active telomerase (Hiyama et al., 1995d). This is true of each leukocytic subset, including granulocytes, T cells (Allsopp et al., 2002), and monocytes/B cells (Broccoli et al., 1995; Iwama et al., 1998). Activity may therefore offer less diagnostic leverage than in other malignancies.

Teleologically, baseline (or rapidly inducible) telomerase activity is required to meet the formidable demand for hematopoetic cell turnover. Telomerase may be required for sustained growth in solid tumors (Shay et al., 1996); it is a quotidian requirement in normal hematopoesis. Required or not, its presence raises the specter of of carcinogenesis. Indeed, activity increases measurably in most hematologic malignancies (Leber and Bacchetti, 1996; Ohyashiki et al., 2002). Curiously, however, the leukocytes in patients with chronic lymphocytic leukemia (CLL) show lower than normal activity early and fairly normal levels again late in their course (Counter et al., 1995). Telomere length may also play a role in CLL (Ishibe et al., 2002). In myelodysplastic syndrome (MDS), activity increases (compared to that in normal marrow) and this correlation is even more evident in patients with acute myeloid leukemia (AML), although the increase is not necessarily associated with telomere maintenance (Liu et al., 2001b; Ohyashiki et al., 2001), perhaps explaining an occasional lack of protection against leukemic instability (Serakinci et al., 2002).

Telomeres shorten progressively in almost all hematologic malignancies (Leber and Bacchetti, 1996; Ohyashiki et al., 2002). Telomere lengths are not maintained in early CLL (and to a lesser degree, MDS), but are maintained later in the disease (Counter et al., 1995). This is assumed to represent the critical point for telomere maintenance in leukemic cells, having already undergone extensive premalignant division (Engelhardt et al., 1997).

Telomerase activity has diagnostic, prognostic, and hence potential therapeutic value in leukemias (Shay et al., 1996). Activity was found in 16/16 (100%) of acute leukemias and distinguished normals from leukemics when bone marrow or circulating mononuclear cells were used (Engelhardt et al., 1997); higher activity is typical of leukemic cells (Ma et al., 2002a). Moreover, remission correlated with decreased activity, suggesting prognostic value in predicting success or failure, relapses, and general clinical response (Engelhardt et al., 1998). Compared with telomerase, telomeric-repeat binding factor proteins (TRF1 and TRF2) change reciprocally. As telomerase rises in acute leukemia, TRF1 and TRF2 fall; the reverse occurs if differentiation is induced. Normal cells maintain higher TRF levels than acute leukemic cells, human malignant hematopoietic cell lines (Yamada et al., 2000), or breast cancer cells (Kishi et al., 2001). Absence of such telomere-regulating proteins may become useful markers (Aragona et al., 2000c, 2001; Lazaris et al., 2002).

Chronic myeloid leukemia is a clonal expansion of stem cells (Jorgensen and Holyoake, 2001; Holyoake et al., 2002) with specific cytogenetic changes due to the Philadelphia (Ph) translocation (Kalidas et al., 2001). There is disagreement regarding telomere lengths and their diagnostic implications, if any. Recently (Brummendorf et al., 2000), chronic-phase telomere lengths predicted disease progression and were shorter during blast phase. An earlier study (Ohyashiki et al., 1997b) found no such correlation. The TRAP assay shows that CML patients have age-independent activity elevation (not simply expression) and high telomerase correlates with further cytogenetic changes. Activity increases even further during blast phase (Ohyashiki et al., 1997b). Half of blast-phase patients show at least 10 times the normal activity and the remaining patients show significant elevations. Chronic myeloid leukemia patients treated with interferon-alpha (IFN-α) had fewer blast crises and better prognosis, correlating with telomere length maintenance (TRFs) and absence of activity (Iwama et al., 1997). Telomere lengths reflect patient response to imatinib (Brummendorf et al., 2003).

Results are similar in acute leukemias. Increased activity may correlate with leukemic type or phase. Acute myeloid leukemias, as well as accelerated and blastic phases of CML, have 10- to 50-fold elevated telomerase activity. Chronic-phase CML, chronic lymphocytic leukemias, polycythemia veras, and MDS, as well as normal hematopoetic cells during the first week of ex vivo culture, have only two- to five-fold elevations (Engelhardt et al., 2000); myeloproliferative disease correlates with accelerated granulocyte telomere loss (Terasaki et al., 2002). Not all patients show an increase, although different assays may be responsible. Activity was elevated in the peripheral cells of 45/55 (82%) patients with AML and 16/23 (70%) patients with acute lymphoid leukemia (ALL). Activity did not correlate with telomere length but with leukocyte count, extramedullary involvement, disease type (French-American-British subtype), cytogenetic damage, prognosis, relapse, and remission (Ohyashiki et al., 1997a). In patients with AML, telomerase was not only present, but associated with poor chemotherapeutic response and prognosis. In vitro, human T-cell leukemia virus type II (HTLV-II) induces activity and up-regulates Bcl-2 (Re et al., 2000).

Plasma cell dyscrasias have been considered. Although telomerase activity is not elevated in monoclonal gammopathy of undetermined significance (MGUS), it appeared during the malignant transformation to multiple myeloma in which 21/27 (78%) patients had elevated activity. Activity was elevated in 4/4 (100%) of patients with plasma cell leukemia (Xu et al., 2001b).

Pulmonary Cancer

Lung cancer, the most common fatal malignancy of both sexes in the United States, carries a mean 5-year survival rate of, at best, 15%. Early diagnosis, increasing survival to almost 60%, might save more than 100,000 patients per year in the United States alone (Landis et al., 1999). There is no widely accepted early screening exam. Most strategies (Petty, 2000) are unlikely to yield clinical benefits in the near future (Frame, 2000). The computed tomography helical (CT) scan has considerable potential (Henschke et al., 1999; Medical Letter, 2001c; Mahadevia et al., 2003), but long-term studies are pending. Effective molecular screening would have immeasurable clinical and human value (Montuenga and Mulshine, 2000; Zochbauer-Muller and Minna, 2000). Not surprisingly, some (Hiyama et al., 1995d; 1998c; Hiyama and Hiyama, 2002) suggest telomerase activity as a diagnostic test.

Telomere lengths are, predictably, not predictive. Long telomere lengths may be associated with poor prognosis, but the relationship is nonlinear (Shirotani et al., 1994) and may be bimodal, with long or short lengths associated with shorter survival than intermediate lengths (Ohmura et al., 2000). Altered telomere lengths were seen in 16/60 (27%) of primary lung cancers: most (14/16) were shorter, 2/16 were longer. There was simultaneous loss of *p53* and Rb genes in 10/16 cases; the other 6 retained normal alleles of both genes (Hiyama et al., 1995f). This finding offers marginal support for the suggestion that p53 and Rb inactivation is responsible for the increased cell divisions and consequently shorter telomeres in some adenocarcinomas.

To a degree, hTERT activity correlates with hTR expression. There may be a spectrum of telomerase dysregulation as cells move down the path from normal to bronchogenic carcinoma, with "intense focal localized hTR expression" indicative of tissue invasion (Yashima et al., 1997a), but data supporting this suggestion are so far unimpressive.

The presence (and activity) of hTERT, however, is another matter. In a series of 92 lung cancers and 32 normal lung tissue samples, hTR was present in 92/92 (100%) of the lung cancers and 94% of normal tissues. In the same samples, however, hTERT was expressed in 82/92 (89%) of the lung cancers and 1/32 (3%) of the normal samples, making it a far better diagnostic marker for lung cancer. TEP1 was, predictably, more reliably present in normal samples (32/32; 100%) than in cancer tissues (86/92; 93%), but differences were neither significant nor diagnostically promising. Although this study found good concordance (77%) between hTERT expression and activity (Arinaga et al., 2000), activity remains the more valid and useful parameter.

Telomerase activity, and the difference between that found in lung cancer and normal lung tissue, varies widely in published studies. In one study, activity was seen in 109/136 (80%) of primary lung cancers but in 30/68 (44%) of adjacent, normal pulmonary tissues (Zhang et al., 2000). Paralleling these results, more recent work reported activity in 31/38 (82%) of lung cancer samples and in only 7/35 (20%) of adjacent non-neoplastic lung tissue samples, but activity was found in 3/7 (43%) of benign parenchymatous lesions (Wang et al., 2001e). Most disagreements are over the frequency of activity in normal lung tissue. While some of this may hinge on small sample sizes, much may be due to small but significant differences in sensitivities of different laboratories in measuring activity.

In contrast to the studies cited above, and for whatever reason, many studies have found a low incidence of activity in normal pulmonary tissue. For example, 16/23 (70%) of lung cancer patients, but only 1/13 (8%) of normal lung samples, had activity (Xinarianos et al., 2000). A separate study found 25/38 (66%) of lung cancer samples to be positive for activity; the only normal positive sample was from a single tubercular patient (Freitag et al., 2000). In perhaps the lowest percentage of activity in lung cancer samples published to date, activity was found in only 34/68 (50%) of samples from patients with non–small cell lung cancer (Komiya et al., 2000). In a study looking at p53, herpes papilloma virus, and telomerase, activity was found in only 19/22 (86%) lung cancer samples while it was present in 22% of normal lung samples (Niyaz et al., 2000). In most studies, normal tissue is rarely positive for activity and, when present, may be due to leukocytes (Dejmek et al., 2000), inflammation (Sen et al., 2001), and chronic infectious disease (Freitag et al., 2000).

At least two questions arise if we consider telomerase activity useful in diagnosing lung cancer: (1) is there a valid distinction between normal and cancerous cells, and (2) can we measure it reliably? Data suggest that there is such a distinction, but that it is neither absolute nor (at least between laboratories) reliable. Overall, most studies find a correlation between activity and lung cancer, with little or no background activity in normal tissue (Dejmek et al., 2000). To a degree, activity has become the default standard in assessing tumorigenicity (Lau et al., 2000). Activity may be a useful adjunct to histology (Xinarianos et al., 2000), but the wide variance in published data gives the lie to optimistic hopes that it deserves our clinical reliance in the near future as the pathognomonic test for lung cancer.

Although technique may explain some of the differences in published activity figures for lung cancer, many studies give no clear data on the grade or type of lung cancer involved. If telomerase activation is a late event or if it varies with tumor type, then data that merely consider activity only as a mean value may be not only unimpressive but superfluous. Activity may be more defining when cancer type and progression are factored into the data (Ohmura et al., 2000). A study looking at hTERT activity and type of lung cancer found activity in 107/115 (93%) lung carcinomas, but no activity in adjacent noncancerous, normal lung tissue. Moreover, hTERT activity was higher in small-cell carcinoma than in other histologic types and higher in poorly differentiated than in well-differentiated squamous cell carcinomas or in adenocarcinomas (Kumaki et al., 2001). This latter finding, that telomerase expression—and its variance—depends on tumor type, is supported in other studies. Within adenocarcinoma, expression correlates inversely with differentiation (Fujiwara et al., 2000).

Surgically resected, primary, small-cell lung cancers show telomerase activity in 11/11 (100%) of samples. In 125 patients with non–small cell lung cancers, however, activity ranged unpredictably from undetectable to high activity. Non–small cell lung cancers apparently comprise (predominantly) mortal cancer cells and a smaller percentage of immortal cells with high activity (Hiyama et al., 1995e). Animal studies support the suggestion that telomerase correlates with tumor aggressiveness (Volm et al., 2000). Unless future advances in measurement techniques prove otherwise, activity might become diagnostic if used within specific types and stages of lung tumors, but it is unlikely to become diagnostic for lung cancers generically.

Lung cancer is suspected from history or chest radiograph and confirmed by biopsy (via needle, surgical, or bronchoscopic specimen) or sputum. In this context, telomerase probably adds little to the diagnostic value of the current histological approach. Besides direct needle or surgical biopsy, other diagnostic approaches have been considered. Pleural fluids (effusions), for example, were positive in 3/3 (100%) of patients with adenocarcinoma (Hiyama et al., 1995e), although unselected effusion samples (Braunschweig et al., 2001b) have a much less impressive sensitivity—19/27 (70%)—and may be a poor diagnostic approach (Braunschweig et al., 2001a), although more recent results have supported its efficacy, particularly when coupled with conventional cytology (Hess and Highsmith, 2002). Bronchial washings have been considered (de Kok et al., 2000). In one study, bronchial washings detected 18/22 (82%) of known lung cancers using the combined results of two TRAP assays. Standard cytologic examination (using Papanicolaou staining) detected cancer in only 9/22 (41%) of the same patients ($p = 0.0061$). The TRAP assay was not affected by (central versus peripheral lung) tumor location (Yahata et al., 1998). Sputum samples have been looked at and showed good diagnostic sensitivity (82%), specificity (100%), and diagnostic accuracy (87%), with the bronchial washings in this same study showing fairly good sensitivity (68%), specificity (100%), and diagnostic accuracy (77%). This study found good correlations ($p < 0.01$) between staging and sputum, bronchial washings, and biopsy samples (Sen et al., 2001). A preliminary but more intriguing and potentially useful approach employed simple blood specimens to detect circulating carcinoma cells. In this technique, circulating epithelial cells were segregated from other blood cells by means of immunomagnetic separation, followed by telomerase assay. Activity was absent in 30/30 (100%) of normal donors, but present in 11/15 (73%) patients with stage IIIB or IV non–small cell lung cancer (Gauthier et al., 2001). These findings suggest the utility of activity as an adjunctive but not pathognomonic marker for malignant lung disease, using any number of standard and potential diagnostic approaches.

Breast Cancer

Breast cancer is a major cancer medically, humanly, and politically. Globally, breast cancer kills half a million people annually (Johnston and Stebbing, 2000). Most of those diagnosed will die. Prognosis is related to age, extent, and estrogen receptor expression. The mammary gland is distinct in its pattern of growth during the reproductive lifetime and this distinct pattern may have implications for mammary gland cancer (Wiseman and Werb, 2002). Although enlargement during lactation is normal among mammals, the relative size of the post-pubertal human breast, independent of lactation, is anomalous. Its unmatched size per body mass variance compared to other adult organs suggests that evolutionary stability has not occurred. These factors may explain a portion of its predilection for cancer. Malignant progression is typical, beginning with ductal hyperplasia and progressing from in situ, through local invasion, to metastasis (Russo and Russo, 2001).

Clinical diagnosis is supplemented by imaging techniques (e.g., mammography), pathology (e.g., needle or surgical biopsy), and genetic characterization (e.g., estrogen receptor status and HER2/neu overexpression). New markers are being tested (e.g., Zhou et al., 2001), but none have proven diagnostically satisfactory. With an untreated median survival of 12 months (Cold et al., 1993), diagnosis or treatment advances promise substantial impact on morbidity and mortality. Telomerase and telomere maintenance are central to indefinite cell division and unregulated growth of human mammary epithelial cells (Elenbaas et al., 2001; Nonet et al., 2001; Yang et al., 2001a; Kim et al., 2002a). The role of telomerase in breast cancer (Mokbel, 2000) has therefore become a target for clinical as well as basic research (Lebkowski, 1997).

Telomere length appears unrelated to disease state or tumor type overall. No significant length difference is found between papillotubular, solid tubular, and scirrhous breast tumors (Takubo et al., 1998), nor between telomeric DNA and size, grade, or stage. Similar results are found in canine mammary tumors (Yazawa et al., 2001). Nonetheless, human breast tumors containing the lowest amounts of telomeric DNA are far more likely aneuploid ($p < 0.002$) and metastatic ($p < 0.05$) than those with higher amounts of telomeric DNA (Griffith et al., 1999b). The latter two associations, themselves correlated to prognosis in invasive breast carcinoma, may imply that measurement of telomeric DNA content may have prognostic value. Telomere lengths may also decrease with age, although not significantly (Takubo et al., 1998).

Independent of activity, hTERT expression correlates with the clinical behavior of breast cancers. hTERT gene amplification occurs in roughly a quarter of breast cancer specimens (Zhang et al., 2000), perhaps explaining increased expression. Most breast tumors, in one study in 101/134 (75%), are hTERT positive and this correlates negatively and significantly ($p = 0.017$) with relapse-free survival (Bieche et al., 2000). Beyond mere presence, hTERT levels correlate with receptor status, including estrogen ($p = 0.002$) or progesterone ($p = 0.048$) receptor negativity, aggressiveness, and Myc overexpression ($p = 0.007$). In estrogen receptor–positive breast cancer cells, estrogen (specifically, 17 β-estradiol) increases hTERT expression and activity. Although recommendations remain in dispute (Kyo et al., 1999c), long-term hormone replacement in postmenopausal women correlates with increased risks (Nelson, 2002; Nelson et al., 2002), particularly breast tumors (Chen et al., 2002a), although meta-analysis suggests a protective effect in colorectal cancer (Grodstein et al., 1999).

Expression also correlates with progression, appearing early in preinvasive stages of tumorigenesis and increasing in amount of telomerase expressed per cell and percentage of cells expressing telomerase per tumor (Kolquist et al., 1998). To a lesser degree, tissue staging correlates ($p < 0.05$) with hTR expression. Even cells from normal epithelium and nonproliferative fibrocystic tissue have a low incidence of hTR expression, though this is not true of stromal cells even from fibroadenomatous tissue. Expression of hTR is elevated in some metaplastic apocrine and atypical hyperplastic cells and even more prominently in cancer cells, whether from in situ or invasive samples, suggesting at least a weak predictive value as a marker for tumor development and invasion (Yashima et al., 1998d). Recent work employing PCR has yielded impressive results. In this case, hTR and hTERT were detected in peripheral blood samples from patients with breast cancer. In patients with breast cancer, 17/18 (94%) of the tumors and 5/18 (28%) of the corresponding serum samples were positive for hTR, while 17/18 (94%) of the tumors and 4/16 (25%) of the corresponding serum samples were positive for hTERT. Neither hTR nor hTERT was detectable in tissues or sera from 21 normal subjects (Chen et al., 2000d).

As in other tumors, activity was expected to be more reliable than length or expression. To a degree, this is borne out (Herbert et al., 2001b; Simickova et al., 2001; Saito et al., 2002). The TRAP assays find a good correlation with disease type (e.g., benign versus malignant) and histopathologic severity (in malignant disease). High activity is absent in benign breast disease: only 1/7 (14%) samples showed even low activity. Fibrocystic disease showed activity in 0/17 (0%) of samples (Hiyama et al., 1996a). In fibroadenomas, activity is more common, found in anywhere from 9/20 (45%) of the samples (Hiyama et al., 1996a) to 4/6 (67%) of the samples tested (Yashima et al., 1998d). In breast cancer cells, activity was easily found in 11/12 (92%) of samples from carcinoma in situ and in 16/17 (94%) of the samples from invasive breast cancers (Yashima et al., 1998d), while another study found activity in 25/38 (66%) breast cancers and none in 16 noncancerous samples (Saito et al., 2002). Staging correlates with activity. PCR assays found activity in 68% of stage I primary breast cancers, 73% of cancers smaller than 20 mm, and 81% of axillary lymph node–negative cancers. Telomerase detection was particularly high (95%) in advanced-stage breast cancer, but misses 19%–32% of less advanced breast tumors and was found in only 2/55 (4%) of adjacent noncancerous tissue (Hiyama et al., 1996a). Comparing cancerous to noncancerous breast tumors, quantitative PCR-ELISA (TeloTAGGG Telomerase PCR ELISA(PLUS)) has a sensitivity of 73% and a specificity of 93% under optimal conditions (Simickova et al., 2001). Fine-needle biopsy results may be sensitive, finding telomerase in 14/14 (100%) of samples in one study (Hiyama et al., 1996a), all of which were surgically confirmed as having malignancy. Other studies, while supporting the diagnostic value of activity, showed a sensitivity rate of only 78/83 (94%), even when combined with cytologic detection (Jin et al., 1999).

Telomerase activity in needle biopsies matches the findings from gross tissue biopsy in 95% of cases and is probably "sensitive and accurate" (Pearson et al., 1998). Using TRAP assay, fine-needle biopsy found that 17/19 (90%) of cancers were positive for activity, whereas gross tissue biopsy found activity in 15/18 (83%) of samples. Using the same approach, fine-needle biopsy found activity in 9/16 (56%) of samples, whereas gross tissue biopsy found activity in 8/15 (53%) of samples. Most surgically resected breast cancers are positive for activity, in one study in 130/140 (93%) (Hiyama et al., 1996a). The same group has continued to extend this work in breast (and other) cancer. They find the diagnostic accuracy of activity of a fine-needle aspirate slightly higher than that of cytology (86% vs. 70%). They suggest that activity can serve as a protection against false-negative or indeterminate cytology results (Hiyama et al., 2000a). Other studies have found similar results (Jin et al., 2000), supporting these conclusions.

As in other solid tumors, margin definition is important to surgical excision. Largely for ensuring survival, it is also important for the cosmetic and emotional implications. Histology alone has not been perfect in this regard, resulting in both recurrence and overexcision. Telomerase is sensitive, but not perfect. Serial sections from surgical margins showed that 31/34 (91.2%) of breast cancer samples had activity. Although telomerase was found as much as a centimeter beyond the histologically determined margins of excised tumor, these cells may not represent false positives, but malignant cells that escaped histologic criteria. Surgical use of telomerase assay may increase the accuracy of excision margins (and survival), while conserving breast tissue (Hara et al., 2001b).

Male Genital Cancer

Of the most common male genital malignancies, prostate and testicular cancers (Epperly and Moore, 2000), testicular cancer is more apparent on routine examination (Moore and Topping, 1999), thus lowering its mortality (Foster and Nichols, 1999; Lawton and Mead, 1999; Toklu et al., 1999). Prostate cancers are difficult to detect. The relative efficacy of current screening strategies is unknown (Ross et al., 2000).

Prostate cancer is the most common nondermatologic cancer and the second most common cause of male cancer death in the United States (Middleton et al., 1995). Risk factors, including age, androgens, and free radical damage, have been identified (Ripple et al., 1999), but their diagnostic or therapeutic worth is unclear (Zietman et al., 2001). Annual prostate-specific antigen (PSA) tests depend on relative rise, not absolute value; their worth is unproven. Although prostate cancer death rates have declined in the United States since 1992, this is most prominent in regions with the lowest rates of PSA testing (Wingo et al., 1998). Globally, there is no consistent relationship between up-to-date diagnostic tests for prostate cancer and mortality (Wilt and Brawer, 2000). Reliable markers (Rubin et al., 2002) are desired.

Initial data on telomere lengths suggest a correlation with mortality, recurrence, and malignant transformation. If confirmed, it might differentiate patients with indolent prostate malignancy, in whom watchful waiting is warranted, from those with rapidly progressive malignancy, who require an aggressive approach. Indeed, in 18 men with prostate cancer, mortality and recurrence were highly correlated ($p < 0.0001$) with reduced telomeric DNA content in prostate cells (Donaldson et al., 1999). In 25 men with prostate cancers, telomere lengths were shorter in tumors than in normal or adjacent BPH tissue and appeared to be a useful marker for prostate malignancy (Sommerfeld et al., 1996). This may be especially true in the earliest stages of prostate malignancy (Meeker et al., 2002b). While various measures of telomere length (e.g., telomeric signal intensity and telomere restriction fragment lengths) may yet distinguish cancer from normal, adjacent prostate cells (Ozen et al., 1998), the correlation needs replication in large samples and severe malignancy.

Telomerase (Uemura et al., 2000) is the central question. Expression correlates with oncogenesis, though not necessarily with stage, perhaps because activity requires, but is not equivalent to, expression. Prostate cancer's slow progression has been dissected into a number of genetic and cellular abnormalities, including genetic loss (8p, 10q, 16q, and 18q), gain (7q31 and 8q), or amplification (c-*Myc*), and changes in chromatin texture, cell cycle status, and proliferative indices, as well as telomerase activity (Ozen and

Pathak, 2000; Sakr and Partin, 2001). These changes probably interact with telomerase and each other. A putative interaction between steroids (e.g., 17β-estradiol and dihydrotestosterone) or antagonists (e.g., tamoxifen and bicalutamide) and telomerase activity has been examined (Aldous, 1998; Bouchal et al., 2002). Additionally, hsp90-related chaperones have shown a potential role in regulating nontranscriptional activity in prostate cancers (Akalin et al., 2001) and may regulate telomerase activity through regulation of assembly. Among prostate cancer patients, 19/33 (58%) overexpressed Myc and 22/33 (67%) expressed hTERT. Although Myc and hTERT expression were correlate ($p = 0.0024$), neither correlated significantly with tumor stage (Latil et al., 2000).

Studies using PCR assays find the same relationship between prostate cancer and activity as for its expression. Most noncancerous samples do not have activity, although (based on rat data) this might be expected to vary with specific location and cell type in the prostate (Banerjee et al., 1998a) and seminal vesicle (Banerjee et al., 1998b). In human prostates, TRAP assay found no activity in 46 patients with benign hypertrophy (Caldarera et al., 2000). Strong activity was, however, found in 21/25 (84%) of cancers (and in metastatic lymph nodes), weak activity was found in 3/25 (12%) samples from adjacent hypertrophic (benign hypertrophy) tissues, and no expression was found in the corresponding normal samples. This suggests that activity may be a useful marker "for distinguishing prostate cancer from normal and benign prostate tissues" (Sommerfeld et al., 1996); other studies disagree (Straub et al., 2002). TRAP assays of biopsy specimens have produced similar results, with 25/30 (83%) of cancer specimens being positive for activity, while only 1/9 (11%) of the normal samples was (Wang et al., 2000g). In a later study, the same group found that 32/35 (91%) cancer patients were positive for activity, but only 1/8 (13%) of normal tissues was (Wang et al., 2001f). Other laboratories have produced less impressive figures. In one study, activity was seen in only 14/24 (58%) of cancer samples and in 0/12 (0%) of the normal samples (Meid et al., 2001). If telomerase activity is linked to androgen stimulation, at least in androgen-sensitive tumors (Soda et al., 2000), this might help explain why some tumors lack activity.

Poorly differentiated and metastatic tumors (Wymenga et al., 2000) and those with greater mass have higher telomerase activity (Wang et al., 2001f). Among poorly differentiated tumors 8/9 (89%) expressed activity, while only 6/15 (40%) of the moderately or well differentiated cancers did so (Meid et al., 2001). These figures (89% vs. 40%) show that sensitivity is highest in those tumors with the greatest clinical hazard. Activity can be detected in voided urine or washings after prostatic massage (Meid et al., 2001), although some reviewers doubt sufficient sensitivity for reliable diagnosis (Konety and Getzenberg, 2001). Ejaculate from patients with prostate cancer is usually negative for telomerase and cannot be regarded as a good source for diagnostic specimens (Suh et al., 2000). When obtained from prostatic fluid, however, activity does correlate with PSA and might offer additional accuracy to this standard clinical test (Wang et al., 2000g), which has come under some criticism as a prognostic indicator (Stamey et al., 2002; Vastag, 2002). Overall, and with some caveats (Zhang and Klotz, 2000) regarding specimens, telomerase may offer additional diagnostic value.

Testicular cancer stands apart. Although the diagnosis is usually made earlier than is the case for ovarian cancer (the corresponding female gonadal malignancy), testicular cancer is more aggressive than prostate cancer. Testicular cancer may not show a reliable correlation between telomerase activity and prognosis or chemosensitivity to agents such as cisplatin (Cressey et al., 2002).

Finally, though far less common than prostate cancer, penile cancer has been found to have activity in 3/3 (100%) patients with verrucous carcinoma, 41/48 (85%) of invasive carcinomas, 9/11 (82%) of adjacent noncancerous skin, and 8/10 (80%) of adjacent noncancerous corpus cavernosum tissue. Although there is a high frequency of telomerase expression in adjacent tissue from those with penile cancers, all of the skin and corpus cavernosum samples from patients with prostatic carcinoma were negative for activity (Alves et al., 2001).

Female Genital Cancer

Female genital cancers encompass a variety of tumors, including cancers of the cervix, uterine endometrium, and ovary. Cervical cancer is the most common fatal malignancy of women in developing countries and ranks fifth in the United States (Shroyer, 1998). Mortality is directly attributable to the difficulty in diagnosing an aggressive malignancy, effectively hidden from discovery during routine examination. Although cytology-based (using the standard Papanicolaou smear) screening programs have proven to be of value for diagnosing cervical cancer, even here, technical requirements and costs limit their use (Goldie et al., 2001; Wright et al., 2002). To have any impact on mortality, a more sensitive test for these malignancies is required (Keating et al., 2001).

Telomere lengths (TRFs) show increasing variance with malignant progression, but offer little diagnostic or prognostic value in cervical cancer. There is no significant correlation between telomere length and clinical staging, histologic type, history of human papilloma virus infection, tumor recurrence, tumor size, or invasiveness (Zhang et al., 1999a).

Although numbers and percentages vary by technique and tissue source, hTERT expression is seen in about 90% of cervical biopsies from known malignancies (Yashima et al., 1998a), with some studies suggesting far higher percentages. Normal cervical cells, by contrast, express telomerase between 0% (Gorham et al., 1997; Zheng et al., 1997a; Takakura et al., 1998; Wisman et al., 2001) and 25% (Yashima et al 1998a). Combining the results from seven cervical cancer studies (Kyo et al., 1996; Anderson et al., 1997; Gorham et al., 1997; Pao et al., 1997; Zheng et al., 1997a; Takakura et al., 1998) representing 104 malignant biopsy samples and 40 normal biopsy samples, telomerase was expressed in 94/104 (88%) of the malignant cervical biopsy samples and 5/40 (13%) of the normal cervical biopsy samples. In a similar summary of studies (Shroyer, 1998), expression was found in 21/21 (100%) of cervical carcinoma samples and only 8/38 (21%) of normal cervical mucosal cells.

The results of cervical smears parallel those of biopsies. Known cervical carcinomas demonstrate telomerase expression in 50% (Gorham et al., 1997) to 100% (Zheng et al., 1997b) of smear samples. This range is slightly broader, but with the same mean as biopsy specimens. Summing the results from five studies (Gorham et al., 1997; Kyo et al., 1997b; Zheng et al., 1997b; Iwasaka et al., 1998; Yashima et al., 1998a), expression was found in 65/69 (94%) of cervical smears from patients with known carcinoma, but in only 24/265 (9%) of normal tissues.

Intermediate grades of cervical cancer have intermediate results. In three early studies of cervical intraepithelial neoplasia tissue biopsies (Pao et al., 1997; Zheng et al., 1997a; Yashima et al., 1998a), telomerase expression was found in 4/12 (33%) of the low-grade intraepithelial neoplasia samples and 12/25 (48%) of the high-grade samples.

In summing data from five studies looking at intraepithelial cervical smears (Gorham et al., 1997; Kyo et al., 1997b; Zheng et al., 1997b; Iwasaka et al., 1998; Yashima et al., 1998a), expression was found in 21/87 (24%) of low-grade intraepithelial neoplasia samples and 46/87 (53%) of high-grade samples. The correlation with cervical dysplasia is similarly suggestive, but not impressive statistically (Reesink-Peters et al., 2003). In one study, expression was seen in 13/22 (59%) samples of mild dysplasia, 10/10 (100%) samples of moderate dysplasia, and 12/13 (92%) samples of severe dysplasia (Shroyer et al., 1998). Broken down by cervical intraepithelial neoplasia grade (CIN I–III), results are better. Telomerase was found in 3/16 (19%) of normal cells, 8/25 (32%) of CIN I samples, 3/6 (50%) of CIN II samples, 18/30 (60%) of CIN III samples, and 21/23 (91%) of invasive cervical cancers (Nagai et al., 1999). Overall, most authors find that telomerase presence correlates with tumor grade (Nair et al., 2000a) and invasiveness (Kyo et al., 1996).

Findings are technique-dependent. For example, the spectrum from normal tissue, through cervical intraepithelial neoplasia (CIN I–III), to cervical cancer is correlated with the homogenous presence of hTERT mRNA ($p < 0.01$) and with hTR as measured by in situ hybridization ($p < 0.001$), but not with hTR as measured by PCR (Wisman et al., 2000), presumably because hTR is expressed more or less constitutively even in normal cervical tissue and a more sensitive assay reflects this presence (Wisman et al., 2001). Overall, up-regulation of hTERT (if not hTR) mRNA expression occurs early in cervical oncogenesis, apparently (and predictably) prior to detectable telomerase activity, which is in turn triggered by other unknown factors (Nakano et al., 1998).

Activity follows a pattern similar to expression (McDougall and Klingelhutz, 1998). The results from five studies of activity in cervical cancer (Kyo et al., 1997b; Zheng et al., 1997a, 1997b; Yashima et al., 1998a; Wisman et al., 2001) were that 120/144 (83%) cervical cancers demonstrated activity, whereas only 24/220 (11%) normal tissue samples did. Cervical smears are less sensitive, having shown activity in 4/13 (31%) of cervical cancers and 1/9 (11%) of smears from normal cervices (Wisman et al., 1998). Intraepithelial samples typically demonstrate activity in about 10/25 (40%) of cases (Zheng et al., 1997b), although when distinguishing between the low- and high-grade cervical intraepithelial neoplasias (Kyo et al., 1997b; Yashima et al., 1998a), activity was found in only 12/29 (41%) of low-grade samples but in 27/45 (60%) of the high-grade samples. Other data are less sensitive, with activity in only 3/26 (12%) of cases with CIN I, 8/35 (22%) of cases with CIN II, and 18/62 (29%) of cases with CIN III (Wisman et al., 1998). Almost all studies concur that cervical intraepithelial neoplasia grade and cervical cancer grade correlate with activity, regardless of the assay sensitivity. While not all data support the generalization (Wisman et al., 2001), activity may correlate with staging, histologic type, and invasiveness (Zheng et al., 1997b; Kyo et al., 1998a) and is generally not found in benign proliferative lesions, such as leiomyoma, condyloma acuminata, or simple endometrial hyperplasia (Zheng et al., 1997a). Attempts to quantify activity suggest a significant rise overall, but not significantly or predictively within intermediate stages (Nagai et al., 1999). Overall, evidence suggests an increase in activity paralleling that of cervical cancer (Sakamoto et al., 2000; Wang et al., 2001b). There are reservations, however, about sensitivity and specificity in clinical use, where activity may lack reliable diagnostic or prognostic value in early stages (Wisman et al., 1998, 2001).

Herpes papilloma virus (HPV) infection, particularly types 16 and 18, is implicated in cervical oncogenesis (Southern and Herrington, 1998, 2000; Keating et al., 2001;

Schlecht et al., 2001) and can apparently activate telomerase cell phenotype–specifically (Klingelhutz et al., 1996; Pillai and Nair, 2000; Cerimele et al., 2001). This might be via deletion of an hTERT transcription repressor on chromosome 6 (Steenbergen, et al., 2001), although this is at variance with results in HeLa cells in which chromosome 6 may not repress hTERT (Backsch et al., 2001) and in which expression alone is not sufficient to prevent experimentally induced senescence (Goodwin and DiMaio, 2001). Papilloma virus infection prompts constitutive expression of E6 and E7 proteins, which may (however indirectly) induce hTERT expression. Experimental inhibition of E6 and E7 expression suppresses cell proliferation (while activating p53 and Rb and down-regulating Cdc25A), but effects on hTERT expression are unclear (Moon et al., 2001). Nonetheless, inactivation of the p53 tumor suppressor protein by the E6 protein is associated with altered expression of the apoptotic regulatory genes *bcl-2* and *bax* and with telomerase activation and proliferation (Pillai and Nair, 2000). Other data likewise suggest an antiapoptotic pathway through which telomerase is up-regulated in response to DNA damage (Sato et al., 2000b). In some studies, presence of papilloma virus correlates with activity (Kawai et al., 1998; Snijders et al., 1998; Wisman et al., 2000), while others (Yashima et al., 1998a) find no correlation. Expression has been discussed as a potential (but insufficiently specific) diagnostic marker for papilloma infection (Keating et al., 2001). The presence of papilloma virus may be critical in this context (Nair et al., 2000a) but depends on a cofactor, although teasing out and proving such cofactors is frustrating (Rapp and Chen, 1998; Anttila et al., 2001; Zenilman, 2001). Many argue that the activation of telomerase remains an independent (and late) event in the transition from papilloma-infected to malignant cervical (Walboomers et al., 2000) or epithelial cell (Shen et al., 2001). True or not, experimentally induced expression of the E2 protein not only represses expression of E6 and E7 oncogenes and induces senescence but is accompanied by a predictable decrease in expression (Goodwin et al., 2000). How papilloma infection relates to c-Myc expression is unknown, but there is good correlation between the expression of c-Myc and hTERT in cervical cancer (Sagawa et al., 2001), probably independent of E6 function (Gewin and Galloway, 2001). Increased mutagenesis may play a role in telomerase dysregulation, as amplification of the hTERT gene is reported in roughly a third of cervical cancer biopsies (Zhang et al., 2000).

Herpes papilloma virus has been used as a screening marker for cervical cancer, but telomerase activity is more diagnostically accurate (Reddy et al., 2001). Evidence from human cell lines (Kang and Park, 2001) suggests that this may be because HPV merely permits the cell to bypass the senescence checkpoint (and enhance the mutation rate), whereas telomerase permits continued cell division and hence indefinite survival of malignant cells. In this study, biopsy material, Papanicolaou smears, herpes papilloma, and activity were looked at in 88 patients. Activity was detected in 97% of cervical tumors and 69% of premalignant cervical scrapings, but not in controls. Telomerase assays had a diagnostic accuracy of 95.8% in tissue samples, 79.1% in scrapings, and 91.2% overall. In contrast, herpes papilloma (subtypes 16 and 18) testing had a diagnostic accuracy of 89.5% in tissue samples, 70.5% in scrapings, and 82.1% overall. Activity might be a good screening test in early cervical cancer. Nonetheless, there are data suggesting that senescence induced by HPV repression is not necessarily associated with short telomeres or low activity (Goodwin and DiMaio, 2001).

Overall, the literature suggests that while quantitative measurement of telomerase activity may be useful diagnostically, mere expression of telomerase components is not.

The issue is not expression, but activation, perhaps by regulatory factors (Harada et al., 2001). Herpes papilloma virus might be such an activating factor in some cervical cells (Southern and Herrington, 2000; Nowak, 2000). Data suggest that telomerase activation occurs via phosphorylation (Yu et al., 2001) and nuclear translocation; hTERT levels may be uninformative (Liu et al., 2001a). This jibes with clinical data suggesting that mere hTERT presence may have no diagnostic value, while the onset of hTERT activity may be defining. This may explain data showing that hTERT expression may not immortalize some cells, which require expression of other genes (O'Hare et al., 2001) that might play roles in activation. In any case, telomerase activation and inactive components remain tantalizing and relevant to the understanding of oncogenesis. The bulk of the evidence suggests that using activation, especially adjunctively with routine pathological markers (Kyo et al., 1997b) including other genetic markers (Ma et al., 2000), will enhance diagnostic sensitivity, if not necessarily specificity.

Level of telomerase activity in endometrial (as opposed to cervical) tissues varies with menstrual phase (Kyo et al., 1997c, 1999a; Tanaka et al., 1998b). Telomerase RNA (hTR) and telomerase associated protein (TEP1) mRNA are constitutively expressed in normal and malignant endometrium. hTERT mRNA is found in most endometrial cancers, but in normal endometrium only during specific phases of the menstrual cycle. Activity was present in 12/13 (92%) of endometrial cancers (Kyo et al., 1996), but activity (and hTERT expression) occurred in normal endometrium only during the proliferative phase. In late proliferative phase, hTERT expression in normal tissue matches that of endometrial cancer. Activity localizes to epithelial glandular (rather than stromal) cells and is found in 20/21 (95%) of endometrial samples (Kyo et al., 1997c). hTERT is not elevated in the secretory phase and only 8/19 (42%) secretory samples demonstrated activity (Kyo et al., 1997c). No endometrial cyclicity occurs for TEP or hTR. Activity decreases in postmenopausal endometrium; in 8/19 (56%) samples activity was demonstrated and with antiestrogen drug therapy (Kyo et al., 1997c). Using postmenopausal endometrium as a control, results were similar for hTERT expression and activity in endometrial cancer. hTERT expression was found in 35/36 (97%) of endometrial cancer tissues, but only 1/9 (11%) of normal postmenopausal samples was positive and mean level of expression was fivefold higher in malignant tissues. hTERT activity was found in 34/36 (94.4%) of endometrial cancer samples, but only 3/9 (33%) of normal postmenopausal samples were positive and mean level of activity was as much as 150-fold higher (Oshita et al., 2000).

These results fit nicely with data showing that estrogen directly binds to the hTERT promoter region (Kyo et al., 1999c; Misiti et al., 2000), although cultured epithelial cells may not show estrogen effects on telomerase activity (Tanaka et al., 1998b). In some colon cancer cell lines, estrogen receptor-β agonists promote expression and can overcome the inhibition caused by tamoxifen (Nakayama et al., 2000). Progesterone may have a more complex effect, varying with duration of exposure and blocking estrogen effects on hTERT expression (Wang et al., 2000f). In summary, constitutive expression in endometrial cancer, coupled with phase-dependent expression in normal endometrium, limits the value of hTERT expression as a diagnostic marker in endometrial cancer. Nonetheless, growing data suggest the value of hTERT activity as a diagnostic and prognostic indicator of endometrial cancer. Activity is higher in primary tumors with lymph node metastases (Sakamoto et al., 2000) and a significant ($p < 0.0002$) independent indicator of tumor progression and recurrence (Bonatz et al., 2001).

Ovarian tumors are the most deadly gynecological tumors (Rosenthal and Jacobs, 1998; Sekine and Tanaka, 2000). Lethality derives jointly from inherent malignancy and concealed location. Prolonged growth often occurs without detection or suspicion. Although the 5-year survival rate of stage I disease is 90%, three-quarters of patients are past stage I at diagnosis (Thigpen, 1999). Comparable testicular tumors are readily examined and fatality rates reflect the inequity. In developed nations, more than 50% of ovarian (but less than 5% of testicular) cancer patients die. Despite advances (Petricoin et al., 2002), particularly in imaging, genetic markers (Menon and Jacobs, 2000; Yaziji and Gown, 2001), and other potential biomarkers (Kim et al., 2002e), ovarian cancer is badly in need of a diagnostic breakthrough (Lea and Miller, 2001). There is no effective screening test (Markman, 2000).

Ovarian cancer was the first clinical cancer in which telomeres were the focus (Counter et al., 1994b). Telomere lengths were short but maintained in metastatic cells and tumors, but not in matched, nonmalignant tissue expressing telomerase. Other studies have usually (Idei et al., 2002), though not uniformly (Wang et al., 2002), confirmed that ovarian cancer cells have shorter telomeres than those of normal ovarian cells. In addition, cancer cells express hTR and most (10/11 specimens) have higher (mean 3.2-fold) telomerase activity (Kiyozuka et al., 2000b).

Telomerase expression is a more sensitive indicator of ovarian cancer than peritoneal fluid cytology. Fully 37/42 (88%) of ovarian carcinomas expressed telomerase, but only 27/42 (64%) were diagnosable by cytologic markers (Duggan et al., 1998). Telomerase was detected in 2/43 normal control specimens, both cytologically negative for cancer. Five patients with known ovarian carcinoma were falsely negative cytologically and by expression. hTR and TEP mRNA are expressed in more than 80% of ovarian cancers (Kyo et al., 1999b), but these components are also found in low-potential malignancies, ovarian cysts, and normal ovarian tissue. hTERT, however, showed expression only (and activity almost only) in ovarian cancers. Expression, not activity, best distinguished normal fibroblasts from ovarian cancer cell lines; hTR and TEP blur this distinction. In ovarian cancers (as elsewhere) p53 appears to regulate expression and correlates with malignancy (Akeshima et al., 2001).

Telomerase activity has been investigated even in the earliest studies (Counter et al., 1994b). Approximately 90% were telomerase positive; refinements are in keeping with this and with other human cancers. Perhaps 43/49 (88%) gynecologic tumors in general and 18/21 (86%) ovarian cancers demonstrate activity (Kyo et al., 1996), as well as 2/2 (100%) tubal cancers and 1/1 (100%) vulvar cancers. Benign ovarian cysts and premalignant lesions are less likely to express telomerase (the latter weakly) and there is no clear relationship between expression and tumor characteristics except invasiveness. That ovarian tumors demonstrate activity has been substantiated by other studies that find activity in 80% to 90% of ovarian malignancies (Zheng et al., 1997a; Kyo et al., 1999b). Histologic subtype may be relevant: clear cell adenocarcinomas show lower activity than other subtypes, especially endometrioid adenocarcinoma (Sakamoto et al., 2000). There is no significant correlation between activity and age at diagnosis or menopause.

Telomerase activity in ovarian cancer is at least three times that of nonmalignant tissue and correlates with clinical staging (Kyo et al., 1998b). Using a normalized scale (maximum = 100), activity was measured in 36 ovarian cancers (mean activity = 51), 5 low-potential lesions (mean = 7), 10 ovarian cysts (mean = 10), and 12 normal ovaries (mean = 10). Without exception, only ovarian cancer tissues had activity above 30.

Later work (Kyo et al., 1999b) also found hTERT activity predominantly in ovarian cancers with rare activity in normal tissue, cysts, and low potential lesions.

Peritoneal washing cytology is reasonably sensitive and specific; telomerase activity may have equal accuracy. In 50 patients with cervical cancer and 47 with benign uterine leiomyomas, conventional cytology had 96% sensitivity and 100% specificity; telomerase had 100% sensitivity and 90% specificity. False negatives were 4.7% for cytology and 6.9% for telomerase (Tseng et al., 2001). Looking at the prognostic value of telomerase in 29 patients with sex-cord stromal ovarian tumors, there was a trend toward earlier death, shorter disease-free interval, and more surgeries with telomerase-positive tumors, but not significance (Dowdy et al., 2001).

Renal and Urinary Tract Cancer

The urinary tract and kidneys are as hidden as the ovaries, but have the advantage of regularly providing us with diagnostic samples. Bladder cancers are diagnosed by urinary cytology and molecular markers, followed by fiberoptic biopsy. Cytology remains the gold standard, with long history, easy availability, and familiarity (Brown, 2000), but other urinary markers (Alvarez Kindelan et al., 2000; Konety and Getzenberg, 2001; Smith et al., 2001) may help in diagnosis of urothelial neoplasia. New approaches have uncertain reliability and validity (Ozen and Hall, 2000; Ross and Cohen, 2000). Telomerase compared favorably in two recent reviews of available tests for bladder cancer. One (Ross and Cohen, 2001) gave a 77% sensitivity and 85% specificity; the second (Lokeshwar and Soloway, 2001) a range from 70% to 86% for sensitivity and 60% to 90% for specificity. Looking at tumors throughout the upper urothelial system, some investigators (Wu et al., 2000a) have claimed sensitivities as high as 100% and lower sensitivities for other studies, including urine cytology (15%) and washing fluid cytology (53%); most differences are probably attributable to tumor type and technique. Poor standardization may limit utility, but clinical enthusiasm remains (Liu and Loughlin, 2000).

Bladder tumors (but not adjacent normal tissues) demonstrate high telomerase activity (Kyo et al., 1997a; Gelmini et al., 2000; Lancelin et al., 2000), but correlations between hTERT expression and staging, pathologic grade, recurrence, or multiplicity of tumors are disputable. hTERT was expressed in 2/12 (17%) normal samples and 33/37 (90%) urothelial cancers; activity also occurred in 2/12 (17%) normal samples, but in all 37/37 (100%) urothelial cancers (Ito et al., 1998a). hTR and TEPs were expressed in all samples. If urine rather than biopsy is used for screening (as practical screening must), telomerase must be present and stable in urine. Several studies have found that urine and bladder washings offer diagnostic information. In situ hybridization can use hTR to distinguish bladder cancer from normal specimens with exfoliated cells. Of the malignant specimens, 11/12 (93%) had high hTR; 5/6 (83%) of the normal specimens had low hTR (Maitra et al., 2001). hTERT activity correlates with urine ($r = 0.650$, $p < 0.001$) and bladder washings ($r = 0.410$, $p < 0.05$). Although this suggests that urine was useful or even "preferred as a diagnostic marker" (Gelmini et al., 2000), direct samples should better this moderate correlation. Nonetheless, other studies find TRAP assay of urine superior to cytology. Urine (73.6%) and specificity (92.7%) were better than those (53.2% and 81.8%, respectively) of cytology (Arias et al., 2000).

Other data disagree. In 50 patients, urinary telomerase activity had a sensitivity of only 57% and poor predictive sensitivity for recurrence (Wu et al., 2000b). Low sensitivity has been echoed in other studies that find it "insufficiently sensitive and reliable" for diagnosis (Arai et al., 2000). Although urinary hTERT activity can be accurately quantified (de Kok et al., 2000), urinary hTR is more labile (Muller et al., 1998).

Lability and technique may explain studies (Bialkowska-Hobrzanska et al., 2000) suggesting that hTERT expression is more sensitive (and less specific?) than activity in diagnosing bladder cancer. The normal versus malignant cutoff chosen in semiquantitative studies of activity determines sensitivity and specificity. In one study (Cheng et al., 2000a), a low cutoff value resulted in a diagnostic accuracy of 88%, sensitivity of 82%, and specificity of 91%. Cutoffs should optimize accuracy while factoring in the risk of false negatives and positives, as well as the impact of parallel tests (cytology, biochemical markers, etc).

At least in urine samples, TRAP assays for telomerase activity may be less sensitive, detecting only 2/30 (7%) cancers, than PCR-based assays, which detected 25/30 (83%) cancers. This parallels other studies, in which hTERT mRNA (by PCR assay) was found in 26/33 (79%) of patients with known bladder cancer but only 1/26 (4%) of patients without cancer (Ito et al., 1998b). Some patients with known bladder cancer and negative urine cytology were positive for hTERT, which suggests at least an adjunctive diagnostic role for this assay. In many developing countries, *Schistosoma haematobium* (bilharziasis) infections are a significant cause of bladder cancer. Expression correlates with tumor stage and is increased in bladder cancer cells, although apparently not to as great a degree as in non-bilharziasis bladder cancers (Abdel-Salam et al., 2001). Whether this is due to different pathology, sampling size, or technique is unknown.

Renal cell carcinomas, less common than prostate or bladder cancers, have a higher mortality rate—above 35% (Van Poppel et al., 2000). Renal cell carcinomas commonly have a deletion on chromosome 3; reintroduction restores cell senescence in these immortal, cell lines (Ohmura et al., 1995). Chromosome 3p contains one or more genes inhibiting telomerase expression in these and other cells (Newbold, 1997). Renal cell carcinomas typically display a number of anomalies, including trisomy of chromosomes 7 and 17, sex chromosome loss, and deletion of von Hippel–Lindau suppressor gene (Van Poppel et al., 2000). The latter is responsible for hemangioblastomas, which are low-grade, capillary-rich tumors, typically in the central nervous system (CNS), but that contribute to preclinical renal lesions. They differ from renal cell carcinoma in hTR expression: 5/5 (100%) renal cell carcinomas expressed hTR, but 0/10 (0%) of the hemangioblastomas did (Brown et al., 1997a). This is peculiar in that hTR and TEPs are constitutively expressed in tumor and normal tissues. hTERT was expressed in 29/36 (80%) renal cell carcinomas but not in normal tissues (Kanaya et al., 1998).

Compared to expression, hTERT activity is both more important in permitting and more useful in diagnosing malignancy. hTR is constitutively present in both cancerous and normal renal tissue, although at higher mean levels in normal tissue. hTERT is not much better: 18/20 (90%) of cancer samples expressed hTERT, as did 15/20 (75%) of normal samples, and neither predicted activity. hTERT and hTR expression notwithstanding, all normal and some cancerous renal tissues lack hTERT activity. This implies that activity is regulated not by expression or threshold availability but by post-transcriptional modification, inhibitor inactivation, or other activating factors (Rohde et al., 2000; Harada et al., 2001).

Activity may also correlate with staging, but studies disagree. In 23 renal cell carcinomas (and four normal kidneys), activity (but not expression) correlated with stage and degree of nuclear grade of the tumor (Hara et al., 2001a). In a larger study, activity was found in 40/56 (71%) renal cell carcinomas, but in 0/56 (0%) normal kidneys. Telomere restriction fragments were shorter in most (but not all) of the 16 renal carcinomas that were telomerase negative. There was, however, no significant correlation between activity and histological grade, tumor staging, DNA ploidy, or clinical outcome (Mehle et al., 1996).

Wilms tumors are congenital malignancies that are usually diagnosed in early childhood. In these tumors and normal embryonic renal tissue hTR expression was found, especially in immature epithelium, but not in mature tubules, glomeruli, or renal stroma, nor in differentiated tissue taken from the kidneys of post-therapy Wilms patients (Yashima et al., 1998c). Angiomyolipomas, a benign tumor of the kidney, apparently lack telomerase, but stable cell lines have been derived (by sequential introduction of SV40 large T antigen and hTERT) for research use (Arbiser et al., 2001).

Gastrointestinal Cancer

Diagnostic use of telomerase has proceeded faster for gastrointestinal cancer (Dlugosz and Ciechanowicz, 1998) than elsewhere, although the reasons for this are unclear. Undergoing unseen initial growth and invasion, these tumors have relatively low survival rates because of inherent delays in diagnosis.

Esophageal cancer, predominantly adenocarcinoma (Blot and McLaughlin, 1999), has a rising incidence in developed countries (Heath et al., 2000; Pera, 2000) and is difficult to diagnose early (Chen et al., 1999). Little is known of telomerase in esophageal adenocarcinoma, but it is one of several newer diagnostic approaches (Moreto, 2001). While some studies have concentrated on telomerase and telomere dynamics in esophageal cancer cell lines (Hu et al., 2000; Kiyozuka et al., 2000a), an increasing number of studies (de Kok et al., 2000; Koyanagi et al., 2000; Lord et al., 2000) are focusing on hTR, hTERT, and activity as diagnostic markers. Results are promising. One study found that "100% of esophageal adenocarcinomas and high-grade dysplasias were strongly positive" for hTR, and expression correlated with transition from low- to high-grade dysplasia (Morales et al., 1998b). hTERT expression has likewise been linked to malignant progression and proposed as a marker in esophageal cells (Shen et al., 2002). Activity, however, is more disappointing. Normal esophageal mucosa have high baseline activity. While 27/31 (87%) esophageal carcinomas had detectable activity, so did 21/92 (23%) normal esophageal mucosa. No correlation was found between activity and stage or outcome (Takubo et al., 1997). Recent work is more sanguine, finding activity in 37/45 (82.2%) esophageal tumors and only 2/40 (5%) normal epithelia (Li et al., 2002).

Gastric cancers, though in decline, remain a major cause of death. They are linked to genetic changes (Yokozaki et al., 2001), diet, and infectious agents, predominantly *Helicobacter pylori* (Graham, 2000), although there is evidence for viral (e.g., Epstein-Barr virus) etiology in some patients (Lo et al., 2001). Early detection has improved survival, but more than 80% of patients still have advanced cancer at diagnosis (Roukos, 2000); Only Japan has been able to improve this statistic through early diagnosis (Palli, 2000). Linked to at least one etiology of gastric cancer (Fang et al., 2001), telomerase is a target for early diagnosis (Kuniyasu et al., 2000; Yasui et al., 2000), but limited data are available. hTR (Hur et al., 2000) and hTERT (Suzuki et al., 2000; Tahara, 2000) are expressed in gastric cancer. Expression of TEP1, hTR, or hTERT probably offer far less diagnostic leverage than does activity (Kameshima et al., 2000, 2001). Studies largely agree on the high percentage of activity in gastric carcinomas: 18/21 (86%) in one study (Furugori et al., 2000), 35/39 (90%) in another (Kakeji et al., 2001), and 56/66 (85%) in a third (Hiyama et al., 1995c). Of tumors in the latter, 8/66 (12%) were early stage, hence more important in defining diagnostic value of telomerase. Unfortunately, 10/66 (15%) of gastric tumors were undetectable by activity, but gastric lavage cytology is even less sensitive. Even with gastric wall invasion, cytology was positive in 9/20 (45%) patients and activity in 10/20 (50%)—not a significant improvement (Mori et al., 2000).

Activity is frequently but not always present and expression may occur too late to improve survival as a diagnostic marker. Nonetheless, correlation between activity and metastasis (and aneuploidy) may help define staging and prognosis. There is a trend for patients with higher activity to have lower survival (Okusa et al., 1998). These studies suggest that evidence of activity offers additional prognostic information (Kakeji et al., 2001) and help in preoperative assessment or staging (Okusa et al., 2000).

Hepatic cancers are common globally (Ulmer, 2000), especially in the Far East. Hepatocellular carcinoma is linked to viral hepatitis of all types (Matsuzaki et al., 1999), although mechanisms go beyond simple infection (Zhao et al., 2000b). Rising incidence in the United States may be attributed to increasing viral hepatitis. That hepatic cancer is a leading cause of death in Japan (Kakizoe, 2000) may explain the plurality of literature on telomerase and hepatic cancer from Japanese laboratories.

The most common liver cancers are hepatocellular carcinoma, cholangiocellular carcinoma, and metastatic colorectal cancer. Current therapy (Ulmer, 2000) for hepatocellular carcinoma (surgical resection, limited resection, transplantation, transarterial catheter embolization, ethanol injection, and microwave coagulation) has limited success with high recurrence, costs, and risks. Therapy for cholangiocellular carcinoma is limited by frequent and extensive lymphatic involvement. Therapy for cancers with liver metastases is likewise suboptimal (Kamohara and Kanematsu, 2000). There is considerable impetus for earlier diagnosis and more effective therapies, plausibly gene therapies, in the near future. Understandably, early results suggesting that telomerase expression might improve staging and diagnostic reliability (Ide et al., 1996) or provide an effective therapeutic target have prompted considerable further work.

Overall, literature suggests that hTERT expression is not pathognomonic of liver cancer but a useful diagnostic adjunct (Erlitzki and Minuk, 1999). Hepatocellular carcinomas usually express telomerase (Ide et al., 1996; Golubovskaya et al., 1997; Miura et al., 1997; Nishimoto et al., 1998; Thorgeirsson and Grisham, 2002). Published expression figures, based on a variety of approaches, range from a low of 38% (Nouso et al., 1996) to a high of 100% (Nakashio et al., 1997; Sheu, 1997; Kishimoto et al., 1998). Regarding hTERT activity, combined data from these and other (Tahara et al., 1995b; Ohta et al., 1996; Kojima et al., 1997; Huang et al., 1998; Park et al., 1998; Nagao et al., 1999; Kanamaru et al., 1999; Hsieh et al., 2000) published studies show activity in approximately 84% of hepatocellular carcinomas. These data are, to a degree, not comparable: some count only "high" activity, others nodules only <3 cm.

Some authors use semiquantitative hTERT activity measurements in high-grade hepatic lesions (Kanamaru et al., 1999), which (though employing idiosyncratic scales) are intriguing. Tumors ≤ 2 cm have approximately half the activity of larger tumors.

Attempts at using Edmondson-Steiner staging criteria suggest an increase between stages I and II (out of four stages) but founder on enormous standard errors (Kojima et al., 1999). Quantitative measures of activity should allow better comparisons and improve diagnostic (Suda et al., 1998) and prognostic (Ohta et al., 1997) accuracy. Pending reliable quantitative measurement, much (Nouso et al., 1996; Urabe et al., 1996; Kanamaru et al., 1998) but not all of the hepatic cancer data (Tahara et al., 1995a; Ide et al., 1996; Ohta et al., 1996; Huang et al., 1998; Park et al., 1998) suggest that activity correlates with staging. Semiquantitative activity increases with tumor stage, from well differentiated to poorly differentiated (Nakashio et al., 1997, 1998; Kishimoto et al., 1998). The same association occurs between activity and histological grade, portal vascular invasion, and intrahepatic metastasis (Kanamaru et al., 1999), although perhaps not with size of hepatocellular nodules (Tahara et al., 1995b; Ide et al., 1996).

Fair sensitivity and poor quantitation are not the only diagnostic issues. Specificity is blurred by viral hepatitis and cirrhosis, both associated with hepatic cancer. Normal liver essentially lacks hTERT activity (Tahara et al., 1995b; Ide et al., 1996; Nouso et al., 1996; Nakashio et al., 1997, 1998; Park et al., 1998), except from infiltrating lymphocytes. Yet hTERT activity occurs in normal liver tissue just beyond tumor margins (Ide et al., 1996; Ohta et al., 1996; Kojima et al., 1997; Sheu, 1997; Huang et al., 1998; Kanamaru et al., 1998, 1999; Nagao et al., 1999), with an overall incidence approximating 18%. This is attributed to currently unappreciated tumor cells, gross portal invasion, or infiltration of the fibrous capsule. Telomerase activity occurs in various hepatic diseases (Nouso et al., 1996; Nakashio et al., 1997; Ogami et al., 1999). Hepatitis alone causes activity (Ogami et al., 1999) in 50% of cases (Tahara et al., 1995b). Cirrhosis likewise causes false-positive activity (Ogami et al., 1999) in one (Park et al., 1998) to three-quarters (Tahara et al., 1995b) of samples. Activity is occasionally attributed to adenomatous hyperplasia (Miura et al., 1997), although it is higher in carcinoma (Kojima et al., 1999). Finally, precancerous nodules have been found positive for hTERT activity (Kitamoto and Ide, 1999).

The diagnostic value of hTR or hTERT expression or telomere length (TRF) has also been examined. hTR increases during hepatocarcinogenesis (Ogami et al., 1999), but potential diagnostic value in vivo is uncertain. hTERT expression might be useful (Wada et al., 1998). In tissue studies it distinguishes tumor from normal tissue, but clinical data are needed (Hisatomi et al., 1999). There is no diagnostic value in telomere length: TRFs change, but not in a way that predicts presence of hepatocellular cancer. TRF lengths fall in some studies (Urabe et al., 1996; Miura et al., 1997; Nishimoto et al., 1998). Other studies find that some TRFs lengthen, others shorten (Kojima et al., 1997; Huang et al., 1998). As cancer progresses, TRFs become predictably and markedly more variable (Nakashio et al., 1998). Increasing variance may reflect a gradual progression from normal cells, through hepatitis or cirrhosis, to cancer (Urabe et al., 1996; Miura et al., 1997; Hytiroglou et al., 1998), similar to colorectal cancer progression (Narayan et al., 2001).

What practical diagnostic benefit do telomerase-related measures offer? The specter of catching only 85% of hepatocellular carcinomas (and missing one patient in eight) is alarming, but consider the context: current techniques are worse. Alpha fetal protein (sensitivity 21%) or angiography (sensitivity 13%), for example (Nakashio et al., 1997), are no better and are easily surpassed by quantitative telomerase assay (Higashi et al., 1998). hTERT activity is imperfect, but useful nonetheless.

Needle biopsy and peritoneal tap (for ascitic fluid) are alternatives to surgical biopsy. In measuring telomerase activity, needle biopsy may be comparable to surgical biopsy (Nouso et al., 1996; Miura et al., 1997), especially if contaminating leukocytes are removed (Kishimoto et al., 1998). In one small study, peritoneal ascitic fluid had 76% sensitivity and 95.7% specificity compared to cytology with 40% sensitivity and 100% specificity (Tangkijvanich et al., 1999). It correctly identified 13/16 (81%) peritoneal carcinomatosis, compared to 9/16 (56%) by cytology. It identified 6/9 (67%) hepatocellular carcinomas, compared to 1/9 (11%) by cytology. When the issue is malignant versus nonmalignant ascites, hTERT activity may more sensitive than cytology.

Prognosis is important to patients and oncotherapy planning. Telomerase activity correlates negatively with disease-free survival rate ($p < 0.01$; Kanamaru et al., 1999) and overall patient survival ($p < 0.039$; Kishimoto et al., 1998).

The other major primary hepatic cancer is cholangiocarcinoma. In cholangiocarcinomas induced by carcinogens in animals, telomerase activity parallels carcinogenesis (Iki et al., 1998). Human data are scant and consider only hTR and TEP; approximately 17/20 (85%) patients with cholangiocarcinoma were positive (Ozaki et al., 1999), with no correlation with histologic subtype. Telomerase associated protein and hTR, not found in normal livers, occur in biliary dysplasia, suggesting progression from normal to biliary dysplasia to cholangiocarcinoma.

Pancreatic cancer, the fifth leading cause of cancer death in the United States, is linked to tobacco, diabetes, obesity, and lack of physical activity, perhaps via hyperinsulinemia and insulin resistance (Michaud et al., 2001). Pancreatic cancer has a poor survival rate, largely due to delayed diagnosis and unresectability; less than 5% of patients survive more than 5 years (Gapstur and Gann, 2001). Molecular markers (such as hTERT) in the blood, urine, stool may improve survival by improving diagnosis but have not been well evaluated (Tascilar et al., 1999). Telomere length may be a valuable marker (van Heek et al., 2002). In pancreatic cancer cell lines, activity correlates with other markers for malignancy, such as K-*ras* (Omata and Tada, 2000), and to clinical behavior, including angiogenesis and metastasis (Sato et al., 2000a).

Using tissue, 6/8 (75%) pancreatic malignancies were diagnosed by hTERT expression; 5/8 (63%) were diagnosed by cytology (Morales et al., 1998a). Together, no malignancy was missed, but false positives occurred with each technique. Real-time pancreatic fluid assays provide "accurate quantitative measurement of hTERT expression" and may have diagnostic potential (de Kok et al., 2000); quantitative comparisons of hTERT and TEP1 (Yajima et al., 2000) might be better. In contrast to many other tissues, some workers (Buchler et al., 2001) suggest that hTERT expression is more sensitive than activity in pancreatic cancer tissues. Expression occurred in 10/20 (50%) normal tissues, 31/36 (86%) chronic pancreatitis tissues, and 26/29 (90%) pancreatic cancer tissues; activity occurred in 0/21 normal, 1/36 (3%) chronic pancreatitis, and 10/29 (35%) pancreatic cancer tissues. Expression may have greater sensitivity (90%) than hTERT activity (35%), but also less specificity (50%) than hTERT activity (100%). Nonetheless, quantification improved sensitivity of hTERT expression and may offer additional diagnostic value. Another approach has been to use activity in conjunction with another marker, such as K-*ras*. hTERT activity occurred in 11/12 (92%) and K-*ras* mutation in 9/12 (75%) of pancreatic cancers. Not found in normal samples, activity and K-*ras* mutation were found in chronic pancreatitis. Combining the two methods resulted in 100% specificity (Myung et al., 2000).

Telomerase activity in fine-needle aspirate biopsies appears useful in diagnosing pancreatic cancer (Pearson et al., 2000). Activity in pancreatic juice (endoscopic retrograde pancreatography) identified 9/12 (75%) ductal carcinomas, using a retrospectively chosen threshold (Suehara et al., 1997). Another study identified 13/15 (87%) pancreatic cancers by activity (Iwao et al., 1998). A larger study found activity in 41/43 (95%) pancreatic cancers, 0/11 benign pancreatic tumors, but also in 1/3 pancreatitis samples (Hiyama et al., 1997b). Activity occurred in 5/3 (14%) putatively normal pancreatic tissues, but from patients with pancreatic cancer, which may reflect occult microinvasion. Ex vivo brushing samples showed activity in 8/8 (100%) pancreatic cancers; but in 0/4 benign lesions (cystadenoma and pancreatitis). Activity might be useful in diagnosing pancreatic cancer, particularly preoperatively (Iwao et al., 1997; Inoue et al., 2001), but experience is early.

Rarer pancreatic endocrine tumors, including insulinomas (Lam et al., 2000), have activity in 3/10 (30%), but small sample size offers little to extrapolate from. Relatively indolent pancreatic endocrine tumors demonstrated activity in only 3/30 (10%) cases; more aggressive acinar cell carcinomas are more frequently positive (Tang et al., 2002).

Biliary tract cancers had activity in 4/10 (40%) bile samples assayed by fluorescence-based TRAP, but in 6/10 (60%) in situ tissue samples (Itoi et al., 1999). Cytology and in situ TRAP assay may be effective, but other diagnostic markers, for example p53, may be more accurate. Activity occurred in 13/16 (81%) malignant biopsies (percutaneous transhepatic cholangioscopy), but achieved 100% sensitivity combined with p53 overexpression. Specificity was 100% for either method in this small sample (Itoi et al., 2000).

Colon cancer is the second leading cause of cancer mortality in the United States (American Cancer Society, 1998). Heritable single gene mutations of *MSH2, MLH1, PMS2,* or *MSH6* (Lynch and De La Chapelle, 1999; Kolodner, 2000; Lamers et al., 2000) that result in hereditary non-polyposis colorectal carcinoma (HNPCC) allow us to screen for predilection, but occurrence (in this or other colon cancers) is another matter. Screening is limited not merely by sensitivity but by patient noncompliance for recurrent examinations (Frazier et al., 2000). There is a strong correlation between sensitivity — fecal blood testing, double-contrast barium enema, and colonoscopy — and patient anxiety for the particular examination. In addition, the most sensitive exam, colonoscopy, is most expensive.

Early work (preceding even ovarian cancer studies) found telomeres to be shorter in colon cancer cells than in normal cells from the same patient (Hastie et al., 1990). Subsequent work showed, as expected in tissues undergoing regular cell division, that telomeres shorten with age in normal and cancerous colon cells (Zhang et al., 2001a; Kim et al., 2002c). Nonetheless, cancer cell telomeres shorten faster, losing 50 bp per year, compared with normal losses of 44 bp per year (Nakamura et al., 2000). Lengths in familial adenomatous polyposis-associated desmoids do not correlate significantly with cytology (Middleton et al., 2000), not surprisingly, given the above discussion, and narrow stage desmoids may represent. In vitro drug-resistant colorectal cells have activity and longer telomeres (Kuranaga et al., 2001). In vivo, expression appears early, even preinvasively, and increases pari passu with tumor progression, in amount of hTERT per cell and percentage of expressing cells (Kolquist et al., 1998).

Early studies found telomerase activity in colorectal carcinoma, though not in adenomatous polyps (Chadeneau et al., 1995a), representing an early stage in loss of growth control and not in normal mucosa (Yoshimi et al., 1996). This finding suggested that expression began after adenomatous polyps but prior to frank carcinogenesis, consistent with telomerase being necessary for prolonged divisions but not for initial transformation. Not all studies concur: activity may occur in 33/50 (67%) colorectal biopsies and correlate with bcl-2 expression but not with staging (Iida et al., 2000). In other studies, depth of invasion correlates with telomerase index (logarithm of relative activity) but not with other clinical indices, including age, gender, histologic type, location, lymph node metastasis, lymphatic infiltration, or Dukes stage (Shoji et al., 2000). Studies employing competitive reverse transcription polymerase chain reaction (RT-PCR) suggest gradual progression of expression and activity during transformation from normal, to adenomatous, to malignant cell (Niiyama et al., 2001). Others would stage patients on the telomerase ratio between normal and colorectal cells (Gertler et al., 2002). One intriguing approach separates circulating colon carcinoma cells from blood, followed by telomerase assay. Activity was absent in 30/30 (100%) normal donors, but present in 8/11 (72%) stage C or D (Dukes classification) colon cancer (Gauthier et al., 2001). Stool studies have not been published, but might offer better sensitivity.

Telomerase activity has been found in all cell lines of gastric and colorectal cancers, as well as in 17/20 (85%) primary gastric carcinomas and 19/20 (95%) primary colorectal carcinomas, regardless of staging or type. Nodal and peritoneal metastases and recurrent gastric cancers were likewise positive. Of precancerous lesions, 10/10 (100%) colorectal tubular adenomas were telomerase positive, as were 3/13 (23%) gastric intestinal metaplasias and 1/ 2 (50%) gastric adenomas. Corresponding normal gastric and colorectal mucosa were negative (Tahara et al., 1995a). Moreover, and contrasting with the lack of activity found in early studies of adenomatous polyps, these and other results (Mizumoto et al., 2001) suggest that telomerase activation occurs early in gastric and colon carcinogenesis. Some workers suggest that activity may be so crucial to tumor progression that agents suppressing tumors, such as indomethicin in mice, may act by suppressing activity (Ogino et al., 1999a, 1999b). Whatever the mechanisms, activity correlates with clinical colorectal outcome, if not with staging (Tatsumoto et al., 2000), offering independent prognostic information.

Central Nervous System Cancer

Central nervous system tumors are suspected clinically and diagnosed radiologically, although other modalities play increasing diagnostic roles. Like other fluids that can be aspirated (Cunningham et al., 1998), cerebrospinal fluid (CSF) obtained via lumbar puncture offers diagnostic information. Telomerase expression, and hence malignancy, can be found on the basis of as few as 10 cells and despite high protein levels or the presence of leukocytes (Kleinschmidt-DeMasters et al., 1998a) that might themselves express telomerase. A variety of central nervous system tumors express telomerase, including medulloblastomas, lymphomas, oligodendrogliomas, and glioblastomas (Kleinschmidt-DeMasters et al., 1998b). Significant expression is likewise seen in metastatic tumors, albeit with wide variance and little apparent prognostic implication (Kleinschmidt-DeMasters, 1998c).

The central nervous system comprises numerous cell phenotypes but, to the surprise of many, glial cells predominate, followed distantly by neuronal cells. Of glial cell tumors, the most invasive, refractory, and deadly are malignant gliomas (Rich et al.,

2001). Gliomas escape growth constraints early, especially those imposed by epidermal and other growth factors, bestowing a selective growth advantage (Nagane et al., 2001). Not surprisingly in rapidly dividing cells, telomerase activity was (initially) demonstrated in 19/19 (100%) oligodendrogliomas and 38/51 (75%) glioblastoma multiformes, though in only 2/20 (10%) anaplastic astrocytomas (Langford et al., 1995). Other studies, however, find activity more common, with 9/19 (47.4%) found in the latter (Chen et al., 2001b). This is borne out by studies finding expression in 5/11 (45%) anaplastic astrocytomas (WHO grade III) and 3/9 (33%) low-grade astrocytomas (WHO grade II). Activity was present in 75% of oligodendrogliomas, but in fully 36/41 (89%) glioblastoma multiformes (WHO grade IV). Normal cell samples showed no (0/4) activity. Percentage of cells with activity correlates with malignancy stage (Le et al., 1998) and type (Kleinschmidt-DeMasters et al., 1998b). Recent work suggests that the degree of activity may predict the course of astrocytomas (Fukushima et al., 2002). Finally, TRF1 expression is heterogeneously expressed in meningiomas (12/14 samples at varying levels) but is absent (0/6 samples) in anaplastic astrocytomas (De Divitiis and La Torre, 2001).

Neuroblastomas, in young (median age 2 years) children, are of neural origin but typically grow in the abdomen or pelvis (Alexander, 2000). The outcome is surprisingly unpredictable (Shah and Ravindranath, 1998; Maitra et al., 1999): some regress spontaneously, some disseminate and are fatal. Gradual improvement in survival over past decades is partially attributable to distinguishing malignant from benign neuroblastomas (Berthold and Hero, 2000), fitting therapy to disease. Oncologists prefer treating malignant cases aggressively, avoiding invasive therapies (and inherent complications) in benign cases.

While malignancy correlates with classical markers, such as ploidy (Kaneko and Knudson, 2000), telomerase activity appears to effectively distinguish benign from malignant cells, particularly in work by Hiyama and colleagues. Initial work measured telomere lengths and, not surprisingly, found variability (1.1 kb to more than 23 kb). Nonetheless, shorter telomeres correlate with advanced malignancy, poor prognosis, and increased percentages of dividing cells. The most interesting diagnostic implication was presence of a subset of advanced tumors with short telomeres and low divisional capacity that regressed spontaneously (Hiyama et al., 1992). While there was no hTERT activity in normal adrenal tissues or benign ganglioneuromas, there was activity in 94/100 (94%) neuroblastomas. Moreover, those with high activity had more unfavorable outcomes than those with low activity, while three neuroblastomas lacking activity regressed (Hiyama et al., 1995a). They also found that of 105 untreated neuroblastomas, 23 (22%) had high activity, 78 (74%) had low activity, and only 4 (4%) had no activity. Genetic alterations (MYCN amplification or 1p32 loss of heterozygosity [LOH]) correlated with high activity. Low-activity tumors were generally aneuploid, with trk-A and Ha-ras expression. Consistent with previous results, three of four tumors without activity regressed spontaneously. Hiyama and colleagues proposed that the correlation between aggressiveness and expression (along with genetic alterations) could be useful to predict prognosis (Hiyama et al., 1997a). Similar results prompted speculation that telomerase, independent of genetic alterations, might be a "non-morphologic marker" for neuroblastoma (Joshi and Tsongalis, 1997), particularly in prognosis, allowing therapy to be tailored to the tumor.

Although work focuses on activity, there is a strong interest in genetic correlates of telomerase. The assumption is that the genetic switches controlling hTERT expression may be of as much interest as (and a prime determinant of) activity. One example is the correlative presence of hTERT splice variants (Krams et al., 2001). In cancer, the implications of genetic markers correlating with telomerase may strike both directions, implicating both the causes of expression and independent risk factors for malignant transformation. Whatever the implication, patients with routine neuroblastomas and amplification of *MYCN* gene (detected by differential PCR) and high hTERT activity have a poor prognosis (Hiyama et al., 1999). Amplification of the hTERT gene, by contrast, appears rare, occurring in roughly one in eight lung cancers (Zhang et al., 2000). Mere expression correlates with high activity and poor prognosis. Nonradioisotopic PCR-based protocols "are rapid and reliable and are likely to be useful" to clinicians in predicting neuroblastoma outcome (Hiyama et al., 1999). Multifocal neuroblastomas, however, have more "favorable biological features" and none (0/8) had c-*myc* gene amplification or high activity (Hiyama et al., 2000a).

Overall, hTERT activity is probably a useful predictor of outcome in most neuroblastic tumors, including neuroblastomas, ganglioneuroblastomas, and ganglioneuromas. High expression correlates with aggressive behavior; low expression correlates with tumors of "limited capacity for progression and a favorable prognosis" (Maitra et al., 1999). Clinicians may lower morbidity and mortality by reserving effective, though hazardous, interventions for patients in whom aggressive therapy is the lower risk.

An olla podrida of nervous system tumors has been examined for telomerase. In relatively benign tumors, such as well-differentiated oligodendrogliomas, 5/5 (100%) were telomerase negative. More malignant tumors have a higher likelihood of expression: 100% of glioblastoma multiformes, 2/3 (67%) anaplastic oligodendrogliomas, and 10/14 (71%) high-grade astrocytomas (although the latter were heterogeneous across multiple regions). Of anaplastic astrocytomas, 2/3 (67%) had at least one positive region. Within oligodendrogliomas, expression correlated with tumor grade. Overall, in adult glial tumors, expression correlated with grade, age, and vascular endothelial proliferation, each of which may have implications for using antitelomerase agents in these cancers (Kleinschmidt-DeMasters et al., 1998b).

Until now, accurate meningioma prognosis was perplexing "because no clear-cut correlation exists between aggressive clinical behavior and histological features or karyotypic abnormalities" (Langford et al., 1997). The TRAP assay detected telomerase activity in 26/52 (50%) meningiomas, but detection rose to 95% in cases classified as malignant, atypical, or with poor outcome. Of morphologically benign tumors, 3/5 (60%) telomerase-positive tumors regrew rapidly after initial resection. Moreover, there was a significant correlation ($p = 0.0002$) between activity and prognosis. In another study of meningiomas, activity occurred in 4/13 (31%) malignant meningiomas but in only 1/49 (2%) benign meningiomas ($p = 0.006$). Telomere lengths were similar: longer telomeres (TRFs) were seen in 6/13 (46%) malignant tumors but in only 1/48 (2%) benign tumors ($p = 0.0002$). Nevertheless, malignant meningiomas tend to have long telomeres while lacking activity (all those with long telomeres lacked activity) or significant activity with short telomeres (75% with activity had short telomeres). Malignant meningiomas apparently require either long telomeres or activity, yet rarely have both (Chen et al., 2000b, 2001b). Although chromosomal abnormalities (deletion of chromosome 22, 1p, 14q, or 10q, or ring and dicentric chromosomes) are classical meningiomas findings, these may be due to telomeric or centromeric instability, precipitating "progression of chromosome aberrations" (Sawyer et al., 2000).

While morphology suffices for prognosis of some (particularly the benign) ependymomas, others evade current criteria altogether. Initial work suggests that grade III ependymomas are more likely ($p = 0.0.0015$) to express hTR than lower-grade tumors (Rushing et al., 1997). In a single study, telomere length but not activity appears to predict the course of schwannomas (Chen et al., 2002b).

Other Cancer

Remaining organs are few, data modest. These studies include investigations of osseous, sarcomatous, adipose, and retinal tissue. There is almost no information on telomerase as a genetic marker in osteoblastic tumors and that little lacks stochastic significance (Radig et al., 1998).

Most human cancers are epithelial; published studies reflect this. Tumors with nonepithelial, connective tissue origins, such as sarcomas, are difficult to categorize and are given short shrift. Nevertheless, data suggest that telomerase may have diagnostic value: 30/37 (81%) primary sarcomas samples (and 0/12 controls) had positive activity (Aogi et al., 2000).

Of 36 malignant and 7 benign liposarcomas in 34 patients, 25/36 (69%) malignant tumors had telomerase activity. None of the seven (0%) benign tumors expressed telomerase and there was no correlation with age. Poorly differentiated liposarcomas expressed telomerase; myxoid and round cell liposarcomas had higher activity than classic low-grade analogs. Tumors expressing telomerase had higher proliferation and 8/8 (100%) recurrent tumors expressed telomerase (Schneider-Stock et al., 1998b, 1999). Activity and increased c-Myc expression may be "helpful molecular markers for characterizing tumor progression in myxoid liposarcoma" (Jaeger et al., 1999).

Retinoblastoma protein (Rb) is a well-known tumor marker. The eponymous tumor is a childhood eye cancer easily seen clinically with an ophthalmoscope, even when small. Cells expressing Rb protein often express telomerase, a correlation that may be less common in other cancer cell lines. Despite long telomeres, only 17/34 (50%) cell lines express telomerase, and telomeres were ($p = 0.0008$) longer in telomerase-negative tumors. This is presumably due to initially long telomeres (these are embryonic tumors), as well as presence of (marginally) sufficient telomerase activity to maintain but not lengthen the telomere (Gupta et al., 1996). If telomerase is a relatively late acquisition, it may have little clinical value.

Head and neck tumors have increased hTERT expression (Soder et al., 1997; Gisselsson et al., 2002) and probably activity as well (Koscielny et al., 2000a; Zhang et al., 2001c; Patel et al., 2002). Activity occurred in 10/11 (91%) head and neck tumors and may correlate with malignant transformation (Henderson et al., 2000b). Squamous cell carcinomas in this region are probably typical in progressing from genetic damage, to loss of cell cycle control, to expression and cellular immortality (Scully et al., 2000). In one series, 25/27 (92%) squamous cell carcinomas had high activity ($p = 0.009$) and progression correlated with increased activity (Soria et al., 2001). Other studies are more equivocal, finding activity in only two-thirds of squamous cell carcinomas of pharynx and larynx, but suggesting that recurrence correlates with expression (Koscielny et al., 2000b). An interesting animal model (Chang et al., 2000b) indicates that expression increases with progression. Most workers postulate that telomerase has adjunctive (rather than diagnostic or prognostic) value (Curran et al., 2000).

Investigation of oral tumors and metastases suggests that activity is a good diagnostic tool (Yao et al., 1999; Sumida et al., 2000; Shimamoto, 2001; Sumida and Hamakawa, 2001).

In nasopharyngeal tumors, expression and level of activity correlate well with carcinoma: 25/29 (86%) of nasopharyngeal carcinomas had activity. Telomerase, in a majority of nasopharyngeal cancers and a smaller percentage of metaplastic samples, may be a useful diagnostic adjunct (Chang et al., 2000a).

Thyroid neoplasia data are scant, but there is a fair correlation between expression and malignancy. Using fine-needle aspiration, hTERT was present in 2/7 (29%) hyperplastic nodules, 1/1 (100%) Hashimoto thyroiditis sample, 3/8 (38%) follicular adenomas, 3/8 (38%) Hurthle cell adenomas, ¾ (75%) follicular carcinomas, 2/2 (100%) Hurthle cell carcinomas, and 11/18 (61%) papillary carcinomas (Siddiqui et al., 2001). Noncancerous thyroid cells probably lack activity, except through lymphocytic infiltration. While many malignant thyroid cells, follicular and papillary, were telomerase positive, variance was high and some cancer cells lacked activity, even with sensitive assay. Moreover, telomere lengths were often long in telomerase-negative malignant thyroid cells, indicating that these cells may employ an alternative pathway to telomere maintenance (Matthews et al., 2001). Some investigators go further, suggesting that nontelomeric mechanisms, such as *RAS*-oncogene, play a central role in thyroid malignancy (Jones et al., 1998). Such results may undercut the reliability of telomerase in thyroid malignancy diagnosis but overall suggest a role in conjunction with other markers, if not independently (Suzuki et al., 2002).

Initial data on parathyroid tumors (Kammori et al., 2002a) suggest an excellent correlation between malignancy and telomerase activity and a fair correlation with telomere length as well.

Prognosis

Diagnosis is a tool, not a product. Its value lies in furthering prognosis and intervention; it is difficult to know course and treatment without identification. Prognosis in cancer derives from a substantial observational database. We greatly narrow prognostic variance using demographic, clinical, and histological data. Certain data, such as lymph node status and metastasis (Sumida et al., 2000), account for much of the variance. Does telomerase (whether expression or activity) account for substantial prognostic variance? The answer depends on how telomerase correlates with outcome in either of two senses. It might be an independent factor or a more easily measured stand-in marker for another predictive but difficult-to-assess factor. In the latter case it might, for example, allow us to infer metastatic status without surgical exploration or expensive scanning techniques (Sumida et al., 2000). Except experimentally, only a modicum of data justifies either prospect (Mokbel et al., 2000).

As an independent prognostic marker, there are some grounds for optimism (Urquidi et al., 1998). Telomerase expression (or level of expression) may not only enable us to distinguish between benign and malignant tumors (as in neuroblastomas), but it will help to assess finer gradations of malignancy. This might permit accurate assessment of risks and benefits of specific surgical approaches (e.g., total versus subtotal mastectomy), as well as specific radiation and chemotherapy protocols.

In lung cancer, survival inversely correlates with activity (Kumaki et al., 2001), but despite claims that it is independent (Komiya et al., 2000), the correlation might be attributable to comparing poorly differentiated lung cancers (with low survival rates and high activity) to well-differentiated lung cancers (with higher survival rates). Other studies confirm the correlation between activity and tumor type (Fujiwara et al., 2000) with similar prognostic implications. However, within sample of patients with a single type of lung cancer (e.g., stage I–III non–small cell), activity may not offer additional prognostic information (Hirashima et al., 2000). Despite this, activity may have prognostic significance in some malignant tissues, such as breast cancers (Simickova et al., 2001). Other markers may be more direct, but telomerase may be more easily assessed and practical.

In AML, data suggest that telomerase may serve as both a pre-therapy prognostic marker and post-therapy efficacy marker (Li et al., 2000c; Preisler et al., 2000), especially for differentiating chemotherapeutic agents (Zhang et al., 1996). Activity increases as preleukemic marrow cells increase in proliferative potential (Li et al., 2000b) and level of activity correlates with prognosis. In one study of 78 patients, the 5 with high telomerase levels had a poor prognosis ($p < 0.05$) and activity declined in those with complete remission, most to normal levels. Two patients who maintained low to moderate activity relapsed. Relapsed patients generally had increased telomerase. Of the relapsed patients, 2/13 (15%) retained high activity, and 11/13 (85%) had normal to moderate activity (Ohyashiki et al., 1997a).

This pattern may hold for other telomerase-positive human tumors. Survival rates for gastric tumors with telomerase activity are lower than those without activity (Hiyama et al., 1995c). Prostate tumor activity correlates with differentiation and metastasis and may distinguish the "relatively good from the ugly" prognosis (Wymenga et al., 2000). In prostate cancers grown on immunodeficient mice, down-regulation of activity (along with c-Myc and Bcl-2 expression) predicts 9-nitrocamptothecin (9NC)-induced regression (Chatterjee et al., 2000) and might reasonably be effective in humans. Telomerase may be a good prognostic indicator in neuroblastomas (Hiyama et al., 1997a). Telomere length is probably less reliable than expression or activity, but in a wide sample of cancers, short telomeres imply poor prognosis (Hiyama et al., 1998a).

Prognosis includes assessment of interventional efficacy (Terashima et al., 2000). In vitro, chemotherapeutic efficacy correlates with declining telomerase activity. After therapy, residual activity may reflect residual tumor cells. Tumor cells resistant to chemotherapeutic agents, such as temozolomide or doxorubicin, show no decline in activity (Faraoni et al., 1997). If this result is typical, activity may predict chemotherapeutic efficacy and disease status.

Besides being an independent marker, telomerase might serve as a dependent indicator of standard prognostic markers, including metastasis. In AML, activity not only correlates with known prognostic markers (French-American-British subtypes, cytogenetics, leukocytosis) but also with extramedullary involvement (Ohyashiki et al., 1997a). Metastasis is an issue commonly raised in solid tumors. Theoretical considerations suggest that telomerase might predict chromosomal instability, metastatic potential, and invasiveness (Pandita et al., 1996). This is supported by in vitro data correlating telomere amplification with invasive and metastatic potential in human and murine cells (Multani et al., 1999b) and in pancreatic cancer lines (Sato et al., 2001). Clinical correlations have been found in gastric and in colorectal carcinomas: all measured nodal and

peritoneal metastases were positive for telomerase (Tahara et al., 1995a). A more detailed look at data (e.g., Rudolph et al., 2001) indicates that expression supports chromosomal stability in normal cells (Cui et al., 2002b) as well as early in carcinogenesis
(protecting against malignant transformation), but indefinite cell proliferation late in
carcinogenesis (permitting malignant survival).

Expression in a small series of metastatic nodes and lymphomas has excellent correlation ($p = 0.0002$) with malignancy. All histologically malignant nodes (17 metastases,
nine lymphomas) expressed telomerase. Metastatic cancer cells had high expression;
germinal centers of secondary follicles had lower telomerase levels, ascribed to activated lymphocytes (Yashima et al., 1997b). Longer telomere lengths, found in some
lymphomas, raised concern regarding use of telomerase in therapy (Remes et al., 2000),
and the use of expression as an indicator of prognosis. In most cases, B-cell non-Hodgkin
lymphomas express telomerase; activity correlates ($p < 0.001$) with proliferative index.
Moreover, activity correlates with aggressiveness within each subcategory of lymphoma
(Ely et al., 2000), suggesting utility for prognosis. In Hodgkin disease, activity is frequently increased and cells typically have longer telomeres (Ohshima et al., 2001), although prognostic reliability is unclear.

The utility of telomerase as a marker for prognosis (or therapeutic response) remains
unsettled. Initial data are suggestive but scant and unimpressive. It is likely that expression and activity will have prognostic value in a substantial number of malignancies.

Therapy

The goal is not diagnosis, but prevention or termination of malignancy. This is much
the same goal—albeit with species, not individual survival in mind—that evolution faces
in selecting mechanisms outlined above. The path to malignancy is barred by a series of
defenses, each of which a malignant cell must overcome, but each defense is also an
opportunity for intervention. Therapeutic research can aim at any of these processes
(Aragona et al., 2000b; Livingston and Shivdasani, 2001), including intracellular targets such as DNA damage, cell cycle control, growth control mechanisms (Pietras et al.,
1998; Wilson et al., 1999; Pegram et al., 2000), signal transduction pathways, apoptosis,
and telomere stability (Mergny et al., 2001), as well as extracellular targets such as
angiogenesis (Barinaga, 2000; St. Croix et al., 2000; Fyfe, 2000; Hood et al., 2003),
immune function (Pawelec et al., 1999d; Hurwitz et al., 2000), metastasis (Kwon et al.,
1999), and interactions within the extracellular matrix (Boral et al., 1998).

If cancer cells are distinguished by aberrant *p53*, for example, then perhaps it can
be distinguished therapeutically as well (McCormick, 1999a, 2000). Antibodies attack-
ing cells with aberrant *p53* and ignoring normal cells offer enormous therapeutic implication: apocryphal magic bullets becomes real technological bullets. There are many
features distinguishing cancer from normal cells, each a potential point of therapeutic
intervention. Which of these points are the most effective, safe, and achievable (McCune
et al., 2001)? Cell senescence has several theoretical advantages.

Two points deserve emphasis. The first is that telomerase does not cause cancer.
Telomerase is "not an oncogene" (Harley, 2002). If telomerase permits cells to progress
to clinical malignancy, it is late and permissive, not early and causal. Telomerase is
required for telomere maintenance and continuing cancer cell viability (Hahn et al.,

1999b; Oulton and Harrington, 2000). This raises the second point: telomerase has two conflicting roles in carcinogenesis (Hackett and Greider, 2002). Expression (and activity) not only does not cause cancer, but telomerase is protective under certain circumstances, particularly early in the course toward malignancy when genetic stabilization is critical (Kim and Hruszkewycz, 2001). The genetic instability resulting from critical telomere shortening permits cancer cells to acquire the multiple genetic aberrations characteristic of malignant progression (Fouladi et al., 2000), including telomerase expression (Delhommeau et al., 2002). Early telomerase activity *protects* the cell against genetic instability and subsequent clonal expansion (Elmore and Holt, 2000). Caveats notwithstanding, the potential of telomerase for protecting against these intracellular mechanisms of oncogenesis stands out. In this, telomerase inhibition may allow unprecedented specificity and efficacy (Harley et al., 1994; Morin, 1995; Seachrist, 1995).

Alternative pathways to telomere maintenance (Reddel et al., 2001) may play a role in normal cell maintenance in yeast (Teng and Zakian, 1999), mice (Blasco et al., 1997a, 1997b), and probably many eukaryotes (Stewart and Weinberg, 2000). One such pathway may explain why dominant negative telomerase inhibition is spontaneously overcome in murine cell lines (Sachsinger et al., 2001). Generically, these alternative lengthening of telomeres (ALT) pathways may include recombination (Harley et al., 1982; Bryan and Reddel, 1997; Kass-Eisler and Greider, 2000; Cerone et al., 2001) and copy switching (Dunham et al., 2000), retrotransposition (Reddel, 1998b), or other mechanisms (Bryan et al., 1997a; Reddel et al., 1997; Hoare et al., 2001). Defects in mismatch repair, such as those demonstrated in hereditary non-polyposis colorectal cancer, may enhance survival in cancer cells using such alternate pathways (Rizki and Lundblad, 2001), such as colorectal (Takagi et al., 2000) or gastric cancers (Kim et al., 2002d). This may permit malignant progression in the absence of telomerase (Kucherlapati and DePinho, 2001; Gan et al., 2002). While recombination may maintain telomere length (Wang and Zakian, 1990b; Chambers et al., 1998; Slijepcevic and Bryant, 1998) by removing the weakest-link problem, i.e., which chromosome has the shortest telomere (Tan, 1999; Hemann et al., 2001), the expression level of telomere recombination genes is unaffected by telomere shortening (Teng et al., 2002) and its result is a greater heterogeneity in telomere lengths. If exogenous telomerase expression occurs in cells using the ALT mechanism, then telomeres are lengthened, but heterogeneity and rapidly fluctuating telomere lengths remain characteristic. The ALT mechanism remains functional even with demonstrated telomerase activity (Grobelny et al., 2001; Henson et al., 2002). However, when ALT-positive cells are fused with cells expressing telomerase, the ALT mechanism is abolished, although apparently not by any direct effect of telomerase (Perrem et al., 2001). It is difficult to understand how ALT might function in the long run (when, fluctuations notwithstanding, all chromosomes share equally short telomeres), except in conjunction with telomerase (Pluta and Zakian, 1989). One possibility is that excessive recombination may offer a selection advantage, permitting some cells to extend their replicative lifespan, allowing further recombination to bypass other barriers to cell division (Shammas and Shmookler Reis, 1999; Klein and Kreuzer, 2002).

While senescence might be signaled by shortest telomere (Hemann et al., 2001) or mean telomere length (Martens et al., 2000b), the mechanism is likely more complex than either (Ouellette et al., 2000a). Moreover, telomere lengths may be more heterogeneous in rapidly dividing, telomerase-positive cells, and mechanisms may be independent of those responsible for length increase (Londono-Vallejo et al., 2001). The degree to which recombination is significant in human cells (Newbold, 1999; Dunham et al., 2000), and particularly cancer cells, remains uncertain and adds uncertainty to therapies aimed at inhibiting telomere maintenance (Henson et al., 2002). While some human cancer cells lack activity, the mechanisms maintaining telomere length are unknown (Reddel, 1998b) and it is arguable whether they can divide indefinitely by such mechanisms. Barring serendipity, optimal therapeutic efficacy requires thorough understanding of telomere function and the protection telomerase affords dividing cells (Blackburn, 2000a).

Whether the siren promise of telomerase inhibitors will ever be fulfilled (Senior, 2000), its appeal is sans pareil (Dhaene et al., 2000b) as a potential generic oncotherapy (Hiyama et al., 1997d; Lees and Weinberg, 1999). Its importance in extracellular defenses, notably immune surveillance, is less apparent. Many tumors have characteristic antigen markers (Pawelec et al., 1999b), but others are immunologically "invisible" (Pawelec, 1999c; van Elsas et al., 1999; Allison, 2000). Markers notwithstanding, effective surveillance requires immune competence, which declines with age and cell senescence (Effros and Valenzuela, 1998). Theoretically, telomerase induction (Liu, 1999) might improve T-cell performance in identifying and destroying cryptic malignant cells. Telomerase inhibition, by contrast, is efficacious for reasons given above (Cowell, 1999). Inhibition has been approached in creative ways (Kelland, 2001; Helder et al., 2002; Maser and DePinho, 2002), inhibiting expression, activity, or promoters, or by telomerase cleavage.

Expression is regulated predominantly as a transcriptional event. Understanding of telomerase regulation may be crucial to development therapies (Zhao et al., 2000a; Chatziantoniou, 2001; Tollefsbol et al., 2001). In a series of papers, Kyo's laboratory suggested that regulation might be assigned to a 400 bp silencer of the hTERT promoter (lying between -776 and -378 upstream of the proximal core promoter). Predictably, inhibition increases as cells differentiate. Mutating the sites increases transcription. A myeloid-specific zinc finger protein 2 (MZF-2) binds to and down-regulates hTERT transcription and therefore activity (Fujimoto et al., 2000). A number of metals, zinc and perhaps cadmium and copper, modulate activity in some human renal cell carcinoma (NRC-12) and prostatic cancer (DU145) cell lines (Nemoto et al., 2000).

Lack of normal growth factor response, typical of malignant cells, correlates with telomerase activity. Predictably, at least one growth factor, autocrine transforming growth factor beta, directly targets hTERT promoter, inhibiting activity and reinstituting senescence in colon and breast cancer cells (Yang et al., 2001a), perhaps by forcing differentiation. In an opposite example, glioblastoma cell lines (in 50%, epidermal growth factor receptor is overexpressed, amplified, or both) transfected with an antisense epidermal growth factor receptor show down-regulated activity, shorter telomeres, and inhibited tumorigenicity (Tian et al., 2002).

Chemotherapeutic agents affecting transcription might inhibit hTERT transcription. Histone deacetylase inhibitors, such as sodium butyrate, induce differentiation and lower hTERT activity. The effect is probably not mediated directly (Nakamura et al., 2001a) but by reciprocal effects on c-Myc and Mad1, which may be responsible for activation (in proliferating cells) and repression (in differentiated cells) of hTERT gene (Xu et al., 2001a). Differentiating agents, e.g., amifostine and interleukin 4, cause decreasing activity, correlating with clinical response (Preisler et al., 2000). Another example is all-*trans* retinoic acid (RA) and granulocyte-macrophage colony-stimulating factor that together suppress hTERT expression in myeloblastic leukemia cells (Mano et al., 2000). Retinoic acid (and analogs all-*trans* RA, 9-*cis* RA, and 13-*cis* RA) can likewise inhibit growth in some human breast cancer lines, probably mediated by down-regulation of hTERT expression and activity; there is no effect on hTR or hTEP1 (Choi et al., 2000). Likewise, other chemotherapeutic agents, such as tamoxifen, inhibit expression (Aldous, 1998; Nakayama et al., 2000; Christov et al., 2003).

Predictably, *p53*, which is perennially involved in cell senescence (Vaziri et al., 1997; Milas et al., 1998 Velicescu and Dubeau, 2002), may regulate telomerase expression. Penclomedine (a synthetic pyridine) may kill telomerase-positive as well as *p53*-defective tumors in vitro (Pandita et al., 1997) and the latter effect is implicated in the former. Promiscuity of *p53* in cellular events may mitigate any specific importance for expression, yet recombinant transfection of wild-type *p53* (not control vectors) down-regulated hTERT mRNA expression and repressed its promoter, followed by decreased activity (Kanaya et al., 2000). That growth inhibition and apoptosis followed hTERT repression (rather than the reverse) does not prove causation. Unwitnessed and unmeasured intracellular events are the rule: hTERT repression may occur after (and because) the cell commits to growth inhibition and apoptosis, but before growth inhibition and apoptosis become apparent.

Although events modulating telomerase expression are largely unknown, some evidence implicates a growth hormone releasing factor antagonist (MZ-5-156) down-regulating expression. The compound had no effect on hTR or TP1 in a glioblastoma cell line (U-87MG) and may offer no clinical leverage in over telomerase (Kiaris et al., 1999).

There is literature (e.g., Falchetti et al., 1999; Horikawa et al., 1999) on interactions between telomerase and various proto-oncogenes, specifically c-*myc*, a known promoter (Cerni, 2000) and one that, at least in some tumors (Sagawa et al., 2001) and tumor cell lines (Wang et al., 2000b), correlates with hTERT expression. Using 15-mer antisense c-*myc* oligonucleotides in three human leukemic lines (HL60, U937, and K562), antisense c-*myc* decreased activity in experimental but not control lines, treated with c-*myc* sense oligomers (Fujimoto and Takahashi, 1997). Controlling expression requires exploration and is likely a promising avenue for intervention (Kyo et al., 2000a).

Once expressed, there are two approaches to intervention: increasing turnover (e.g., cleavage) or activity inhibition (Hahn and Meyerson, 2001). Hammerhead ribozyme, "teloRZ," specifically cleaves synthesized hTR. When tested on cell extracts from HepG2 or Huh-7 (human hepatocellular carcinoma lines), teloRZ inhibited activity, suggesting its potential (Kanazawa et al., 1996). Hammerhead ribozyme transfection decreased activity in breast tumors in vitro, as did ribozyme-expressing adenovirus; both increased sensitivity to topoisomerase inhibitors (Ludwig et al., 2001). Direct application and transfection were effective in vitro against melanoma cells, causing loss of activity and (in transfected cells) delayed doubling (Folini et al., 2000). Although telomeres lengths may be unaffected, these and other results (Yokoyama et al., 2000; Qu et al., 2002) support hammerhead ribozyme inhibition.

One hesitates to portray telomerase inhibition as the usual approach at such an early stage (Mu and Wei, 2002), yet despite criticisms (Bearss et al., 2000; Ohyashiki et al., 2002), it is a major avenue of investigation (Kelland, 2000; Herbert et al., 2001b; Kyo and Inoue, 2001). Research focuses on screening techniques to identify inhibitors

(Gourdeau et al., 2002; Naasani et al., 2002) as well as assays for expression (Keith et al., 2002; Salonga et al., 2002) and activity to measure inhibition (Double and Thompson, 2002), by fluorescent (Aldous et al., 2002), TRAP (Burger, 2002; Ohyashiki and Ohyashiki, 2002), PCR (Emrich et al., 2002; Emrich and Karl, 2002; Nakayama and Ishikawa, 2002), and other methods (Sun, 2002). Early publications found that telomerase inhibition limited division of malignant ovarian cells without affecting normal ovarian epithelial cells (Feng et al., 1995). Some inhibitors, e.g., heavy metals including arsenic (Chou et al., 2001), platinum (Blasiak et al., 2002), and lead (Cui et al., 2002a), are nonspecific and induce damage to chromosomal ends. This highlights the current foci, which are not efficacy but specificity, stability, and safety. Succinctly, the hurdle is going from in vitro to in vivo performance. In vitro (van Steensel et al., 1998; Wang et al., 1998a; Karlseder et al., 1999) performance is impressive and expected given the role of telomerase in tumor viability (Herbert et al., 1999; Zhang et al., 1999a).

Transfection of a competitive mutant employs an ineffective, mutant telomerase gene that kills tumor cells (Hahn et al., 1999b), for example, hepatoma cells (Zhang et al., 2002b). Human cancer cell work shows efficacy at stemming cell proliferation and tumor growth despite simultaneous wild-type activity and stable telomere lengths (Hodes, 2001; Kim et al., 2001c). A dominant negative mutant of telomerase suppressed ($p < 0.025$) spontaneous immortalization of breast epithelial cells from women with Li-Fraumeni syndrome (Herbert et al., 2001a).

Direct inhibition, in which a specific telomerase inhibitor is added to the cell medium, is more common (Herbert et al., 1999). Telomerase inhibitors cover a wide gamut including peptide nucleic acids, 2'-O-MeRNA oligomers (Corey, 1998), antisense telomeric RNA (Cowell, 1998), and serendipitous inhibitors (antibiotics, chemotherapeutic agents, etc.).

One such inhibitor, antisense phosphorothioate oligonucleotide (PTO) used on human prostate cancer cells (Schindler et al., 2001), reduced cancer cell viability but required 2 weeks of continual in vitro cell exposure. Oligonucleotide N3'→P5' phosphoramidates have been used against human breast cancer cells and showed slow but significant inhibition (Brittney-Shea et al., 2002). Similarly, 2'-O-alkyl (e.g., 2-methoxyethyl) oligonucleotides (Chen et al., 2002d), complementary to the hTERT RNA template region, have shown long-term (7-day) inhibition in cell extracts and may be tried clinically (Elayadi et al., 2001; Corey, 2002). In a slightly different approach, antisense oligonucleotide to hTR induces apoptosis of prostate tumor cells, but not normal fibroblasts. In mice, this induced apoptosis and suppressed tumor growth (Kondo et al., 2000), with parallel results for in vivo tumors (Cowell, 1999). Antisense hTR oligonucleotides were also effective in ovarian cancer cells (Yatabe et al., 2002), gastric carcinomas (Yang et al., 2002a), and nasopharyngeal carcinomas (Zhang et al., 2002e). Similarly, a 19-mer antisense hTR reduced viability in seven human bladder cancer lines without affecting normal human fibroblast growth. The compound induced (caspase-dependent) apoptosis in human bladder cancer cells grown subcutaneously in mice (Koga et al., 2001b). The stability and efficacy of oligonucleotides support their oncotherapeutic potential (Dapic et al., 2002).

Peptide nucleic acids (PNAs) take telomerase out of circulation by mimicking telomeres, binding hTR, and inhibiting the activity of telomerase molecules that would otherwise bind normal telomeres. Depending on the sequence, they can inhibit activity in the picomolar to nanomolar range. They are 10- to 50-fold more efficient than analogous phosphorothioate oligomers. Not surprisingly, some sequences are ineffective (Villa et al., 2000a). Despite early work on mice, oligonucleotides (Brand and Iversen, 1996) may be less effective than PNAs. As a class, PNAs have higher affinity and better specificity than oligomers (Norton et al., 1996; Hamilton et al., 1997) and are effective (Autexier, 1999). Tumor suppression is controllable, indeed reversible, confirming efficacy. Moreover, when the template is block by complementary PNA oligomers, immortal cells revert to senescent growth arrest (Shammas et al., 1999).

Antisense nucleic acids and oligonucleotides (Delihas, 2001) have been used with the same rationale, though with limited results. In vitro, this approach effectively ($p < 0.001$) suppressed spontaneous immortalization in breast epithelial cells from women with Li-Fraumeni syndrome (Herbert et al., 2001a). Using a retrovirus containing UUAGGG (complementary to the hTR template), immortalized murine fibroblasts, human HeLa cells, and human kidney carcinoma cells showed at least 75% inhibition, but in only half the cell lines. Although correlating with characteristics of cell senescence (morphology, proliferation capacity, growth rate and telomere content), unreliability precludes clinical use (Bisoffi et al., 1998). However, a 2', 5'-oligoadenylate antisense oligonucleotide against hTERT RNA inhibited in vitro ovarian cancer cells without affecting normal ovarian epithelial cells (Kushner et al., 2000). This was effective against human glioma cells in vitro, especially paired with conventional cisplatin therapy (Kondo et al., 2001). Cisplatin itself shortens telomeres but may have little direct effect on telomerase (hTERT, hTR, or TEP1) components, at least in human hepatomas (Zhang et al., 2002d). Normal-sense telomere oligonucleotides alter the telomeric structure and may also have a therapeutic role (Pandit and Bhattacharyya, 2001). These telomere-mimicking oligonucleotides inhibit tumor growth in telomerase-positive tumor cell lines; efficacy correlates with oligonucleotide length (Saeki et al., 1999).

Current chemotherapeutic agents work through a plethora of mechanisms. As some restrict cell proliferation, they may predictably disrupt telomere maintenance or affect inhibition (Huang et al., 2001). The two effects are separable: genistein (4,5,7-trihydroxyisoflavone) appears to have no effect on activity, but enforces telomere shortening in cancer cells by preventing hTERT access to the nucleus (Alhasan et al., 2001). In some, though not all (Kubota et al., 2000b; Vietor et al., 2000), cases, these may prove to be the primary mechanism of action. Certain pro-apoptotic agents (staurosporine, thapsigargin, anti-Fas antibody, and some cancer chemotherapeutic agents including ara-C) cause telomere cleavage and aggregation, arrest cells in G2/M phase, fragment DNA, and induce apoptosis (Multani et al., 2000). Some agents may disrupt telomere maintenance, but many differentiation-inducing and antineoplastic agents inhibit activity (Pathak et al., 1998; Li et al., 2000b; Preisler et al., 2000). Widely used chemotherapeutic platinum compounds, for example, probably inhibit telomerase (Blasiak et al., 2002); other heavy metals have inhibitory (lead) or protective (selenium) effects on activity and telomere maintenance (Cui et al., 2002a). Declining telomerase activity often predicts response to standard oncotherapeutic agents (Faraoni et al., 1999; Preisler et al., 2000). In ovarian cancer cells, hTR expression correlates with sensitivity to chemotherapeutic agents, including cisplatin, etoposide, CPT-11, and cyclophosphamide/ifomide (Kiyozuka et al., 2000b; Kikuchi, 2001). There is no correlation between chemotherapy response and prior activity or mean telomere lengths. Of ovarian cancers failing, however, 7/11 (58%) showed increased hTERT expression (Takahashi et al., 2000).

At least one demethylating agent, 5-azacytidine, transcriptionally represses a promoter (Kitagawa et al., 2000). Bromodeoxyuridine represses telomerase (without altering telomere lengths) and induces multiple markers of cell senescence, including β-galactosidase, fibronectin, collagenase I, p21(wafl/sdi-1), and mortalin (Michishita et al., 1999). Other currently used agents inhibiting telomerase include 6-mercaptopurine, 6-thioguanine, and abacavir (Tendian and Parker, 2000). Telomerase inhibition may be more prevalent than we appreciate. Antineoplastic compounds may include natural telomerase inhibitors, such as the epigallocatechin gallate in tea (Naasani et al., 1998), or verbascoside, a phenylpropanoid glucoside extracted from *Pedicularis striata Pall* (Zhang et al., 2002a). Such compounds and their synthetic derivatives (Seimiya et al., 2002) are not standard chemotherapeutic agents but are known to have antineoplastic effects and concomitantly inhibit telomerase.

Azidothymidine and carbovir, which are reverse transcriptase inhibitors, can block telomerase function (Kazimirchuk et al., 2001). Indeed, these drugs (especially azidothymidine) induce cell senescence in some cultures and immortal murine fibroblasts and macrophages, though not immortal 3T3 Swiss cells (Kazimirchuk et al., 2001). Although these drugs cause telomere shortening in certain human tumor lines (U-937 and MeWo), they do not result in cell senescence. Cells undergo initial crisis, become resistant, and replication resumes. High activity correlates with resistance to reverse transcriptase inhibitors (Yegorov et al., 1999).

Cisplatin and TMPyP4 (a porphyrin-derived compound) may interfere with telomerase activity (Grand et al., 2002). Prior to treatment, MCF7 breast cancer cells had one-third the activity of a reference HeLa cell line. Telomere lengths showed enormous variance but did not correlate with telomerase levels. Perhaps implicating an alternative pathway for telomere maintenance, it might imply only significant variance (with declining lengths) in malignant cells not expressing telomerase and equal variance (with maintained lengths) in malignant cells that do. Whatever the implication, attempts to assess the efficacy of telomerase inhibition in terms of simple telomere lengths (Remes et al., 2000) are misguided; efficacy must be practical, e.g., retardation of cancer cell growth. Cisplatin and TMPyP4 down-regulate activity in these cancer cells and appear to prevent cell proliferation (Raymond et al., 1999). TMPyP4 effects appear unrelated to known antiangiogenic properties of porphyrins (Izbicka et al., 2000). Despite clinical utility, cisplatin has no apparent effect on telomere length in nasopharyngeal tumors (Wang et al., 2001d) but causes direct telomere loss in *Saccharomyces cerevisiae* (Ishii et al., 2000). In combining cisplatin with telomerase induction to target human glioma cells in vitro, the two approaches may be complementary and may target semi-independent mechanisms, perhaps including apoptosis (Kondo et al., 2001).

Radiation therapy can have similar effects on telomerase activity in some cancers in vivo. In rectal cancer, activity fell in 8/10 (80%) patients, remained constant in one, and went from no to weak activity in one patient (Kim et al., 2000). The mechanism is unknown, but some data suggest a strong negative correlation between telomere length or stability and radiation sensitivity in breast cancer and normal patients (McIlrath et al., 2001). This is reminiscent of the effects of telomerase in preventing chemotherapeutic efficacy in agents inducing double-stranded DNA breaks (Lee et al., 2001c).

Some antibiotics (currently "lead compounds" rather than therapeutically useful) inhibit telomerase. These antibiotics include rubromycins and analogues, especially β- and γ-rubromycin and purpuromycin (Ueno et al., 2000), distamycin (Zaffaroni et al.,

2002), doxorubicin (Zhang et al., 2002c), and adriamycin, which induces senescence by inhibiting both telomere function (Elmore et al., 2002a) and telomerase (Kunifuji et al., 2002).

Many feel that "the stage is now set for the chemist" (Cech, 2000), and computer modeling of telomerase inhibitors is in progress (Jenkins, 2000; Ren et al., 2002). One target is the G-quartet, unique structural features of quadruplex telomeric DNA (Han and Hurley, 2000; Read and Neidle, 2000; Koeppel et al., 2001; Mergny et al., 2001) which bind telomere-associated proteins (Parkinson et al., 2002) and block telomerase action. Not surprisingly, given the importance of structural shape (Shafer and Smirnov, 2001), binding depends on stearic factors (Kettani et al., 2000; Izbicka et al., 2001; Tuntiwechapikul and Salazar, 2001). This may render telomerase inhibition based on stabilizing the quadruplex structure sensitive to oxidative changes (Szalai et al., 2002). Quadruplex-stabilization compounds have good in vitro efficacy, including 3,6, 9-trisubstituted (Read et al., 2001) and other (Alberti et al., 2001) acridines. Numerous small molecules (Newbold, 2002) ranging from anthraquinones to porphyrins, acridines, and complex polycyclic, aromatic chromophores (Neidle and Read, 2000–2001), and quinolines (Riou et al., 2002) inhibit activity, even at submicromolar concentrations, by stabilizing this guanine-rich structure (Neidle et al., 2000; Gowan et al., 2001, 2002) and their inhibition is detectable by TRAP assay (Gomez et al., 2002). In some cases, inhibition occurs through suppression of c-*myc* (Simonsson and Henriksson, 2002). Some (Kerwin, 2000) suggest that direct binding to quadruplex telomeric DNA (e.g., perylene diimides that may be noncytotoxic, G-quadruplex–selective, telomerase inhibitors) might result in quicker antiproliferative effects and faster clinical response. Response time has been raised repeatedly and data support an advantage for quadruplex-binding telomerase inhibitors (Raymond et al., 2000; Rezler et al., 2002).

Identification of telomerase-positive cells allows not merely inhibition but targeted killing based on this defining feature. This supposes that exceptions (telomerase-positive normal cells and telomerase-negative malignant cells) will not be clinically significant, an expedient supposition, but one requiring evaluation. If we reintroduce susceptibility to apoptosis, e.g., if hTERT gene promoter is used as such a marker for a caspase-8 expression vector, then the results would demonstrate in vivo (in mice) and in vitro (without measurable effects on normal fibroblast cells) tumor inhibition via induced apoptosis of cancer cells (Koga et al., 2000). The same laboratory employed a similar technique with caspase-6 (Komata et al., 2001b) and with Fas-associated protein with death domain (FADD; Koga et al., 2001a). In a parallel approach, hTERT promoter induced expression of transfected *Bax* gene, causing tumor-specific apoptosis in vitro (Gu et al., 2000). Similarly, hTERT promoter induced expression of FADD in malignant human glioma cells transfected with hTERT/FADD construct. Overexpression normally induces apoptosis, regardless of surface expression of Fas. Experimentally, it kills hTERT-positive malignant glioma cells, sparing normal, hTERT-negative cells (Komata et al., 2001a).

A second approach, targeting telomerase-positive cells for cytotoxic immunity, assumes that telomerase approximates a "universal" tumor antigen (Greener, 2000; Rousseau and Soria, 2000; Schultze et al., 2001). Precursor cytotoxic T lymphocytes are antigenically stimulated with telomerase (Heiser et al., 2000; Morse and Lyerly, 2000; Vieweg, 2000) or hTERT-derived peptides (Arai et al., 2001). Monoclonal antibodies can also be produced in mice immunized with telomerase from breast tumor cells (Kaur et al., 2001). Immunologic approaches have been proposed for plasma cell dyscrasias, including multiple myeloma and Waldenstrom macroglobulinemia (Treon et al., 2000). Precursor cytotoxic T lymphocytes, stimulated with telomerase peptides from prostate cancer cells, lyse human cancer cells in vitro. In vivo, hTERT-specific cytotoxic T lymphocytes have been generated in transgenic mice (Minev et al., 2000). hTERT-specific lymphocytes are found in prostate cancer and normal patients, but in vivo efficacy of univalent antigen therapy is unproven. Polyvalent antigens may lyse more effectively than univalent antigens, e.g., in prostate cancer (Heiser et al., 2001b). Superior efficacy of multiple antigens for dendritic cell stimulation has been shown in renal cell carcinomas (Nair et al., 2000b; Heiser et al., 2001a). hTERT-specific cytotoxic T lymphocytes, however, are active against multiple unrelated tumors. Murine cytotoxic T lymphocytes lyse melanoma and thymoma tumor cells, as well as inhibiting many other tumors; human cytotoxic T lymphocytes not only lyse cells transformed by Epstein Barr virus (EBV), but also renal and prostate cancer cells (Nair et al., 2000b). Even here, however, polyvalent antigens were more effective than hTERT alone. Claims of a universal cancer vaccine are premature and exaggerated, but deserves the research it will doubtless inspire.

A third approach makes hTERT expression lethal. An expression vector for diphtheria toxin was linked to hTR and hTERT transcriptional regulatory sequences in bladder and hepatocellular cancer cells. Protein synthesis correlated inversely with hTR or hTERT transcription (Abdul-Ghani et al., 2000). Similarly, herpes simplex virus thymidine kinase gene controlled by hTERT promoter (a hTERTp/TK cassette) sensitizes human osteosarcoma cells to ganciclovir. Osteosarcoma cells expressing this cassette were eradicated from mice by ganciclovir (Majumdar et al., 2001).

Current interventions are tantalizingly, yet only partially, effective. Specific telomerase inhibitors are likely candidates for cancer intervention. Remaining obstacles fall into two categories: technical and clinical. It is technically difficult to identify effective agents that can be reliably delivered to malignant cells. Clinical use requires not only efficacy but relative safety in living patients. Clinical efficacy has been demonstrated in oncotherapeutic agents that, serendipitously, inhibit telomerase. Varying widely in efficacy and safety, their clinical profiles are known, but whether their efficacy depends significantly on telomerase inhibition is not. Current use grants them retroactive cachet in regard to clinical efficacy. Cachet does not, however, extend to new telomerase inhibitors. Telomerase inhibitors may be strikingly effective in vitro (Hahn et al., 1999b; Sasaki et al., 2001) without being stable, safe, and effective in vivo.

Drug kinetics depend on several variables, notably absorption, distribution, degradation (or excretion), and (in some compounds) metabolism from inactive to active moiety. Useful agents must be deliverable, survive for a sufficiently long period in the face of enzymatic degradation, liver metabolism, and/or renal excretion, not interfere with other cellular and intercellular activity, and enter the cell wall and nuclear membrane with good solubility. Binding coefficients, mode of action (irreversible or merely competitive), and hTERT turnover rates all affect pharmacokinetics, and while these may be smaller problems than we fear (Neidle and Kelland, 1999; Damm et al., 2001), only data, particularly in vivo, can address these concerns.

Pure pharmacokinetics is not the central timing issue, however. Effective inhibition might require high intracellular concentrations for weeks or months, as telomeres erode sufficiently to induce crisis. Bluntly stated, even given optimal pharmacokinetics, will the compound kill the cancer before cancer kills the patient? The rapidity with which a candidate telomerase inhibitor can kill tumor cells is crucial. Given the little we know, time courses are likely to be weeks to months rather than days to hours. Cancer cells must senesce sufficiently to undergo cell crisis. This is not likely to occur rapidly (Sidorov et al., 2002), compared to the pace of current chemotherapy. Onset of many chemotherapeutic regimens correlates with time to initial cell division, rather than time to senescence. The dependence of telomere shortening on cell division suggests that inhibitors may be more effective on faster-growing, more malignant tumors (Sidorov et al., 2002). The question is not speed of drug action or rate of cell division, but the ratio between the two, a match we know next to nothing about. Ironically, some data suggest loss of telomere capping, rather than telomere shortening, might be the critical effect. Human ovarian cancer cells, transfected with a ribozyme against hTERT, die rapidly prior to significant division or telomere loss, perhaps by apoptosis. This fast-track mechanism may have clinical relevance (Saretzki et al., 2001); its effect on the ratio of malignant death to malignant growth will remain unknown pending clinical trials (Lavelle et al., 2000). None of the above establishes inhibitors as a magic bullet (Soria et al., 1998), or more prosaically, tells us their therapeutic ratio.

Nor do we know the incidence of side effects on germ line cells, stem cells (Rubin, 2002a), and other cells (such as lymphocytes) that, as telomerase-positive normal cells (Burger et al., 1997), are hypothetically at risk (Fossel, 1996, 1998c; Sasgary et al., 2001). In advanced-cancer patients, immune changes inhibit lymphokine-activated killer cells, as well as telomerase activity and population doublings (Minami et al., 2001). Such curious findings aside, theoretical considerations suggest that risk may be minimal (Holt et al., 1996b): normal somatic cells probably have longer telomeres than cancer cells and normal stem cells express telomerase transiently (not constitutively) upon stimulation (Englehardt et al., 1997). Telomerase inhibitors used against telomerase-positive cancer cells (Zhang et al., 1999b) might be administered over limited spans (hours to weeks?), limiting the impact on telomerase-positive somatic cells (Holt et al., 1996b). Somatic cell telomeres might shorten more than usual, but cancer cells have shorter lengths than normal, bordering cells (Shay and Gazdar, 1997). Cancer cells are on the edge of senescence. Telomerase inhibition should (even with equal division rates) preferentially kill cancer cells.

Unfortunately, not all cancer cells have shorter telomeres, nor is there a simple or necessary correlation between length and stage of malignancy (Pandita et al., 1996). Some lymphomas (Remes et al., 2000) and prostate cancers (Ozen et al., 1998) have longer telomeres (TRFs) than normal fibroblasts. Prostate cancer cells demonstrate hTERT activity, stronger telomere signals, and lower apoptotic indices than normal surrounding cells. (Ozen et al., 1998). Longer telomere lengths raise the issue of whether telomere inhibition will be effective in such cells (Remes et al., 2000).

Even the lack of telomerase in most somatic cells does not mean telomerase inhibitors may not harm them. Penicillin, which inhibits bacterial β-lactam cell wall production, causes seizures in contact with mammalian cortex. The effect is unrelated to the primary action and intent of penicillin. Equally, telomerase inhibitors may have unpredictable side effects on somatic cells, unrelated to their effect as telomerase inhibitors. Initial data (Rha et al., 2000) confirm unexpected effects from a G-quadruplex interactive porphyrin (TMPyP4).

Collectively, these issues raise the question of coordinate therapies: surgery, radiation, and standard chemotherapy. Telomerase inhibition might function without adjunct, but is more likely to be employed adjunctively, e.g., "mopping up" after surgical excision or debulking, or increasing efficacy of other chemotherapeutic regimens (Helder et al., 1999; Villa et al., 2000b; Ohyashiki et al., 2002). This is a characteristic shared with other potential therapies, e.g., growth factors (Slamon, 2000) or p53 (McCormick, 2000). In vitro, chemotherapeutic agents are more effective when combined with telomerase inhibitors (Misawa et al., 2002).

Nonetheless, telomerase inhibition has remarkable potential and, while conservative prediction is appropriate, may become the most effective oncotherapy. Even fulfilling its promise, success would be balanced against costs (Newbold, 1999). Current oncotherapeutic regimens incur substantial clinical costs. We must watch for the risks and trade-offs of telomerase inhibitors (Faraoni and Graziani, 2000; Sasgary et al., 2001), despite theoretical considerations suggesting risks are minimal. Context is important: not simply risks and benefits, but risks and benefits relative to current—significant and daunting—oncotherapies. We cannot scoff at the risks, but there is considerable room for improvement.

The opposite intervention, telomerase induction, deserves comment here. This issue is raised by the remainder of this text, which considers the potential use of this intervention in other age-related diseases. Senescence is normally dominant (Loughran et al., 1997) and immortalization requires subversion of dominantly acting genes (Parkinson et al., 1997). If shortening telomeres can arrest cancer cell division, what is the risk of lengthening telomeres therapeutically? If we extend telomeres to prevent cell senescence and associated age-related diseases, do we increase the risk of malignancy? To an extent, concern over telomerase induction arises through a misperception. Perhaps required for malignant cell survival, telomerase does not cause malignancy. This is most clearly seen in studies of hTERT immortalized human keratinocytes (Matsui et al., 2000), fibroblasts, and retinal pigmented epithelial cells that still retain normal growth controls (Jiang et al., 1999; Dickson et al., 2000; Franco et al., 2001) and exhibit no characteristics of malignant cells (Bodnar et al., 1998; Beeche et al., 1999). hTERT expression has no effect on growth potential or the cell cycle checkpoints (Cerni, 2000), nor on normal cellular responses to viral infection (McSharry et al., 2001).

The initial landmark paper (Bodnar et al., 1998) showed that telomerase transfection effectively extended human cell lifespan without malignant transformation, evidenced by karyotype, contact inhibition, growth in low-serum, and other gross phenotypic or morphologic changes. This same point has been addressed repeatedly since that time (e.g., Harley, 1998a; Jiang et al., 1999; Franco et al., 2001). Results remain uniformly negative, other than extended cellular lifespan. Malignancy is often associated with genomic instability (O'Hagan et al., 2002), but hTERT immortalized human fibroblasts maintain normal genomic stability, as evidenced by DNA mismatch mechanisms (Roques et al., 2001). The same effect is seen in renal carcinoma cells, in which hTERT activity correlates with genomic stability, DNA ploidy, and telomere lengths (Izumi et al., 2002). Malignant transformation requires additional viral or chemical mutagens (Hahn et al., 1999a; Gonzalez-Suarez et al., 2001). Telomerase may be necessary, but is not sufficient for malignant transformation.

In fact, telomere shortening and senescence may increase risk of carcinogenesis (Campisi, 1997a), independent of immune aging. Predictably, telomerase expression with cell immortalization should lower intracellular risk of malignant transformation by stabilizing the genome (Counter et al., 1992). Experimentally, hTERT immortalization confers and is correlated with genetic stability (Amit et al., 2000). The opposite, greater genetic instability, occurs when human bronchial cells are transformed by human papillomavirus type E6 and E7 genes (Coursen et al., 1997), although this technique immortalizes human retinal (and other) cell lines without affecting stability (Roque et al., 1997). hTERT immortalized cells, however, have a predictable increase in genomic stability (Counter et al., 1992; Golubovskaya, 1999). Suggestions to the contrary notwithstanding, telomerase increases genetic stability, arguably lowering risk of clinical malignancy.

Our knowledge of cell senescence offers two final benefits to cancer patients, via monoclonal antibody production and marrow transplantation. First, multiple inherently unstable cell lines produce commercial monoclonal antibodies for cancer (as well as other) therapy. Telomerase promoters would extend cell line survival of normal B cells, avoiding instability and unpredictability problems in hybrid-cell sources (Krupp et al., 2000a, 2000b). Epstein-Barr virus transformation of B cells may occasionally result in immortalization and drastically increased telomerase expression, but also yields chromosomal instability (Okubo et al., 2001). Second, bone marrow transplant is employed for severe aplastic anemia (Molee et al., 2001) or in radiation or chemotherapy. Marrow cells (or circulating stem cells) are harvested, then returned after radiation or chemotherapy to reconstitute immune and/or hematopoetic function. Reconstitution requires cell division, hence accelerates cell senescence (Shay, 1998b), typically the equivalent of 40 years of additional aging of marrow cells (Moore, 1997; Wynn et al., 1998), although with considerable variance (Schroder et al., 2001). Stem cell proliferative potential may not be significantly compromised (Mathioudakis et al., 2001). Initially accelerated telomere loss, with wide fluctuations during the first year (Thornley et al., 2002b), returns to normal within two decades (de Pauw et al., 2002). Telomerase might increase the take of marrow transplantation or permit serial marrow transplantation, and the use of selected stem cell populations for this procedure appears to prevent telomere attrition, presumably through cytokine-induced telomerase expression and subsequent telomere maintenance (Roelofs et al., 2003).

Despite understandable eagerness to employ telomerase inhibition in human cancers, there is much we do not understand (Robinson, 2000; Bibby, 2002). These gaps include mechanism (Saretzki et al., 2001) and clinical outcome. Efficacy, even if unarguable in vitro and then proven unambiguously in vivo, is only one facet in determining a drug's clinical value (Double, 2002). We have substantial theoretic reasons to suspect that telomerase inhibition will be clinically effective (Meyerson, 2000; Perry et al., 2001; Granger et al., 2002), but we lack clinical proof or clinical assessment of safety (Newbold, 1999; Steenbergen, et al., 2001). This is not a cause for suspicion, but further investigation. Measured enthusiasm is warranted; celebration is not.

CHAPTER 6

Parasitic Disease

Pathology and Incidence

Save cancer, most diseases discussed in this text are those in which senescing cells result in human age-related pathology. Parasitic disease, however, results from cells that maintain telomeres and avoid senescence. Here, alone among all others discussed, the cells involved are not human, but invaders. The parallel with cancer remains valid, the more so in sharing a potential intervention: telomerase inhibition.

The shortness of the chapter is no reflection of the significance of parasitic disease—global in scope, high in incidence—but of the paucity of interventional data on cell senescence in parasitic disease. Much may be inferred, little is known. The notion that cell senescence has a role derives not from parasites undergoing senescence but from unicellular parasites not doing so. With two caveats, we might treat parasitic infection by enforcing cell senescence in unicellular parasites (Fossel, 1996; Cano et al., 1999).

The first caveat is that bacteria, technically unicellular parasites, are irrelevant to this discussion. Their ring (not linear) chromosomes do not have, let alone lose, telomeres and the cells do not senesce. Unfortunately, considering the morbidity and ubiquity of bacterial infections, this removes them from this discussion.

The second caveat is that many common parasites are not unicellular, but multicellular. These share many of the mechanisms of linear chromosome replication with larger organisms, such as vertebrates, including somatic cell senescence and organismal aging. To the extent that this is accurate, telomerase inhibitors will offer few therapeutic benefits. Our discussion ignores multicellular ones, despite their incidence and clinically significance. This excludes platyhelminthine (flatworm) parasites such as trematodes (flukes) and cestodes (tapeworms such as *Taenia* and *Echinococcus*), despite their clinical importance. Worldwide, trematodes such as *Schistosoma mansoni* (the intestinal fluke), *S. japonicum* (the blood fluke), and *S. haematobium* (the liver fluke) infect about two hundred million people. *Schistosoma haematobium* infection (bilharziasis) causes bladder cancer in Egypt and other developing countries (Abdel-Salam et al., 2001). Lung flukes (*Paragonimus westermani*), tapeworms, roundworms (*Nematode* diseases, as in onchocerciasis), pinworms, hookworms, whipworms, thorny-headed worms, guinea worms, *Wuchereria*, *Loa*, *Trichinella*, and arthropods (scabies, lice, etc) are all excluded.

Is there anything left? Despite these caveats, this leaves a robust category of disease and human suffering. Unicellular parasites with linear chromosomes comprise some of the most common and daunting diseases of humankind. Each one is protozoal. They include malaria, trypanosomiasis (African sleeping sickness), and lesser-known parasites. They are global and comparatively untouched by effective clinical interventions.

Entomoeba, infecting about 10% of the world population (Markell and Voge, 1976, p 50), causes amoebic colitis, amoebic abscesses, and amoebic dysentery. Naegleria causes meningoencephalitis, usually within a week of infection. Mastigophoric infections, including *Giardia lamblia* and *Trichomonas vaginalis*, are endemic and common diagnoses even in the higher socioeconomic strata of developed nations. Leishmaniasis is endemic in many tropical parts of the world: visceral leishmaniasis is 90% fatal. *Balantidium*, *Isospora*, *Toxoplasma* (toxoplasmosis), *Babesia* (babesiosis), *Pneumocystis* (causing pneumocystis pneumonia in HIV+ and other immunocompromised patients), and Chaga disease (a trypanosomiasis affecting perhaps 20% of residents in parts of South America) together cause disease in every populated continent, country, and ethnic group. Some trypanosomes cause cattle sleeping sickness—nagana—preventing ranching (for local food and profitable export) in much of Africa (Markell and Voge, 1976, p 126; Basch, 1978, p 64).

The most universal, significant, and tempting parasitic disease target is malaria. This blood-borne protozoal disease is caused by four species (falciparum, malariae, vivax, and ovale) varying in virulence and distribution. Annually, these four, but especially falciparum (Le Bras et al., 1998), kill approximately 0.43–0.68 million children aged 0–4 in Africa alone (Snow et al., 1999). The World Health Organization reports 300–500 million cases and 1.5–2.7 million annual deaths, with 2.3 billion people at risk. Often ignored by developed nations, malaria annually kills the equivalent of 1% of the United States population. The risk is highest in Africa, with an incidence of 700 cases per 1000; South America and Asia have risks of only 4 to 5 cases per 1000; risk is negligible in Europe and North America (Danis and Gentilini, 1998). This excludes indirect mortality as infected patients succumb to other, unrelated diseases (Molineaux, 1997). The entire world budget for parasitic disease research is less than that for heart disease in the United States.

Finally, fungal diseases also have linear chromosomes, maintained with telomerase, and are therefore targets for telomerase inhibition. Fungal disease has always been common, indeed ubiquitous, but associated mortality has grown with the advent of modern medicine (particularly immunosuppressive therapy) and HIV disease. The common denominator is identical: immunosuppressive therapy and HIV disease permit fungal organisms, otherwise held in check by human immune mechanisms, to proliferate and kill. Though seldom a major cause of death compared to bacterial etiologies, fungal infections are the daily fare of most modern hospitals in developed nations and might likewise respond to telomerase inhibition.

These parasites, amoebic and fungal, share a dependence on telomerase activity. Whether this dependence is an academic triviality or a clinical Achilles heal remains unknown.

Cell Senescence and Intervention

The possibility of using telomerase inhibition to treat parasitic disease was first raised informally in the early 1990s by Michael West, then at Geron Corporation. The first published discussion addressed the potential of cell senescence in treating human disease, including malaria, sleeping sickness, river blindness, and fungal disease (Fossel, 1996). The potential hinges on telomerase maintenance in unicellular parasites. Telomerase is active in such organisms, for example, *Trypanosoma brucei*, *Leishmania* major, and *Leishmania tarentolae*. Though supporting telomerase as "a new target for chemotherapeutic intervention" (Cano et al., 1999), telomeric mechanisms (Cano, 2001) and subtelomeric organization (Stern et al., 2001) may be more complex than first guessed.

A variety of organisms share similar telomere sequences, but with subtle differences. Malaria, for example, has a heptad telomeric repeat, TTTAGGG, instead of the human hexad repeat, TTAGGG (Blackburn, 1990b), and other subtle alterations in telomeric organization (Scherf et al., 2001). These differences may prove useful. Polymerase chain reaction assays aimed at the telomere sequence of *Leishmania donovani*, for example, show diagnostic promise (Chiurillo et al., 2001).

Despite subtle differences in telomere sequence, telomerases share a common shape (Chen et al., 2000c). Therapeutic intervention is likely to aim at telomerase, not telomeres, to enforce parasite telomere attrition. To the extent that these observations are accurate, use of telomerase inhibitors in parasitic disease should overlap use in cancer. Oncologic therapies interfering with telomere maintenance are appropriate and enticing candidates for testing in unicellular parasitic disease.

Acceptable risks and side effects depend on the disease: regulatory hurdles for acne therapy are appropriately high, those for melanoma, low. In parasitic disease, the diseases are often fatal; current therapies are costly, often risky, seldom totally effective. Therapies for parasitic infection, not expensive by standards of developed nations, are often beyond the means of patients most at risk. Given limited funding, public health investment often focuses on vector control, not pharmacology. Mosquito nets, drainage ditches, insecticides, and other measures are cheap and common. Unfortunately, efforts to control parasites or vectors, despite historical bursts of optimism, have suffered recurrent failures (Molyneux, 1997, 1998). There is a growing understanding that developed nations have an economic self-interest in the public health of underdeveloped nations (Brundtland, 2002). The potential of telomerase inhibitors in treating unicellular parasitic infection is not academic, but addresses a global and growing need. Whether this need can be met remains to be seen.

PART II

The Aging Organism

There are certain queer times and occasions in this strange mixed affair we call life when a man takes this whole universe for a vast practical joke, though the wit thereof he but dimly discerns, and more than suspects that the joke is at nobody's expense but his own.

Herman Melville
Moby Dick, 1851

If aging is cell aging, then age-related disease may be attributable, directly or indirectly, to aging cells. This is not equivalent to ascribing all diseases to cell aging nor age-related diseases solely to cell aging. Neither statement is likely accurate and neither here defended. Nonetheless, there is good reason (supported by clinical pathology) to suppose common diseases of aging, such as atherosclerosis, may be driven by changes in gene expression and cell behavior occurring as critical cells senesce.

Diseases are the result of causes, entire cascades of contributing risk factors culminating in pathology. We cannot, like the old doctor in de Maupassant's story, simply throw up our hands, proclaiming we have, "no idea, no idea at all. He died because he died, that's all" (de Mauppassant, 1980). In discerning causes of disease, we sometimes simplistically choose one cause over another as though they were mutually exclusive. Was his heart attack the result of smoking, high cholesterol, dietary fat, genes, lack of exercise, or high blood pressure, or was it diabetes? In reality, high cholesterol may have played a role, but diet fed into it, many genes permitted it, lack of exercise left the low-density lipoprotein (LDL) level high, smoking allowed the cell damage that began the inflammation, ad infinitum. If we try to ask a question about how much a given risk factor contributed, we stumble unless we understand what we mean. We might better phrase the question as one of intervention. If we normalize cholesterol, what percentage of patients will not have atherosclerosis that would otherwise? If we normalize blood pressure, what percentage do not die of heart attacks? If they had never smoked, what percentage would not have angina? These questions, while devilish to answer, speak to practical intent. How can we prevent disease?

In treatment, the same reasoning pertains. If we have a large group of patients with stenotic coronary arteries and we lower cholesterol with drug X, or they stop smoking, or we can lower the blood pressure, what percentage will avoid cardiac death over what time period? These questions are more useful than are misleadingly simple issues of cause, because they untangle conceptually difficult strands of causation and rewind them into a tangible skein we can work with. We also avoid illusory contradictions about whether diseases are caused by A or B. Often, reality is A and B, and dozens of other interacting variables. Hypertension, for example, is simultaneously a risk factor and a protective variable for mortality in the elderly (Satish et al., 2001). Clinically difficult pathologies accompanying old age epitomize this complexity. We should assume complex cascades of causation, while assessing relative efficacy of various points of clinical intervention. We cannot assume, like our fictional doctor, that an older patient "just died because he died."

Yet, it is a common solecism that age-related diseases "just happen" because "things wear out" or "damage accumulates." These explanations don't go far enough. Things that wear out are often sophisticated and technical: mitochondria, genes, lipid bilayers, and protein chains. Accumulations of cholesterol, lipofuscin, foam cells, and neurofibrillary tangles are well documented and consistent. Equally facile pronouncements were taken seriously one and a quarter century ago in explaining away infectious disease. "Subtle metabolic poisons" and "rural miasmas" (Porter, 1997) lay at the root of cholera, tetanus, puerperal fever, anthrax, and cellulitis. Old names, such as blood poisoning and malaria, remain tokens of our ignorance, but we forget the lessons that Pasteur learned in his attic above the Rue des Fleurs. Aging diseases are treated as an olla podrida of pathologies. The assumption that these diseases are linked only by chronology goes unstated, but equally unsupported. That aging is cell aging and that age-related diseases share this common denominator explains much that was puzzling and provides a common ground to understand age-related human pathology.

Age-related diseases have their etiology in genetics (Rose and Archer, 1996; Martin, 1997a) and epigenetics (Caspary et al., 1999; Tzukerman et al., 2002), specifically cell senescence (Fossel, 1996; Kipling and Faragher, 1999). There has been a profound lack of understanding of the mechanisms involved, their implications, and limitations of the model. The lack of coherent formulation has resulted in, on the one hand, naive criticism and unwarranted disbelief and, on the other, naive claims and an equally unwarranted faith.

Cell senescence is not, in some simplistic sense, the cause of all age-related disease. To the contrary: cell senescence operates upon a substrate of genetic diathesis. We do not get atherosclerosis because we age, we get it because we age in the context of specific inherited genes. Cell senescence is a background effect, a subtle, pervasive trend that alters the pattern of gene expression and therefore the pattern of disease expression. Most diseases, are in a sense, caused by genetic problems, but they unfold and are accentuated by the alterations in gene expression incumbent upon cell senescence. Hypertension may occur as sporadic genetic disease neonatally or in childhood (Dluhy and Lifton, 1999; Prince et al., 1999; Su et al., 2000) as well as with aging; the effects of cell senescence are overlaid on the genetic diathesis of particular alleles.

This extends our current understanding of disease. In atherogenesis, the usual suspects (hypertension, diabetes, hypercholesterolemia, tobacco use) remain indicted, but we now discern a ringleader behind the pathology. Cell senescence not only explains the anomalies (such as atherogenesis in progeric children, who lack the usual risk factors) but offers new and potentially profoundly more effective approaches to intervention. Just as tetanus was once "prevented" with hygiene and "treated" with wound cauterization, we prevent heart disease with diet, drugs, and behavioral change and treat heart disease with angioplasty, transplantation, and other procedures. An understanding of immunization allowed us to effectively prevent tetanus; an understanding of cell senescence would allow us to more effectively treat age-related disease.

Emerson once remarked that "old age seems the only disease, all others run into this one" (Beck, 1968), yet to some, the concept of aging as a disease is ludicrous (Hayflick, 1998c). We die of myocardial infarction, not of aging or high cholesterol. We die of cancer, not of aging or tobacco. None of us dies of aging, but of disease. The central question is not denotation (what is a disease?), but intervention (what can we do about clinical problems?). Should we replace atheromatous coronary arteries or lower the high cholesterol that underlies atherogenesis? Disease or not, high cholesterol is an independent variable whose manipulation can prevent disease. Risk factors may be superb therapeutic targets.

The same may be, a fortiori, true of cell senescence. It may be universal in age-related disease and without equal as a therapeutic target. Arguments about whether aging is a disease are disingenuous (Clarfield, 2003) and collateral. We don't question whether hypercholesterolemia is a disease but whether lowering cholesterol prevents atherosclerosis and death. The number of angels that can fit on the head of a pin is important only when our problems are caused by a glut of microangels.

In this context, the question of whether cell senescence causes aging is neither useful nor interesting. As in Talmudic tradition, there is more value in whether a medicine works, than in the underlying theory of why it works (Steinsaltz, 1976). Our goal is alleviating human suffering; all else is merely a tool to achieve this end. If the tool is optimal, so much the better, as we are more likely to succeed. Current therapy for atherosclerosis is partially effective, but there may be more effective, fundamental, and universal therapies. Does the role of cell senescence imply such a therapy?

Arterial endothelial cells and chondrocytes show telomere shortening, lung fibroblasts senesce, and senescent vascular, hormonal, or neural changes may lie behind a host of other age-related changes, such as sarcopenia. In each case, cell senescence does not contradict what we know of pathology but extends current theoretical underpinnings and implies tantalizing suggestions for novel interventions. In osteoarthritis, for example, the accumulated pressure stress upon cells within the joint result in increased cell loss, cell turnover, and hence cell senescence. That chondrocytes do, indeed, demonstrate senescence raises the question of what happens if we reset gene expression via telomerization. Would such joints gain a new lease on life, allowing cells to meet the needs imposed upon them? What of hepatic cirrhosis, coronary artery disease, and other pathology? We are on the verge of answering these questions (Hornsby, 2002).

Clinical interventions are legion, but some are more effective and operate at more fundamental levels than others. We might treat traumatic hemorrhage by continual transfusion, but prefer closing the disrupted vessel. Some interventions are not only more effective but more cost-effective. Treatment of tetanus 150 years ago was inadequate; treatment of current aging disease is likewise inadequate. As we improved our understanding of microbial disease, we achieved more effective interventions for tetanus. Broader and more fundamental understanding of age-related pathology may permit more effective (and cost-effective) therapy for age-related disease.

Aging is not theoretical, but tangible. An 87-year-old, asked if she would take a pill that would reverse aging, said "No, I'd let nature take it's course." Reminded about the scar on her chest (a coronary artery bypass graft), her swollen knuckles (arthritis for which she, ineffectively, took ibuprofen), and why was she in the hospital, she said, "I have pneumonia and need an antibiotic. Oh, wait a minute. . . . Forget what I said. I'd take the pill." Once there is potential for intervention (Kirkland, 2002), aging becomes a disease. In the second half of the book, we review aging in each tissue and organ, how normal cells behave in these structures, how they go awry, and the role that cell senescence may play. And in every case, we do so with an eye toward intervention.

CHAPTER 7

The Progerias

What They Are

In a book on cell senescence in human disease, it is negligent not to discuss progerias, yet from what perspective? Does cell senescence cause progerias? Do the progerias cause cell senescence? Are "progeroid syndromes" (Brown, 1995) related to cell senescence at all (Greally et al., 1992)? These echo older questions clinicians have asked regarding progerias, viz., do these diseases have anything to do with "real" aging (Reichel et al., 1971)? Shorn of sophistry, we don't know.

Progeric syndromes haunt us—conceptually enticing, they are clinically tragic reminders of our abiding and powerless ignorance. Few who have known a child with progeria are not struck with the certainty, however ineffable the defense, that progeria must have something to teach us about aging. Over the past two decades, we have come to realize that this intuition is at least partially correct. What they have to teach us appears largely within the domain of genetic function and cell senescence, hence their inclusion here.

Perhaps a dozen syndromes have been included over the past century within the rubric of progeria; only two—Werner and Hutchinson-Gilford—will be discussed here. Others (Neill and Dingwall, 1950; Martin, 1977c; Brown, 1995), such as Wiedemann-Rautenstrauch (Korniszewski et al., 2001), Donohue, Cockayne's (Cockayne, 1936), Down, Klinefelter, Seip, Rothmund (Thannhauser, 1945), Bloom, and Turner (and Ullrich-Turner) syndromes (Kveiborg et al., 2001a), ataxia telangiectasia, cervical lipodysplasia, myotonic dystrophy, acrogeria, metageria (Gilkes et al., 1974), acrometageria (De Groot et al., 1980; Greally et al., 1992), and other similar but poorly characterized cases (e.g., Ruvalcaba et al., 1977; Suter et al., 1982; Pallota and Morgese, 1984), as well as possible animal analogs for progeria (Pearce and Brown, 1960a, 1960b), will be largely ignored for no more reason than the space and time required for such discussion.

Werner syndrome (WS) is seen in adults; Hutchinson-Gilford is in children. Werner's patients typically die in their fifth decade; Hutchinson-Gilford children, early in their second decade. Both share the mask of aging. Whether these patients share other, deeper similarities, such as a common genetic instability (Martin and Oshima, 2000; Simbulan-Rosenthal et al., 2000), which will ultimately explain their course, remains uncertain. Progerics look old; they die of the diseases of old age. Despite this, neither is true aging; both have exceptions. Worse, each hides a series of diseases behind its eponym. Werner's is not one disease, but a collection of helicase alleles. Hutchinson-Gilford is probably not one progeria, but a set of syndromes that we are unable to tease apart (see Greally et al., 1992; Matsuo et al., 1994). Acrogeria (in which children retain head hair, lack the coronary risk, and live longer than progeric children) and metageria (representing a midground between pro- and metageria) may represent forme frustes of classic progeria or more limited, cell-line mosaic diseases (see below) than progeria. If we observe carefully and avoid preconceptions, each of the progerias probably has much to teach us about aging.

Werner Syndrome

Werner syndrome (Werner, 1904) is adult-onset progeria caused by a rare autosomal recessive inheritance (Faragher et al., 1993; Martin et al., 1999) of one of several mutant alleles of (Oshima et al., 1996b; Yu et al., 1997) a specific helicase gene (Yu et al., 1996). Bloom syndrome also displays an altered helicase (Ellis et al., 1995; Karow et al., 1997; Kaneko et al., 2001). The diagnosis of Werner's is usually made in the third decade (Epstein et al., 1977) with a mean age at death of 47 years. Growth retardation may be present during the second decade (Blau, 1962). Death is usually due to cardiovascular disease, although diabetes, cancer (10% incidence), and other less significant clinical problems, including poor wound healing, cataracts, gray hair, sarcopenia, osteoporosis, and hypogonadism, are common (Cohen and Shelley, 1963; Zalla, 1980; Brown, 1995). There are no predictable or uniform endocrine abnormalities; extensive endocrine examination can be normal (Samantray et al., 1971). The frequent cardiac pathology may not necessarily be accompanied by atherosclerosis, but may in some cases represent a primary cardiomyopathy (Tri and Combs, 1978). Alzheimer dementia is not typical. Patients show early onset of subtle immune changes (Nakao et al., 1980) typical of immune senescence (Goto et al., 1979, 1982), which might, along with the genetic abnormalities discussed below, explain the high malignancy rate in these patients (Tao et al., 1971; Kobayashi et al., 1980; Hrabko et al., 1982). Clinical observations suggest that Werner's is a form of premature aging (Epstein et al., 1965; Brown et al., 1985), or more aptly a segmental progeria (Faragher et al., 1993), in that only a limited subset of the normal findings of aging are observed (Herstone and Bower, 1944; Brown, 1995; Martin, 1997b). For example, risk for atherosclerosis is higher in Werner patients than age-matched normals, but lack a correspondingly increased risk for Alzheimer disease (Faragher et al., 1993).

Epidemiologically, these patients are scattered worldwide, although there are clusters of patients, as occurs in Japan (Epstein et al., 1977; Castro et al., 1999). A genetic basis was proposed early (Comfort, 1961) and was intimated by familial clustering (Boatwright et al., 1952) and existence of forme fruste types (Jacobson et al., 1960), but early work failed to find crude chromosomal abnormalities (Fraccaro et al., 1962; Learner et al., 1962; Motulsky et al., 1962). There has been dispute as to whether sister chromatid exchange rates are normal (Darlington et al., 1981) or increased (Elli et al., 1983).

The genetic defect in Werner syndrome (Yu et al., 1996) is an abnormal *WRN* gene in the RecQ family of DNA helicases (Moser et al., 1999; Mohaghegh and Hickson, 2002) mapped to chromosome 8 (Goto et al., 1992). In Werner patients (but not murine analogs), the helicase is found predominantly within the nucleolus (Marciniak et al., 1998). The *WRN* gene causes not only genetic (Gray et al., 1997; Balajee et al., 1999; Wang et al., 1999) and cellular (Gray et al., 1998) but clinical abnormalities of Werner syndrome, for example, myocardial infarction (Ye et al., 1997). Mouse models are available (Treuting et al., 2002) and *WRN* gene has been transfected into mice with results parallel to Werner's (Wang et al., 2000d). There are polymorphisms (Castro et al., 1999), each with variable risks of cardiovascular or other nominally age-related clinical outcomes. DNA synthesis is retarded in Werner syndrome (Goldstein, 1969; Martin et al., 1970; Tanaka et al., 1980), perhaps due to the helicase abnormality, although this has been ascribed directly to cell senescence (Fujiwara et al., 1977).

The known role of other RecQ helicases in DNA repair, coupled with unstable karyotype and a mutator phenotype of WS cells (Gahan and Middleton, 1984; Gebhart et al., 1988; Fukuchi et al., 1989), prompted suggestions that WS cells might have a defect in DNA repair (Huang et al., 1998), as do fibroblasts from Hutchinson-Gilford progerics (Brown et al., 1976, 1978). Hence, they accumulate DNA damage, perhaps inducing the early cell senescence seen in fibroblasts from Werner patients (Beckman and Ames, 1998; Kirkwood, 1999). Alternatively, the effect might make use of silencing proteins, as happens in yeast where mutation of the *SGS1* helicase gene alters Sir3 location from the telomere to the nucleolus (Guarente, 1997b; Sinclair et al., 1997). It has become clear that the SGS1 and WRN proteins play a role in telomere maintenance (Johnson et al., 2001a; Opresko et al., 2001; Orren et al., 2002), perhaps via TRF2 (Opresko et al., 2002; Stavropoulos et al., 2002). These may bind the G-quadruplex structure of the telomere or affect the ALT (non-telomerase) mechanism of telomere maintenance (Li et al., 2001).

In normal human fibroblasts, senescence is triggered by telomere shortening (Harley and Sherwood, 1997a; Bodnar et al., 1998; Counter et al., 1998a; Vaziri and Benchimol, 1998), without evidence of accumulated DNA damage, but the suggestion that this might be an independent path to (telomere shortening and hence) cell senescence remained viable. If so, telomerase should not affect senescence in WS cells. It was therefore surprising when forced telomerase expression (using an amphotropic retrovirus expressing hTERT) postponed (or perhaps even prevented) WS cell senescence (Wyllie et al., 2000) as it does in normal cells (Bodnar et al., 1998; Vaziri, 1998), although without fully resetting the mRNA expression pattern of those cells (Choi et al., 2001).

In normal humans, T lymphocytes retain the ability to up-regulate telomerase in response to proliferative stimuli. Since the T lymphocytes of Werner patients likewise up-regulate telomerase, then these lymphocytes should have approximately normal cellular lifespans, which they do. These finding have been claimed as support for the notion that *WRN* mutations affect telomere maintenance directly (James et al., 2001).

For example, a simple but not exclusive hypothesis is that *WRN* mutations lead to increased peritelomeric deletions, causing early cell senescence. Available results have prompted additional speculation regarding chromosomal mechanics and cell senescence (Hisama et al., 2000). For example, it is possible that helicases "activate" telomeres for extension by telomerase (Cech and Lingner, 1997). Another possibility is that the accelerated rate of telomere loss in Werner patients occurs because the helicase mutation causes a longer telomeric overhang. The length of overhang correlates directly with the rate of telomere loss per division (Huffman et al., 2000) and could effectively explain accelerated telomere shortening in Werner's. It is consistent with telomerase's efficacy in reversing accelerated cell senescence in these patients (Wyllie et al., 2000). Unfortunately, other than the potential effects of helicase, the factors regulating overhang length are relatively unexplored. Curiously, Werner B-lymphoblastoid reach senescence with a much wider variance among their telomere lengths than do corresponding normal cells (Tahara et al., 1997), suggesting that some additional factor beyond telomere length per se (perhaps the length of the telomeric overhang) precipitates senescence. Whatever the mechanism of helicase abnormalities, the telomerase results suggest that, were it technically feasible and with theoretical reservations, telomerase might have therapeutic potential in Werner syndrome (Choi et al., 2001).

In vitro fibroblasts from Werner patients senesce more rapidly than normal cells (Nakao et al., 1978, 1980). Though starting off with normal replicative ability, they soon fall behind. Normal fibroblasts typically have 60 population doublings, Werner fibroblasts, about 20 (Faragher et al., 1993). The accelerated senescence (Epstein et al., 1965; Holliday et al., 1974; Kill et al., 1994) has been linked to the clinical progeroid phenotype and the kinetics of this phenomenon have been explored. Current evidence (Faragher et al., 1997a) suggests that it is not an overexpression of senescence-specific proteins in Werner cells that triggers senescence. At each cell division, there might be an increased proportion of cells that stop cycling and become senescent compared to the far lower risk of turning senescent inherent in normal cells, which has been attributed to "unstable telomere dynamics" in these patients (Sugimoto, 1998). In keeping with these observations regarding cell senescence, telomere lengths at birth are comparable to normal lengths, but their rate of DNA base loss is accelerated.

Curiously, Werner syndrome appears to result less from the alteration of helicase than its lack of expression. Many of the mutated WRN proteins demonstrate helicase activity (Moser et al., 2000), but their expression is markedly impaired. The activity of the WRN promoter, whose absence of TATA and CAAT boxes suggests that it is a so-called constitutive promoter, is dramatically reduced in cells from these patients (Wang et al., 1998b). Cells from patients with Werner syndrome express reduced amounts of WRN protein and have reduced helicase activity (Moser et al., 2000).

Disruptions of cell function are diffuse and almost ubiquitous (Oppenheimer and Kugel, 1934; Boyd and Grant, 1959; Ishii and Hosoda, 1975). The altered c-fos regulation (Oshima et al., 1995; Yan et al., 1996), thermolabile enzymes (Brown and Darlington, 1980), calcium-dependent potassium currents (Faragher et al., 1997a), euploidization of hepatocytes (Gahan and Middleton, 1984), changes in isomerases (Tollefsbol et al., 1982), and excessive urinary excretion of hyaluronic acid (Kieras et al., 1986), as well as steroid metabolism (Bauer and Conn, 1953) are presumably (as with chromosomal instability; Gebhart et al., 1988) but not definitively linked to the known helicase abnormalities. Overall, these changes tend to parallel changes seen in normally senescent cells of similar phenotype and may reflect those changes in the pattern of gene expression that underlie normal cell senescence, albeit in an aberrant genetic context. In the same vein, the poor healing, postsurgical and otherwise (Jonas et al., 1987), observed in these patients may be linked to the actions of the helicase mutation, perhaps via their accelerated (though aberrant) cell senescence. As in the senescence occurring in normal cells, there is no evidence that the abnormalities found in Werner cells are the result of abnormal superoxide dismutase (CuZn or Mn forms), catalase, or glutathione peroxidase (Marklund et al., 1981).

A general model in which alterations in telomerase maintenance can be expected to result in the clinical syndrome has been proposed. Invocation of this model (Ostler et al., 2002), in which wrn-mediated, peritelomeric deletions affect replicative cell lifespan, explains telomerases correcting the abbreviated lifespan in Werner fibroblasts and the absence of such abbreviation in T cells (which separately up-regulate telomerase expression). Whatever the mechanisms and despite the likely differences between Werner and normal aging, the syndrome has considerable conceptual value as we try to understand the aging process (Goldstein and Singal, 1974; Holliday et al., 1974; Martin et al., 1999).

Hutchinson-Gilford Syndrome

Hutchinson-Gilford progeria, often simply called progeria (DeBusk, 1972, 1979), was first described by Hutchinson (1886) and then Gilford (1897). "Progeria," meaning early aging, was coined by Hutchinson (Gilford, 1904), relegating Werner syndrome to being merely "the adult-onset form." Since approximately 1950, the term *progeria* was applied to Hutchinson Gilford syndrome with some exclusivity (Gabr, 1954), although the spate of recent research on Werner syndrome has partially reversed this. Hutchinson-Gilford syndrome, here *progeria*, is presumptively inherited as a sporadic, autosomal dominant disease (Badame, 1989; Brown, 1992; but see Maciel, 1988; Khalifa, 1989), although the possibility of its being an autosomal recessive has received some limited support (Mostafa and Gabr, 1954; Goldstein and Moerman, 1978). Contrary claims notwithstanding (Bowles, 1998), there is no evidence of the helicase abnormality (Oshima et al., 1996a) now felt to define and underlie Werner syndrome. Although the genetic basis remains unknown, there is a slight correlation with elevated paternal age at conception (Jones et al., 1975; Brown, 1992), and several recent articles attempt to explain the etiology (De Sandre-Giovannoli et al., 2003; Lewis, 2003).

Epidemiologically, these children are predominantly found in developed nations, although this is likely due to increased survival, diagnosis, communication, and registry in developed nations with more extensive medical infrastructures. Although the incidence is estimated at one in eight million live births, the uncertainty caused by those cases which escape diagnosis and tabulation, especially in medically underdeveloped areas of the world, undermines the accuracy.

To those of us working with Hutchinson-Gilford children, the children appear so shockingly similar in body habitus and facies that most (researchers, clinicians, and family members alike) agree that they look like siblings (Fig. 7–1) (Mitchell and Goltman, 1940; Rosenthal et al., 1956). Children are typically diagnosed within the first few years of life (Gabr et al., 1960; Brown, 1995), though occasionally perinatally

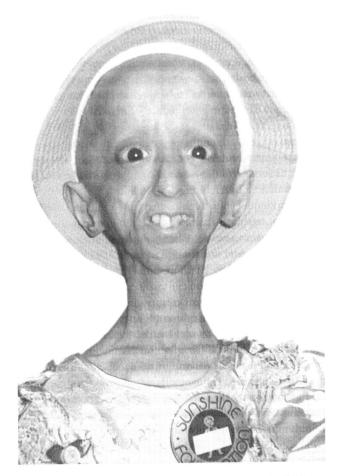

Figure 7–1 Progeric child (13-year-old Vietnamese child). Progeric children resemble other progerics (and an aging phenotype) more than those with similar ethnic, racial, or familial genotypes.

(Runge et al., 1978). Diagnosis is commonly triggered by a failure to thrive (Omar, 1982) and general growth retardation (Cooke, 1953) or as a result of the specific abnormalities described below. The disease mechanisms are presumptively operating prior to birth (Faivre et al., 1999) and at least five apparently neonatal cases have been reported (Zucchini et al., 1986; Rodriguez et al., 1999).

Progeric children die at a mean age of 12.7 years (Sephel et al., 1988). The maximum confirmed age at death was 21 (personal case observation). A few longer-lived (but likely not truly progeric) individuals have been reported in the literature (Ogihara et al., 1986; Corcoy et al., 1989; Parkash et al., 1990). Death is overwhelmingly due to atherosclerotic pathology (Baker et al., 1981) including disease in cardiac (Baldzhiev et al., 1984; Dyck et al., 1987), cerebrovascular (Meme et al., 1978; Naganuma et al., 1990), renal (Riedel, 1980), and other organs. Several tissues may demonstrate accelerated aging, including heart (Makous et al., 1962; Ha et al., 1993), central and peripheral arteries (Sivaraman et al., 1999), the skin (Badame, 1989; Gillar et al., 1991; Wollina et al., 1992), and eyes (Moehlig, 1946; Gupte, 1983; Iordanescu et al., 1995). Bones (Monu et al., 1990; Fernandez-Palazzi et al., 1992; Le et al., 1999a) demonstrate characteristic changes including early osteoporosis, osteolysis (Ozonoff and Clemett, 1967), dysplastic skeletal changes, avascular necrosis of the femoral capital epiphysis, and hip dislocation. Bone healing is markedly delayed (Moen, 1982). Some authors (Curtin and Kotzen, 1929; Gamble, 1984) report frequent joint problems; others (Moen, 1982) find stiffness, but suggest that joints are otherwise normal, and autopsy findings frequently support this (Rosenthal et al., 1956; Gabb et al., 1960). Progeric children are almost uniformly sarcopenic and bald, and have thin skin devoid of subcutaneous fat. Scalp (and frequently other) veins are prominent. Clinical concerns voiced by the parents are predictable and fairly uniform, including problems with skin, bones (and joints), teeth (too many in small jaws, often with permanent teeth crowding decidual teeth), and frequently hyperacusis and ocular photosensitivity. Poor healing, cardiovascular risks, and airway abnormalities can make these patients poorer surgical risks (Chapin and Kahre, 1979). The general underdevelopment of the lower face and particularly the jaw (micrognathism) has been repeatedly observed and confirmed by careful measurement (Rosenthal et al., 1956).

Despite the severity of their atherosclerotic disease, these children seldom display known risk factors, such as hypertension, diabetes, or tobacco use. Cholesterol is usually though not always (Rosenthal et al., 1956; Jyoti et al., 1981) normal. Subfractions have not been well explored: in one proband, high-density lipoprotein (HDL) was abnormally low (a known risk factor for atherosclerosis) compared to siblings and parents (Szamosi et al., 1984). Dietary restriction of saturated fats has been unsuccessfully attempted (MacNamara et al., 1970). Other sequelae of cardiovascular disease, such as aneurysms (Green, 1981), may have a higher incidence.

Curiously, some tissues may be relatively (or even completely) unaffected (Badame, 1989). The nervous system, for example, is not primarily affected, although cerebrovascular disease is common. Intelligence is normal (Atkins, 1954) or above normal, although subnormal intelligence has been reported (Moehlig, 1946). As with many rare genetic diseases, the mean and variance of intelligence may be typical for a cohort of children (with genetic errors unrelated to cortical development) whose diagnosis and reporting are skewed by having access to quality medical care. The immune system is likewise normal (but see Harjacek et al., 1990). There is no defect in HLA antigens or immune function. HLA expression and inheritance are normal and there is no association between HLA type and progeria (Brown et al., 1980). Malignancy (King et al., 1978), cataracts, and dementia are rare (Brown, 1995). As a segmental progeria, it is a useful but imperfect model of aging (Brown et al., 1980a; Brown, 1995). Many of the tissues affected in progeric children are known to display cell senescence during normal aging (Wolf and Pendergrass, 1999), including the immune system, lens (cataracts), and bones (osteopenia/osteoporosis). Cell phenotype–specific data are not available for progerics, although cells from progeric children have long been known to show abnormal in vitro growth and early senescence (Danes, 1971; Goldstein et al., 1975).

Standard laboratory studies are usually normal (Badame, 1989; Wisuthsarewong and Viravan, 1999) and offer little diagnostic aid. Although other suggestions have been offered (Goldstein, 1969; Singal and Goldstein, 1973), the only known diagnostic marker is elevated urinary hyaluronic acid (Tokunaga et al., 1978; Kieras et al., 1986; Zebrower et al., 1986a; Brown, 1992). The cause or implications of this elevation are unknown. Hyaluronic acid increases in normal aging, although not to the same degree seen in Hutchinson-Gilford or Werner syndromes (Zebrower et al., 1986b). Hyaluronic acid and hyaluronidase are both elevated in bladder cancer and are used as two of many potential diagnostic markers (Lokeshwar and Soloway, 2001). In progerics, elevated hyaluronic acid may reflect several possibilities: early hepatic senescence (Appel et al., 1979), vascular insufficiency (Feinberg and Beebe, 1983), a compensatory angiogenic response (Lokeshwar and Block, 2000) to vascular insufficiency, arthritic inflammation (Wollheim, 1999), or other unsuspected processes.

Despite early claims to the contrary (Gilford, 1913), hormonal levels are often normal (Plunkett et al., 1954) and, when abnormal, are not reliably diagnostic. Suggestions that testosterone might play a role in the pathology of progeria (Selye et al., 1963) are not supported. Growth hormone levels are normal, but insulin-like growth factor 1 (IGF-1) is below normal and there is decreased sensitivity to these factors in progeric and normally senescent cells (Harley et al., 1981). At least one case has been reported (Briata et al., 1991) of a progeric child with an absence of insulin receptors; insulin resistance is common (Rosenbloom et al., 1983). Although basal metabolic rates are higher than normal (Villee et al., 1969; Brown, 1992), progeric cells, like normal senescent cells, produce more lactate, consistent with higher energy demands or perhaps less efficient oxidative phosphorylation (Goldstein et al., 1982). The mitochondria may be structurally and bioenergetically adequate, but have altered morphology (Goldstein and Moerman, 1984) and decreased functional competence (Goldstein and Korczack, 1981). Progeric mitochondria are thinner and have more cystic blebs, apparently due to a weaker inner membrane. Osmophilic inclusions, particularly lipofuscin granules and autophagic vacuoles, are increased.

Trials of supplementary growth hormone have been undertaken. Brown (1992) found an initial increase in growth in two patients, although without other clinical improvement. He questioned the form of growth hormone available or possible interactive effects of hyaluronic acid in inhibiting angiogenesis. Other trials have been equally ineffective (Abdenur et al., 1997).

With the possible exception of urinary hyaluronate, diagnosis is clinical. Diagnosis is frequently questionable or arguably confused with other progeroid (or even nonprogeroid) syndromes (e.g., Ogihara et al., 1986; Corcoy et al., 1989; Parkash et al., 1990; Greally et al., 1992). The problem may lie in our propensity to define diseases as distinct entities, rather than as spectrums of pathology. Those accustomed to seeing Hutchinson-Gilford progeric patients occasionally find the diagnostic categories an ill fit for what is observed clinically. Discrepancies may be resolved by cellular or genetic data, but current diagnosis is largely by clinical recognizance.

Much is known about cellular dysfunctions in progeria, without corresponding clarity of mechanism. The most visible abnormalities are in skin. Histology shows an excessive network of abnormal dermal elastic fibers, with a thickened basement membrane (Colige et al., 1991b). Although the pattern of the collagen polypeptides is normal, elastin and collagen (especially type IV) synthesis are elevated (Colige et al., 1991b; Giro and Davidson, 1993; but see Sephel et al., 1988). Fibronectin, collagen (Maquart et al., 1988), and elastin (Davidson et al., 1995) show secretory increases and accumulate in the matrix. Tropoelastin production is elevated six- to ninefold at the protein and mRNA levels (Sephel et al., 1988). Glycoprotein accumulates in the dermal connective tissue, perhaps reflecting abnormal glycosylation (Clark and Weiss, 1993, 1995). Such data have prompted suggestions that progeria is, at least histologically, a "connective tissue disease" (Ishii, 1976).

Mitogenic responses to growth factors are diminished. Elastin response to tumor growth factor beta 1 (TGF-β1) is almost absent (Giro and Davidson, 1993). Progeric cells do not respond normally to epidermal growth factor (EGF), despite normal receptor affinities and numbers. Above 10 population doublings, progeric cells appear senescent and display a decline in collagen synthesis as well as total loss of further inhibition by EGF (Colige et al., 1991a). Responses of progeric cells to cell stimulation are typical of normal senescent cells (Chen et al., 1986). The changes found in lymphocytes and fibroblasts (Chapman et al., 1983), for example, parallel those seen in normal elderly patients. Hutchinson-Gilford fibroblasts constitutively (and abnormally) express platelet-derived growth factor (PDGF) A-chain mRNA and PDGF-AA homodimers and have an impaired response. The gene is neither amplified nor rearranged. While receptor numbers and autophosphorylation are normal, induction of c-fos mRNA is not (Winkles et al., 1990). Progeric fibroblasts from probands (but not parental controls) have increased expression of c-*myc*, a proto-oncogene. There is no amplification or translocation of the gene and expression of other proto-oncogenes is normal (Nakamura et al., 1988).

Within cells, protease activity is sharply decreased and sensitivity to trypsin-catalyzed hydrolysis increased. Suggestions that turnover is increased are supported by finding increased tropoelastin synthesis, without detectable change in net tropoelastin stores (Sephel et al., 1988). The cellular changes in isomerases (Tollefsbol et al., 1982), metalloproteinases, inflammatory responses, and connective tissue remodeling are similar in progeria and normal aging (Millis et al., 1992). Turnover abnormalities have prompted speculation that rapid accumulation of altered proteins might cause progeria (Prokofeva et al., 1982), although if so, it is not due to incorrect synthesis. Fidelity of protein synthesis is normal in progeric cells (Brown and Darlington, 1980; Harley et al., 1980; O'Brien et al., 1998), as in normal senescent cells (Wojtyk and Goldstein, 1980). This lack of defects in protein synthesis undercuts attempts to portray progeria as resulting from protein error accumulation, as in the error catastrophe theory.

Despite apparently normal capacities for net RNA production (e.g., type IV collagen and elastin messenger RNAs), most investigators (though not all; Sephel et al., 1988) find decreased net mRNAs (Colige et al., 1991b; O'Brien and Weiss, 1995). The serum-induced activity of CCAAT binding protein for thymidine kinase declines with population doublings and is absent in progeric cells (Pang et al., 1996). DNA repair decreases (Brown et al., 1978; Matsuo et al., 1994; Sugita et al., 1995), although whether this is primary or merely secondary is unknown (Epstein et al., 1973). Variance is large, but the finding is reliable and the difference diverges increasingly from normal cells as divisions accrue (Epstein et al., 1974). Despite early reports to the contrary (Regan and Setlow, 1974), lower DNA repair rates are not due to in vitro conditions (Brown et al., 1980b) and are reversed by coculturing with normal cells (Brown et al., 1976). The enhancement of DNA repair normally occurring prior to scheduled synthesis is absent in progeric cells and temporal control of DNA repair is impaired (Lipman et al., 1989). Ultraviolet-induced unscheduled DNA synthesis is decreased. Progeric cells are less capable of repairing ultraviolet excision damage and less than half as likely as normal cells to survive the damage (Wang et al., 1990, 1991). Some workers report that progeric cells are more easily damaged by gamma ray exposure than normal cells, although not as easily damaged as ataxia telangectasia cells (Arlett and Harcourt, 1980). Others find progeric cells to be just as capable of repairing gamma ray damage as normal cells, no increase in the rate of spontaneous or X-ray–induced chromosomal aberration, and normal polymerase function (Prokofeva et al., 1982). Perhaps as a consequence of DNA repair abnormalities, while the frequency of aneuploidy is normal in early passage progeric fibroblasts, it is markedly elevated (particularly in the X chromosome at interphase) in late-passage progeric fibroblasts (Mukherjee and Costello, 1998). Cell cycle regulation of base excision repair remains normal (Cool and Sirover, 1990).

Hutchinson-Gilford fibroblasts have the morphology and cellular responses characteristic of normal senescent cells (Chen et al., 1986; Winkles et al., 1990) and early senescence as assessed by replicative ability (Goldstein, 1969, 1990; Allsopp et al., 1992; Mukherjee and Costello, 1998). They demonstrate perhaps a third as many divisions as fibroblasts (Colige et al., 1991b). Like normal cells (Shay et al., 1993; Jha et al., 1998), both Hutchinson-Gilford and Werner fibroblasts are immortalized by SV40 transfection, normalizing DNA repair (Saito and Moses, 1991). Telomerase transfection, accomplishing the same end, immortalizes Werner fibroblasts (Ouellette et al., 2000b; Wyllie et al., 2000), but has not yet been attempted in Hutchinson-Gilford cells. If shortened telomeres play a role in progeria, it is ironic that one of the earliest articles (Gilford, 1913), predating the 1938 coinage of the word *telomere*, called progeria "ateleiosis."

As a segmental progeria, Hutchinson-Gilford progeria might be the result of segmental accelerated senescence of a limited number of cell phenotypes. Affected cells include dermal fibroblasts, arterial endothelial cells, chondrocytes, and perhaps other phenotypes. Unaffected cells should then include glial, neural, and lymphocytic cell lines, corresponding to the lack of clinical findings in these tissues. Unfortunately, available data focus on fibroblasts. While these cells show evidence of shorter telomeres (Allsopp et al., 1992) and correlative early cell senescence (Goldstein et al., 1983), dermal abnormalities are only a small part of Hutchinson-Gilford progeria.

It is true that progeric fibroblasts are less responsive to insulin than normal fibroblasts, as well as having more abundant tissue factor (a procoagulant), and this might contribute to progeric atherosclerosis (Goldstein and Harley, 1979). What of other relevant cell phenotypes? Parental concern (appropriately) and risk have prevented acquisition of arterial wall biopsies and the most clinically relevant cell phenotypes. Limited information is available on lymphocytes, although immunosenescence is not a feature of progeria and would not be expected to display abnormalities. Their telomere lengths and telomerase activities (from only two progerics) were predictably normal (Shay and Fossel, unpublished observations). Werner syndrome fibroblasts, but not lymphoblastoid cells, show an analogous but different distinction in their DNA mismatch repair. Lymphoblastoid cells have normal repair, whereas fibroblasts are deficient (Bennett et al., 1997). This parallel is intriguing, but perhaps serendipitous.

The data are consistent with Hutchinson-Gilford progeria originating as an epigenetic mosaicism: a defect in specific cell lines that occurs during fertilization or early prenatal development, altering telomere lengths and accelerating cell senescence. Beckwith-Wiedemann syndrome is epigenetic (albeit not a mosaic), raising the question of whether progeria might also be due to defective chromosomal methylation (Caspary et al., 1999; Tilghman, 2000). In progeria, however, the defect occurs only in specific cell lines (hence being a mosaic disease), such as skin fibroblasts and (presumptively) vascular endothelial cells, chondrocytes, osteoclasts, etc. Some cell lines—cardiac myocytes, for example—are not directly affected while other cell lines—leukocytes, hematopoetic stem cells, neurons, for example—are unaffected. This finding suggests accelerated senescence (extensive prenatal division?) in some cells but not others, probably due to nonhereditable (e.g., viral infection, toxic, etc) events affecting a few key cell lines. The alternative, a heritable, genetic abnormality, requires an alteration in telomere maintenance (through effects on gene expression or enzyme activity) occurring only in specific cell lines, perhaps triggered by differential gene expression in specific cell phenotypes. Affected cell lines—fibroblasts, vascular endothelial cells, etc.—may be more sensitive to altered telomere dynamics. A similar effect occurs in the tissue-specific pathology seen in early generations of telomerase-negative mice (Blasco et al., 1997a). In such (mTR–/–) mice, telomere lengths fall with each successive generation (Hande et al., 1999a), but even in the earliest generation we find defects in neural tube closure (Herrera et al., 1999a) as well as in highly proliferative tissues, affecting spermatogenesis and hematopoesis (Lee et al., 1998c). As discussed previously, tissue-specific defects might result from errors in resetting linkage and gene expression. Progeric cells may likewise display early cell senescence because of subtle errors in linkage position or inaccurate resetting of gene expression during fertilization.

A genetic etiology was recently supported by lamin-A defects in progeric children (De Sandre-Giovannoli et al., 2003; Eriksson et al., 2003). This finding may be misleading, however. Lamin-A defects cause nuclear envelope interruptions, partial chromatin extrusions, and gene silencing on such extrusions (De Sandre-Giovannoli et al., 2003), such as the string of three collagen genes at 1q32 (PRELP, Fibromodulin, Opticin), indirect outcomes which may underlie the Hutchinson-Gilford phenotype (Lewis, 2003). Here again, progeria may be epigenetic in etiology.

Whatever the etiology, progeria is mosaic in expression, affecting the onset, but not rate of cell senescence. Histologically, specific cell lines approach their replicative limits and senescence in early perinatal development. Clinically, progeric children display age-inappropriate pathology and die early in their second decade.

CHAPTER 8

The Skin

Structure and Overview

Skin integrity is critical; without it we die. Although we often ignore its importance, relegating it to the merely cosmetic, the error is brought home when skin fails. Third-degree
burns prevent most normal skin functions and, with a moderate percentage of total body
surface area affected, can be fatal. Death is usually due to infection or fluid and protein
losses. Burns are horrendously difficult to treat even in the best specialized burn units at
the start of this millennium. Skin is far more than a "bag that holds us together."

Although aging is far more insidious and subtle than an acute thermal injury, aging
nevertheless alters clinical skin function fundamentally and decisively. To characterize a concern for aging skin as petty cosmesis is inappropriate and betrays an unbe-
coming ignorance of pathology. Aging skin is not as dramatic or well publicized as
cancer or atherosclerosis, but nonetheless causes morbidity and mortality. Malignancy,
heart attacks, and strokes inflame our fear; decubitus ulcers, sepsis, hypothermic stress,
and poor healing remain quiet and anonymous bit-players in human suffering.

Though underappreciated, skin is publicly apparent. We see aging skin in grocery
store aisles, on television, and on the faces of our friends, even when we have no idea of
the corresponding states of their arteries, joints, or brains. Arterial aging is insidious
and may be expressed in varying clinical presentations (McDermott et al., 2001), but
too often becomes apparent with sudden, unforeseen disaster, such as myocardial infarction. Our skin lacks such misleadingly sudden disasters, but we see it obviously in
the mirror and watch its subtle progression.

The gross and microscopic anatomy of human skin has become known over several centuries and even at the ultrastructural level, skin histology (e.g., Bloom and

Fawcett, 1975), has been well characterized for more than a generation. The past several decades have shifted our focus down to the physiology, genetics, and complex cell–cell interactions of the skin. Skin is a continuous layer of external cells, but simplicity ends there. Normal skin is almost always more than a single sheet of identical cells. Corneal epithelium and fetal epidermis are simple layers of few cells (Griffith et al., 1999c), but normal skin consists of multiple layers with multiple distinct cell phenotypes, sophisticated intracellular interactions, and a plethora of "immigrant cells" (developmentally, as in neurons and melanocytes, or recurrently, as in mast cells) serving diverse and critical functions.

Even excluding glandular (sudoriparous, sebaceous, and mammary) and follicular structures, skin is sufficiently complex to require exposition. Its complexity reflects multiple functions. Ignoring excretion, skin provides mechanical protection, thermal regulation (as a passive barrier and an active regulatory system), sensory reception, and immune defense.

There are three basic layers. Outermost is the epidermis, composed almost exclusively of keratinocytes of ectodermal origin and forming a stratified squamous cell layer whose primary function might be characterized as gradual collective suicide in defense of the underlying dermis and body. These cells produce and accumulate keratin until the cell is nothing but a sheet of protein—much like a shingle—sloughed away in preference to loss of the living cells beneath it.

The underlying dermis is a more complex and busy layer, full of blood vessels and sensory organs, actively responding to and meeting environmental stresses and invasions. The major indigenous cell of the dermis, the fibroblast, is of mesenchymal origin. Dermis is a stratified columnar layer in which most of the vascular, immune, and sensory structures are located and it is in this layer (as contrasted with the simpler changes of the epidermis) that we see multiple and more demonstrable changes as human skin ages.

The deepest layer is more passive, made up of subcutaneous fat and loose collagen, and more concerned with insulation and holding us together structurally than with actively responding to the threats from the outside world. This loose connective and subcutaneous adipose tissue is followed in turn by deep fascia, periosteum, or mesenchymal tissues.

Together the skin (and the cornea) covers the entire external surface of the body. In the average adult, the skin has a surface area of slightly less than two square meters. It makes up approximately 16% of body weight, is capable of holding 25% of the body's blood supply (Balin et al., 1997), and axons of its sensory organs, which run to the spinal cord, form a substantial portion of the ascending tracts to the brain. Skin is not trivial functionally, nor is its dysfunction trivial as it ages.

Epidermis is characterized by renewal and loss in a gradient from the basal layers of proliferative keratinocytes, through a finely regulated transition of terminal differentiation, to dead, cornified, keratin-filled cells sloughed off approximately 28 days after initial division. Cells in the germinative, basal cell layer are generally locked in G0, but divide in response to cytokine stimulation (Peacocke et al., 1989). Cycle time and response to growth factor stimulation, such as epidermal growth factor (EGF) or keratinocyte growth factor (KGF), varies with body location (Liu et al., 1998), nutritional status, and age (Stanulis-Praeger and Gilchrest, 1986). Although keratinocytes make up more than 90% of the epidermal cells, melanocytes (2%–4% of cells), and

Langerhans cells (1%–2% of cells) are also present (Kaminer and Gilchrest, 1994). Keratinocytes serve as mechanical protection via production (of keratin) and division (by constant basal renewal and superficial sloughing). Melanocytes provide electromagnetic (especially ultraviolet) protection by producing melanin (Xu et al., 2000b) for keratinocytes (Bandyopadhyay et al., 2001). Photons (visible and ultraviolet) directly and indirectly (via free radical production) damage complex molecules. Blocking and absorbing photons, melanin decreases DNA and other damage in epidermal and dermal cells. This lowers the incidence of dysfunction in individual cells (which can be replaced) and the risk of malignant transformation that might kill the organism. Found in increased numbers in sun-exposed areas of skin, melanocytes decrease by 10%–20% per decade, independent of the degree of ultraviolet (UV) exposure among individuals or between exposed (e.g., hands) versus non-exposed (e.g., buttocks) skin. Langerhans cells provide initial and limited immune protection within the epidermis. Found especially in the perivascular areas of the underlying dermis, they recognize and present antigens to other immunocompetent cells.

The dermal–epidermal junction, between the dermis and epidermis, is no simple plane, no merely arbitrary boundary between two flat sheets of adherent cells. To the contrary, it is almost indecipherably corrugated. This junction, the "plane" along which blisters form and older skin sloughs free in minor trauma, is tightly held together in young, healthy skin by both cell–cell adhesion and an interdigitated architecture. The deeply rugose valleys and mountains form a landscape between epidermal and dermal cells preventing easy separation by shape, independent of adherence. The boundary is easily defined by function and distinctive staining in all ages. While separating easily in the elderly, it is almost impossible to force apart through shear stress in the young.

Dermis is an active layer, metabolically and functionally. It is complex, not only for its spectrum of indigenous cells but the wealth of adscititious cells and structures commuting through and often residing within this layer. Epidermis is well ordered, dermis is not. Although epidermal cells progress from a deep, proliferative layer to the superficial dead husks of keratinocytes, dermis lacks such terminal progression. It is a vital and active structure full of multiple types of cells, vascular structures, nerves, and an extracellular matrix consisting of collagen (synthesized by fibroblasts) and elastin fibers embedded in ground substance. Even the matrix is complex. Collagen comes in at least 11 different types (or more, especially if we include other species; e.g., Li et al., 1993), though always consisting of three separate chains of protein wound tightly together in fibrils, collectively forming collagen fibers. These form a jungle gym of structural elements throughout the dermis, binding apposing layers and constraining structures and cells within the dermis. Through the warp of collagen a weft of elastin is woven, adding flexibility and resilience just as collagen provides strength. Although apparently random, most collagen and elastin fibers imprecisely parallel the overlying surface, defining wrinkles and the preferred direction of surgical incision for optimal wound healing. The dermal–subcutaneous junction has no sharp frontier, either intellectually or histologically. Gradually, with vague interdigitation, dermis gives way to subcutaneous adipose tissue and deeper fascia, without a well-defined boundary.

Skin is not simply a set of local cells with local purposes but an encompassing organ with functional implications for distant cells and organs throughout the organism. Young epidermis is substantially invested with free nerve endings (sensory axons) that enter from the deep subcutaneous layers and ascend through dermis and arborize throughout epidermis, especially in deeper, germinative layers, providing information about light touch and pain. Free nerve endings are ubiquitous, while more specialized sensory structures, such as Pacinian corpuscles, Meissner's corpuscles, Ruffini endings, Krause end bulbs, Golgi-Mazzoni receptors, and Merkel's cells (Moll et al., 1984) are restricted to the dermis and deeper structures (Mather, 1985). The skin is likewise a major arena for immune defense, as a large portion of potential pathogens gain access through its layers. Skin is an organ for body temperature control. While subcutaneous adipose tissue is a passive insulator (and a caloric storage area, cushion, and dimorphic secondary sexual characteristic), its vascularity and regulated control of dermal capillary beds make it the major active player in body temperature regulation (Hardy and Bard, 1974). Above all, skin is a mechanical barrier, not only through its collagen and elastin webbing and its ability to sacrifice superficial cells, but through its permanent cellular elements and their adherence. Faced with tangential force, young skin stretches or abrades rather than separating.

Aging and Other Pathology

Many organs fail with age. Superficially, the problem of skin aging is not that it doesn't work, but that there isn't much of it. Old skin is thin. Skin appears to evaporate with age as subcutaneous fat disappears, cells become fewer, and layers grow thinner and more fragile.

Nonetheless, this observation is misleading. Epidermis, for example, maintains much of its thickness. Moreover, at the gross level we see redundant skin hanging in loose folds. Rather than having too little skin (in top-to-bottom thickness), from side to side, older skin elongates, becoming loose and inelastic, prompting plastic surgeons to cut away the apparent excess to regain youthful appearance. The critical problem of old skin is neither thinness nor redundance but loss of function. To a degree, this reflects aging in underlying tissues (Selmanowitz, 1977) upon which skin is dependent, such as muscles, bones, and especially deep vascular beds. Yet skin also ages intrinsically and independently of underlying tissue changes.

The failure of aging skin is ubiquitous. If cells should divide and replace others, they do so less frequently. If they are to provide melanin, they do so less effectively and less reliably. If they are to produce collagen, their production is deficient and defective. Glands become fewer and more erratic, hair follicles fail, capillary beds diminish (Kalaria, 1996; de la Torre, 1997; Bemben, 1998; Roffe, 1998) and vascular regulation becomes erratic (Kaminer and Gilchrest, 1994). In each case, to varying degrees and in different ways for each cell phenotype, aging skin cells fail in their cell-specific roles.

Young skin is a mechanical barrier and a tough protective layer—a characteristic lost progressively with age. Old skin becomes thin and tears easily. The loss of thickness is visible to the eye and confirmed by measurement. Each layer shares in this loss to some degree. At the cellular level, extensive changes occur, including decreased keratinocyte lifespan (i.e., from final division to sloughing). Young epidermis constantly turns over, as new cells move outward and slough. By the eighth decade, turnover time shrinks by approximately 50% (Kaminer and Gilchrest, 1994), paralleling epidermal thinning. Dermis changes in the same fashion, becoming thinner, more acellular, and more avascular (West et al., 1989). Perhaps the most striking finding however, and one with profound mechanical consequences, is the flattening of the epidermal–dermal junction. The loss of complexity of the dermal–epidermal junction is startling and explains the clinical observation that aging epidermis sloughs with only trivial tangential traction. With little impediment to lateral shear stress, the junction separates easily along a single smooth plane, allowing epidermis to separate from underlying dermis (Fig. 8–1). Once elastic and capable of resisting tangential forces, skin now transmits such force directly to this simplified and now poorly adherent junction. Large sheets of aging epidermis slide free with less and less force from increasingly minor events.

Other mechanical changes occur progressively with age and have clinical consequences (Gilchrest, 1990). Skin that once was thick and resistant now permits the easy transmission of axial forces to underlying vessels, resulting in ecchymosis as vessels tear and bleed. There is concomitant and significantly increased damage to deeper structures. Once cushioned by subcutaneous fat and thick dermis, bones now receive concentrated impacts, as do nerves, major arteries, and organs. The result is an increasing incidence of fractures, neuropathies, vascular injuries, and organ damage. We bruise, we injure underlying structures, and we lose protective epidermis wholesale with trivial forces.

Changes at the histological level are apparent, but changes within cells are at least as robust and underlie histological change. The major indigenous skin cells, fibroblasts and keratinocytes, show age-related population decrease, but are not alone. Melanocytes decrease, increasing UV damage, as well as malignant transformation, cell stress, and perhaps cell turnover in the dermis and epidermis (Herzberg and Dinehart, 1989), thus accelerating cell senescence (Smith et al., 2000a).

As melanocytes decrease, skin cells fall back upon cellular immune defense and intracellular repair. Unfortunately, cellular immunity is compromised. Langerhans cells decrease by as much as 40% with age (Rogers and Gilchrest, 1990), with a gradual loss of delayed sensitivity (Sunderkotter et al., 1997). Overall loss of immune function decreases skin immune surveillance, allowing tumor cells to survive in increasing numbers (Rogers and Gilchrest, 1990). Mast cells decrease by as much as 50%, further undercutting immune defenses (Kaminer and Gilchrest, 1994). Macrophages alter, becoming less effective (Sunderkotter et al., 1997). Coupled with a smaller capillary bed

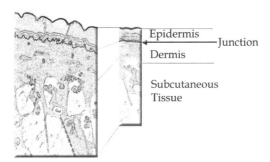

Figure 8–1 Aging skin. Histologically, older skin not only has thinner layers but a far less complex dermal–epidermal junction; interdigitations are absent, microbullae become common, and trivial force will separate the two layers.

(Kalaria, 1996; de la Torre, 1997; Bemben, 1998; Roffe, 1998), decreasing immune cell (e.g., T cell) access, age-related impairments jeopardize (and explain the failure of) immune function (Sunderkotter et al., 1997).

Skin cells change both numerically and functionally. Response to normal growth signals decreases, response to growth inhibitors increases. Stem cells of the basilar epidermis (Harle-Bachor and Boukamp, 1996) become less abundant (Michel et al., 1997). Keratinocytes have increasing mitochondrial dysfunction (Maftah et al., 1994). Fibroblast membrane composition alters, as does adhesion, extracellular matrix production, and secreted enzyme activities (Yaar and Gilchrest, 1990). Many studies have looked at baseline gene expression and changes in gene expression in response to stimuli. Fibroblasts and keratinocytes from older donors show limited or inappropriate responses to intercellular signals and environmental change (Yaar, 1995). For example, normal chronological and photoaging increase c-fos inducibility, while aging increases the baseline expression of SPR2 and interleukin-1 (Garmyn et al., 1992). Compared to neonatal keratinocytes, adult cells are less responsive to hypothalamus-derived mitogen KGF (200- vs. <75-fold cell number increase), as well as to KGF and EGFs in combination (Gilchrest, 1983a). Similar changes are typical in comparing young with old skin cells. Comparing responses to stimuli, many differences occur in cell protein production and gene expression (Gilchrest and Yaar, 1992). Proliferation-associated gene (*cdc2* and *E2F-1*) mRNAs are down-regulated in senescing keratinocytes, which express genes normally specific to differentiating squamous cells, such as cornifin (Saunders et al., 1993; Yaar et al., 1993). Response defects are probably not in signal reception but late in the response mechanism. Senescent human fibroblasts, for example, have impaired response to tumor necrosis factor (TNF), yet two to three times the receptors of younger fibroblasts, with identical affinities. Even activation of nuclear transcription factor (NF-κ B) is identical (Aggarwal et al., 1995).

While aging cells are apparently less careful in which genes they express and may appear to express phenotypically inappropriate genes, it is possible that this represents a teleologically intentional and appropriate response to other age-related changes in the cell and its environment. We cannot be sure whether aging is merely chaotic or an increasingly complex and unstable attempt at cellular homeostasis (Wright and Shay, 2002). Where hubris infers chaos, humility admits incomprehension.

Skin is not merely collected cells, but interdependent cells surrounded by specific and complex cell products. Matrix, largely an organic framework of protein products, shows progressive dysfunction in several parameters (Tan et al., 1993). Matrix is the product of the two basic metabolic variables defining turnover: an anabolic variable (synthesis) and a catabolic variable (degradation). Although equal in stable matrices, their linked rates (and hence turnover) may vary, altering the quality and makeup of the matrix protein pool (see Chapter 3). Even with a stable overall pool size, the composition may vary, one protein proportion rising, another falling correspondingly. Likewise, the percent of damaged proteins can vary. Pool size, while easier to measure, is an inadequate measure of function; it ignores protein proportions, percent damaged molecules, and turnover rates. Most known changes involve changing ratios and types of matrix proteins, particularly collagen (Tan et al., 1993).

Genes responsible for components of the extracellular matrix show alterations when comparing human keratinocytes and fibroblasts from donors of varying ages. Tan et al. (1993) used cells from individuals between 18 and 65 years of age and found that the older keratinocytes showed a four- to fivefold increase in the mRNA for type XVII collagen, although there was no observable change in the more common type IV collagen. Looking at fibroblasts from individuals between 17 and 74 years of age, they found that there were reliable age-related decreases in the expression of specific type I collagens. Likewise, younger cells were almost twice as responsive to a collagen promoter (TGF-β) than were cells from older donors, which expressed less intrinsic promoter. Although they drew cells from varying ages and "minimized the effects of in vitro cellular aging and senescence," the same effect has been seen in studies of in vitro senescence (see below).

Other matrix-related changes in gene expression have been observed. There is an increasing overexpression of tissue-type plasminogen activator (t-PA), whose activity should lead to progressive disruption of extracellular matrix maintenance (West et al., 1996). Moreover, in vitro, the senescent cells exhibit a more constitutive pattern of gene expression and are less responsive to environmental signals that should prompt altered gene expression. Specifically, senescent lung and skin cells show constant expression of urokinase-type plasminogen activator (u-PA) and plasminogen activator inhibitor-1 (PAI-1). In the face of serum deprivation, younger cells showed an appropriate decrease in their secretion of PAI-1 and in the resulting level of this inhibitor in the extracellular matrix pool. The authors suggest that fibroblast senescence "is associated with an altered expression of several genes regulating tissue maintenance that, in turn, could lead to degenerative changes in tissue in age-related disease(s)." A related problem with baseline gene expression in senescent dermal cells is seen not in the invariant but in the increased baseline expression of differentiation-associated SPR2 and interleukin 1 receptor antagonist (IL-1ra) genes, although the UV inducibility of these (and many other) genes apparently remains intact (Gilchrest et al., 1994).

A clear decline in the baseline expression, with potential problems for pool size and percentage of damaged proteins as a result of decreased turnover, is found in dermal collagen, the most prominent protein in dermal matrix. Among collagen's functions is providing anchoring fibrils, predominantly, if not exclusively, type VII collagen. Dermal fibroblasts show an age-dependent decrease in expression of their type VII collagen gene. Although expression is appropriately enhanced upon stimulation by transforming growth factor-beta (TGF-β), aging dermal cells have a decreased response to pro-inflammatory cytokines interleukin-1 beta (IL-1β) and TNF-α, which normally increases type VII collagen mRNA levels dose-dependently (Chen et al., 1994).

The age-related loss of the normal up-regulation of collagen synthesis in the face of inflammation could reasonably cause an overall decrease in the quantity of collagen within the matrix pool or an increased proportion of dysfunctional proteins within that pool. These two cytokines continue to cause elevated collagenase gene expression even in aging cells, supporting the first possibility. Moreover, baseline collagenase expression and collagenase in the matrix are elevated in aging cells. These effects are found in older cells in vivo (Burke et al., 1994) and in senescent cells in vitro (West et al., 1989). The impact of such changes in cellular response are likely manifold. Consider elastin alone, whose expression is modulated by multiple peptide growth factors, steroid hormones, and phorbol esters, including TGF-β, which acts as a post-transcriptional regulator (Davidson et al., 1995). Not only the synthesis of matrix proteins but the entire process of protein turnover is likely affected by tissue processes in aging skin. Inflammation might contribute to increased protein degradation, increased proportion of protein damage, or both effects. Collagen synthesis and degradation are affected by aging skin cells, with a lower rate of incorporation of new collagen paired with a higher rate of matrix degradation. Either outcome might contribute to age-related losses of normal dermal function, to observable age-related changes in dermal appearance, or to both.

The suggestion that the aging matrix is merely deficient in collagen or the result of increased "synthesis of adhesion molecules" (Giacomoni and Rein, 2001) drastically misrepresents the complexity of the situation. Not only are there fewer epidermal cells and a weakening of the intracellular matrix, but the character of the matrix changes. Even as the dermis shows an increase in the deposition of elastic fibers, there is a loss of the elasticity of those fibers: aging elastin is abnormal and dysfunctional. These changes are usually exacerbated by concomitant photoaging, in which there is hypertrophic repair, increased melanogenesis, collagen degeneration, and a twisted, dilated microvasculature (Gilchrest, 1996).

Clinical functions of skin result from of all of these. Poorer wound healing (Krohn, 1962), for example, is likely due to the relative dearth of cells, their poorer response to growth factors, slower rate of cell division, decrease in matrix, and gradual mechanical failure. Wound healing is slower and all phases are affected. Inflammatory and proliferative responses are delayed. Remodeling is less extensive and complete and collagen formed in older wounds is qualitatively different (Gerstein et al., 1993). Nor are these complex, intrinsic dermal changes the only cause of poorer wound healing. Increasing microvascular insufficiency and peripheral nerve loss (sympathetic and sensory) have been implicated as contributors (Khalil and Merhi, 2000). Not only is there an overall loss of capillary beds (Kalaria, 1996; de la Torre, 1997; Bemben, 1998; Roffe, 1998), but a striking impairment in vascular regulation (Kaminer and Gilchrest, 1994). As human skin ages, there is a substantial loss of such specialized sensory structures, whose population may decrease by two-thirds (Kaminer and Gilchrest, 1994). This loss of sensory input plays a possible role not only in wound healing but in the increased risk of inadvertent and unappreciated skin damage in older skin.

Not all changes are necessarily evident when averaged in a tissue comprising billions of cells. Although cells from neonatal, young, adult, and old skin may show a continuous spectrum of gradual change (often an unexpressed assumption), there may be sudden, quantal changes in individual aging cells, hidden in averaged data, frequently all that is available. Studies often extrapolate from neonatal versus mature or young versus old skin cells to aging tissues or vice versa, without regard for whether such comparisons are conceptually appropriate or justified by extant data. Some changes may represent gradual, generic aging changes, whereas others may pertain solely to individual cells or may be quantal, stochastic events. The interpretation of data on tissue aging in general, and skin aging in particular, may be warranted, but should be done with caution and a healthy degree of suspicion.

The Role of Cell Senescence

As the first of the chapters on aging organs, some prefatory comments are necessary regarding the role (and common misunderstandings of the role) of cell senescence in aging organs. Misconceptions abound. We might, for example, assume that the model implied that all cells, or an overwhelming percentage of cells, are senescent in old organs.

Neither assumption is supported by data. To the contrary, the model does not even imply that there are fully senescent cells in aging organs. There is substantial variability in the degree of senescence and few if any fully senescent cells, but a significant degree of altered gene expression within a percentage of partially senescent cells. The degree of alteration in gene expression, as we shall see, may be modest yet result in tissue dysfunction.

The critical requirement, if cell senescence is to play a role in aging organ function, is that a sufficient percentage of cells undergo alterations in gene expression sufficient to alter the function of the surrounding tissue. The key question, in an academic and a clinical sense, is whether the observed degree of cellular change can reasonably result in the observed degree of tissue dysfunction (Fig. 8–2).

A major consideration in tissue function, particularly in the function of dermal tissue, is the intracellular matrix. We must therefore address not only changes within cells but the resultant changes that occur among cells. As elsewhere, the dermal matrix comprises several protein pools, including elastin, several different collagen species, etc. And as in any protein pool, whether within a cell or in the matrix, the key question is the rate of protein turnover. As discussed above (Chapter 3) in some detail, it is the rate of protein turnover that critically determines the percentage of available proteins that have incurred damage in a given pool. Small changes in rate of turnover can have large effects in percentage of damaged proteins, even without change in protein pool size (see Chapter 3) or increased damage rate. In dermal aging, we must consider evidence not only for alterations in cell function, but for even minimal changes in production of exported cell proteins, such as collagen and elastin. With these caveats, we shall consider evidence for cell senescence in skin.

The question is not whether cell senescence occurs in vivo, for it does so, but to what extent in vivo cell senescence results in age-related pathology and changes—physiological and histological—that occur in aging skin. The ongoing senescence of dermal cells may be reflected in changes in gene expression and thereby cell function, but is cell senescence responsible for dermal aging or are the changes in gene expression merely appropriate secondary cellular responses to some other aging process occurring in dermal

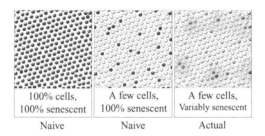

100% cells,	A few cells,	A few cells,
100% senescent	100% senescent	Variably senescent
Naive	Naive	Actual

Figure 8–2 Naive versus actual skin aging. A naive view of aging skin suggests that either all cells become totally senescent or even if only some skin cells are senescent they are totally senescent. This neglects both the gradual nature of senescence in cells as well as the interactive effects upon other cells. A realistic view suggests that a modicum of cells display varying degrees of senescent change. Senescence is not all-or-nothing histologically, nor in the individual cell, nor in secondary effects on other cells.

cells? While the known accumulation of senescent fibroblasts and keratinocytes in aging skin might cause compromise in function, such accumulating cells may have "long-range, pleiotropic effects—degradative enzymes, growth factors, and inflammatory cytokines" more central to explaining the loss of function in aging skin (Campisi, 1998b). These changes—the mere presence of senescent cells and alterations in gene expression that have long-range effects on an entire tissue—are worth consideration.

While gene expression changes with aging and age-related disease, mere iteration and confirmation do not address the question. Changes in gene expression may be secondary and appropriate responses to pathology rather than necessarily reflecting a fundamental process of aging. Similarly, the bald correlational finding of senescent cells in aging skin does not prove their etiology in any clinical outcome. Contrarily, however, a finding that only a minority of cells were senescent does not disprove the hypothesis that these dysfunctional cells drive dermal aging and are responsible for the age-related changes discussed above. Not surprisingly, the suggestion has been made that cell senescence may cause at least a portion of dermal aging (Yaar and Gilchrest, 1998), but do data support an even stronger and more conclusive statement?

If cell senescence and telomere maintenance are causally related to dermal aging (Roupe, 2001; Yaar and Gilchrest, 2001), we might expect pathology when these processes go awry. The possibility that cell senescence contributes to dermal aging is supported by work showing that telomere maintenance plays a role in the dermal pathology seen in several known diseases. Scleroderma patients, for example, have shortened telomeres and increased chromosomal instability, which correlates with the presence, though not the duration, of the disease (Artlett et al., 1996). Similarly, telomerase abnormalities in fibroblasts may underlie systemic sclerosis (Ohtsuka et al., 2002). Inappropriate or abnormal dermal cell senescence may be responsible for the altered cell and matrix function, resulting in the characteristic clinical outcome seen in these patients. Psoriasis patients, who are at increased risk of malignancy, particularly lymphoproliferative cancers (Margolis et al., 2001), might be predicted to have abnormal cell senescence. Keratinocytes taken from psoriatic plaques do have elevated telomerase levels (Nickoloff, 2001). Whether this is an explanation of or (more likely) a response to psoriatic pathology is unknown.

While elevated telomerase expression is found in chronic, radiation-induced skin ulcers (Zhao et al., 1999), this may be simply a normal and generic response of some cell lines to low-level radiation exposure (Finnon et al., 2000). The location of telomerase-expressing cells has been of considerable interest (Yasumoto et al., 1996). It is interesting to note that interventions (such as down-regulation of 14-3-3σ) associated with keratinocytes remaining within the stem cell compartment rather than becoming differentiated into stratified epithelia result in telomerase expression (Dellambra et al., 2000). While differentiated keratinocytes do not express telomerase (Lee et al., 2000a), the proliferative basal cells of the epidermis express telomerase (Harle-Bachor and Boukamp, 1996), presumably to allow indefinite cell division and replacement of the continually sloughing epidermal cells.

A more interesting pathological model, linking telomere shortening to human disease (Marciniak et al., 2000; Weng and Hodes, 2000; Ruggero et al., 2003), is dyskeratosis congenita (DKC). Patients with this rare genetic disease typically die of bone marrow failure or pulmonary complications. If we compare the different subtypes of DKC, the mean age at death correlates with the degree of residual telomerase function.

For example, patients with the most severe form, the dominant, X-linked form (who show approximately 20% of normal telomerase activity) have lifespans approximately 20% of the lifespans of unaffected individuals. Those with the recessive, autosomal form, with approximately 50% of normal telomerase activity, have lifespans approximately 50% of the lifespans of unaffected individuals. The disease is attributed to one of several missense mutations (Heiss et al., 2001) of the dyskerin gene (putatively a pseudouridine synthase), which interferes with normal telomerase subunit assembly and results in less hTR (Mitchell et al., 1999; Shay and Wright, 1999; Vulliamy et al., 2001a). Reduced telomerase and shortened telomeres (Vulliamy et al., 2001b; Alter, 2002) limit proliferative capacity of not merely rapidly dividing but specific somatic cell lines (Heiss et al., 2000), particularly hematopoetic stem cells, leukocytes, and epithelial cells (Shay and Wright, 1999; Vulliamy et al., 2001b). The predilection for these cell lines may explain the typical clinical findings of alopecia, nail dystrophy, abnormal skin color, precancerous cells in the mucous membranes, pulmonary fibrosis, GI abnormalities, high risk of skin cancer, fragile bones, and undeveloped testes. These patients make telomerase, but it is more unstable and ineffective in telomere maintenance. Dyskeratosis congenita leukocytes, for example, cannot maintain their telomere lengths and demonstrate an age-dependent increase in chromosomal rearrangements, such as fusions, dicentrics, Robertsonian translocations, and ring chromosomes. The telomerase dysfunction in DKC patients results not so much in early cell senescence as in telomerase instability and hence a "chromosomal instability syndrome" (Shay and Wright, 1999).

If cell senescence plays a role in normal dermal aging, then we might expect more subtle indications than those of genetic disease. Correlational evidence abounds for cell senescence in dermal aging. As expected, initial data showed that tissue-specific rates of telomere shortening occur in normal, aging skin cells (Lindsey et al., 1991; Nakamura et al., 2002a) and are significantly higher in rapidly dividing cells of the epidermis (mean 2.5 kb shorter) than in more slowly dividing cells of the underlying dermis (Wainwright et al., 1995). More recent work continues to support the conclusion that the telomeres of in vivo human keratinocytes taken from normal, healthy individuals shorten with advancing age (Matsui et al., 2000; Kang et al., 2002). Telomerase activity decreases with the age of dermal cell donor, as well as with serial passage of such cells in vitro (Kang et al., 1998; Matsui et al., 2000). Younger skin cells not only have longer telomeres, but are more likely to express telomerase. The epidermal basal cells from newborn foreskins, for example, express hTR at moderate levels. In sun-protected areas at least, most adult skin cells, however, do not express hTR. Epidermal basal cells from sun-exposed areas are more likely to show hTR expression, as do basal psoriatic cells, basal cells in patients with dermatitis, and in the proliferative cells of the anagen hair bulb (Ogoshi et al., 1998). Epidermal cells from sun-exposed areas are more likely to express hTERT (Ueda, 2000).

A recurrent question has been the percentage of senescent cells in aging skin and, even if it increases with age, if it can be sufficient to explain dermal aging. An extreme, and conceptually untenable, position is that since a percentage of nonsenescent skin cells are found in skin samples taken from even the most elderly patients, cell senescence can't play a role in dermal aging. The logical parallel is to argue that since a large percentage of perfectly normal cells are found in patients dying of cancer, malignancy can't play a role in cancer deaths. The arguments are parallel, but faulty logically and clinically.

The key theoretical question is not the *presence* of normal cells in aging skin, but the degree to which the *function* of the tissue is disrupted by senescent cells. Aging skin does have a significant and increasing percentage of senescent cells, but we must ask if such senescent cells can (and do) interfere with overall dermal function in a manner that can (and does) explain the clinical outcome.

The working hypothesis is that senescent keratinocytes and fibroblasts underlie the dermal changes and age-related pathology found clinically (Smith et al., 2000a). Dermal cell senescence results, in turn, from the repetitive, lifelong occurrence of cell division to replace losses due to quotidian, gross, and thermal trauma, UV exposure, infection, toxin exposure, and vascular insufficiency, among other factors. Testing this hypothesis is more difficult than might first appear. One approach is to show that senescing cells affect tissue function deleteriously and significantly, the other, to experimentally intervene in cell senescence with a resultant intervention in skin aging. As we shall see, both approaches have supportive experimental data.

Within the purview of the first approach are related issues. The major issues are to show that skin cells senesce in significant numbers, that such senescence is then accompanied by changes in cell function, and that such changes have a detrimental impact on skin, characteristic of clinical aging.

Although many tissues have cell phenotypes that exhibit little or no cell division, the skin is exposed to continual degradation and hence requires continual cell replacement. Such replacement is the province of dermal stem cells. Although most of the cells are telomerase negative, there is an actively dividing subset of hTERT-positive stem cells in the basal layer of the epithelium (Kolquist et al., 1998). Human basilar stem cells may transiently express telomerase at cell division (Ramirez et al., 1997; Shay and Bacchetti, 1997), thereby slowing telomere erosion and extending their cellular lifespan, in keeping with the need for dermal cells over a century or more. This expression is probably tightly controlled, but responds to extrinsic stimuli, such as EGF (Rea and Rice, 2001) and retinoic acid (You et al., 2000.

Hair follicles likewise demonstrate stem cells, in the bulge of the follicle. During anagen (active hair formation) phase, these cells repopulate the dermal papilla from which the hair strand grows, beginning the hair cycle (catagen, telogen, anagen) anew (Rusting, 2001). As in hematopoetic tissue, the reserve stem cells may define the lifespan during growth phases (Oshima et al., 2001). The follicle cells (not the reserve stem cells of the bulge) then senesce during the catagen phase, when there is no telomerase expression, even in the stem cells of the follicle. During the telogen phase, changes in the gene expression of the remaining, senescent follicle cells (Gupta and Fuchs, 1999; Fuchs and Segre, 2000) may prompt transient telomerase expression in the reserve stem cells (Ramirez et al., 1997). Curiously, such expression is more prominent in the bulb-containing fragment of the hair follicle than in the bulge area (the intermediate fragment where the stem cells are more common) or the gland-containing fragment of the follicle. Parenthetically, note that among progerics (but not acrogerics), whose dermal fibroblasts demonstrate short telomeres, baldness is almost universal (Fossel, personal observation).

Telomerase may be present (at least transiently) in basilar skin stem cells, but older skin has fewer stem cells and their decrease correlates with the number of cell divisions in culture (Michel et al., 1996). Telomerase expression is not sufficient to maintain length: telomere erosion continues to occur in these cells and, along with it, changes in gene expression. A priori, however, the attribution of such change is unclear and easily arguable. Barring data to the contrary, the existence of changes in gene expression with age does not automatically imply that cell senescence underlies these changes, nor that there is a functional relationship between the two processes. Other causes of aging might be equally (or even totally) responsible for altered gene expression.

Experimental data support the conclusion that cell senescence, and specifically changes in telomere length, drives such changes in gene expression. This conclusion derives from studies that measure patterns of gene expression before and after the insertion of an hTERT gene into human dermal fibroblasts (Shelton et al., 1999). If the senescence-associated pattern of gene expression is the product of changes in telomere length, then we must go further and ask how dermal aging in turn may be the product of changes in the patterns of gene expression.

The changes in gene expression during dermal aging are characteristic. Within aging human skin, there is an increase in the production of inflammatory factors (Shelton et al., 1999). There is an up-regulation of inflammatory genes and changes in the cellular response to inflammatory cytokines (Ly et al., 2000). Although there is down-regulation of many genes that regulate the cell cycle and cell division (Ly et al., 2000), there is constitutive expression of other cell cycle genes (Shelton et al., 1999). The inflammatory pattern, reminiscent of that seen in inflammatory wound repair, is typical of in vivo senescent human skin fibroblasts (as distinct from other cell phenotypes) and is found in vitro (Millis et al., 1992). This apparently differs from the in vivo pattern in chronic wound fibroblasts (Stephens et al., 2003). Additional aging changes, such as the predictable changes in elongation factors, energy metabolism, lipid turnover, are found, but, again, vary among cell phenotypes. The overall pattern for aging cells is one of diminished function and efficiency, but the specific pattern of senescence-associated gene expression varies among cells.

Gene expression changes in a specific and characteristic way in skin cells from aging donors. This is not to imply that there is a parallel and uniform change in the expression of every gene. To the contrary, while some genes may show increased expression and others a decline, the expression of certain genes may be unaltered by donor age. For example the expressions of TGF-α (Compton et al., 1995) or TGF-β 1 (Compton et al., 1994) show no pattern of decline with donor age. Other genes (*EPC-1*) may show nonlinear patterns of change, or alterations early in the donor lifespan (perhaps related to growth and maturation), but not during postmaturational aging (Tresini et al., 1999).

Many genes change expression with age, however, and these drive further changes in cell function. In keratinocytes from hair follicles taken from donors of varying ages, for example, glutathione reductase (GSSG-RD), glutathione-*S*-transferase (GSH-S-T), gamma-glutamyl transpeptidase (γ-GT), and glucose-6-phosphate dehydrogenase (G6PDH) decrease with age (Kermichi et al., 1990). There is a decrease in sensitivity to insulin-like growth factors in cells from old donors and in cells that senesce in vitro, as well as in cells from progeric fibroblasts (Harley et al., 1981). While a myriad of other changes occur during in vitro cell senescence (Younus and Gilchrest, 1992) and in cells from older donors, a few specific markers and altered patterns of gene expression deserve special attention in regard to cell senescence in the aging skin. Several cell and tissue-specific senescence–associated gene expression patterns have been characterized. Markers have been proposed—for example, monoclonal antibodies (SEN-1, SEN-2, and

SEN-3) specific to senescent human diploid fibroblasts were isolated and may help identify senescent epidermal keratinocytes and mammary epithelial cells (Porter et al., 1992).
The possible roles of p15, p16, p21, and p53 in keratinocyte senescence have been considered (Parkinson et al., 1997; Sayama et al., 1999). While some suggest that p16
(Loughran et al., 1996; Chaturvedi et al., 1999; Fuxe et al., 2000) or p21 (Kallassy et al.,
1998; Sayama et al., 1999) may be critical in cell senescence, others (Tunstead and
Hornsby, 1999) find that neither is unique, nor a useful marker. Indeed, it may be merely
an artifact of the feeder layer on which the cells are grown (Ramirez et al., 2001).

For better or worse, however, β-galactosidase has become a (relatively and perhaps arguably) specific marker for cell senescence (Dimri and Campisi, 1994a; Dimri
et al., 1995; Campisi, 1998b; Matsunaga et al., 1999a). Although β-galactosidase might
be an appropriate marker for senescence in human skin fibroblasts or even in retinal
pigmented epithelial cells, two naive usage errors are common.

The first mistake assumes that β-galactosidase is 100% specific and sensitive for
fibroblast senescence. It probably is neither (Severino et al., 2000). Part of the problem
is that it is such a good marker that we can identify β-galactosidase–positive cells among
a population of cells, some senescent and some probably not. That senescent tissue is a
mosaic of cells of different degrees of senescence (Mikhelson, 2001) leads some investigators to suggest that β-galactosidase is not a good marker because not all skin fibroblasts in aging skin are positive, but not all skin fibroblasts in aging skin are senescent.
β-galactosidase may not be a perfect marker for cell senescence (Yegorov et al., 1998),
but even if it were, it would show a mosaic of positive cells in aging skin. We should
not reasonably expect to find no staining (fetal skin?) or 100% staining of all cells. Experimental results are consistent with a sophisticated understanding of β-galactosidase
as a marker for cell senescence: it is a fairly accurate marker for senescence in individual human skin fibroblasts and useful as a marker for fibroblast cell senescence in
populations of human skin cells. Predictably, telomerase-expressing DS-1 cells do not
show significant β-galactosidase staining (Funk et al., 2000).

The second error extends β-galactosidase use to all cell phenotypes. Cells differ
and, almost by definition, their differences are caused by and associated with differences in gene expression. β-galactosidase is no exception. In cells that express
β-galactosidase constitutively (Yegorov et al., 1998) or even in non-fibroblast cell phenotypes that may increase their expression during cell senescence (Matsunaga et al., 1999a),
we cannot expect that expression should necessarily parallel those changes occurring
in senescing dermal fibroblasts. That β-galactosidase does not necessarily function as a
marker for senescence in all cell phenotypes does not detract from its usefulness as a
marker within specific cell phenotypes.

By extension, there are other markers that may work equally well (or far better) in
other cell phenotypes. As technical advances allow us to portray cells in terms of large-
scale gene arrays (King and Sinha, 2001), the appropriate question is no longer how a
specific marker changes with senescence, but how the pattern of gene expression changes
with aging. In the same sense that the array varies among cell phenotypes, so too does
the array vary as cells senesce and this change can be used to adequately characterize
senescence. Just as we can now define a cell's phenotype solely by its pattern of gene
expression, we could define senescence solely by the shifting pattern of gene expression for that cell phenotype. Done consciously and with due caution, the gene array may
change from our marker of senescence to our standard definition.

At issue, however, is not merely the panoply of changes in gene expression, but their putative effect upon tissue function. In short, do such changes have an impact on the dermal matrix, other cells, or dermal function? At the gross histological level, functional changes are attributable to gradual thinning. Senescent cells divide and differentiate more slowly, and their responses to intercellular signals changes (Koizumi and Ohkawara, 1996; Norsgaard et al., 1996). Human epidermal keratinocytes from older donors, for example, not only have a poor proliferative response to mitogens but an increased response to growth inhibitors, such as interferon (Peacocke et al., 1989). Fibroblasts show similar changes, becoming resistant to fibroblast growth factor due to post-receptor changes in the cellular response, specifically an impairment in tyrosine phosphorylation (Garfinkel et al., 1996). As cell senescence occurs, one result is a slower rate of cell replacement. Although cell "production" slows, cellular losses do not. A constant, perhaps accelerated, loss of cells occurs with age as dermal tissues become less functional. In humans, for example, sensory losses alone result in more accidental burns, abrasions, and pressure losses as aging progresses. As the balance of cell replacement and cell loss shifts, the result is a smaller population of dermal cells at any moment. Cells are fewer and tissues layers are thinner as aging occurs. This is evident in human skin and reflected in the long observed thinning of the epidermal, dermal, and subcutaneous fat layers in aging human skin.

But dermal aging is more complex than the mere thinning of major identifiable skin layers. At the microscopic and functional levels, there is a parallel reduction in rete ridges, vascularity, mast cell number and function, vitamin D production, dermal epidermal junction convolutions, Langerhans cells, healing rates, dermal epidermal adhesion, sensory receptors, heat conservation, and tear resistance. The dermal epidermal junction not only becomes less convoluted and less well bound, but the result is an increasing propensity toward bullae formation and sloughing along tissue planes with age. The decrease in stem cells may be an explanation for the slower rate of healing in older skin (Michel et al., 1996). Indeed, such cells gradually become less responsive to trophic factors, such as EGF, that stimulate telomerase activity and prevent the loss such cells from the stem cell compartment (Rea and Rice, 2001).

While melanocytes expressing hTERT maintain stable telomere lengths and have an extended replicative lifespan, normal melanocytes, like normal fibroblasts, show typical cell senescence. Telomere shortening triggers their replicative senescence. Although melanocytes and fibroblasts exhibit common changes during senescence (e.g., increased binding of cyclin-dependent kinase inhibitor [CDK-I] p16(INK4a) to CDK4, down-regulation of cyclin E protein and loss of cyclin E/CDK2 activity, underphosphorylation of retinoblastoma protein, and more E2F4-RB repressive complexes), there are characteristic differences between the two cell types. In senescent melanocytes, in contrast to senescent fibroblasts, CDK-Is p21(Waf-1) and p27(Kip-1) are down-regulated (Bandyopadhyay et al., 2001). With aging, there is poorer control of melanocyte division and localization, and melanocyte population diminishes by 10% to 20% per decade, accelerating UV damage to dermal cells. This last process is typical of the vicious cycle of damage within aging tissues: the diminution of one function causes an acceleration of cell damage and cell turnover, thereby accelerating cell senescence, which decreases cell function and so accelerates the initial problem.

Many changes are attributable not to having merely fewer cells but to changes in cellular function. Dermal fibroblasts not only senesce (Gilchrest, 1983b; Dimri et al.,

1995), but in vitro studies have shown clear constitutive overexpression of collagenase, stromolysin, and elastase (Grey and Norwood, 1995; Zeng and Millis, 1996), while metalloproteinases (TIMP 1 and TIMP 2) are reduced (Millis et al., 1992). Fibronectin is produced in a less effective, less adhesive form (Sorrentino and Millis, 1984), and proteoglycan synthesis decreases (Hubbard and Ozer, 1995) as does contractility (Bell et al., 1979), while cell permeability increases (Macieira-Coelho, 1983). The major components of the intercellular matrix, collagen and elastin, show "degeneration consistent with the overexpression of proteolytic activity" (West, 1994). Although altered synthesis and proteolysis may be responsible, likely the complete explanation is more complex. Senescent dermal fibroblasts may overexpress metalloproteinases, which may play a role (West, 1994), but there are likely other pertinent changes in gene expression. In vivo dermal fibroblasts from aging donors show changes in genes regulating collagen synthesis (Tan et al., 1993; Furth et al., 1997) and turnover (Chen et al., 1994), as well as changes in genes for other proteins that make up the extracellular matrix. In vitro, senescent fibroblasts show parallel changes (West et al., 1989; Martin et al., 1990; Choi et al., 1992), with increasing matrix degradation (Cristofalo et al., 1998b) and collagenase synthesis (Millis et al., 1989; West et al., 1996), as well as other changes in the expression of mRNAs encoding proteins involved in connective tissue remodeling (Millis et al., 1992).

Although a hodgepodge of data are consistent with cell senescence being responsible for dermal aging, no firm and proven data show this the most likely, let alone proven, explanation. As a hypothesis, it is elegant and consistent, but scarcely held down by the weight of careful arranged and inescapable data. Nonetheless, the hypothesis does receive additional support from a more direct approach.

While the hypothesis that cell senescence results in dermal aging can be approached by the consideration of observational data, it can, as mentioned initially in this section, be approached more forcefully by interventional experiments. Even without clarification of the intermediate mechanisms, we might directly intervene in cell senescence and observe the outcome. This has usually been accomplished using telomerase (e.g., transfection of an hTERT gene), which resets telomere length and hence cell senescence. Such an approach has thus far been done in vitro and ex vivo, but direct in vivo experiments are now technically feasible.

The first of the in vitro experiments was published in 1998 (Bodnar et al., 1998) and showed the clear mutability of cell senescence in human dermal (and other) fibroblasts. The study was immediately followed by other studies (e.g., Vaziri, 1998; Vaziri and Benchimol, 1998) that affirmed and extended these initial results. These results have been discussed in the first section of this book and do not, of themselves, speak to the issue raised here: does cell aging drive tissue aging?

While the in vitro results were crucial (and startling to many), the ex vivo approach comes closer to providing definitive support for the issue at hand. Human skin comprises two major indigenous cell phenotypes: keratinocytes and fibroblasts. Respectively, these cell types predominate in the epidermis and dermis, where they are accompanied by a variety of other indigenous cells (e.g., melanocytes, hair follicle cells, glandular cells) as well as cells of nondermal origin (e.g., lymphocytes and vascular endothelial cells).

In the key experiment (Funk et al., 2000), these two cell types were grown on an immune-compromised mouse. Using this model (Wang et al., 2000a; Casasco et al.,

2001), human keratinocytes and fibroblasts will routinely layer out over the course of 2 weeks and form an "organotypic human skin equivalent" that closely matches the normal human dermal architecture. This dermal tissue has many of the defining characteristics of human skin, such as an epidermal layer, a dermal layer, and dermal–epidermal interdigitations between these two layers.

Skin reconstitution from early-passage (20 population doublings) cells that had long telomeres demonstrated good adhesion, complex dermal–epidermal interdigitation, and good resistence to sheer stress. There were no microbullae or splitting between the two layers. These results were equivalent to results observed clinically in young skin.

Late-passage (85 population doublings) human dermal cells that had short telomeres showed poor dermal–epidermal adhesion, simplified interdigitations, and a high sensitivity to sheer stress. There was extensive splitting and blistering (microbullae) along this junction. These results are equivalent to results observed clinically in older skin.

If the same senescent cells are then transformed using an hTERT-expressing retrovirus and passaged an additional 20 population doublings beyond senescence, their telomeres relengthen and resultant skin reconstitution is again morphologically equivalent to young skin. At the ultrastructural level, the early-passage and transformed cells were equivalent, showing normal hemidesmosomes with filamentous connections from the epidermal cells to the dermal fibroblasts. Only in cells with relatively long telomeres and normal gene expression do we observe normal filamentous connections. Ultrastructural filament loss corresponds to increasing clinical instability along the dermal–epidermal tissue plane. Changes in gene expression in senescing cells correspond to tissue dysfunction in aging skin. While hTERT resets the dysfunctional gene expression, normalizing changes are not found in cells transformed with an hTERT-negative control retrovirus. Insertion of hTERT is the determining variable that results in morphologically young skin reconstitution.

Changes in gene expression paralleled the changes in dermal morphology, with a rough equivalence between measures of gene expression in young or transformed cells. For example, β-galactosidase expression increases with serial passage, but is not found in the hTERT-transformed cells. In the same model, DNA microarrays confirm that hTERT transformation resets gene expression to that characteristic of young (early-passage) cells (Shelton et al., 1999). Senescent fibroblasts show a relative overexpression of numerous genes, including those involved in cell cycle regulation, inflammation, matrix degradation, wound repair, and oxidative stress. Senescent fibroblasts likewise show a relative repression of genes involved with the deposition and maintenance of the extracellular matrix. In hTERT-transformed cells, the majority of markers showed a return to levels characteristic of early-passage cells. Most changes in gene expression associated with cell senescence are reset by hTERT expression. There are exceptions. While collagen production is restored to levels seen in young cells by hTERT expression, elastin production is not (Funk et al., 2000).

The exceptions beg an interesting question that remains unanswered—i.e., the reason for the failure of hTERT to reset all gene expression in these fibroblasts. One possibility is simply that senescence has caused immutable changes that cannot be undone by hTERT or by relengthening telomeres. A second possibility is that the degree of success depends on the degree of senescence. We might expect better results from mid-passage (50 population doublings) fibroblasts than those from late-passage (85 population doublings) fibroblasts. This recalls the issue raised in Chapter 3: is senescence an all-or-nothing or a gradual change in cell behavior? A third possibility is that just as gene expression may take time to occur, so too might resetting take time after hTERT activity begins. The additional 20 doublings after retroviral transformation used in this experiment might be insufficient to reset the pattern of gene expression, which took four times that long to induce. Some genes may reset, while others may require a longer time period or other additional stimuli. These results are in only a single cell phenotype and may not reflect results in endothelial, glial, or dozens of other cell phenotypes, each of major clinical concern. These experimental results are startling, yet much remains unclear regarding the degree to which hTERT can cause a reversion of gene expression in senescent cells and implications for tissue aging. At issue here is not merely the astonishing result and its explanation, but the implications for tissue aging and our approach to aging experimentation.

As in atherosclerosis, dermal aging is probably caused by several variables. One major contributor to dermal aging is photoaging. Photoaging is not a simple phenomenon and its cellular effects vary by location on the body (Bhawan et al., 1992). Nonetheless, as it contributes to dermal aging, we might expect it to contribute to (and be mediated by) cell senescence, which it does (Gilchrest, 1979; Gilchrest et al., 1983), perhaps through a process of reactive senescence (Faragher et al., 1997b). Photoaging, however, is not the only contributor to dermal aging. Additional causes include repetitive trauma such as shear forces, pressure, heat, infection, etc. Other factors play a role, including tobacco use, diabetes, and a host of genetic diseases. It is difficult (and probably unnecessary) to strictly distinguish local factors from vascular causes; likely there is enormous interaction between vascular aging and dermal aging. The cell senescence view of aging not only regards strict apportionment of such local and distant factors as unrealistic but further regards such interactive effects as the heart of the process. Aging, in any organ, dependents on not only local factors that drive cell senescence but bidirectional or multiple interactional effects between local and more distant cells and tissues.

The process does not stop at the genetic, intracellular, and intercellular levels. Culmination of the process is clinical dysfunction. At the gross level, the result is wrinkles, poor healing, decubiti, and heat loss. The result is universal, the cause subtle and poorly understood. It is not simply a matter of photoaging through UV exposure, nor is it mere trauma, toxic damage, or reactive oxygen species (ROS) production. It is not even solely the shortening of telomeres, the slowing of cell division, the alteration of gene expression, or some other single factor. However defined or understood, though, the practical question remains: can it be altered? In a sense, there are already a multitude of therapies to slow skin aging or hide its outcomes. Entire commercial ventures are founded on no more than retinoids, face lifts, moisturizers, sun blocks, and similar approaches to avoiding the tread of time. But is there evidence that we can intervene in this process at a more fundamental level?

Intervention

Many regard aging skin as a merely cosmetic issue, in which wrinkles become evident. Vast amounts of money are applied to modify superficial appearance to appease social vanity. Surprisingly to many, aging skin can result in mortality, usually via infection, ulceration, or heat loss. Our understanding of the pathology of ulceration in aging skin is imperfect, as is our ability to prevent and treat such disease (Thomas, 2001).

Skin aging is a significant problem in the aging population and often manifested in poor (or non-) healing of lacerations, infected (and occasionally fatal) decubitus ulcers, an increasing risk of infection, and poorer thermal homeostasis. Skin becomes a less effective barrier to trauma, heat loss, microbes, and other assaults. We may predict which patients may succumb to the problems of skin aging, such as pressure ulcers (Allman, 2001; Berlowitz et al., 2001; Margolis et al., 2002), but have surprisingly little to offer as a clinical intervention. Caloric restriction, at least in mice, is effective in slowing senescence in dermal fibroblasts (Pendergrass et al., 1995), although normalization of the diet may be necessary to translate such effects into improved skin healing (Reed et al., 1996).

Our current interventions to slow the course of dermal aging are less than impressive. Despite claims (and fervent wishes) to the contrary, optimal diet, exercise, topical agents, vitamin and other dietary supplements, and sun screens may at best delay (Perricone, 2000) but do not prevent skin aging. Dermal aging is not the same as photoaging (Yaar and Gilchrest, 1998) and their patterns of gene expression differ (Garmyn et al., 1995), but photoaging does accelerate dermal aging and is probably responsible for many visible changes. Efforts directed at preventing dermal aging should deal with photoaging (Gilchrest, 1996; Griffiths, 1999). The use of sun screens against the near (UVA) and far (UVB) ultraviolet spectrum are the first line of defense against skin aging and our only effective clinical intervention in this area.

For skin already aged, current interventions include antioxidants, α-hydroxy acids, or topical retinoids, which may have some effect on wrinkles and other markers of dermal aging. Retinoids, and perhaps retinol or tretinoin (all-*trans* retinoic acid) in particular, have beneficial effects on photoaged skin and may slow or prevent photoaging (Gilchrest, 1997; Griffiths, 1999), but prophylactic dietary supplementation with tocopherols does not (Werninghaus et al., 1994) and retinol may increase the risk of osteoporosis (Denke, 2002; Feskanich et al., 2002). Nonetheless, in multicenter, double-blind trials, tretinoin improved photodamaged skin within 4–6 months of daily use. Histologically, long-term use results in "reconstitution of the rete pegs, repair of keratinocyte ultrastructural damage, more even distribution of melanocytes and melanin pigment, deposition of new papillary dermal collagen, and improvements in vasculature" (Gilchrist, 1996). Retinoic acid has been shown to maintain telomerase activity in human oral keratinocytes (You et al., 2000). Although the effects on telomerase are unknown, similar clinical results, if less impressive and substantiated, are seen with α-hydroxy acid therapy (Gilchrest, 1996).

Botulinum toxin (Botox) has achieved recent notoriety solely for its apparent effect: the reduction of skin folds due to the paralysis of the facial muscles that underlie such folds (Medical Letter, 2002). Glabellar, nasolabial, and frontal folds, for example, are due to the basal tone of subcutaneous facial muscles that draw on multiple diffuse fibrous attachments to the overlying dermal tissue. The paralysis of such muscles results in the relaxation of major planes of the face, easing the visible valleys we associate with aging, the result of habitual facial expression. Although there is a prominent and growing market for the cosmetic use of botulinum toxin, no data support any benefit of this intervention for dermal health or aging. Caveats notwithstanding, however, the public responds better to cosmetic than functional concerns. Arch attempts to condemn the preference are jejune and unprofitable.

As skin, like other organs, has repair ability, merely preventing further UV exposure may be enough to promote repair (Gilchrest, 1996). Nonetheless, healing decreases markedly with age. Our approaches to optimizing wound healing, especially in the elderly, are largely unchanged from those of a century ago. Perhaps the only truly novel addition to our armamentarium is growth factors, although the clinical trials have so far been disappointing (Bello and Phillips, 2000).

Cell senescence is likely to play a central role in skin aging, and approaches that intervene directly in this process have considerable promise. Although current supportive data are circumstantial and clinical potential difficult to predict (Deveci, 1999), the initial work using telomerase to intervene in dermal aging has been impressive. The earliest, in vitro work showed that dermal fibroblasts can be prevented from senescing by using hTERT transfection (Bodnar et al., 1998). More recent work has used an ex vivo model, in which human fibroblasts and keratinocytes reconstitute dermal tissue on an immunocompromised mouse. Senescent cells, transformed with hTERT by a retroviral vector, will reconstitute what may be histologically (Funk et al., 2000) and genetically (Shelton et al., 1999) young human skin. These experiments offer considerable support for the value of intervention in cell senescence as a potentially effective intervention in dermal aging, but by no means prove clinical efficacy. Contradictory data (Stephens et al., 2003), in which researchers "reversed the senescent cellular phenotype," resulted in cells with "inhibit[ed] extracellular matrix reorganizational ability, attachment, and matrix metalloproteinase production and . . . impaired key wound healing properties": the authors predict that telomerase would be ineffective in treating chronic wounds. Data can scarcely argue that reversal of senescent phenotype is ineffective if not actually accomplished.

Nevertheless, difficulties are substantial, including practical and theoretical issues. We are only marginally capable of transfecting the telomerase (or any) gene into an in vivo model. Likewise, we could scarcely treat an experimental subject by removing their skin and then replant transfected autologous or homologous skin cells. The costs of sufficient gene production are high, the delivery mechanism uncertain, and our ability to treat large areas of skin only theoretical. Moreover, even if telomerase induction were sufficient to prevent (or to an extent reverse) cell senescence in some cellular components of the skin, such as dermal fibroblasts, the effect may not carry over into other equally important dermal cells. While fibroblasts have been immortalized by induction of telomerase expression and, despite occasional claims to the contrary (MacKenzie et al., 2000), may have indefinite lifespans with otherwise normal cell function (Bodnar et al., 1998; Jiang et al., 1999), some groups (Dickson et al., 2000; McDougall, 2001) have claimed that keratinocytes (along with mammary epithelial cells) are not immortalized by hTERT induction alone, but require an additional abrogation of the p16(INK4a) cell cycle control mechanism and perhaps employ the ALT mechanism for telomere maintenance (Stoppler et al., 1997; Opitz et al., 2001; Reddel, 2001; Rheinwald et al., 2002; Tsutsui et al., 2002). Paralleling this observation, down-regulation of 14-3-3σ (specifically expressed in human stratified epithelial cells) prevents keratinocyte differentiation and reserves these cells to the keratinocyte stem cell compartment. These cells escape replicative senescence and maintain telomerase activity, and show a down-regulation of the *p16(INK4a)* tumor suppressor gene (Dellambra et al., 2000). Whether this down-regulation is required, however, is not clear.

The suggestion that *p16(INK4a)* is required for keratinocyte immortalization may prove merely artifactual (Ramirez et al., 2001) or simply one of several ways of inducing hTERT (Oh et al., 2001b; Sashiyama et al., 2001; Veldman et al., 2001), yet the principle remains: an effective therapeutic intervention might require not only hTERT (Harle-Bachor and Boukamp, 1996; Guo et al., 1998; Liu et al., 2000a; Fujimoto et al., 2001) but perhaps also other additional and independent mechanisms (Farwell et al., 2000). Clinical use of hTERT might have drawbacks, including carcinogenesis (see Chapter 5), inadequate keratinocyte differentiation (Alani et al., 1999), inadequate "rescue" (Kanzaki et al., 2002), or other unexpected consequences. Even if we overcome the difficulties and find minimal drawbacks, skin is not an isolated tissue. It depends on the function of other tissues, including investing vascular trees and nerve branches. It will avail little if we renormalize keratinocyte and fibroblast cells, while vascular and neurological function remains impaired.

A final parenthetical observation must be made regarding baldness, particularly male pattern baldness, if for no other reason than aging men find the issue important. There is no firm, and little suggestive, evidence that male pattern baldness is even partially attributable to cell senescence. Testosterone, to the contrary, has excellent support, in terms of observational and interventional data, as a major (though perhaps only a permissive) cause of male pattern baldness. Nonetheless, the observations on progeric children, as well as what data we have on cell senescence and telomerase expression in human follicles (Ramirez et al., 1997), might reasonably serve as suggestive support for cell senescence, perhaps driven or triggered by the integral of lifetime testosterone exposure. Absent data, intuition suggests that telomerase intervention might be effective in restoring hair growth in elderly males.

In our venue, baldness has another, strictly analogical value. One of the major conceptual mistakes, stressed repeatedly throughout this text, is to consider aging as strictly a matter of wear and tear, instead of the failure of the cells to maintain themselves in the face of wear and tear. Consider the analogy to baldness. Baldness is not simply a matter of losing hair because of wear and tear. Hair does not abrade away. Brushing hair or wearing a hat does not cause baldness, despite the repeated wear and tear involved in these actions. Wear and tear may remove individual hairs, but does not cause baldness. To the contrary, baldness is a failure to adequately maintain hair growth (anagen) to compensate for hair loss. Even then, the competition is not between anagen and trauma, but between anagen and catagen. Baldness, like aging, occurs because changes in gene expression undermine the ability to maintain the status quo, and not merely because of wear and tear. We do not stop growing hair because we become bald, we become bald because we stop growing hair. And we do not fail because we age, we age because we fail.

Despite the obstacles and potential risks, the results of intervention in skin cell senescence are startling and clinically intriguing. They firmly support the hypothesis that cell senescence underlies aging and that aging is clinically modifiable. Initial work suggests that our knowledge of cell senescence in aging can be translated into clinical interventions for aging and age-related disease.

CHAPTER 9

Cardiovascular System

Structure and Overview

Most deaths worldwide are the result of vascular aging (Mehta and Yusuf, 2000). Only a century ago, this statement was true of only developed nations, while death due to infectious disease led in undeveloped nations. By the end of the millennium, however, cancer and vascular pathology had become the two leading causes of death in almost all nations, developed or otherwise. Where once we died young of infection (Yoshikawa, 2001), we now die in old age of atherosclerosis and cancer.

Although myocardial infarction is among the most common causes of death (and has a 25% mortality rate per event; Mehta and Yusuf, 2000), the myocardium is seldom the primary pathology. Myocardium is usually healthy barring insufficient coronary artery flow. The primary pathology is arterial vessels, usually relatively obstructed prior to the acute event. The event is often precipitated by a thrombotic "plug" of the diseased vessel, critical to continued survival of the pathologically innocent heart muscle. As we shall see, the origin of most vessel pathology is, in turn, attributable to changes in the endothelial cells that line atherosclerotic vessels.

The heart is a large, muscular, cycling pump with four chambers controlled by humeral, nervous, and local pacer-cell inputs, and supplied by major arterial vessels. The right atrium accepts the initial venous return from the body and passes it through a one-way valve (the tricuspid) into the right ventricle that then pumps blood through another one-way valve (the pulmonary valve) to the lungs for oxygenation. The left atrium accepts blood back from the lungs, passes it through a one-way valve (the mitral) into the left ventricle that then pumps it through another one-way valve (the aortic) to the entire body, exclusive of the lungs. The left ventricle is, understandably, the most muscular chamber of the heart and, perhaps because of its importance, the site of most fatal myocardial infarctions. It receives its only blood supply not directly from the blood in its chamber, but through two coronary arteries that branch from the aorta immediately beyond the aortic valve and that provide flow to the entire heart muscle only during diastole. These two major coronary arteries divide into smaller supplying branches and are the vessels replaced surgically when patients undergo coronary artery bypass grafts because of atherosclerotic coronary artery disease. As the left ventricle contracts (systole), blood flows throughout the vascular bed of the body. Its flow and pressure are further controlled by the pressure of the (non-coronary) vessel walls, supplied by muscular and elastic elements.

The thickness and complexity of an arterial wall correlate with the luminal area. The aortic wall is thick and complex; capillary walls are thin and simple. Where the aorta may have thousands of cells and tough, fibrous layers for strength and elasticity, the capillary wall may have only individual endothelial cells with a single, flattened layer of external pericytes (Carmeliet, 2000). The area of this endothelial surface is estimated at 1000 square meters in the adult human (Muller and Griesmacher, 2000). The aorta is classically considered as having three layers: the innermost endothelial layer, smooth muscle layer, and outer fibrous layer. The predominant respective cells in each layer are, predictably, endothelial cells, smooth muscle cells, and fibrocytes. Elastin and collagen fibers are found throughout the outer layers, but especially between layers. Such layers, particularly of elastin, are particularly prominent in large arteries, such as the aorta, and less prominent in smaller vessels. In the young adult, this elastic property of large vessels allows them to distend during systole and rebound during diastole. This enforces a more constant and less episodic blood flow despite sudden surges of systolic blood from the heart. The rheologic "smoothing effect" of elastin in young arteries lessens the sudden acceleration/deceleration shear forces that stress the endothelial cells lining the arteries. More distant, smaller arteries are less elastic, but more muscular and adjust the blood pressure as well as the differential flow to specific organs. The smallest arteries, the arterioles, have the greatest integral volume, surface area, and (consequently) friction to blood flow. This friction serves as the greatest factor in maintaining normal blood pressure (Bloom and Fawcett, 1975).

Although arteriolar pathology may play a defining role in age-related disease in many peripheral organs, especially muscles (McDermott et al., 2001), major pathology occurs in the large vessels, especially the aorta and coronary arteries. It is appropriate to focus on their anatomy rather than anatomy of the far smaller and far more numerous arteries of the body. The aorta and coronary arteries are thick, although less so in proportion to their luminal area than are the smaller, more muscular arteries. The innermost endothelial layer comprises a continuous sheet of polygonal cells with no clear directional orientation. Beneath (centrifugal to) these cells lies the intermediate layer, largely composed of elastin fibers, collagen fibers, fibroblasts, and smooth muscle cells. Normally, the smooth muscle cells are flattened, branched, and arranged circumferentially. The outermost layer is thin, comprising mostly fibroblasts and collagen matrix.

Aging and Other Pathology

Three centuries ago, the English physician Thomas Sydenham (1624–1689) observed that "a man is as old as his arteries" (Brallier, 1993). Although the most apparent cardiovascular change is atherosclerosis (in large elastic and small peripheral arteries), other changes contribute to morbidity and mortality. These include the loss of arterial wall elasticity, causing greater work for the heart and consequent hypertrophy and failure (Lakatta, 1994), as well as changes in shear stress (and shear stress fluctuation) on arterial endothelial cells (Kohara et al., 2000). In addition, there is a loss of volume, complexity, and function of the capillary beds in end-organs (Kalaria, 1996; de la Torre, 1997; Bemben, 1998; Roffe, 1998), as well as changes in endothelial cells lining such capillaries (see below). Peripheral arterial disease, resulting from atherosclerosis, is common in many older patients (Ouriel, 2001), especially those with concomitant large-vessel disease, though fine-vessel disease is often unsuspected, undiagnosed, and untreated (Hirsch et al., 2001). Age is an independent risk factor for peripheral arterial changes and resulting clinical diseases that incur substantial morbidity and mortality (Ness et al., 2000a). The extent to which such a decreased capillary supply might cause end-organ pathology is addressed in specific chapters dealing with each organ.

Frank ischemia and infarction are only one type of pathology that occurs in end-organs. Although myocardial infarctions and aneurysms are the more dramatic, congestive heart failure is the more common clinical diagnosis, with significant morbidity and mortality (Martins et al., 2001b) and arguable intervention (Nohria et al., 2002; Poole-Wilson, 2002). Congestive heart failure is the result of the heart's inability to pump sufficient blood for the body's requirements. While failure can result from mechanical cardiac dysfunction (e.g., valvular dysfunction), our interest lies in the archetypical failure of myocardial tissue. We know much about the progression from tissue failure, through cardiac hypertrophy (Lewis, 2001), to the classic clinical stigmata of failure (Mercadier, 2000), and our diagnostic acumen is improving (Morrison et al., 2002). Although the loss of functional myocytes is the common denominator of clinical heart failure, our knowledge of the factors that prompt this loss is imperfect at best (Rubin, 2000). The pathophysiology of this failure is assumed to be the result of intracellular changes in the cardiac myocytes, often attributed to changes in gene expression (Hwang et al., 2001a), especially inflammatory changes, and mast cell function particularly (Hara et al., 2002), or mitochondrial dysfunction (Guertl et al., 2000). In turn, this is assumed to result from external factors, including humoral (Cody, 2000), neural (Colucci, 2000), or mechanical signals (Carabello, 2000; LeWinter et al., 2000; Sharpe, 2000) and ischemic damage (Weber and Sun 2000). Independent of disease, the aging cardiomyocyte undergoes a gradual loss of contractile protein, while the tissue undergoes an increase in connective tissue protein. At least in part, this alteration is regulated pre-translationally within the aging cell (Lakatta and Boluyt, 2000).

Ironically, even though the heart is the most critical part of the cardiovascular system, it shows the fewest intrinsic effects of aging. Nevertheless, it suffers severe secondary damage due to atherosclerotic supplying vessels, rather than to primary dysfunction (Fig. 9–1). Aside from gross atherosclerotic changes in its coronary arteries, it is almost impossible to determine the age of the heart from a postmortem pathologic examination (Arking, 1998). There are few intrinsic clinical changes associated with the aging myocardium, as opposed to the extrinsic clinical changes due to supplying vessels. Even subtle changes in electrical excitability, such as the increasing risk of atrial fibrillation with age (Go et al., 2001), might be secondary rather than intrinsic. The myocardium does change, of course, whatever the cascade of causes. There are a variety of age-correlated changes, such as an increase in ventricular wall thickness (correlated with increased systemic blood pressure) that may occur with disease (Roffe, 1998), but the

Myocardial infarction results from

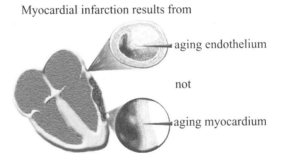

aging endothelium

not

aging myocardium

Figure 9–1 Myocardial infarction. Myocardial infarctions are secondary to primary pathology occurring in coronary arteries. The age-correlated pathology occurring in the myocardium—infarction—is profound (and often lethal), but results from senescence of endothelial cells in the arterial wall and not from senescence of myocardial cells in the heart.

only cardiac change known to be relatively specific to aging myocardial cells is an accumulation of lipofuscin pigment (Helenius et al., 1996; Kohn, 1977; Roffe, 1998; Terman and Brunk, 1998b). More recent work suggests that there may be other, more subtle changes in gene expression within the myocardial cells (for example, the increased expression of cyclooxygenase-2 in rat myocardium), which result in changes in their ability to handle oxidative stress (Kim et al., 2001b).

Since myocardial cells do not usually divide, they offer few of the changes that we expect to see in senescent cells. The lipofuscin accumulation may be due to chronic free radical damage (Muscari et al., 1996; Lee and Wei, 1997; Terman and Brunk, 1998a), but in at least in some species it appears to respond to antioxidant supplementation (Ma et al., 1996; Marzabadi and Llvaas, 1996). Other studies suggest that it is actively turned over (Monserrat et al., 1995), prompting the question of whether lipofuscin accumulation is an aging problem or merely a dietary one. In some species, lipofuscin accumulation can even decrease in response to hormonal stimulation. In aging rat adrenocortical cells, a 7-day course of adrenocorticotropic hormone supplementation decreases lipofuscin deposits (Cheng et al., 1999), suggesting that age-related lipofuscin accumulation is not irreversible. Lipofuscin may be the product of "reactive senescence" in cells (Faragher et al., 1997b), rather than a simple chronological accumulation. Telomere shortening occurs in some rat myocytes, apparently as a result of myocyte replacement rather than myocyte division (Kajstura et al., 2000). An additional possibility is that the relative loss of myocytes and compensatory hypertrophy of remaining myocytes seen in some aged hearts is an example of primary cardiac aging, perhaps (as might be lipofuscin) due to accumulated free radical damage rather than systemic hypertension. Changes in the degree of cell phospholipid saturation and in cardiac myocyte hydrogen peroxide and oxygen-radical scavenger enzyme levels are in line with this suggestion (Muscari et al., 1996), but might equally be a response to diminished coronary artery perfusion.

While myocardial infarctions and cerebrovascular disease are the most striking outcomes of atherosclerosis, peripheral arterial disease is the more ubiquitous. The effects are more subtle than the sudden events of heart attack and stroke but affect all organs and become progressively more common with age. Unfortunately, the definition of peripheral arterial disease is inherently open to disagreement and technically more difficult to assess than is large-vessel disease (Newman, 2000). Consequently, clinical disease that results from this form of atherosclerosis may not always be assigned to this cause. It is difficult to know how much of organ dysfunction can be attributed to this age-associated disease rather than to intrinsic organ aging. Peripheral arterial disease causes muscle dysfunction, normally in leg muscle, and classically intermittent claudication. Even in this case, however, the common diagnosis—claudication—along with extensive, but independent comorbidities—diabetes, neuropathy, and spinal stenosis—overshadow the more common and more extensive but less appreciated quotidian impairments caused by peripheral arterial disease (McDermott et al., 2001). Patients with aging peripheral arteries are less active, slower, and less capable of performing many tasks than are those without arterial problems.

Intermittent or poor peripheral circulation can result when there is a transient decrease in central pressure (insufficient to maintain flow in the face of high peripheral pressure in diseased capillaries) or increase in end-organ demand. The latter case can occur when behavioral events, such as exertion in the heart, prompt a mismatch between metabolic demand and available capillary oxygen. The result, angina, is common not only in the heart but in other organs. In the gastrointestinal tract, for example, the stress of a simple meal may be enough to induce intestinal angina—bowel ischemia with the associated risk of intestinal infarction. In other organs, although seldom going by the same epithet, similar mismatching may equally occur, with resultant risk of end-organ infarction to the brain, kidney, adrenal gland, etc.

The most apparent, and arguably most critical, pathology is not within capillaries but the largest arteries. This is especially true of not only the aorta, in which aneurysms are dramatic reminders of pathology (Herron et al., 1991; Herron, 1996), but of the coronary arteries, although the intramyocardial portions of the coronary arteries are spared, likely because of rheologic and mechanical factors (Scher, 2000). Atherosclerosis underlies most adult deaths worldwide and usually expresses itself as death due to cardiac or central nervous system failure, i.e., heart attacks or strokes. Although other disease processes contribute to morbidity and mortality in the aged, the overwhelming cause of organ failure is an inadequate arterial supply; the overwhelming cause of this failure is, in turn, atherosclerosis. The major outline of the pathology has been understood for more than a century, indeed since Sydenham's time three centuries ago, and over the past half-century has become characterized at the gross, microscopic, and ultrastructural levels.

Histologically, the entire pathology of atherosclerosis lies within the arterial walls. Within these walls, in turn, endothelial cells are now regarded as the trigger in the cascade of atherosclerosis (De Caterina, 2000a and b; Muller and Griesmacher, 2000). The endothelial cells, lining the arterial system, not only demonstrate morphological changes, becoming more irregular in size and shape (Arking, 1998), but become more dysfunctional with age (Kimura et al., 1999; Britten and Schachinger, 1998), perhaps in part due to hypertension and shear stress (e.g., Taddei et al., 1997). Several researchers (Kalaria, 1996; DeJong et al., 1997; Robert et al., 1997; Shah and Mooradian, 1997; Degens, 1998) have found thinning of the endothelial cells, loss of endothelial mitochondria, thickening of and inclusions within the basement membranes, and changes in the blood–brain barrier in the aging vascular system. Moreover, such endothelial cells participate actively in regulating arterial pressure (Dzau et al., 1994). While classically

true of resistance arteries, pressure is actively regulated through endothelial modulation of elasticity and compliance in the subendothelial layer. Endothelial cells in older
patients show a diminished response to vasodilators, such as acetylcholine (Andrawis
et al., 2000), as well as suffering the results of a reduced synthesis and/or increased
degradation of vascular nitric oxide (NO) (Cooke and Dzau, 1997). In capillaries, which
have little else but endothelial cell elements, such changes may be critical to altering
function, as in peripheral vascular disease. Aging capillary walls reveal a general deterioration, underlying the decline in vascular function and a chronic hypoperfusion to
end-organs (Kalaria, 1996).

Despite endothelial cells, historically, the classic histologic changes of atherosclerosis were better attested to in the deeper layers, underlying the endothelium.
Typical atherosclerotic lesions consist of a patchy, irregular thickening of the intermediate layer marked by intra- and extracellular deposition of lipid ("fatty streaks")
and calcification (hence "hardening of the arteries"). It has long been clear that smooth
muscle cells proliferate, alter their morphology and function (Lindop et al., 1995),
and even migrate into the inner layers of the vessel (Bloom and Fawcett, 1975), but
monocyte-derived foam cells proliferate, matrix changes (Robert et al., 1998), and
inflammation increases (Danesh, 1999; Koenig, 2001; Selzman et al., 2001). The inflammation typically begins with macrophages and progresses to lymphocyte infiltration; this progression correlates with plaque morphology (Okimoto et al., 2002). Most
inflammatory cells derive from the circulation and in this their function resembles mer-
cenaries. Machiavelli once devoted an entire chapter to the damage caused by mercenary troops in a republic (Machiavelli, 1513); the damage caused by monocytes in an
arterial wall is no less fatal. "Disorganized, undisciplined, ambitious, and faithless" is
an apt description of mercenary soldiers and monocyte inflammation. Inflammation may
be the cause of much of the arterial pathology and first becomes apparent with the proliferation of monocytes.

Cell proliferation of monocytes and indigenous cells of the arterial wall cells,
coupled with fatty deposition and excessive formation of collagen and other changes in
the extracellular matrix, results in the thickening of the vessel wall and its progressive
intrusion into the arterial lumen. Additional complications often include hemorrhage
and cell necrosis, abetting the inflammation and calcification. Overall, elastic and smooth
muscle layer thickness may increase by up to 40% (Arking, 1998) and the bulk of this
increase occurs at the expense of the lumen rather than an increase in external arterial
wall diameter. In coronary arteries, lesions less than perhaps 90% (as a three-dimensional
reconstruction; 70% by coronary angiography) are seldom considered clinically significant. Nonetheless, obstruction due to thrombus becomes increasingly likely as the lumen
narrows. The final event is usually sudden and often fatal.

The pathology of atherosclerosis has long been (and appropriately) thought of as a
cascade of events, influenced independently and interactively (Mehta et al., 1998) by a
myriad of risk factors (Arbustini et al., 1999; Kadar and Glasz, 2001). Among the most
well-known risk factors are hypertension, hypercholesterolemia, hyperglycemia, and
tobacco use, but they are not alone (McGill and McMahan, 1998) and about half of all
patients with myocardial infarction lack these classic risk factors (Koenig, 2001). Additional risk factors have been identified over the past few decades (Steinberg and Gotto,
1999) and include diet, alcohol, obesity, lack of exercise, homocysteine levels, individual cholesterol fractions and ratios, apolipoprotein E4 (Hazzard, 2001), estrogen

levels, tocopherol levels (Cherubini et al., 2001; Mezzetti et al., 2001), prothrombotic mutations (Psaty et al., 2001), C-reactive protein levels (Koenig, 2001; Patel et al., 2001; Ridker et al., 2001), myeloperoxidase (Zhang et al., 2001b), stress (Nordstrom et al., 2001), dental infections (Valtonen, 1999; Slavkin and Baum, 2000), and arterial wall DNA and RNA viral (e.g., herpesvirus, cytomegalovirus, coxsackievirus) or bacterial (e.g., *Chlamydia, Helicobacter,* etc.) infection (Mattila et al., 1998; Muhlestein, 1998; Movahead, 1999; Shor and Phillips, 1999; Smith, 1999), and inflammatory biomarkers in general (Pradhan et al., 2003). In a general way, we might divide these factors into two major types of risks: extrinsic and intrinsic factors. The former include behavioral factors such as diet, exercise, alcohol, and tobacco. The latter include not only broadly genetic processes (Hoeg, 1996) such as diabetes, immune function, hypertension, and disorders of lipid metabolism, but "intrinsic aging processes" (Bierman, 1994) and at least one rare, but illuminating genetic disorder, Hutchinson-Gilford syndrome (early-onset progeria). In this latter case, all of the normal risk factors are lacking, yet the atherosclerotic pathology is nonetheless severe and inexorable.

Curiously, the cascade of pathology does not begin in the intermediate layers, despite their pathology and inflammation. Underlying this classic histology of atherogenesis we find the endothelial cells. This should come as no surprise, considering their location and vulnerability to intravascular insult. Endothelial cells line arteries and lie between the arterial lumen and resultant gross pathology. If serum cholesterol, hypertension, hyperglycemia, and circulating tobacco products contribute to atherosclerosis, we might expect mediation of such pathology through this intervening layer and first-line cellular defense.

Equally, that cholesterol deposition may be a central feature of, but is not the primary culprit in, atherogenesis should come as no surprise, given the epidemiological exceptions to the rule. Hutchinson-Gilford syndrome is but one example. While the correlation between cholesterol and atherosclerosis is excellent, there are numerous exceptions on both sides of this correlation. Some patients with high cholesterol may have little clinical disease; others with low or normal cholesterol may have striking pathology. The subordinate role of cholesterol metabolism is borne out repeatedly in laboratory studies as well as in the epidemiological data.

Blocking cell proliferation is sufficient to block atherogenesis, even without altering serum cholesterol. In normal vascular grafts, for example, restenosis is a routine and recurrent clinical problem (Sopko, 2002). Cell division can be blocked, however, by the use of antisense oligonucleotides. This arrests vascular cell cycle progression in the vascular grafts while preserving normal endothelial phenotype and function. The result is that occlusive disease does not recur in these cases, as it does in normal grafts (von der Leyen et al., 1996; Mann and Dzau, 1997; Mann et al., 1997a). Such grafts remain free from macrophage invasion, foam cell deposition, and other classic hallmarks of atherosclerosis, whether provoked by ischemia (Poston et al., 1998) or with high-lipid diets that ordinarily induce accelerated vascular disease (Dzau et al., 1996). In short, cholesterol may commonly play a role and is effective as an interventional dietary variable, but it is not a necessary feature in arterial disease. Emphatically, none of this should be taken as an argument that cholesterol is unimportant nor as an argument against clinical intervention in cholesterol or lipid metabolism. These and other observations only suggest (and support the view) that more occurs in atherogenesis than mere passive accumulation of overly abundant serum cholesterol.

In summary, the cardiovascular system shows almost ubiquitous age-related pathology. The arteries suffer classic age-related atherosclerotic disease. The capillary bed undergoes changes that are less well understood, but that may be inherent in the epithelial cells and may have profound implications for disease in multiple end-organs. The heart is a special end-organ, lying within the cardiovascular system. While demonstrating little inherent age-related pathology, extensive secondary pathology due to atherosclerosis of its coronary arteries is responsible for a large proportion of deaths worldwide.

The Role of Cell Senescence

Cardiovascular disease is the result of well-understood vascular pathology that, in turn, is increasingly understood to hinge upon endothelial cell dysfunction (Forgione et al., 2000; Herrmann and Lerman, 2001). These cells divide and demonstrate senescent changes; it is to these cells that we must turn to understand the bulk of cardiovascular disease. Although the cascade was once felt to begin within the smooth muscle layers of the arterial wall, evidence over the past decade has implicated the endothelial cell layer lying upstream in the etiology (Cooper et al., 1994). This has been extended by the correlative observations of Harley's group (Chang and Harley, 1995), who found that cells in areas of high vascular stress showed telomere shortening prior to onset of vascular disease and these data have been extended (see below). The circumstantial evidence of death due to atherosclerosis in progeric children is likewise consistent with the model that endothelial cell senescence not only underlies atherosclerosis but is an effective interventional target (Minamino and Komuro, 2002).

As a hypothesis, the model is easy to outline. The causes of endothelial cell senescence (e.g., circulating toxins, hypertension, lipids, hyperglycemia) are understood. Endothelial injury is followed by cell loss and replacement, telomere shortening, and changes in endothelial gene expression. This in turn results in secondary changes (including the classic ones of cholesterol accumulation) in the intermediate layers, followed by a gross reduction in the luminal area. Simultaneously, the endothelial surface acquires pathological changes in adhesiveness and other characteristics, increasing the likelihood of thrombus formation and arterial blockage. It is here, within the endothelial layer, that cell senescence appears to play a pivotal and impelling role in atherogenesis.

The model is supported. Vascular endothelial cells undergo chronic and repetitive injury (Lefkowitz and Willerson, 2001). Endothelial cells are not only exposed to circulating infectious agents and toxins such as tobacco products, oxidized low-density lipoprotein, and free radicals (from the oxidation of homocysteine and other substances), but to the direct effects of fluctuations in shear stress during systole (Malek et al., 1999) as well as to hypertensive stresses (for an interesting variant on this theme, see Aviv and Aviv, 1999). The result of such stress is endothelial cell apoptosis and direct cell loss. Several circulating factors have toxic, apoptotic, or damaging effects on the endothelium (Vapaatalo and Mervaala, 2001), and effects of aging may hasten these effects dramatically (Kunz, 2000). While high-density lipoprotein may be protective, apoptosis is induced by oxidized low-density lipoproteins, angiotensin, and oxidative stress, as well as secondary increases in Bax and Fas, triggered by subendothelial changes (Rader and Dugi, 2000; Choy et al., 2001).

Of all risk factors, the major four are tobacco, hypercholesterolemia (and lipids), hypertension, and hyperglycemia. Tobacco by-products, as well as alcohol and other circulating toxins, directly affect the endothelial cells (Najemnik et al., 1999; Kunz, 2000; Vapaatalo and Mervaala, 2001) and are responsible for continual cell losses in those patients exposed to such products. In this same context, homocysteine, a common clinical marker for (or causative factor in) atherosclerosis (The Homocysteine Studies Collaboration, 2002; Wilson, 2002), is known to accelerate telomere erosion and other markers of cell senescence in human vascular endothelial cells in vitro (Xu et al., 2000a).

Lipid peroxidation plays a classic role in atherogenesis (Morel et al., 1984; Steinberg et al., 1989) and has been causally linked to cell senescence (von Zglinicki et al., 2000a). Atherogenic lipids include cholesterol, particularly oxidized low-density cholesterol, and can cause changes in endothelial cell function within hours of exposure (Adams et al., 2000). The abnormal endothelial cell function found in hyperlipidemia (Dugi and Rader, 2000) has been attributed to abnormal NO metabolism (Landmesser et al., 2000), probably due to increased production of superoxide in hyperlipidemia (Warnholtz et al., 2001). Hypercholesterolemia results in altered endothelial cell function (Libby et al., 2000). Normalization of endothelial function is considered a major goal of therapeutic interventions in lipid metabolism (Chilton, 2001; Puddu et al., 2001) and may provide novel therapeutic targets (Barton, 2000).

Hypertension—not merely diastolic, but systolic, mean arterial, and pulse pressures (Domanski et al., 2002)—is a major risk factor for atherosclerosis, probably through endothelial cell–mediated changes in arterial elasticity and compliance (Glasser, 2000), as well as through direct effects caused by distending pressure (Arnett et al., 2000). Though the direction of causation is argued, endothelial cell dysfunction is considered to precede and probably cause the changes in arterial wall smooth muscle that underlie essential hypertension (Raitakari and Celermajer, 2000; Taddei et al., 2000). Aging endothelial cells show blunted and atypical reactions to changes in arterial pressure (Britten and Schachinger, 1998). In response to shear stress (Ohno et al., 1995) and arterial pressure, endothelial cells actively regulate arterial smooth muscle tone via NO, prostacyclin, endothelin-1, several prostanoids, angiotensin, superoxide anions, and other factors (Pearson, 2000; Puddu et al., 2000; Goodwin and Yacoub, 2001). Reciprocally, hypertension causes further vascular damage and specifically endothelial cell damage (Kimura et al., 1999) via shear stress and other mechanisms (Contreras et al., 2000; Gimbrone et al., 2000). Similarly, smooth muscle cells respond to increased intraarterial pressure with changes in gene expression (Tamura et al., 2000), as well as with pathologic cell proliferation. At least in spontaneously hypertensive rats, telomerase is activated in these cells. Telomerase inhibition prevents smooth muscle cell proliferation and induces apoptosis. Telomerase may be critical for increased vascular smooth muscle proliferation (Cao et al., 2002b). As with cancer, telomerase does not cause but may be required to maintain cell proliferation.

Diabetes (generically, hyperglycemia) is an independent risk factor for atherosclerosis, interactively with hypertension. Both accelerate atherogenesis and cause endothelial cell dysfunction (Cosentino and Luscher, 2001). Hyperglycemia is believed to trigger endothelial cell changes by modifying lipoproteins, forming advanced glycation end-products and lipoprotein immune complexes, altering the NO pathway, and elevating homocysteine (Najemnik et al., 1999), thereby accelerating endothelial cell loss.

As a consequence of stresses to intimal cells, endothelial cells frequently die; the transient denudation is subsequently repaired by division of surviving, neighboring endothelial cells. Precise turnover rates of in vivo endothelial cells are unknown, but are high relative to similar cells elsewhere in the vascular system (e.g., venous walls) and to other cell types underlying intima. This is confirmed by measures of telomere lengths in arterial endothelial cells compared to venous wall cells (Chang and Harley, 1995): telomere lengths are shorter in areas of high vascular stress and atheroma formation than in areas of low stress and in which gross pathology is uncommon. As expected, human vascular endothelial cells show telomere attrition and increasing aneuploidy in vivo and these measures of cell senescence correlate with donor age (Aviv et al., 2001).

To the extent that the endothelial cells undergo replication, we anticipate changes in gene expression. Changes in gene expression occur in vitro and in vivo (Cooper et al., 1994; Hwang et al., 2001a; Monajemi et al., 2001). As in the classical model, as a result of such changes, events then progress downstream, with a rapid onset of inflammatory changes (Akishita et al., 2000), cholesterol deposition, foam cells, smooth muscle proliferation, thrombus formation, and general atheromatous change (Lefkowitz and Willerson, 2001). However, these changes are not merely passive (e.g., passive lipid accumulation). They are the active response of subendothelial cells to an altered pattern of trophic factors, secreted by endothelial cells, on which they depend for normal function. The pattern of gene expression in senescing endothelial cells is specific to this cell phenotype (Shelton et al., 1999). This dysfunctional change defines endothelial cell activation (see the parallel discussion of microglial activation in Chapter 13), a key event in atherogenesis (Keaney, 2000; Kinlay et al., 2001; Tedgui and Mallat, 2001). Endothelial cell activation in atherogenesis is expressed in key changes: a loss of vascular integrity, an increased expression of cell adhesion molecules, a bias in favor of vascular thrombosis, an increase in cytokine production, and an up-regulation of HLA molecules (Hunt, 2000). Moreover, there is a progressive inactivation of the gene for the estrogen α-receptor, most prominent in areas of atherosclerotic plaque (Post et al., 1999). More recently, data have been accumulating that imply a tight relationship between cell senescence and atherosclerosis.

In comparing young normal human aortic endothelial cells to senescent endothelial cells and endothelial cells immortalized with hTERT, we find differences. Compared to young endothelial cells, senescent endothelial cells show a decreased expression of endothelial nitric oxide synthase (eNOS), as well as a decreased production and activity of NO, changes critical in atherogenesis and hypertension. Similarly, senescent endothelial cells demonstrate increased monocyte adhesion, again implicated in atherogenesis. This difference in adhesion is accentuated further by exposure to TNF-α. In all cases, these differences are ameliorated or normalized by hTERT immortalization. Endothelial cell senescence results in decreased NO activity and increased monocyte binding. Contrarily, hTERT expression results in human aortic endothelial cells that revert to a pattern of gene expression typical of a younger phenotype (Matsushita et al., 2001).

Similarly, strong β-galactosidase staining is found in vascular endothelial cells within atherosclerotic lesions of the coronary arteries, but not in similar cells within the internal mammary arteries. In vitro induction of cell senescence in human aortic endothelial cells results in changes implicated as central to atherogenesis. Not only has there been confirmation of the decrease in the expression of eNOS in senescing endothelial cells, but intercellular adhesion molecules (ICAM-1) are increasingly expressed. More importantly, when hTERT is used to extend the endothelial lifespan, these changes are inhibited. Together, these results indict cell senescence as contributing to human clinical atherogenesis (Minamino et al., 2002).

Perhaps unexpectedly, endothelial cells that line vessels and mural cells (smooth muscle cells and pericytes) that give strength to vessels may derive from the same stem cell lineage (Yamashita et al., 2000). Their specific differentiation depends on their differential exposure to specific growth factors (Carmeliet, 2000), not on a different stem cell origin. Endothelial cells and vascular smooth muscle cells may therefore have parallel fates in their rate of cell senescence. In any case, although endothelial cells proliferate in response to cell loss, proliferation is more notable in the subendothelial cells. At the histological level, atherosclerosis is largely a disease of cell proliferation within the vascular wall (Braun-Dullaeus et al., 1998). The smooth muscle proliferation, resembling in this respect a benign neoplasm (Bonin et al., 1999), is monoclonal (Benditt and Benditt, 1973; Murry et al., 1997). Interference with cell division at any of several levels (Mann and Dzau, 1997; Tomita et al., 1998) can arrest atherosclerosis independent of alterations in dietary or other standard risk factors. The central role of cell proliferation in atherogenesis has prompted investigation into potential therapies based on inhibition of cell cycling (Hsueh and Law, 2001) and cell division.

Like fibroblasts, vascular smooth muscle cells (the other major cell type indigenous to the subendothelium) demonstrate cell senescence and replicative lifespans in vitro (Moss and Benditt, 1975; Bierman, 1978). Moreover, and again similar to most neoplasms, the clonal expansion is accompanied by a propensity to express telomerase, especially in restenosis of human coronary arteries, in which plaque regrows after therapeutic removal (Gupta et al., 2000). As in neoplasm, telomerase expression may be necessary but not sufficient; the result but not the cause of such transformation.

Although the changes induced in the subendothelial arterial wall are histologically clear, much of this derives from immigrating cells, the result of the adhesion and attraction of such cells. Interactions between platelets and endothelial cells are poorly understood, but central to atherosclerosis (Sachais, 2001). Changes in adhesion, resulting in thrombus, are determined by location, arterial wall topology, and flow characteristics (Scher, 2000). As endothelial cells become dysfunctional, adhesion is one of the most prominent changes. To a degree, this is a local phenomenon involving endothelial cell adhesion, but involves increased adhesion among circulating platelets and leukocytes (Amoroso et al., 2001), apparently from circulating endothelial factors.

Inflammation, mediated through increased endothelial cell adhesion as well as the release of cytokines, chemokines, tissue-destroying metalloproteases (Newby and Zaltsman, 2000; Shah, 2000), and reactive oxygen species (Maytin et al., 1999; Touyz, 2000; Aviv, 2002a, 2002b), is the hallmark of atherogenesis (Sullivan et al., 2000; Selzman et al., 2001) and may be laid at the door of endothelial cell senescence. The inflammation begins with endothelial cell dysfunction (Fichtlscherer and Zeiher, 2000) and is characterized by the infiltration of inflammatory cells, predominantly monocytes (Vorchheimer and Fuster, 2001). Vascular smooth muscle cells migrate to and divide within the atherogenic lesion. The monocyte response is signaled by chemotactic factors (e.g., monocyte chemotactic protein-1 and angiotensin), while smooth muscle cell migration is signaled by ligand-induced activation of receptor tyrosine kinases (Kraemer, 2000). Smooth muscle proliferation occurs, triggered by angiotensin (Dzau, 1994a;

Braun-Dullaeus et al., 1999) and can be experimentally blocked using promising genetic approaches (Mann et al., 1995; Morishita et al., 1995b, 1997). Parallel to the role of chemotaxis in monocyte infiltration is the role of cell adhesion molecules, largely glycoproteins, in permitting monocytes to glom onto and enter the vascular wall (Huo and Ley, 2001; Krieglstein and Granger, 2001). The control of cell adhesion, and hence of leukocyte migration, is vested in the endothelial cell (De Caterina, 2000a, 2000b). Inhibition of cell immigration has become the basis for potential interventions, including inhibition of monocyte migration (Hsueh and Law, 2001).

Although atherosclerosis may correlate with endothelial cell senescence and consequences of changing gene expression, there have been attempts to measure telomere lengths of (far more available) leukocytes from atherosclerotic patients. There is significant correlation between shorter telomere lengths in circulating leukocytes and coronary artery disease, equivalent to 8.6 years of aging (Samani et al., 2001; see also Nowak et al., 2002) and higher mortality from heart disease (Cawthorn et al., 2003). Hypertensive patients show correlation, although inverse: the shorter the telomere, the greater the pulse pressure (Jeanclos et al., 2000). The authors suggest that this correlation is somehow causal, although it is difficult to see how. The correlation is no surprise, as these (and many other variables) might form a constellation of factors playing a role in cardiovascular disease, immune senescence, and aging.

Like atherosclerosis, cardiac failure may ultimately be due to the effects of altered gene expression (Hwang et al., 2001a) and cell senescence within the coronary arteries, although primary myocyte senescence (Kajstura et al., 2000) and changes in gene expression (Helenius et al., 1996) occur to a limited degree. In myocardial failure and as a result of microvessel disease, vascular supply no longer matches cardiac demand and a relative hypoxia ensues. Regional hypoxia can potentially trigger cardiomyocyte apoptosis (Sabbah et al., 1998). In either case, the result is a progressive loss of cardiac muscle and function.

One frequent question, largely unanswered, is the degree to which cardiac myocytes divide and therefore senesce. In many species, such as the rat, telomerase activity may be developmentally regulated. Cardiomyocytes proliferate dramatically after birth, but telomerase activity falls off soon thereafter, as does myocardial cell division (Borges and Liew, 1997), accounting for the stability of telomere in adult cardiomyocytes (Takubo et al., 2002). In the adult rat, cardiomyocyte replacement occurs via satellite or stem cell division, with continued and telomere attrition in 16% of adult myocytes and changes in gene expression even in cells with no measurable telomere loss (Kajstura et al., 2000). In rats, estrogen may affect telomerase expression and hence have a direct effect on the rate of myocyte loss, higher in males than in females. With little other supportive evidence, the suggestion has been made that this may underlie the longer lifespan and decreased incidence of heart failure in women (Leri et al., 2000).

Humans, however, may be a markedly different matter. Although the functional significance is uncertain, human myocardial cells have been shown to divide in response to losses incurred in myocardial infarction (Raman et al., 2001). Myocardial stem cells migrate into the damaged heart from unknown sources (Bolli, 2002; Quaini et al., 2002). Whatever the sources and practical impact (if any), these findings suggest that replacement of human myocardial cells may occur throughout the human lifespan as a result of stem or satellite cell division. To the extent that this is true, it may explain primary age-related changes in myocardial function. It remains far more likely, however, that the overwhelming majority of age-related myocardial dysfunction is attributable to more distant changes within the endothelial cells that line the arteries that supply the myocardium. It is to these cells, and perhaps other cell types within the arterial walls, that we must assign the blame for most clinical cardiovascular disease.

We have shown evidence consistent with a model in which cell senescence plays a central role in atherogenesis. The model, while complex, offers the advantage of explaining much of the complexity of the pathology. Within this same purview, the reason that progerics have heart disease becomes explicable. Although lacking the standard four major risk factors—hypercholesterolemia, smoking, hypertension, and diabetes—their endothelial cells probably partake of the same abnormally early cell senescence found in their skin fibroblasts (Counter et al., 1995), that is, shortened telomeres. Likely, their senescent endothelial cells have senescence associated gene expression at birth, hence an altered pattern of trophic factor production, on which cells in the media depend, hence the otherwise remarkable onset of atherosclerosis in their first decade of life, resulting in rapid death due to stroke or myocardial infarct. Whether this explanation, while consistent, is accurate remains unproven. To date, we have no progeric donation of arterial endothelial tissue and remain unlikely to obtain any in the near future. Assays of telomere length and cell senescence in progerics have thus far been restricted to skin fibroblasts and leukocytes (see below).

Whether the observed changes in gene expression and cell senescence associated with routine clinical atherogenesis are the primary pathology, merely secondary reactions to endothelial cell senescence, or even more distant effects of the primary pathology (i.e., reflecting compensatory cell responses) is arguable and will remain so pending in vivo interventional studies. The undoubted experimental importance is, however, a distant second to the immense clinical importance of this question. The most tangible benefit of the cell senescence model of cardiovascular disease is its potential for offering an additional point of therapeutic target. As already stressed, the aim is not delineation of causation but identification of the most effective and efficient target for intervention. Cell senescence, particularly at the level of the vascular endothelial cell, may offer such a target.

Intervention

None of the work on cell senescence in atherogenesis is germane but for the possibility of effective intervention. Classic interventions (diet, exercise, stress reduction, etc) have varying effectiveness (Keysor and Jette, 2001; Lee et al., 2001b; Tice et al., 2001), some surprisingly so (Ornish et al., 1998). Current drug and surgical interventions have reliable efficacy, particularly the angiotensin-converting enzyme (ACE) inhibitors, which have potent and fundamental effects on the mechanism of atherosclerosis (Diet et al., 1996; Dzau, 1998). Newer and potentially more effective interventions (Pratt and Dzau, 1999), based on a better understanding of the biology of atherosclerosis (Dzau, 1994b, 2001) and genetics of the cardiovascular system (Dzau et al., 1995; Dempsey et al., 2001), are only beginning to demonstrate their promise (Francis et al., 2001).

Despite initial (Grady et al., 1992) and some continued (Hayashi et al., 2000; Wagner, 2000) enthusiasm for estrogen as cardioprotective in postmenopausal women, a more careful review of data suggest that it may be ineffective (Herrington et al., 2000), detrimental (Hulley et al., 1998), especially if used with progestin (Fletcher and Colditz, 2002; Writing Group for the Women's Health Initiative Investigators, 2002), or protective only in patients lacking specific interactive risk factors, such as prothrombotic mutations (Psaty et al., 2001). While estrogen might be beneficial in specific cases, perhaps even after accounting for the possible cancer risks (Van Hoften et al., 2000; Chen et al., 2002a), no unanimity exists regarding claimed benefits of hormone replacement in lowering the atherosclerotic mortality. Early data were ambiguous (Beral et al., 1999; Petitti, 2002), but recent data suggest that hormonal replacement therapy increases cardiovascular risk (Nelson et al., 2002; Waters et al., 2002). Given both cardiovascular and noncardiovascular risks (Hulley et al., 2002; Noller, 2002), current guidelines do not recommend hormone replacement (Mitka, 2001; Grady et al., 2002) and use with progestin is contraindicated (Fletcher and Colditz, 2002; Writing Group for the Women's Health Initiative Investigators, 2002).

Current interventions in atherosclerosis do not affect fundamental cell function. Although heart transplants, coronary artery bypass grafting, endarterectomy, and vascular stenting are effective to a degree, they by no means interrupt the onset or course of the recurrent pathology. Classic interventions have shown efficacy as measured by morbidity or mortality, such as low-dose daily aspirin, particularly among older patients with known coronary artery disease (Gum et al., 2001), yet they are far from universally protective. Although drug alteration of lipid metabolism, dietary changes, exercise, and control of contributory risks (diabetes, hypertension, and smoking) lower the vector of disease progression and do so at a presumptively more fundamental level than the repair or replacement of vessels, they do not strike deeply enough. From a practical perspective, an optimal intervention in atherosclerotic (or, for that matter, any) disease should have four desirable characteristics. Optimal interventions should be

1. cheap (compared to coronary artery bypass grafting, for example),
2. uniformly effective, regardless of genetics, environment, etc.,
3. preventative (as immunization is in infection), and
4. curative (as antibiotics are in infection).

Contrast each characteristic with current and historical treatments.

Coronary artery bypass grafting, endarterectomy, and cardiac transplantation all have a degree of efficacy, yet are expensive compared to the costs of immunization and prevention. Most health plans, most underdeveloped nations, and most uninsured patients cannot afford unlimited use of such technology in treating heart disease. While it is true that post-occurrence therapies may be improved in the near future by the use of innovative techniques, such as revascularization and recovery of ventricular wall function (Sayeed-Shah et al., 1998) and embryonic stem cell replacement of myocytes, there remains prevention as the preferential approach to cardiovascular disease.

Current preventative measures for atherogenesis are more patient-specific than is optimal: antihypertensives, drugs to alter lipid absorption or metabolism, tobacco cessation, and platelet inhibitors vary in their efficacy with genetic background and patient behavior. Again, contrast this specific efficacy with the more uniform applicability of immunization in microbial disease. A century ago, we had no effective way to prevent tetanus; now the rate of tetanus death is limited only by our ability to ensure universal immunization. In a similar vein, we can avoid many but not all atherosclerotic deaths through diet, drugs, and behavioral intervention, but could do far more by preventing cell senescence. The survival rate from tetanus is only 50% with the best of medical care. The survival rate for those with apparent atherosclerosis is poor. We have limited ability to reverse the disease. If cell senescence underlies atherogenesis, then we might be able to reverse the ongoing process prior to end-organ damage.

A key issue is the most efficient point of intervention. Even if we could universally afford to transplant damaged organs (whether hearts, knees, or livers), the most effective (and cost-effective) point of intervention is before transplantation. There is a current tendency to hold sacred those medical approaches relying on prevention rather than treatment. Preventive approaches are often more effective, yet the assumption that prevention is better is usually assumed and seldom analyzed. The value of upstream, or fundamental, or preventive interventions lies *not* in an inherent superiority but in relative efficacy. Such an approach is usually cheaper, more effective, less painful, and easier for all concerned. Likewise, an intervention that employs the prevention or reversal of cell senescence to treat atherosclerosis and its clinical outcomes will be preferable to current therapies not because it is more fundamental, but only to the degree that it is demonstrably more effective. Clinical therapy aimed at cell senescence will be aimed at the more efficient point of intervention in atherosclerotic disease.

Atheromatous damage can not only be prevented but ameliorated, i.e., to some degree reversed. Regression of atheromatous lesions (Davies, 2001) and lowered mortality (Serruys et al., 2002) can be accomplished by drugs such as statins, as well as through diet and behavioral interventions (Ornish et al., 1998). Several promising possibilities (at least in the eyes of the public), such as antioxidant vitamins, have shown only equivocal benefits (Tardif, 2000; Waters et al., 2002), although such supplements have appropriate benefits in patients whose specific deficiencies or suboptimal intakes (especially folate, pyridoxine, and cyanocobalamin) contribute to their pathology (Fairfield and Fletcher, 2002; Fletcher and Fairfield, 2002). Newer and more effective therapies are widely believed to be on the horizon, especially molecular therapies (Gibbons and Dzau, 1996), given a growing understanding of the cell biology involved. Unbridled cell proliferation plays a role in atherosclerosis and revascularization hyperplasia, causing restenosis and angioplasty failures (Gibbons and Dzau, 1994). This cell proliferation has been targeted therapeutically. Antisense oligonucleotides to cell cycle regulatory genes (e.g., cdk 2 kinase) have shown moderate success in preventing proliferation, at least in rats (Morishita et al., 1994). Other targets for inhibiting endothelial cell proliferation and changed gene expression include peroxisomal proliferator-activated receptors (Plutzky, 2001) and E2F. An E2F decoy has been used to successfully prevent intimal hyperplasia in vein grafts (Mann et al., 1999; Ehsan et al., 2001), though overexpression of E2F may bypass some inhibitory agents (Goukassian et al., 2001).

As we come to understand the basic biology underlying atherosclerosis (Leopold and Loscalzo, 2000), new therapeutic targets are being considered (Dzau et al., 1997). Each target involves a critical step in the progression of atherosclerosis, including the reversal of endothelial cell dysfunction (Cooke, 2000), control of apoptosis (Horiuchi et al., 1998), or the prevention of thrombosis, inflammation, or neointimal hyperplasia (von der Leyen et al., 1995; Morishita et al., 2000).

Anticipating cell replacement therapy, distinct cells have been targeted for possible replacement to treat cardiovascular disease. The primary cell targets for replacement are the cardiomyocytes and vascular endothelial cells. Among cells considered as sources for replacement are myogenic cell lines, adult skeletal myoblasts, immortalized atrial cells, embryonic and adult cardiomyocytes, embryonic stem cells, teratoma cells, genetically altered fibroblasts, smooth muscle cells, and bone marrow–derived cells (Kessler and Byrne, 1999). In most cases, however, the limitations of cell senescence suggest that telomerase-based therapies will play a central role in deriving an effective cell lines for clinical intervention.

Primary among the cellular targets for molecular intervention (including telomerase-based therapies) are the vascular endothelial cells (Leopold and Loscalzo, 2000; Parikh and Edelman, 2000; Cajero-Juarez et al., 2002). Proliferation is not the only point of potential intervention. In atherosclerosis as in cancer, the concern is not so much cell proliferation as it is unbridled proliferation of abnormal cells. As in cancer cells, some abnormally proliferating cells from atheromas are telomerase positive and their presence is associated with restenosis (Gupta et al., 2000). Immortalization of human vascular smooth muscle cells, however, does not result in inappropriate proliferation (Loeuillet et al., 2001). As in cancer, pathological cells may express telomerase, but there is no evidence that telomerase causes a pathological transformation in cancer or atherosclerosis. Unbridled cell proliferation is anathema to normal arterial function (as to organ function in cancer), but the prevention of cell senescence may provide unparalleled clinical benefits. The therapeutic intent is not to cause cell proliferation but to renormalize cell phenotype–specific gene expression. The pathology of atherosclerosis is not that cells merely proliferate but that they function abnormally and proliferate without regard for the effective tissue function. Consider the parallel with leukemia, in which cell proliferation is the hallmark, but in which proliferating cells are not only numerous but dysfunctional. While we might approach leukemia by preventing proliferation (as occurs in most chemotherapy), we might better intervene with therapies that reinstitute appropriate cell differentiation and appropriate control of cell proliferation. This is the intent of cell senescence therapy: reestablishment of normal cell growth, appropriate gene expression, and effective control of cell proliferation within the arterial wall, rather than permitting the pathological damage incurred by cell senescence and consequent clinical disease.

Interventions that avert cell senescence may do so using ex vivo (such as in cell replacement raised above) or in vivo approaches (primarily targeting vascular endothelial cells). Arterial catheters have been used for effective in vivo delivery and may have potential in the treatment of vascular disease (Morishita et al., 1995a). Viruses have already been used in vascular tissues to transfect cardiovascular cells. These include adenoviruses (Song et al., 1998; Asfour et al., 1999), herpesviruses (Conway et al., 1999), fusigenic Sendai virus-liposomes (Mann et al., 1997b), and other liposome vectors based on hemagglutinating viruses, which can efficiently transfer genes up to 100 kbp. The latter has been employed to inhibit endothelial cell proliferation, carrying antisense oligodeoxynucleotides against cell cycle genes, double-stranded oligodeoxynucleotide decoys against E2F, and NO synthase (Dzau et al., 1996; Kaneda et al., 1997). Plasmids have been used to effectively transfect oligonucleotides into normal as well as injured nonatherosclerotic or atherosclerotic arteries (von der Leyen et al., 1999). Arterial gene transfer demonstrates the efficacy of local angiotensin in causing hypertrophy and NO in inhibiting cell proliferation (Dzau and Horiuchi, 1996). The same technique results in widespread transfection without known damage to cardiomyocytes (Aoki et al., 1997).

Considering the role endothelial cells in cardiovascular disease and the suggestion that cell senescence underlies all of the changes in gene expression, cell proliferation, and atherogenesis, the most tempting and direct approach is probably in vivo transfection of hTERT. Pending direct human trials, animal models and in vitro data bear consideration. Murine models help us understand the mechanisms of atherosclerosis (Breslow, 1996), but are not directly comparable in assessing hTERT's utility for humans. Mice constitutively express telomerase, humans do not.

When human vascular endothelial cells are transfected with hTERT, they show an indefinite extension of cell lifespan accompanied by normal endothelial gene expression (Yang et al., 1999a). Likewise, they exhibit a normal pattern of endothelial cell surface marker proteins (e.g., CD31/PECAM-1 and $\alpha(v)\beta3$-integrin) and have appropriate LDL receptors (Venetsanakos et al., 2002). Just as in the parallel case of fibroblasts and retinal pigment epithelial cells (Bodnar et al., 1998; Jiang et al., 1999), there is no evidence of malignant transformation. To the contrary, these large-vessel and microvascular endothelial cells demonstrate normal differentiation, karyotype, and functional phenotype. Moreover, such cells demonstrate a normal capacity to form microvascular structures (angiogenic potential) in vitro and upon transfer into animal recipients. This latter potential has been further explored using human dermal microvascular endothelial cells. Retroviral-mediated transfection with hTERT results in cells that form normal microvascular structures in vivo. The cells were then implanted in immunodeficient (SCID) mice and formed normal capillaries and murine–human capillary anastomoses that were stable over time. These capillary cells responded to angiogenic and angiostatic factors with appropriate modulation of vessel densities. This latter approach could be effective in creating "engineered human vascular tissues" for several purposes (Yang et al., 2001b).

Using hTERT, human aortic endothelial cells (HAECs) not only have longer telomeres and considerably longer cellular lifespans, but they show delayed onset of the functional characteristics—decreased expression of eNOS and increased expression of ICAM-1—associated with senescence and atherosclerosis (Minamino et al., 2002).

In comparing young HAECs, senescent HAECs transfected with control vector, and immortalized human aortic endothelial cells containing hTERT, several other effects suggest the potential value of hTERT. Old cells show a decrease in the expression of eNOS compared to that in the young, and this change is blunted in hTERT transfected cells. Shear stress causes an increase in the expression of eNOS in old cells and this response is far more prominent in young or hTERT transfected cells. The production and activity of NO is decreased in old cells compared to that in young or hTERT transfected cells. Normal monocyte adhesion is greater in old cells than in young or hTERT transfected cells and exposure to TNF-α causes an even greater increase in adhesion in old than in young or hTERT transfected cells. In short, hTERT results in endothelial cells that are functionally and phenotypically normal (Matsushita et al., 2001; MacKenzie et al., 2000). Telomerase effectively resets senescence and senescent changes in human endothelial cells, and these are among the changes playing significant roles in clinical atherogenesis.

Although caution is warranted, specific risks (other than those attributable to gene therapy, arterial catheterization, and delivery methods generically) have no supportive data. Obvious risk might accrue from cellular immortalization, but no data support specific risk. As with cancer, cell proliferation must be considered, particularly in light of the proliferation of vascular intimal tissue in atherogenesis. As noted above, however, immortalization of the specific cell phenotype most pertinent to this concern, human vascular smooth muscle cells, does not cause inappropriate proliferation. Moreover, these cells have a normal, conserved phenotype (Loeuillet et al., 2001), consistent with all available data on immortalization of other human somatic cells since the initial work (Bodnar et al., 1998). Similarly, other data on hTERT transfection of human cells from large-vessel and microvascular sites show no effect on their differentiated and functional phenotype or on karyotype. Such cells maintain their angiogenic potential in vitro and are relatively (compared to normal senescent endothelial cells) resistant to apoptosis. These findings support the conclusion that immortalized human vascular endothelial cells may be "highly desirable for designing vascular transplantation and gene therapy delivery systems in vivo" (Yang et al., 1999a).

Vascular endothelial cells may be the origin of most human cardiovascular disease, indeed of the majority of modern age-related human deaths on a global scale, but they are not the only target for therapies whose aim is the correction of cellular senescence. In myocardial infarction, for example, locking the barn door of endothelial cell senescence can offer little to make up for the stolen horse of dead myocardium. Save for cardiac transplantation, current medical therapy has (realistically) nothing to offer, but regenerative medicine approaches might offer much (Tzukerman et al., 2002). In this case, transplantation might be that of myocardial cells rather than of the entire organ. Alternatively, we might encourage endogenous myocardial cell transplantation by using hTERT.

After myocardial infarction, human myocardial cells are locked irreversibly out of the cell cycle. In mice, forced telomerase expression not only results in longer telomere lengths but, histologically, in hypercellularity, increased myocyte density, and increased DNA synthesis. This is followed by myocyte enlargement without evidence of fibrosis or cardiovascular dysfunction (Oh et al., 2001a). Human myocytes immortalized with hTERT, "retained the properties of primary HMF cells, as they expressed fibroblast markers (prolyl-4-hydroxylase, vimentin), cytokines (interleukin 1α, 6, 8), and angiotensin II receptors and were permissive for coxsackievirus B3 infection" (Harms et al., 2001).

Current interventions in cardiovascular disease are not notably effective in comparison with the incidence and severity of the disease. We have only to remember that atherosclerotic disease is the major single killer globally, and specifically in almost all developed nations, to realize how far we are from satisfactory intervention. Malignancy remains the only significant competition as a cause of death. Cell senescence is probably universal in and fundamental to atherosclerosis and its clinical consequences. This possibility, coupled with potential therapy, justifies substantial investment of intelligence and finances in testing cell senescence as an effective point of intervention. Telomerase therapy, whether by transfection or induction, is likely to become the most efficient point of intervention in human atherosclerosis.

CHAPTER 10

Orthopedic Systems

Structure and Overview

Bones are the physical supports that keep us from being shapeless lumps of protoplasm, but they serve other, perhaps equally important, functions. They offer protection (the skull, spinal rings, and rib cage) to critical soft tissue organs, provide lever arms for muscle movement (most bones to some degree), and maintain storage depots of calcium, phosphorus, and other minerals for rapidly shifting and acute metabolic needs. These (and other) functions can be most profitably discussed from the standpoint of aging pathology. In aging humans, bones get brittle and prone to fracture (osteoporosis), while joints degenerate and become inflamed and painful (osteoarthritis).

Our bones (here excluding the marrow and joint structures) are composed of cells, matrix, and minerals. The cells manufacture the matrix, which attracts and tightly holds the minerals. Together the properties of the matrix and ratio of the minerals determine compressive strength, hardness, resistance, and elasticity of bone. Cells determine the nature of the bone but are influenced by diet (e.g., mineral supply), hormonal signals (e.g., estrogen, parathyroid, etc), vascularity, and physical usage.

Bone cells come in two types, osteoblasts and osteoclasts. This cellular duality might be almost Manichean, although the delicate bony balance is not so much between good and evil as between creation and destruction. The Hindu division between Brahma (the creator) and Shiva (the destroyer) is a more apt analogy for living bones: osteoblasts constantly create bone while the osteoclasts constantly destroy it (Travis, 2000). This is current orthodoxy, despite a surprisingly lack of data showing that (with the exception of two specific transcripts) osteoblasts differ from generic fibroblasts or that bone mineralization (as opposed to matrix formation) is controlled by the osteoblast (Ducy et al.,

2000). Nonetheless, however orchestrated, the result is continual turnover as bone is remade moment to moment, which serves to replace the adult skeleton approximately every decade (Manolagas, 2000). As Marcus Aurelius (Staniforth, 1964 p 109) put it so thoughtfully, nature "will change everything . . . and out of their substance will make fresh things . . . renewing of the world's youthfulness." Alas, not entirely, for the rate of renewal slows and the outcome of this "perpetual renewing" becomes less structurally sound over time.

Two variables are paramount and they can change independently in growth, age, or disease. The first variable is the balance between the osteoblasts and osteoclasts. If bone is created and destroyed at the same rate, the result is a constant bone mass, constantly in flux. A slight imbalance and patients have net gain (as in normal childhood growth) or net loss (as in osteoporosis).

The second variable is more subtle: the rate at which bone is turned over. Even if no *net* gain or loss of bone occurs, turnover rates may be rapid (as in healing) or slow (as in hypothyroidism). Rapid turnover provides a good response to damage and exercise, but the cost is a high metabolic demand. Slow turnover is metabolically cheap, but the result is slow healing and mismatch between what our activity demands and what our bones can provide.

Remodeling is constant and responsive to our needs. It adapts rapidly to meet the needs of growth and demands of physical stress on our bones. Even when the body demands a net change in bone, for example, in normal growth when the osteoblasts lead and the balance is unequal, both cells work concurrently to remodel and create functional bone. It is not enough to make more bone; it must be bone that works. Adult bones are not merely more bony than immature bone, they have been remodeled many times over (Manolagas, 2000).

The *osteoblast* is basically a "sophisticated fibroblast" (Ducy et al., 2000) that synthesizes and deposits the extracellular matrix that, once mineralized, is new bone. Osteoblasts therefore create longitudinal bone growth and are crucial to the continual remodeling that maintains our structural integrity and responds to the changing structural requirements resulting from growth, injury, and behavior (e.g., exercise). Nonetheless, the osteoblast and osteoclast are in continual and intimate communication and the interchange, rather than the osteoblast, defines the skeleton and its integrity in the face of time and stress.

The *osteoclast* is a multinucleated cell formed by the fusion of several cells of the macrophage or monocyte family (Teitelbaum, 2000). Maturation of osteoclasts from the macrophage precursor appears to require contact with osteoblasts, as well as two factors that the osteoblasts or other stromal cells must secrete: macrophage colony-stimulating factor (M-CSF) and a receptor for activating nuclear factor κ B ligand (RANKL). Physical cell contact is signaled by osteoprotegerin (OPG), an inhibitory surface molecule on the osteoblast which competes with the aforementioned receptor molecule. Activated T lymphocytes express this same receptor molecule and trigger osteoclastogenesis, which may explain the osteoclastic destruction seen in rheumatoid arthritis. Over the last decade of the twentieth century, the regulatory roles of serum calcium, estrogen, bisphosphonates, and integrins in controlling the osteoclast and its function have gradually become clearer, although some details remain enigmatic.

As a result of changing hormonal, behavioral, and metabolic inputs, the balance between bone destruction and growth is continually in flux. Bony resorption by the osteoclast is a sophisticated version of normal macrophage function. The cell attaches to bone and isolates a small portion. It then dissolves the mineral portion by acidification and degrades the remaining protein matrix. Finally, it endocytoses the resulting products, releases them back into circulation, and moves on to a new site. This cycle typically requires 3 weeks and at any one time, the osteoclasts are destroying approximately one to two million sites in the average adult skeleton. Osteoblastic regrowth, by contrast, requires approximately 3–4 months (Rodan and Martin, 2000).

Aging and Other Pathology

After age 40, the balance between bone destruction by osteoclasts and bone formation by osteoblasts shifts to favor resorption. The end result is age-related disease, especially osteoporosis (Rodan and Martin, 2000). This outcome comprises not only clinical and personal but financial losses. The latter are estimated at $14 billion per year in the United States alone, where at least 10 million patients have osteoporosis (Kiberstis et al., 2000). Nor is osteoporosis the only age-related disease of the skeleton. Bone cancers (primary and secondary) have been covered previously. For a multitude of reasons—osteoporosis primary among them, but including pathological fractures due to cancer, increases in gait instability, sensory dysfunctions, slower reflexes, and vascular problems, and complex interactive effects between each—the older patient is more likely to suffer from fractures. As patients age, they are less able to heal effectively, less tolerant of resultant disabilities in performing daily activities, and therefore less able to function independently. Moreover, to some extent, problems due to bone aging may be minor compared to problems due to joint aging. Aging joints are apt to cause severe and constant pain, as well as inability to perform quotidian activities. Aging joints are especially prone to osteoarthritis but the incidence of rheumatoid arthritis is not far behind, followed by the less dramatic rise in intraarticular fractures. Collectively, these pathologies are outcomes of and underscore changes in the aging skeletal system (Fig. 10–1).

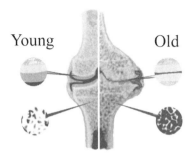

Young   Old

Figure 10–1 Aging orthopedic tissue. In the aging joint (top pullouts), chondrocytes senesce causing gradual thinning and finally a total loss of the cartilage layer, resulting in inflammation and destruction of joint surface. In aging bone, the predominating osteoclast balance causes gradual loss of trabeculae, resulting in decreased strength and increased fracture probability.

Osteoporosis is the most publicized disease of the aging skeleton, largely due to its clinical consequences. Hip fractures alone have a mortality that increases with age and increases more rapidly when accompanied by cognitive impairments, such as Alzheimer dementia (Cree et al., 2000). This observation can be extended into a general rule: risks of osteoporosis are multiplied by concurrent age-related disabilities in other physiological systems, such as vascular pathology, renal dysfunction, etc. Although early surgical intervention in hip fracture has proven valuable, many of the other factors that determine mortality and morbidity remain only partially understood (Hannan et al., 2001). Improvement in our understanding of the pathology is needed, as well as in our consequent ability to treat or prevent it.

Osteoporosis is the loss of minerals, bony matrix, and bone strength as we grow older (Baylink and Jennings, 1994; Chestnut, 1994). The World Health Organization defines *osteopenia* as bone density from 1 to 2.5 standard deviations and osteoporosis as less than 2.5 standard deviations below the normal mean density for young women (World Health Organization, 1994; Medical Letter, 2000b). The loss of mineral mass is documented not only in humans (Lindsay et al., 1992; Rico et al., 1993; Siris et al., 2001) but in other primates, where it correlates with age and may not be related to gonadal or nutritional deficiencies (Colman et al., 1999b), although, as in humans, it is common after menopause (Colman et al., 1999a). Perhaps a third of postmenopausal white women are affected and a fifth of elderly men (Melton, 1995, 1998) and it is probably a largely underdiagnosed disease (Chestnut, 2001). Though thought of as a disease of aging women, the loss of bone density is found in both sexes (Scopacasa et al., 2002). Generically, osteoporosis has been linked to weight loss (Chao et al., 2000), a frequent concomitant of aging in either sex. Elderly men have an age-specific increase in incidence of hip and vertebral body fractures (Kenny et al., 2000; Ravaglia et al., 2000), roughly half that of age-matched women (Khosla et al., 1999).

In women, early postmenopausal bone loss (type I osteoporosis) is considered a direct consequence of estrogen deficiency. Declining estrogen exposure causes an increase in bone resorption without compensatory increase in bone formation. Late postmenopausal bone loss (type II osteoporosis) may be attributable to estrogen deficiency (Khosla et al., 1999), although other age-related factors (independent of estrogen decline) are likely to play a significant role. As bone loss occurs, there is a correlated increase in parathyroid hormone secretion, which should cause increased bone resorption and bone loss.

In men, the etiology of age-related bone loss is argued, but is probably largely equivalent to the process in women. Evidence from a male genetically deficient in estrogen receptor-α and in two males with a genetic aromatase deficiency indicate that estrogen may play a role in bone metabolism in both sexes. Moreover, large epidemiologic studies looking at aging men have found that bone mineral density correlates better with serum estrogen than it does with testosterone (Khosla et al., 1999). While the gradual decline in male serum testosterone may play some minor role in the genesis of osteoporosis (Kenny et al., 2000), estrogen is the primary player (Katz, 2000). Probably, estrogen functions in conjunction with other interacting factors, such as the declining muscle mass (Ravaglia et al., 2000) and increases in cortisol secretion (Raff et al., 1999) that occur with age. Dietary factors may play a role. For example, diets chronically high in retinol may promote osteoporosis (Denke, 2002; Feskanich et al., 2002).

In either sex, whatever the etiology or interactive effects of hormones, muscle mass, diet, and physical activity, the common denominator in all age-related osteoporosis is osteoblast dysfunction (Kveiborg et al., 2001b). This results in the gradual but cumulative loss of bone and bone matrix. Remodeling becomes weighted against the osteoblast and bone formation and in favor of the osteoclast and bone destruction. The outcome is osteoporosis and markedly increased morbidity.

Joints have their own age-related pathology, predominantly *arthritis*, a generic term for inflammatory joint processes. The two major types, osteoarthritis and rheumatoid arthritis, together afflict half of the world's population over 65 years of age (Hagman, 2000). The primary risk factors are injury, obesity, genetic predilection, and age.

Osteoarthritis is an age-related degenerative disease of the joints in which the joint surface is gradually lost to erosion and inflammation. Our understanding of aging suggests that aging and osteoarthritis share common causes (Kirkwood, 1997; Lee et al., 2002a) and aging is linked to the incidence and pathology. The mechanisms of this linkage are unclear. Although ascribed to wear and tear, some individuals incur only little disease and only late in life, whereas others show severe osteoarthritis at an early age. This observation not only underlines the known linkage to cumulative trauma and genetic predisposition (Ingvarsson et al., 2001) but recalls the common thread throughout other organ systems. Aging is not merely wear and tear, but is due to the increasing failure to repair and maintain tissues in the face of such wear and tear as we grow older. In osteoarthritis, the older joint is less capable of self-repair and self-maintenance.

Treatment for osteoarthritis falls into two major categories: joint replacement and agents that interfere with joint inflammation. Of the latter, nonsteroidal agents (such as COX-2 inhibitors) have shown inarguable efficacy in treating the pain consequent upon the disease, but are expensive (Geba et al., 2002) and probably do little to alter the course of the disease. Osteoarthritis is characterized by a gradual but inexorable destruction of the joint surface. The normal joint surface is composed of a glistening layer of intercellular matrix and chondrocytes. These latter cells are specialized fibroblasts that form the cartilage and define the joint. The joint surface is notorious for having a marginal nutrient supply, since capillaries do not extend into the joint surface. Transport of nutrients and oxygen to the chondrocytes is accomplished in a more or less passive fashion as a result of diffusion and fluctuating compression and traction as the joint bears weight and moves. As the joint bears weight and moves, these latter alternating forces act much as squeezing a sponge does in transferring nutrients into and waste products out of the layer of cartilage. The health of the chondrocyte depends on the quality of its vascular supply and activity of the joint. Rather than making chondrocytes independent of aging in the vascular bed, however, the reliance on compressive and diffusive forces leaves the joint surface and chondrocytes that compose it more at risk. The result is that arterial disease and traumatic (or inadequate) physical activity can be, independently, responsible for the genesis of joint disease.

Rheumatoid arthritis increases with age (Pisetsky and St. Clair, 2001), but juvenile forms occur. Despite its increasing prevalence with age, rheumatoid arthritis is often neglected as an age-related disease. Although rheumatoid and osteoarthritis have an inflammatory component, rheumatoid arthritis is considered to be due to immune system dysfunction rather than to other causes. Over the years, the trigger for this immune reaction has been blamed on traumatic injury, microbial infection, and a host of other causes. Whatever may incite the destruction, the immune response is often not restricted to joints but may have widespread manifestations, affecting the entire body and lowering life expectancy (Mikuls and Saag, 2001; Pisetsky and St. Clair, 2001). With some justification, this form of arthritis might be considered a form of immune (rather than joint) dysfunction and therefore properly discussed in the context of immune senescence. The immune system shows profound changes. While healthy individuals maintain a diverse T-cell repertoire, patients with rheumatoid arthritis do not. There are contractions of the T-cell repertoire and of receptor diversity (Koetz et al., 2000), and the emergence of oligoclonal T-cell populations. This restriction in immune response is peculiar to rheumatoid arthritis and is not found in other forms of chronic inflammation, such as hepatitis C. Moreover, it is not limited to memory cells, but occurs in the naive T cells, which suggests that the origin of rheumatoid arthritis lies within the immune system, not the joint. The pathology is not due so much to synovial antigens as it is to intrinsic problems within the immune system, specifically the T-cell population, although mast cells equally play a role (Lee et al., 2002a). The full extent of perturbations and their causes are unknown (Wagner et al., 1998).

The Role of Cell Senescence

The skeletal system, as discussed here, encompasses two sorts of cells: those within trabecular bone and those of the joint surface. If age-related changes in the skeletal system are attributable to cell senescence, then senescent change should be present in cells from both tissues. In the former tissue, we should expect evidence of cell senescence within older osteoblasts (and perhaps older osteoclasts); in the latter tissue, we should expect evidence of cell senescence within older chondrocytes. Moreover, in each case, we should expect that observed changes in gene expression of the indigenous cell type should correspond to pathological changes found clinically in their respective tissues. Current evidence is in keeping with these expectations.

Osteoblasts show considerable change with age and these underlie the poor function seen in patients with osteoporosis. Some changes are generic, such as changes in morphology and increased β-galactosidase activity (Kassem et al., 1997) or a decrease in cell numbers or the rate of cell division (Wolf and Pendergrass, 1999). As in other tissues in which cells continue to divide, telomeres are shorter in senescent osteoblasts and in osteoblasts taken from older patients (Yudoh et al., 2001). Although some investigators report no clear excess of shortened telomeres in osteoporotic patients (Kveiborg et al., 1999), this may be due to (1) an insufficient statistical sample size, (2) an increased variance in such cells, or (3) interacting variables other than osteoblast senescence. For example, two patient samples with equivalent osteoblast senescence but widely divergent estrogen levels might reasonably have different clinical outcomes, making it more difficult to tease out an independent effect of osteoblast senescence.

Osteoblasts demonstrate cell phenotype–specific changes as they senesce, changes that have more direct relevance to the observed clinical pathology. In vitro osteoblasts show reductions in the mRNAs of alkaline phosphatase, osteocalcin, and type I collagen (Kassem et al., 1997; Yudoh et al., 2001). Such changes are not due to a decrease in the calcitriol (vitamin D) responsiveness of the osteoblasts. There is no change in the location or number of vitamin D receptors. Calcitriol effectively induces alkaline phosphatase and osteocalcin expression in senescing osteoblasts. (Kveiborg et al., 2001b). Insulin-like growth factors are known stimulators of osteoblast function and bone formation. Although IGF-2 mRNA remains unchanged in senescing osteoblasts, expression of IGF-1 mRNA falls by 50%. Levels of binding proteins fall: IGF-3 binding protein (IGFBP-3) mRNA falls by 70% and its protein production by 84%; IGFBP-4 mRNA falls by 30%, and IGFBP-5 mRNA by 40% (Kveiborg et al., 2000).

Many other changes in gene expression occur during osteoblast senescence. These changes might, perhaps with less justification, be linked to clinical outcome in patients with osteoporosis, despite scant theoretical and almost no experimental basis for doing so. These additional changes in gene expression include up-regulation in so-called gerontogenes, such as Apo J and GTP- (Gonos et al., 1998). Changes are found in transforming growth factor beta (TGF-β). When calcitriol is present, TGF-β normally induces osteoblast differentiation and formation of bony matrix, but inhibits osteocalcin production, which is necessary for osteoblast differentiation (Kassem et al., 2000). Likewise, there is a dramatic decline in the gene expression for the mRNAs of CBFA 1 (a transcription factor known as polyoma enhancer-binding protein, or PEBP2αA) and topoisomerase I mRNA. Neither decrement occurs in immortalized osteoblasts. While it is clear that the dysfunction that occurs in aging human osteoblasts is paralleled by alterations in gene expression (Christiansen et al., 2000a), the direction of causation is unproven. Extrapolating from what we know of other senescing cells in other tissues, it is most likely that changes in gene expression cause the age-related clinical pathology (osteoporosis). The contrary remains possible: the clinical pathology might cause the observed changes in gene expression.

Osteoporosis and arthritic disease are considered distinct disease processes, but a curious blend of pathology occurs in periarticular bone. Rheumatoid and osteoarthritis often demonstrate osteopenia in bony tissue underlying and surrounding affected articular surfaces. Here again, cell senescence may play a role. Periarticular osteoblasts from patients with rheumatoid or osteoarthritis demonstrate decreased telomere lengths, replicative lifespans, rates of cell proliferation, and common osteoblastic markers (alkaline phosphatase activity, osteocalcin and C-terminal type I procollagen secretion, and cAMP response to parathyroid hormone). While these changes correlate with age, they are more pronounced in patients with osteoporosis and most pronounced in patients with rheumatoid arthritis, suggesting that osteoblast replicative senescence contributes to periarticular osteopenia (Yudoh et al., 2000).

Osteoarthritis depends on normal chondrocyte function. Good evidence exists that chondrocytes senesce during osteoarthritis (Aigner et al., 2002; Martin et al., 2002b). Overall, the correlation between disease and age (between or within species, including humans) is poor, while that between disease and cell senescence is excellent (Yudoh et al., 2000; Martin et al., 2002b). Chondrocyte senescence occurs in vivo in human joints (Parsch et al., 2002). The association supports the hypothesis that chondrocyte senescence plays a role in osteoarthritis (Martin and Buckwalter, 2001b). Osteoarthritis is not related so much to age as it is to other histological measures. These include fibrillation of the articular surface, decrease in the size and aggregation of proteoglycan aggrecans, increased collagen cross-linking, and a loss of tensile strength and stiffness in the matrix. These are the result of changes in chondrocyte function that decrease the ability of the cells to maintain the tissue. As chondrocytes senesce, they demonstrate decreased synthesis, more frequent synthesis of dysfunctional proteins (e.g., smaller, less uniform aggrecans), and a decreased response to chondrocyte growth factors. They show a decrease in telomere length, a marked decline in mitotic activity, and (as do other aging fibroblasts) an increased expression of β-galactosidase (Martin and Buckwalter, 2001a, 2001b; Martin et al., 2002b).

Osteoarthritis is a cascade of failure: the ability of the joint to incur and repair repetitive trauma is limited by the ability of the chondrocytes to replicate and maintain homeostasis. As the chondrocytes senesce, their pattern of gene expression changes. Replication and cell replacement are inadequate to the needs of the articular surface. The matrix becomes less durable and more friable. As daily joint use continues, cell senescence accelerates, as does the loss of tissue function and articular surface. The final outcome is joint destruction; the diagnosis, osteoarthritis.

Rheumatoid arthritis is dependent on immune mechanisms and (periarticular osteopenia aside) might therefore be expected to demonstrate correlations with immune senescence (see Chapter 11). One hypothesis suggests that this is due to alterations in tumor necrosis factor (TNF) in senescent cells (Crew et al., 1998). The role of TNF in this disease has spawned a series of new drugs (see below). Telomerase activity is prevalent in activated lymphocytes, particularly monocytes (Yamanishi et al., 1998), and is found in 60% (28/47) of patients with rheumatoid arthritis, including monoarticular arthritis. This is true of chrondromatosis and osteoarthritis, but not of other forms of joint disease. Telomerase activity has a 96% (52/54) specificity for rheumatoid arthritis (Yamanishi et al., 1999). Moreover, the degree of telomerase activity correlates with the severity of the disease (Yamanishi et al., 1998).

As noted above, receptor diversity is contracted in the lymphocyte population of patients with rheumatoid arthritis. Contraction is characteristic of older patients. For example, the percentage of CD4 T cells containing T-cell receptor rearrangement excision circles (TREC) is markedly reduced in patients with rheumatoid arthritis to levels characteristic of matched control patients who are 20 years older. Even young patients with rheumatoid arthritis show erosion of telomeres in their circulating T cells (de Boer, 2002; Koetz et al., 2000). That this loss correlates with disease presence but not duration or intervention (Koetz et al., 2000) and that naive T cells are equally involved (Wagner et al., 1998) suggests an accelerated lymphocyte turnover in these patients that probably occurs as a direct result of the abnormal autoimmune response.

Cell senescence is far more likely an outcome than a cause of rheumatoid arthritis, although it may play a critical role in how the pathology plays out within the articular tissue. Genetic factors account for one-half to two-thirds of human osteoarthritis and rheumatoid arthritis (Ho et al., 2000). These factors probably play a stronger role than immune senescence, although genetic abnormalities might hasten immune senescence by driving lymphocytic proliferation, for example, in autoimmune dysfunction and continual antigenic stimulation. There appears little doubt that rheumatoid arthritis is more than merely cell senescence, although the expression of specific genetic defects may become more prominent in senescent cells, thereby accelerating the articular damage to increasingly senescent chondrocytes caused by increasingly senescent lymphocytes.

Intervention

As in other tissues, the complexity of the pathology creates a plenitude of targets for therapeutic intervention (Kiberstis et al., 2000; Rodan and Martin, 2000). Although bone density is a primary marker for bone health in the elderly, increasing the density is not the point, nor necessarily an effective point of intervention (Haguenauer et al., 2001). An intervention is useful if and only if it has clinical benefits (e.g., lowering the rate of vertebral fractures). Exercise, for example, may increase bone density (Hagberg et al., 2001; Kohrt, 2001), but has practical value only if it improves or retains bone function. Most interventions in osteoporosis target osteoclasts and bone resorption, rather than osteoblasts and bone formation. These interventions include estrogens, selective estrogen receptor modulators, and bisphosphonates. There are, however, a growing number of drugs that focus on the osteoblasts and bone formation, including particularly the statins, but also recombinant parathyroid hormone segments (Medical Letter, 2003a), novel matrices, signaling molecules, and cultured stem cells (Service, 2000).

Some interventions have interactive effects on other common age-related and often coincident pathology. For example, the most common cause of death among women with osteoporosis is cardiovascular disease (Kado et al., 1999). Interventions, such as statins (Meier et al., 2000; Wang et al., 2000e), aimed at osteoporosis must therefore be assessed in regard to their effect on cardiovascular risk as well as osteoporosis (Cummings and Bauer, 2000).

Until now, osteopenia and osteoporosis have been treated with combined calcium and vitamin D (calcitriol), estrogen, selective estrogen receptor modulators such as raloxifene (Johnston et al., 2000a), bisphosphonates (Reid et al., 2002), calcitonin, HMG-CoA reductase inhibitors (statins), parathyroid hormone and its recombinant segments, isoflavones, and combinations with varying success (Alexandersen et al., 2001; Villareal et al., 2001), costs, and side effects (Altkorn and Vokes, 2001; Hennessy and Strom, 2001; Medical Letter, 2000b; van Staa et al., 2001). Bisphosphonates (e.g., risedronate) have been used in Paget's disease and osteoporosis and may be effective (Harris et al., 1999b; Eastell, 2001; Reid et al., 2002). It may prove more effective at reducing fracture risk than estrogen replacement (Grady and Cummings, 2001).

Ironically, despite calcitriol and calcium being prerequisites for normal osteoblast function (Kveiborg et al., 2000), clinical data do little to show that supplementing these compounds beyond normal adult requirements has substantial benefit. None of these are totally effective.

Hormone replacement has been considered relatively effective in preventing appendicular fractures in the elderly patient and in preventing (but not necessarily treating) the postmenopausal osteoporosis that underlies such fractures (Grady and Cummings, 2001; Torgerson and Bell-Syer, 2001; Nelson et al., 2002). Meta-analysis suggests an additional trend toward decreasing efficacy of fracture prevention with increasing patient age (Torgerson and Bell-Syer, 2001). It may be that the greatest effects from hormone replacement are found only in those age groups with the lowest risk of fracture. If this is so, then the risks of long-term hormone replacement may prove to exceed its potential benefits (Grady and Cummings, 2001). The potential cardiovascular risks and benefits of estrogen have been discussed previously in the chapter on the cardiovascular system. Although some data suggest that hormone replacement increases the risk of breast or endometrial cancer (Chiechi and Secreto, 2000; Chen et al., 2002a), there has been disagreement (Campagnoli et al., 1999; Leslie et al., 1999). Ironically, a minority body of data suggest that hormone replacement therapy may be protective against certain forms of cancer, including ovarian (Ness et al., 2000b) and colon cancer (Crandall, 1999; Grodstein et al., 1999). Extensive and careful review of epidemiological data suggest increased risk from use of estrogen therapy (Noller, 2002) and even higher risk in combination with progesterone (Writing Group for the Women's Health Initiative Investigators, 2002; Fletcher and Colditz, 2002), although others have argued that data are insufficient for accurate assessment (Beral et al., 1999). The overall balanced risk (cancer risk versus osteoporosis risk) remains uncertain and doubtlessly varies with the individual (Boroditsky, 2000; Crawshaw, 2000; Nelson, 2002; Noller, 2002), but hormone replacement is still a standard therapy. The specific hormone replacement, such as estradiol, estriol (Hayashi et al., 2000), or an estrogen analog, that will optimize bone retention with minimal side effects remains an open issue, as does the optimal time to initiate replacement (Cure-Cure and Cure-Ramirez, 2001) and most appropriate (and perhaps safest) dosage (Lindsay et al., 2002). The ligand for the osteoporotic effect of sexual steroids is apparently independent of the ligand in reproductive organs (Kousteni et al., 2002). Although hormone replacement is more effective in lowering osteoporotic risk than selective estrogen receptor modulators, the higher potential (cancer) risks of hormone replacement and possible cardiovascular benefits of selective estrogen receptor modulators (Umland et al., 1999) may make receptor modulators or bisphosphonates (Harris et al., 1999b; Eastell, 2001; Reid et al., 2002) more appropriate clinical choices (Genazzani and Gambacciani, 1999; Grady and Cummings, 2001).

More fundamental interventions remain for consideration. One of the only known interventions in extending healthy lifespan, caloric restriction, fails to prevent osteoporosis in aging male rats (Sanderson et al., 1997). The significance of this observation for aging humans of either sex is obscure.

Intervention in osteoblast senescence is tempting but difficult (Fossel, 1996, 2001b; Yudoh et al., 2001). Prime target for intervention in osteoporotic pathology or not, no data have been published on in vivo intervention (except in mice), although such studies are planned. In vitro, however, such intervention has already demonstrated its efficacy. hTERT gene, transfected into human osteoblastic cells (from donors and from osteoblastic cell strain NHOst 54881), results in significant telomerase expression and activity. Moreover, these cells have elongated telomeres and continued alkaline phosphatase activity and secretion of procollagen I C-terminal propeptide (PICP), thus supporting the need to test this approach as an ex vivo therapy for human osteoporosis (Yudoh et al., 2001). Other published work suggests that hTERT expression (coupled with SV40 T antigen) not only extends the lifespan of osteoblast and osteoclast precursor cells but that the resulting osteoblasts and osteoclasts have normal phenotypes (Darimont et al., 2002).

When human bone marrow stromal cells are transfected with hTERT, they show increased telomere lengths and continue to proliferate even at 10 times the normal number of population doublings. These cells show normal osteoblastic markers, differentiation potential, and karyotypes. Transfected human cells implanted subcutaneously in immunodeficient mice form more bone than normal cells (Simonsen et al., 2002). That such telomerized stromal cells maintain their osteogenic potential and are capable of generating normal mineralized lamellar bone structure and associated marrow suggests that telomerase therapy may be useful in bone regeneration and repair (Shi et al., 2002). While much critical experimental work remains undone, initial data support the possibility that osteoblastic senescence is a key mechanism in human osteoporosis and likely the single most effective point of clinical intervention.

Although the complexity of pathology might be viewed as an opportunity, the numerous roads that lead to human joint degradation, coupled with the extensive and perhaps irreparable articular damage that occurs in osteoarthritis, have prompted some researchers to conclude that a single cure is unlikely (Hagman, 2000). Current therapy (beyond pain relief) devolves into questions of the timing and efficacy of joint replacement. Nonetheless, alternative therapies have been tried (and found wanting) over the years. There is extensive public interest in and a dismissive academic attitude toward glucosamine (with or without chondroitin). The good news is that despite widespread use, there are few known side effects. Surprisingly to many clinicians, the few animal studies are largely supportive of beneficial effects, but initial results of the large-scale, double-blind, human study are unimpressive (Medical Letter, 2001d).

Cell senescence of the chondrocytes is likewise a target. Ignoring senescent chondrocytes may limit the efficacy of other interventions. Transplantation procedures, for example, intended to restore osteoarthritic articular surfaces may, paralleling a like problem seen with bone marrow transplantation, be limited by the replicative lifespan of transplanted chondrocytes (Martin and Buckwalter, 2001b). More fundamental and effective therapy for osteoarthritis is intervention in chondrocyte senescence (Fossel, 1996; Martin and Buckwalter, 2001a). The goal is to ameliorate, prevent, or reverse chondrocyte senescence and thereby intervene in osteoarthritis. Initial trials of transfection of human chondrocytes with hTERT show that these cells have extended lifespans and maintain a normal cell phenotype (Piera-Velazquez et al., 2002). Given these results, telomerase or some telomerase-independent intervention (Martin et al., 2002b) in chondrocyte senescence might be clinically effective. Moreover, the aging chondrocytes of the human joint are more approachable technically than are the aging osteoblasts of the human bone.

Rheumatoid arthritis remains a common and disabling disease. Despite considerable recent progress in treating rheumatoid arthritis (Case, 2001a; Pisetsky and St. Clair, 2001; Wildy and Wasko, 2001), there is room for improvement. Current therapies involve the use of common antiinflammatory medications or the less common and more potent strategy of immune suppression. No nonsteroidal antiinflammatory (NSAID) is consistently more effective than another, although individual patients may derive more benefit from specific nonsteroidals (Medical Letter, 2000a). These drugs work by inhibition of the two isoforms of cyclooxygenase: COX-1 and COX-2. The COX-2 inhibitors cause less gastric toxicity than older, nonselective nonsteroidal antiinflammatory medications (Medical Letter, 2000a; Silverstein et al., 2000), but may simultaneously increase the risk of cardiovascular problems (Medical Letter, 2001a; Mukherjee et al., 2001). Nonetheless, most clinical consultants recommend the use of COX-2 inhibitors in treating rheumatoid arthritis, often in conjunction with other medications (Medical Letter, 2000a). Although COX-2 inhibitors may be effective in osteoarthritis, these drugs are less effective in rheumatoid arthritis.

There is a wide selection of other (often immunosuppressive) drugs that have been used in rheumatoid arthritis and newer agents are coming into use (Case, 2001b). Current disease-modifying antirheumatic drugs (DMARDs) include hydroxycholoquine and other antimalarials, steroids, gold compounds, penicillamine, cytotoxic drugs (azothioprine and cyclophosphamide), sulfasalazine, methotrexate, leflunomide, etanercept, infliximab cyclosporin, and TNF inhibitors, as well as combination therapy and apheresis (Gabriel et al., 2001; Kremer, 2001; Laan et al., 2001). Several agents (infliximab, etanercept, and adalimumab) inhibit TNF-α, which induces fibroblast proliferation and the cascade of inflammation that causes rheumatoid arthritis (Medical Letter, 2003b). Despite gradually increasing clinical optimism, no approach is considered totally effective nor free from side effects (Wollheim, 2001).

In osteoarthritis, chondrocyte cell senescence may be central to the pathology, but this is not likely true of rheumatoid arthritis. Senescent cells are abundant in affected rheumatic joints, but the senescent cells are immune in origin rather than indigenous to the joint. If cell senescence plays a role in rheumatoid arthritis, then that role is predominantly lymphocytic rather than chondrocytic, and secondary rather than primary.

Attempts to intervene in age-related disease in the skeletal system should most profitably focus on osteoblast and chondrocyte senescence, with an eye toward osteoporosis and osteoarthritis, respectively. Senescence of these cells may be central to these ubiquitous diseases.

CHAPTER **11**

Hematopoetic and Immune Systems

Structure and Overview

The hematopoetic and immune systems share a common cellular nursery in the bone marrow and, largely for that reason, are considered here together. Such cells are usually divided into red cells, white cells, and other miscellaneous cells, not all of which are true cells in that they may lack nuclei (e.g., mature red cells) and other intracellular organelles (e.g., thrombocytes). Red cells are responsible for ferrying oxygen from the lungs to distant cells without allowing the molecules to oxidize and damage molecules en route. Conversely, they carry carbon dioxide back from distant cells back to the lungs for exhalation. White cells are largely involved with infection control and what might loosely be termed "janitorial functions," i.e., cleaning up antigens and other insoluble and otherwise unrecyclable molecules throughout the body. Platelets are a primary component of clotting and for this reason a target for drugs (such as aspirin) aimed at lowering mortality in the aged by preventing clots.

Most blood cells are transitory and continuously replaced. Although prenatally much of the blood is made in the liver, by halfway through gestation the balance begins to shift to production within the developing bones. The volume of bone marrow is about the same as the volume of the liver, but the marrow is spread throughout the bones of the body. At birth, the bone marrow is almost uniformly active in all bones, but after birth the marrow becomes less metabolically active and gains fat, becoming less red and more yellow. Adult marrow is less active in producing blood cells, especially within the long bones of our extremities. In the adult, most blood cells are produced within ribs, sternum, pelvis, and vertebral bodies. This shift in marrow activity is reversible and responds rapidly to the need for new blood cells.

Although red blood cells, granular leukocytes, and platelets are each different, they all derive from a common pluripotent stem cell within the marrow. These common stem cells divide, one cell perhaps remaining pluripotent, the other progressing a step further down the road to differentiation. This more differentiated cell, though no longer pluripotent, is still a unipotential stem cell for a single cell line. Thus, there may be separate unipotential stem cells for platelets, erythrocytes, lymphocytes, myelocytes, and monocytes. Each unipotential stem cell remains separate once diverging from the pluripotent stem cell. Each will divide and may differentiate more fully, committing to a particular cell line. Some unipotential stem cells may remain in reserve, while daughter cells differentiate fully and enter peripheral circulation. This process—cell division, cell differentiation, and stem cell reserve—is under complex, active, and exacting control.

Erythrocytes are anuclear "cells" that derive from the marrow and that have a circulation half-life of approximately 20 days in the blood. They are usually removed by the spleen as they finish their 3-week span and become less functional. In erythrocytes, the unipotential stem cells in the bone marrow respond rapidly to transfusion, hemorrhage, high altitude (with the consequent fall oximetry), and other distant changes in the body and in its requirements for erythrocyte transfer of oxygen. Such control of erythrocyte cell-line division is maintained by several mechanisms, the primary among them being erythropoietin, a glycoprotein produced in the kidney and that acts directly upon unipotential erythrocyte stem cells to promote division and differentiation of erythrocyte precursors. Speed and degree of response is dictated by three main variables: erythropoietin stimulation, available nutrients (primarily iron), and capabilities of marrow and its component cells. Healthy adult marrow is capable of increasing erythrocyte production to four to five times the basal replacement rate (Bloom and Fawcett, 1975).

T and B lymphocytes are the major cellular components of the immune system. Like erythrocytes, they derive from hematopoetic stem cells in the bone marrow, but unlike erythrocytes, they retain their nuclei and have no fixed term for cellular survival. Thanks to a complex recombinant system, the lymphocyte can generate an incredible number of antigen receptors, estimated in excess of 10^8 different receptors (Effros and Valenzuela, 1998). The immune system is therefore capable of recognizing far more antigens than could be directly coded for a limited number of available genes, even if they were dedicated solely to antibody generation. This amplification of available diversity allows for the recognition of antigens, even if never previously encountered during evolution. Differentiated lymphocytes and their progeny express multiple copies of a single antigen receptor (Janeway and Travers, 1997). At least as important as antigen receptor generation is clonal selection. The immune system needs to weed out receptors for indigenous antigens (that might otherwise result in autoimmune disease) and clonally expand lymphocytes that recognize foreign antigens (and so prevent infection). These tasks must be performed without flaw; the latter task, clonal expansion, must be rapid and must result in a lifelong recognition (immunity) of foreign antigens.

Aging and Other Pathology

Hematopoesis keeps up with our needs, despite some decrements in performance (Fig.11–1). There is only a slight decrease in the number of circulating activated hematopoetic stem (CD34+) cells, a well-maintained capacity for response to appropriate

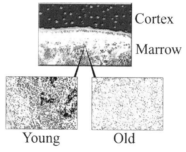

Cortex

Marrow

Young   Old

Figure 11–1 Aging hematopoetic tissue. As aging progresses, there is a correlated, gradual, and increasingly profound loss of bone marrow cells due to accruing senescence among stem and other hematopoetic cell populations of the marrow.

cytokines, and a slight decrease in the ability of leukocytes to produce some cytokines (e.g., granulocyte/macrophage-colony stimulating factor and interleukin-3; Bagnara et al., 2000). In consequence, older patients not only maintain an appropriate numbers of circulating erythrocytes and leukocytes (Sansoni et al., 1993) but preserve a modicum (albeit diminished) ability to respond to stressors, such as blood loss or infection, by producing new cells to match their need. Although there are changes in the erythrocyte supply, these changes are negligible (Effros and Globerson, 2002).

The immune system shows more robust changes with age. There have been attempts to construct models in which the immune system causes aging in the entire organism (Walford, 1969, 1970). While such models have foundered on a lack of supporting and consistent data, the immune system does show pronounced aging changes (Makinodan and Kay, 1980), specifically in lymphocyte function (Globerson and Effros, 2000), and these changes have demonstrable clinical significance in multiple organs (Gardner, 1980; Tarazona et al., 2002). Despite agreement on these findings, the magnitude and, to a greater degree, the mechanisms of immunosenescence are vigorously argued (Bruunsgaard and Pedersen, 1999, 2000). Such changes cannot fairly be characterized as simple failure of the immune system, as though aging were equivalent to other forms of immunodeficiency. It is not. The alterations are not so much quantitative as qualitative, as, for example, in the shift in the relative proportions of immunoglobulins (Igs; in favor of low-affinity autoreactive IgM antibodies) and likewise in proportions of T-cell type (in favor of killer cells) as well as T-cell phenotype and response characteristics (Laux et al., 2000). Although the term *immunosenescence* remains in general use, its simplicity is misleading and ignores the adaptive and complex changes that occur in the aging immune system (Effros, 1998a, 2001a). Many changes remain poorly understood, although major coordinated efforts are in progress to clarify immune system aging (Pawelec et al., 2000b).

Among other changes, autoimmunity (particularly non-organ-specific) increases with age, although this may represent a secondary response to increased cellular damage rather than primary dysregulation of the immune system (Candore et al., 1997). Innate immunity (Ginaldi et al., 1999b) and adaptive (Ginaldi et al., 1999a) immunity suffer with age, though adaptive immunity undergoes the greater losses (Pawelec et al., 2000a). The mechanisms underlying functional losses are argued (Pawelec et al., 1998c, 1999d). Some changes are not so much a matter of aging as of increased immune experience (Franceschi et al., 1999, 2000). With age, we retain fewer naive T cells and achieve a preponderance of memory cells (Ginaldi et al., 1999a; Romaniukha and Iashin, 2001), although with increasing B-cell variance (Breitbart et al., 2002). Moreover, on average, memory cells have shorter telomeres than naive T cells, regardless of donor age (Weng et al., 1995). This shift reflects immunological experience and normal function—not so much loss of naive T cells as of naivete among cells (Hodes, 1997; Linton et al., 1997; Pawelec et al., 2002a). The concomitant loss of CD4+ cells with age, by contrast, occurs irrespective of immunological experience.

Age-related deterioration in innate immune function, though less impressive than in acquired immune function, is significant. Such changes have been reviewed in detail (Ginaldi et al., 1999b) and include changes in granulocyte and natural killer (NK) cell activity, adhesion molecules, and cytokine production. Neutrophils become less capable of phagocytosis, but NK cells show less consistent change and show efficient killing in centenarians. The expression of cell adhesion molecules increases and cytokine network regulation alters, shifting from Th1 to Th2 production and increasing proinflammatory cytokines.

Acquired immune senescence is more dramatic. Although a simple numerical assessment of the circulating blood cells shows few uniform or reliable changes with age, the functional outcome, immunosenescence, is "one of the most dramatic physiologic changes associated with aging" (Effros and Valenzuela, 1998). Indeed, for equivalent infectious diseases the ratio of mortality in the elderly compared to the young adult ranges from approximately threefold in sepsis, meningitis, pneumonia, endocarditis, and septic arthritis to as much as 10- to 20-fold in tuberculosis, urinary tract infections, and appendicitis. To an extent, this is due to barrier losses in the skin, but much of the dysfunction is attributable to immunosenescence (Effros, 2000a). Such changes are found not only in the dermis but in mucosal immune response (Beharka et al., 2001b). Despite these clinical observations, much of the immune system remains unchanged with aging and it is difficult to find functional deficits in phagocytosis, complement activity, and NK cells, although the NK response to cytokines may diminish (Yoshikawa, 2001).

The clinical loss of function (Hodes, 1997) is most dramatically seen in the T-cell compartment (Pawelec et al., 1995, 1997a, 2002a; Miller, 1996) and may be responsible for the increasing morbidity and mortality due to infectious (Effros et al., 1991b; Effros and Pawelec, 1997; Pawelec and Solana, 1997) as well as malignant disease among the elderly (Effros and Valenzuela, 1998; Pawelec et al., 1998b; Effros, 2000a). The same loss of immune efficacy with aging is seen in natural and vaccine-induced influenza immunity in mice (Bender et al., 1998; Klinman et al., 1998) and humans (Bernstein et al., 1999; Remarque, 1999). Functional losses include decreased responsiveness to T-cell receptor stimulation, an impaired T-cell proliferative capacity, a decline in the frequency of CD4+ T cells that produce IL-2, a decreased expression of IL-2 receptors, a decrease in the early events of signal transduction, a decrease in activation-induced intracellular phosphorylation, and a decrease in the cellular proliferative response to T-cell receptor stimulation (Ginaldi et al., 1999a). Although the functional losses may be the more critical, changes do occur in proportions of T-cell subsets (Potestio et al., 1999). For example, the number of CD16+, CD95+/CD28+, and CD95+ lymphocytes increase with age, whereas CD19+ and CD28+ lymphocytes decrease. The latter cells, CD28+, tend to be hTERT positive (Speiser et al., 2001), correlating with the observation that telomerase is less common in circulating leukocytes from older individuals.

With growing (and more careful) data, even immune cells that have not previously been seen as vulnerable to aging problems, such as macrophages, show diminished presentation of antigens and declines in interleukin (IL-1 and IL-6) and tumor necrosis factor (TNF-α) production (Effros et al., 1991a). Evidence for changes in IL-6 remains controversial and recent work suggests no age-associated increase in humans (Beharka et al., 2001a). There is no evidence for age-related changes in mitochondrial DNA with age (Ross et al., 2002). Curiously, caloric restriction has little effect on the impairment of cytokine response, although it does normalize baseline, constitutive cytokine expression (Spaulding et al., 1997a).

Other specific and uncommon diseases have some bearing on aging in the hematopoetic system. The striking absence of immune senescence in Hutchinson Gilford progerics has already been noted, as has the presence of early immune senescence in trisomy 21 (vide supra). Bone marrow transplant recipients have likewise noted on as showing pronounced initial accelerated telomere loss, although this loss becomes asymptotic and therefore has limited clinical consequence. Transplantation with hematopoetic stem cells obviates such risk (Roelofs et al., 2003). Patients with Shwachman-Diamond syndrome show (age-adjusted) loss of telomere length within the leukocyte compartment, which may explain their hematopoietic dysfunction ranging from single-lineage cytopenia to severe aplasia and/or myelodysplasia. The degree of telomere loss does not correlate with severity, suggesting that the disease may be due to an initial (prior to clinically apparent disease) phase of leukocyte stem cell "hyperproliferation" (Thornley et al., 2002a).

The Role of Cell Senescence

When Milton (1652) said those "also serve who only stand and wait," he did so in apposition to the more active of God's retainers: "thousands at his bidding speed, and post o'er land and ocean without rest." Some cells stand and wait, some divide ceaselessly and "post o'er land and ocean without rest." These are the cells of the blood—red and white, hematopoetic and immune—that ceaselessly travel the body, ceaselessly divide, and just as ceaselessly senesce.

The immune system is much like the brain: it starts young, vigorous, and ignorant, it finishes old, slow, and knowledgeable. The senescent immune system has a broad experience with antigens and pathogens, but a contrasting tendency to be sluggish and less specific than is necessary for long-term survival. This lack of specificity includes an increased propensity for autoreactivity and autoimmune disease. Several lines of evidence suggest that cell senescence is involved in immune senescence (Effros and Pawelec, 1997; Pawelec et al., 1997a; Effros, 1998b), but how central a role is arguable (Robertson et al., 2000). The suggestion has even been made that cell senescence, much as it plays a physiologically beneficial role in limiting malignant cell growth, along with apoptosis, may regulate and limit activated T-cell accumulation in the body (Soares et al., 2000).

The major question, however, is not the potential benefits of cell senescence in normal immune function but the potential costs of cell senescence in the abnormal immune function of the elderly (Weng, 2001). One substantially flawed line of argument against cell senescence in immunosenescence—that the longer telomeres of rats and mice should (but do not) preclude immune senescence in such species (Miller, 2000)—unfortunately misrepresents the biology of cell senescence and this error has already been dealt with in earlier chapters and in the literature (Blasco, 2002a). The appropriate variable is not absolute length of telomeres but relative shortening of telomeres compared to the younger animal. The more appropriate and operational question is if changes in gene expression, which accompany and define senescence in immune-related cells, play a causal role in immune senescence. The answer to this more accurately phrased question is the fundamental issue.

Although most immune system cells senesce as do other somatic cells, the presence of stem cells capable of expressing telomerase upon stimulation (Weng, 2002) results in a slower overall rate of aging in the immune system (Edelstein-Keshet et al., 2001) than might be expected from consideration of (*1*) the number of divisions required to produce circulating lymphocytes over the human lifespan or (2) the telomere lengths found in the human hematopoetic stem cell population at birth.

Nonetheless, immune senescence does occur in the elderly and does so in parallel with clear evidence of both telomere shortening (Cawthorn et al., 2003) and cell senescence, particularly in memory (CD8+) T cells (Effros, 2000b). This feature of immune senescence (failing immune memory) is documented clinically on the basis of recurrent herpes zoster infections, poor response to immunization, and high morbidity to influenza infection. Cancer surveillance is impaired in the elderly, putatively due to immune senescence (see below; Effros and Valenzuela, 1998). If we look at lymphocytes directly, the most profound effects of senescence are seen within the T-cell population, profoundly diminishing its ability to defend against not only infections but cancer. T-cell senescence is associated with the loss of expression of critical signaling molecules and has been reviewed by Effros (Effros and Valenzuela, 1998). Although a great many markers do remain invariant with T-cell senescence (surface markers reflecting lineage, adhesion antigens, and receptor structures), CD28, which is responsible for an essential activation signal in these cells, shows a profound decline (Valenzuela and Effros, 2002). In neonates, only 1% of T cells lack CD28, whereas in centenarians, nearly 40% lack the marker (Boucher et al., 1998), making immune senescence one of "the most dramatic cases of examples of in vivo replicative senescence" (Effros and Valenzuela, 1998). CD28 has a multitude of critical functions, but in this context it is worth noting that it is crucial for stimulated expression of telomerase in lymphocytes. Senescing cells lose the ability to express telomerase; senescence accelerates in aging lymphocytes, as they can no longer slow telomere loss.

Paralleling the immune system, the nature and function of the hematopoetic system requires lifelong replacement of cells through cell replication (Weng et al., 1998). The erythrocyte requirements in the average adult may be greater than 10^{12} cells per day (Moore, 1997). The lifetime requirements have therefore been estimated at between 4×10^{15} (2^{52} cells, hence 52 divisions; Lansdorp, 1998) and 4×10^{16} (2^{55} cells, hence 55 divisions; Lansdorp et al., 1997). To provide for these stunning requirements, cell senescence might be delayed (though not necessarily prevented). Although replicative potential falls with age (Jiang et al., 1992), senescence within the bone marrow pleuripotent stem cell compartments is delayed, paralleling their ability to express telomerase in response to proliferative signals (Hiyama et al., 1995d; Chiu et al., 1996). The requirements for maintaining hematopoetic cell division cannot be met within the limits to cell replication imposed on most other somatic cells. It should come as little surprise, therefore, to discover that some stem hematopoetic stem cells express telomerase to stimulation, though not constitutively. Moreover, telomerase activity correlates with the capacity of such stem cells to reconstitute the hematopoetic system: so-called short-term hematopoetic stem cells have lower activity than long-term hematopoetic stem cells (Morrison et al., 1996).

Telomerase in stem cells was first identified within the hematopoetic system (Chiu et al., 1996). Averaging millions of such cells together, telomerase is expressed at a basal level; in reality it is induced in hematopoetic stem cells by cytokine stimulation and down-regulated again with the proliferation and differentiation of hematopoetic cells (Weng et al., 1995; Chen et al., 2000a; Otsuka et al., 2000; Weng, 2002). The intermittent, low level of telomerase activity is insufficient to maintain stable telomere lengths throughout the human lifespan. Although telomere lengths among hematopoetic stem cells may be on the average longer than those found in other somatic cells with an equivalent number of population doublings, stem cells themselves show a slow but significant erosion of telomeres over time (Vaziri et al., 1994; Lui et al., 1998; Effros and Globerson, 2002) as well as an age-related slowing in cell turnover time and a loss in population numbers (Leber and Bacchetti, 1996; Lansdorp et al., 1997; Lansdorp, 1998). There is uncertainty and disagreement regarding the proliferative lifespan of hematopoetic stem cells. Likely candidate cells show a loss of telomere length associated with increased proliferation, which suggests that the proliferative potential of such stem cells is limited and decreases with age (Pawelec, 1999b and c). Although stem cells can be harvested from the elderly patient, they are fewer, have shorter telomeres, and are less effective than those taken from fetal marrow. Among circulating leukocytes, telomeres shorten with age (Hastie et al., 1990; Frenck et al., 1998; Rufer et al., 1999).

Many of the features observed in senescent T lymphocytes (Wolf and Pendergrass, 1999) could plausibly explain immune senescence (Pawelec et al., 1996). In vitro, senescent T cells respond poorly to stress stimuli, are more prone to activation-induced cell death, are less likely to express CD28, are less likely to express or respond appropriately to several interleukins, have shortened telomeres, and lack detectable telomerase (Pawelec et al., 1996; Spaulding et al., 1999). In vivo, T cells likewise show shortened telomeres with age, although they can express telomerase (Allsopp et al., 2002) and tend to have longer telomeres than neutrophils that lack telomerase (Robertson et al., 2000). The loss of the CD28 marker on T cells occurs during normal in vivo aging and may be the outcome of repeated immune stimulation and represent senescence in T lymphocytes (Effros, 1997). This observation and others like it support the suggestion that replicative senescence underlies immune senescence in the elderly (Effros, 1998c; Blasco, 2002a). The mechanism of this relationship is not only unclear but may involve different levels, including defective stem cell maintenance, thymus involution with decreased production of naive T cells (Andrew and Aspinall, 2002), defects in antigen-presenting cells, postmitotic aging in resting immune cells, disrupted activation pathways, or replicative senescence of clonally expanded cells due to extensive antigen-induced activation (Solana and Pawelec, 1998; Pawelec et al., 1999a). The relative contributions are undefined, although likely each plays some role in immunosenescence (Solana and Pawelec, 1998).

Immune cells senesce and lose telomere length in vivo (Frenck et al., 1998; Rufer et al., 1999; Lee et al., 2002b) and many immune functions may decline with age, but are these related phenomena? After all, cell senescence might not be causally related or even correlated with the observed failure of clinical immune function. CD4+ T lymphocytes, CD8+ T lymphocytes, and B lymphocytes all show telomere shortening with age, although at differing rates, and their mean telomere lengths differ (Son et al., 2000), perhaps due to induced telomerase expression (Hathcock et al., 2003).

Senescent T cells are not only dysfunctional but, as might be predicted, they accumulate with age, as well as with chronic infection (Effros and Valenzuela, 1998). Although cloning conditions may play a role in proliferative capacity (Pawelec et al., 2002b), the telomere length of circulating CD+4 T cells decreases with age, as it does during differentiation from naive to memory cell in vivo (Weng et al., 1995) and with cell division in vitro. Overall, telomere lengths correlate with lymphocyte replicative history and with the remaining replicative potential (Weng et al., 1997c).

Inducible telomerase expression (Allsopp et al., 2002) remains observable even in T cells from older patients, although the degree of induced cell activity declines with repeated antigenic stimulation (Valenzuela and Effros, 2000), presumably causing an accelerated telomere loss in this cell population (Vaziri et al., 1993). Although senescent T cells lose replicative response to stimulation (Perillo et al., 1993a), cytolytic activity does not decrease in kind. To the contrary, senescent T cells recognize foreign cells and initiate normal T-cell responses in vitro (Perillo et al., 1993b) and in vivo, including T-cell recruitment during exercise (Bruunsgaard et al., 1999). This suggests that at least in T cells, senescence might not be associated with a generalized loss of function. Even supportive data may be difficult to interpret. For example, there are losses of T-cell function, such as the production of heat shock protein (HSP70), and this failure correlates nicely with senescence but is unrelated to proliferative activity at the time stimulation (Effros et al., 1994b). There remains the possibility that the gradual loss of proliferative response is not directly attributable to cell senescence but to another independent proliferative control mechanism. In some hands (Hooijberg et al., 2000), hTERT is sufficient to achieve T-cell immortalization, while in others, transgenic human CD8+ T lymphocytes which express hTERT and maintain telomere lengths nevertheless demonstrate the same loss of proliferative potential seen in untreated control cells (Migliaccio et al., 2000). Ironically, these last two references were published, with opposing titles, 2 weeks apart in the same journal; the field has far to go. T cells serve as a model for cell senescence (Effros, 1996; Pawelec et al., 1999e), and as we overcome the barriers to in vitro cultivation (Pawelec et al., 1998a), they may help bridge the gap between cell senescence and clinical immune senescence, as well as serve as a screen for future interventional trials (Pawelec et al., 2000b).

The degree of telomerase expression varies within the immune system. It is found in relatively high levels in thymocyte subpopulations, intermediate levels in tonsil T lymphocytes, and low to undetectable levels in circulating, peripheral blood T lymphocytes (Weng et al., 1996). While the role of IL-2 is disputed (Soares et al., 1998; Natarajan et al., 2002), IL-7 appears to stimulate and control telomerase expression within T cells, permitting extrathymic proliferation of certain subpopulations of neonatal T cells and maintenance of the adult T-cell pool despite extensive cell division over a lifetime (Soares et al., 1998). Other leukocytes, such as myelocytes, show similar down-regulation of telomerase (and TRF1) in parallel with differentiation (Otsuka et al., 2000). Although there are species that contain leukocyte subpopulations that constitutively express telomerase (Barker et al., 2001), the same is not true of humans. The human leukocyte stem cell does not express telomerase constitutively, only under limited circumstances. Nonetheless, all leukocytic subtypes appear capable of such expression with appropriate stimulation (Broccoli et al., 1995).

Considering the cited need for cell division, it may be surprising that most hematopoetic stem cells in adult bone marrow are quiescent rather than actively dividing (Lansdorp, 1998; Cheng et al., 2000b). Clinically, the rationale for this relative quiescence has been implied by animal experiments in which stem cell division is artificially accelerated (by interfering with p21, which serves as a brake on stem cell cycling). The result of this acceleration is premature death of the animal via "hematopoetic cell depletion" (Cheng et al., 2000b). In the extreme case, continual cell division can exhaust the stem cell's potential for division.

Although most pluripotent, hematopoetic (CD34+ CD38−) stem cells are found in the marrow, a few are found in the peripheral circulation and their numbers can be increased by using cytokines, which play a role in inducing transient telomerase expression (Chiu et al., 1996; Englelhardt et al., 1997). Stimulation with phytohemagglutinin, for example, increases, telomerase activity by greater than 10-fold. Stimulation of the T-cell receptor (TCR)/CD3 complex and costimulatory CD28 receptor increase telomerase activity. On the other hand, rapamycin (an immunosuppressant that blocks the T cell receptor prevents this increase in telomerase activity (Buchkovich and Greider, 1996).

Upon stimulation with lymphokines, the stem cell transiently expresses telomerase, reextends its telomere, shuts down telomerase expression, then goes through one cell cycle (Feist et al., 1998). Typically, one daughter cell then begins to proliferate dramatically; its offspring "inexorably move toward terminal differentiation" (Cheng et al., 2000b). Simultaneously, these dividing cells become insensitive to further effects of lymphokine stimulation on telomerase expression. They are no longer capable of resetting their telomere lengths, which shorten progressively as in other somatic cells (Vaziri et al., 1993).

The other daughter cell remains a member of the undifferentiated reserve stem cell population and is fully capable of responding to lymphokine stimulation by reexpression of telomerase, although is does not do so constitutively. The mechanisms of arrested differentiation in this reserve daughter cell are gradually being clarified (Fearon et al., 2001). These stem cells may be the "crucial location" of senescence in the immune system (Pawelec, 1999b). Telomerase activity in these cells is sufficient to slow but not halt telomere erosion. Telomere length in this stem cell population continues to degrade, albeit at a far slower rate than is typical of somatic cells.

Contradicting the assumption that such telomerase-expressing cells reside solely within the marrow, a few circulating lymphocytes can express telomerase to stimulation (Counter et al., 1995). Their number or ability to express telomerase falls with age (Vaziri et al., 1993). Overall telomere lengths likewise fall in correlation with donor age (Slagboom et al., 1994) and this correlates with both death from infectious disease and overall life expectancy (Cawthorn et al., 2003). Circulating peripheral blood monocytes demonstrate telomerase activity that declines with age (Iwama et al., 1998). Parenthetically, unpublished data on two Hutchinson-Gilford progeric children showed that the telomerase expression and telomere lengths of their circulating leukocytes were identical to those of a single age-matched normal volunteer (Shay and Fossel, unpublished data).

Regulation of Telomerase Expression

Not only are cell division and differentiation carefully controlled, so is telomerase expression in the stem cells (Hodes et al., 2002). Initial telomerase expression is triggered within specific cells by antigenic or cytokine stimulation. In T cells, the subsequent telomerase expression partially compensates for the telomere loss incumbent upon cell division (Hiyama et al., 1995d; Weng et al., 1997c; Allsopp et al., 2002) and in B cells it may more than compensate for such loss (Weng et al., 1997a; 1997c). As discussed previously, telomerase expression carries a significant though merely permissive risk of malignancy. As a teleological consequence, evolution ensures that telomerase expression is stringently regulated. The regulatory mechanisms are complex and vary with cell type and cell fate. For example, stem cells that remain pleuripotent and resident within the marrow down-regulate telomerase expression through a transcriptional repression pathway. In response to mitogenic or growth factor signaling, these quiescent but telomerase-competent stem cells reenter the cell cycle and reacquire telomerase activity independent of DNA synthesis. In cells that differentiate and leave the stem cell compartment, however, proteolysis alone is the more likely mode of regulation (Holt and Shay, 1999).

Within the stem cell compartment, telomerase activation occurs early in cell proliferation, allowing more effective leverage in telomere maintenance during the ensuing wave of cell division (Bodnar et al., 1996). The RNA component, hTR, is regulated in normal T cells during development and after activation. Although hTR probably plays some role in telomerase regulation within hematopoetic stem cells (Weng et al., 1997b), whether this is merely secondary to hTERT regulation is unknown.

A rewarding distinction can be made between the stem cell's response and its ability to respond to these telomerase-inducing signals. As stem cells age, they stop proliferating (in response to autocrine signals) before losing their ability to do so (as regulated by telomere length). The normal T-cell proliferative response is actively (but not irrevocably) lost because of ill-defined mechanisms prior to being passively (and irrevocably) lost from mere telomere loss. Cultures of aged T cells show well-documented growth cessation (Weng et al., 1995). However, such cells stop replicating and lose the capacity to secrete IL-2, long before they lose their ability to replicate and to respond to exogenous growth factors (Adibzadeh et al., 1995). These cells have not reached critically short telomere lengths and they continue to respond to exogenous signals, but they no longer respond equivalently and they no longer proceed to division. Data showing that telomere lengths decrease during autocrine expansion, and with fewer population doublings in memory than naive phenotype cells, measured autocrine response rather than replicative potential (Weng et al., 1995). It is therefore uncertain and perhaps unlikely that the cessation of growth seen in these cells can be attributable to a blockade of replicative potential secondary to shortened telomeres. There are many steps from autocrine availability to cell proliferation. Autocrine response is a complex product of the stimulation of growth factor secretion, up-regulation of the growth factor receptor, and correct signal transduction, among other things, and is not merely an outcome of telomere length. The potential relationship between telomere shortening and blockade of autocrine proliferation remains unknown (Pawelec, 1999b).

Telomerase induction and subsequent activity are themselves complex. Although telomerase shows initial increase in expression beginning within 24 hours and extending up to 72 hours after stimulation, it then falls again barring restimulation (Yamada et al., 1996). This is sufficient to prevent telomere erosion initially but, perhaps because of subsequent down-regulation, not during long-term culture (Bodnar et al., 1996; Weng et al., 1997).

Optimal induction requires stimulation (via CD3) and costimulation (for example, with CD28). Defects in this mechanism such as age-associated defects in costimulation result in poor telomerase induction. Age-associated loss of telomerase up-regulation may be the result of a decrease in the expression of CD28 or of costimulatory molecules. The mechanisms regulating telomerase expression are incompletely defined; age-related declines may be attributable to changes in poorly understood mechanisms. The result will ultimately be failure of T-cell competence (Pawelec et al., 1997b). This complexity may account for the failure to find a clear correlation between the efficiency of T-cell cloning and donor age (up to 95 years and as long as the donor is healthy). These mechanisms hide the explanation to more striking discrepancies (Adibzadeh et al., 1996). Even from the same donor and under the same conditions, some T-cell clones are capable of generating only 10^5 progeny, while others may generate up to 10^{24} (Pawelec et al., 1999c).

Whatever the mechanisms, age-related failure of T-cell response is not merely due to restrictions of telomere length but is complexly mediated and interacts upstream with the maintenance of telomere length and telomerase expression and downstream with T-cell proliferation and response in general. If cell senescence plays a major role (as appears likely), it does so via relatively early changes in gene expression (potentially attributable to partial telomere loss) rather than via late changes attributable to putatively complete loss of telomere length.

There are a wealth of changes in gene expression, although the causal relationship to the altering proliferative response is uncertain. Characteristic of replicative failure in T cells, c-fos is repressed (Sikora et al., 1992). There are increases in several mitotic inhibitors, including p16-INK4a, p21-WAF, and p27-kip1, relative to control mRNAs, such as β-actin. While these increases do not necessarily imply changes in function and will require further investigation, they do suggest a mechanism that might down-regulate continued proliferation of old T cells (Pawelec, 1999b).

Telomerase activity probably increases during B-cell activation (Weng et al., 1997c), although dynamics may differ from that of T cells (Martens et al., 2002) and less is known about telomerase response trajectory during aging (Effros, 2001b) and differentiation (Jung et al., 2001; Schaniel et al., 2002), or indeed, about how differentiation is controlled in selected long-lived mature B cells (Schiemann et al., 2001; Thompson et al., 2001; Waldenschmidt and Noelle, 2001). Surprisingly, in B cells telomere lengths may increase in some circumstances (Martens et al., 2000a), even without reference to malignant transformation. Such increases have been seen during tonsillar B-cell differentiation and formation of germinal centers in lymphatic nodes (Norrback et al., 2001). The level of telomerase was more than 100-fold higher in germinal center B cells than in naive or memory B cells, correlating with their longer telomeres. Within less active lymphatic nodes, resting lymphocytes retain the ability to up-regulate telomerase activity upon activation (the B-cell antigen receptor in the presence of CD40 engagement and/or IL-4) and this capacity shows no decline with age. This mechanism is presumed necessary in maintaining the replicative potential of B cells in the humoral immune response over the entire human lifespan (Weng et al., 1997a, 1997c).

Cell Senescence in Other Hematologic Disease States

To the extent that stem cells may require telomerase under normal circumstances to keep up with quotidian replacement and minor infectious challenges, they will require it a forteriori under truly pathologic circumstances. A modicum of data on pathologic states bears on this specific issue, including α-thalassemia, myelodysplastic disease, bone marrow transplantation, aplastic anemia, trisomy 21, and HIV. α-thalassemia is a singular anomaly and may involve an increase, rather than a decrease, in telomerase expression and telomere stability. Suggestive evidence attributes the pathology to inappropriate telomerase expression in the germ cell line, resulting in an undesirable stabilization of terminal deletions and loss of critical gene loci (Morin, 1996b).

In myelodysplastic syndrome, for example, in which cell turnover is accelerated, telomere shortening not only occurs but is associated with higher risk of leukemic transformation, perhaps due to increased genomic instability. The increased risk of leukemia is better correlated with telomere length (as measured by telomerase restriction fragments) than with telomerase activity (Ohyashiki et al., 1999). Baseline ability of hematopoetic stem cells to divide and maintain blood cell populations remains intact. However, the ability of hematopoetic stem cells to respond appropriately to hematologic stress, such as massive blood loss, is eroded. The degree to which patients lose the ability to respond rapidly and fully to such stresses depends not only on age but history. A lifetime of prolonged or recurrent infectious disease, for example, may have no effect on baseline hematologic parameters (hematocrit, reticulocyte count, total leukocyte count, neutrophil percentage), while having profound but occult effects upon the ability to respond to further stress. In short, the ability of stem cells to meet hematologic challenges gradually declines with age (Globerson, 1999).

The same effect occurs when senescence is accelerated iatrogenically, as in bone marrow transplantation (see discussion Chapter 5). Here, the marrow is forced to undergo cell division on a massive scale to reconstitute the entire hematopoetic system, with resulting rapid senescence (Podesta, 2001). The number of cell divisions that such stem cells must undergo to replace the blood cells in the recipient is unknown. Cell divisions should be the outcome of the number of cells transplanted and their functional efficacy (e.g., adequacy of HLA-match, survival, ability to divide, response to growth signals, division potential, normal differentiation). Data match these expectations. The telomeres of granulocytes from recipients are shorter than those of matched cells from the donors. The loss of telomere length occurs within the initial year post-transplantation and is stable thereafter (Brummendorf et al., 2001b; Robertson et al., 2001).

One alternative is the use of circulating stem cells ("allogenic peripheral blood progenitor cells") in lieu of bone marrow stem cells, since these CD34+ CD38– stem cells show earlier engraftment and immune reconstitution following transplantation and may therefore be preferred to whole marrow (Lansdorp, 1998). Telomere shortening might occur in either case (Robertson et al., 2001). Although some have argued against the value of stem cells to prevent telomere loss (Sakoff et al., 2002) and despite the substantial replicative stress on the donated stem cells (Thornley and Freedman, 2002), the use of stem cells apparently prevents telomere loss (Roelofs et al., 2003). Regardless, clinical success is not solely a matter of telomeres but of a cell's ability to successfully home to the marrow and seed germinal marrow centers.

Absolute success is another matter, however. In bone marrow rejection, for example, telomere loss and cell senescence accelerate, which may play a causal role in subsequent transplant failure (Multani et al., 2001). Overall telomere shortening occurs in recipients, averaging perhaps 200 kbp in T cells and 300 kbp in neutrophils (Robertson et al., 2001). Various estimates have been published, but the suggestion has been made that marrow transplantation is (by estimates of telomere length) is equivalent to 40 years of in vivo aging (Moore, 1997; Shay, 1998b; Wynn et al., 1998). This places (and explains the) severe limits upon serial autologous marrow transplantation, limits that might be overcome by inducing increased telomerase express in these cells (Allsopp and Weissman, 2002).

In aplastic anemia, the issue of cell senescence should predictably hinge on the cause of the pathology: is the pathognomonic abrogation of cell production secondary to cell senescence or vice versa? We might consider three predictable possibilities:

1. If the pathology is a unique event resulting in wholesale cell loss and consequent cell senescence (as in infection or radiation, with marrow depletion), then telomere shortening should precede conspicuous clinical disease and be found in all diagnosed patients, regardless of how advanced their course. All patients have short telomeres; progressive loss is not characteristic.
2. If the pathology is continual and due to accelerated cell turnover, then cell senescence is a late outcome of the disease process and telomere shortening may or may not be found in patients with frank clinical disease. In this case, telomere lengths in affected cells should correlate with the course. Most patients have short telomeres; progressive loss is characteristic.
3. If the pathology involves the telomere, as in impaired telomere maintenance, then once again telomere lengths will vary in diagnosed patients and correlate with the course of the disease. Most patients have short telomeres; progressive loss is characteristic.

As in the second case, telomere shortening should be (and is) typical of patients with advanced aplastic anemia (Vulliamy et al., 2002). As a curious exception, while granulocyte telomeres of untreated and nonresponding aplastic anemia patients are shorter than normal, successfully treated immunosuppressed patients have approximately normal telomeres. While initially surprising, this finding meets the second prediction given above and is likely due to the suppression of a subgroup of cells that had extensively proliferated (and had shorter telomeres) and repopulation of the peripheral blood by other cells with a less extensive history of cell division (Brummendorf et al., 2001a, 2001c). The accelerated cell turnover has been stopped, allowing relatively quiescent, residual stem cell populations with normal telomere lengths to come out of hiding.

This parallels events occurring in chronic myelogenous leukemia (CML) patients, with marked expansion of myeloid cells, a positive Philadelphia chromosome (Ph+), and hence shortened telomeres. Lymphocytes negative for the Philadelphia chromosome (Ph–), however, have perfectly normal telomere lengths. Moreover, the second prediction above is again validated: the telomere lengths of affected lymphocytes show a continued and significant fall as the disease progresses to late chronic phase (Brummendorf et al., 2001c; Terasaki et al., 2002).

Trisomy 21 patients are examples of the third case, in which telomere maintenance is impaired, although only in specific cell lines, such as leukocytes. Moreover, rescue, in the sense seen in immunosuppressed aplastic anemia patients, is impossible: there are no phenotypically appropriate, residual, unaffected stem cell populations that can reemerge after putative intervention. Shorter leukocytic telomeres are typical of young trisomy 21 patients and length of their telomeres correlates with their immune dysfunction (Vaziri et al., 1993). Although risk of dementia is increased (perhaps due to impaired microglial telomere maintenance?), the bulk of clinical problems typical of trisomy 21 patients are attributable to the abnormally rapid erosion of leukocytic telomeres. They demonstrate leukocyte-derived pathology, with increased infection (typically pneumonia) and hematologic malignancy (typically leukemia) rates. Not surprisingly, solid tumor incidence does not increase, although their risk of leukemia goes up as much as a 56-fold (Hasle et al., 2000).

Additional clinical relevance is found in HIV disease and AIDS. Even in the asymptomatic patient (with HIV infection, but without frank clinical AIDS), estimates suggest that lymphocytes are destroyed at the rate of 1–2 billion cells per day and replaced at the same rate. Given the accelerated (CD4+ T-cell) lymphocyte loss in HIV disease, this might reasonably be expected to imply accelerated cell senescence (Cohen, 1996; Effros et al., 1996; Wolthers et al., 1998). More to the point, such cell senescence might be blamed for the underlying immune failure, the hallmark and clinical problem of AIDS.

Although CD4+ cells reliably decline during the course of AIDS, no clearly correlated senescence occurs among these cells (Wolthers et al., 1996; Wolthers and Miedema, 1998; Richardson et al., 2000). In experimental infections with simian immune virus in primates this appears to be true, although here the outcome appears to result from upregulation of telomerase and stable telomere maintenance. Animals lacking this response rapidly succumb to the immune virus (Bostik et al., 2000). Whether this occurs in humans is unknown. Curiously, however, CD8+ cells do show an apparent acceleration of cell senescence (Effros, 2000c), particularly (and not merely in CD8+ cells) in patients undergoing highly active anti-retroviral therapy (HAART) therapy (Sondergaard et al., 2002). In HIV patients, the length of their telomere restriction fragments approximate those of centenarians (Effros et al., 1996). This difference between CD4+ and CD8+ cells is supported by a twin study, in which HIV patients had CD4+ T cells with longer telomeres, while the telomeres of their CD8+ T cells were shorter. In keeping with this finding, the replicative response of the CD4+ cells was normal. Although it was inducible, constitutive telomerase activity was not found in either cell type. This study (Palmer et al., 1997) and others like it (Tucker et al., 2000) suggest that while cell senescence might play an indirect role through the effect of senescing CD8+ cells on nonsenescing CD4+ cells, not much evidence supports cell senescence as a direct cause of the decline in CD4+ T-cell numbers typical of HIV patients. This does not directly address the tantalizing findings of transient telomerase expression in simians (Bostik et al., 2000), however, which might reserve the importance of cell senescence for normal CD4+ function in HIV.

Supporting the possibility that cell senescence plays some role, albeit indirectly, is a growing body of data showing that therapeutic interventions affects AIDS and various measures of cell senescence. Highly active anti-retroviral therapy, for example, results in an increase in the mean length of the CD8+ T-cell telomeres, as measured by telomere restriction fragments (Aladdin et al., 2001). Younger patients show better CD4+ restoration after HAART than that of older patients (Pomerantz, 2001; Viard et al., 2001), a result that might be attributable to differences in cell senescence between young and old patients. In a study that looked at those who responded poorly (or well) to a year of

HIV therapy, after therapy, poor responders had shorter (3.8 vs. 5.3 kbp) CD4+ telomeres than those who responded well. Poor responders were older, had higher initial CD4+ and CD8+ counts, and after therapy had fewer naive T cells and less thymic tissue (Teixeira et al., 2001). Again, compare these results to the simian data (Bostik et al., 2000) cited above, in which transient telomerase expression maintained telomere lengths and appeared to play a role in surviving viral infection.

Other interesting data support the relationship between cell senescence and HIV disease. The proportion of CD28-negative lymphocytes correlates directly with disease progression (Effros et al., 1996; Wolthers et al., 1996), suggesting that stem cell exhaustion may play a role in progression from HIV+ status to clinical AIDS, although there remains substantial disagreement about this role (Feng et al., 1999). Peripheral mononuclear cells show an inverse correlation between their telomere lengths and progression of immunosuppression. Telomere loss correlated with disease progression and loss of replicative ability of the mononuclear cells, though not with telomerase activity (Bestilny et al., 2000).

These results support suggestions that cell senescence plays a role in clinical HIV disease, although not a simplistic one in which CD4+ cells are killed, their progenitors divide repeatedly, the population progressively senesces, and the result is immune dysfunction. More likely, the mechanisms are more complex, involving transient CD4+ hTERT expression or interactions between several cell populations, with some cell types senescing (e.g., CD8+ cells) and others not (e.g., CD4+ cells), but with an overall loss of effective immune function indirectly mediated through cell senescence.

Just as abnormal human physiology (disease) may teach us something about normal function, so to do animal experiments. The results from knockout animals support cell senescence in immune and hematopoetic aging. Telomerase (mTERT) knockout reduces proliferative capacity in B and T cells, causing abnormal hematology and splenic atrophy (Herrera et al., 1999b). These animals do not respond normally to immunization, perhaps because their germinal centers (in which B lymphocytes normally proliferate during the immune response) are dramatically reduced compared to those in normal animals. As noted above, the telomeres of normal human B lymphocytes may increase in length during immune stimulation (Martens et al., 2000a), as do those in normal mice. In the knockout, however, these telomeres shorten after immunization. These results demonstrate the likely mechanism and importance of cell senescence (and its modulation) to the antibody-mediated immune responses (Herrera et al., 2000).

The hypothesis that cell senescence is central to immune and hematologic aging (and relevant diseases) has strong and growing experimental support. We lack, however, a clear understanding of the mechanisms. The outlines are apparent, details remains uncertain. Only among details will we discover an ability to intervene.

Intervention

In a gentle tack from hematopoetic to merely poetic stem cells, we might quote Shakespeare (Sonnet 19) in hoping that "Devouring time would . . . burn the long-lived phoenix in her blood." So far, his entreaties have had an equal effect to those of modern science on renewing hematopoetic and immune function as aging inexorably "blunt's the lion's paws."

Over the years, several approaches to treating immunosenescence have surfaced. A perennial candidate, caloric restriction has beneficial effects on the normal age-related loss of T-cell proliferative capacity in mice (Grossmann et al., 1990; Pendergrass et al., 1995; Spaulding et al., 1997b). Even if not fundamental in their effects, some approaches, such as estrogen replacement, may prove to have some beneficial effects on immune function. In estrogen, these may include improvements in B-cell numbers, mitogen-induced T-cell proliferation, and induced TNF-α availability (Porter et al., 2001). Other approaches have already been discounted by contradicting data or may be appropriately relegated to the category of grandmotherly advice. To suggest, as some journal articles do, that effective immune function in the aged requires (as an example) adequate nutrition is unarguably true, but nutritional supplementation scarcely speaks to the issue of aging (Graat et al., 2002) nor to the seemingly immutable loss of protective function. The issue at hand is to identify therapies that affect the processes that underlie aging in the immune and hematologic systems and that cause human clinical problems. As these changes are probably related to aging within the cells comprising these systems, we turn our attention to the issue of intervening at the cellular level.

Cell senescence has been studied in long-lived lymphocytes (Siwicki et al., 2000) and a large body of work reflects attempts to intervene in immunosenescence within cells, usually in vitro (Pawelec, 1999b). These have included manipulation of oxidative stress (Flescher et al., 1998), culture conditions (Freedman et al., 1994), CD28 expression (Vallejo et al., 1998), DNA repair (Moritz et al., 1995), apoptosis (Effros and Valenzuela, 1998), costimulatory molecule expression on the T-cell surface (Effros et al., 1994a; Monteiro et al., 1996; Boucher et al., 1998; Vallejo et al., 1998), CD134 and CD154 (Pawelec et al., 1997b; Lio et al., 1998; Weyand et al., 1998), and telomerase expression (Vallejo et al., 1998; Kiyono et al., 1998). As a result of the recent work showing that hTERT can be safely and effectively inserted in human cell lines with good results (Bodnar et al., 1998; Vaziri, 1998), there is a strong interest in moving this approach to ex vivo or in vivo trials (Fossel, 2001b; Lord et al., 2002).

Some authors (Effros and Pawelec, 1998; Effros and Valenzuela, 1998) have remarked on their interest in the hematologic and immune systems as a primary choice for therapeutic trials of interventions in cell senescence. This is largely, though not exclusively, because the technical hurdles are less severe here than they are in many alternative organ systems, such as the nervous system. In blood, for example, we can remove circulating stem cells, transfect them with human telomerase (hTERT), and return them to the body with almost ridiculous technical ease. It is, however, in the simplicity and power of the approach that complications—regulatory, ethical, and human—arise (Fossel, 2003). Capability of intervening in immune aging is one thing; doing so carefully, appropriately, and safely is another.

Human blood cells are eminently available with no more technical difficulty than a sharp, hollow needle to penetrate the skin and a syringe to withdraw a sample. Most cells—erythrocytes—lack nuclei and are unqualified for hTERT transfection. The leukocytes, however, normally about 0.2% of the circulating human blood cell population, are available. Within this population are numerous CD34+ CD38– stem cells, and their numbers can be increased by preparing the patient beforehand with cytokines (Lansdorp, 1998). Once drawn, the sample can be spun down and concentrated. Even without transfection, T cells might serve as a useful measure overall immunosenescence and a marker for potential interventions (Pawelec et al., 2000). Such cells, once transfected, not only express telomerase and maintain their telomeres but have normal karyotypes, normal cytotoxic properties, and no indications of apoptosis or malignant transformation (Rufer et al., 2001). The possibility that hTERT could be used to manipulate T-cell senescence in vitro and that this technique might ameliorate the decline in immune function that characterizes aging (Effros and Pawelec, 1998) explains why this approach to intervention is likely in the near future.

In each of the cases discussed in this chapter—normal immunosenescence, marrow transplantation, HIV, and other diseases—cell senescence (and thereby the clinical problem) might be ameliorated by use of transfection. The Bodnar work (Bodnar et al., 1998) establishes our ability to reset cell senescence. Technically, we are capable of identifying stem cells in peripheral circulation, transfecting them, and replacing them ex vivo. The obstacles to such clinical experimentation on these groups (and trisomy 21 patients for reasons discussed above) are largely ethical, not technical. Do the risks (malignancy, immune dysfunction) justify genetic alteration of circulating lymphocytes? The problem is a catch-22. Healthy patients have no indication justifying the risk; severely ill patients lack time to transfect and reconstitute immune function. The same is true in trisomy 21 patients. In HIV or marrow transplantation, however, the risks of the disease are acutely higher and may justify this sort of immune reconstitution under certain conditions. Telomere-based therapy for immunosenescence (Lord et al., 2002) is not only technically feasible (Effros and Valenzuela, 1998) but justifiable on ethical and clinical grounds.

In terms of our technical ability, we are already at the point where, particularly in immune senescence, we can test the therapeutic utility of the theory that cell senescence underlies age related disease. It remains only to try.

CHAPTER 12

Endocrine Systems

Structure and Overview

The endocrine system is, in most ways, a conceptual conglomeration of several physiologically unrelated and anatomically disparate systems. Nonetheless, the striking parallels in organization, function, and intent of such systems, to say nothing of their subtle interactions, make this notional melting pot an appropriate one, albeit with some caveats.

The endocrine system communicates between and coordinates the functions of 100 trillion body cells. The form of communication is chemical and such hormonal "information packets" are generally, but not exclusively, carried throughout the body by the blood. The exceptions to the vascular medium include local intercellular hormonal messages (e.g., trophic factors), neurotransmitters (between neurons or between neurons and muscles), and intrapituitary hormonal transfer (e.g., hormonal releasing factors from the posterior to the anterior pituitary which employ a specialized, local capillary bed rather than trusting to a more diluted delivery via the entire vasculature). Most hormonal communication is from a few local to the many distant cells, coordinating metabolic functions between cells. For example, insulin is released by the pancreas in response to elevated serum glucose and permits cells to take up and use glucose. Thyroid is released by a gland in the anterior neck to coordinate and regulate the metabolic rate of cells in the entire body. The action of most hormones is not direct and causal but indirect and modulatory. Thyroid hormone, for example, doesn't affect metabolic rate directly; it acts as a signal, ordering the cell to alter its metabolic rate. In so doing, thyroid hormone not only has the effect of raising the metabolic rate but coordinates metabolic rates among different cell phenotypes throughout the body.

In the grander sense, the aim of the endocrine systems is survival of the organism and species. The first is accomplished by optimizing the body's homeostasis, the second by optimizing reproduction success. Hormonal systems accomplish the former by coordinating growth, cell division, energy metabolism, electrolyte levels, cardiovascular function, and immune function. They accomplish the latter if they ensure that sperm or ova are prepared, that menses and pregnancy succeed, and that the organism has sexual, and ultimately parental, success. Genetically, such systems have been selected to maximize individual and species survival and they do so in a complex, interrelated, and effective fashion.

The endocrine systems are not a simple, single organ. They are linked historically and conceptually only in their roughly common teleology (communication and coordination) and mechanism (secretion, excluding interneuronal or neuromuscular contacts usually considered part of the nervous system). They share no single molecular type (protein, glycoprotein, steroid), nor a common anatomic location. The endocrine systems might be and often are lumped together as a single system ("the endocrine system") or might literally (and not altogether irrationally) encompass every cell in the entire body as part of a unified endocrine system. For practical reasons, however, endocrine systems are usually divided into an arbitrary but small number of axes. While other divisions might be (and have been historically) used, one example (Strollo, 1999) divides endocrine systems into nine axes: (1) bone mineralization axis (e.g., parathyroid and other hormonal effects on calcium and phosphorus metabolism), (2) hypothalamic–pituitary–adrenal axis (e.g., glucocorticoids), (3) hypothalamic–pituitary–gonadal axis (e.g., estrogen and testosterone), (4) hypothalamic-pituitary-somatomammotrophic axis (e.g., prolactin and growth hormone), (5) hypothalamic–pituitary–thyroid axis (thyroid hormones), (6) renin–angiotensin–aldosterone axis (e.g., antidiuretic hormone and two natriuretic peptides), (7) erythrocyte mass regulation (e.g., erythropoietin), (8) glucose metabolism (e.g., insulin and glucagon), and (9) the sympathetic system (e.g., circulating epinephrine, norepinephrine, and dopamine). Initially, and arbitrarily, we will divide endocrine axes by anatomic origin. In discussing endocrine systems in aging and pathology, we will focus on those with known relevance to aging and age-related diseases. Some endocrine systems deserve discussion primarily because of public notoriety as putative aging interventions.

Hypothalamic hormones are small polypeptides with effects on the pituitary gland and most distant structures. These include antidiuretic hormone (ADH), oxytocin, thyrotropin-releasing hormone (TRH), corticotropin-releasing hormone (CRH), luteinizing hormone–releasing hormone (LHRH); gonadotropin-inhibiting hormone (GnRH), somatostatin (GIH), growth hormone–releasing hormone (GRH), prolactin-inhibiting hormone (PIH), and prolactin-releasing hormone (PRH). As is apparent from their names, these neuroendocrine hormones have disparate actions ranging from electrolyte maintenance, to metabolic coordination, to the control of menstrual cycling, pregnancy, and labor.

Pituitary hormones are all polypeptides, such as adrenocorticotropic hormone (ACTH), prolactin (PRL), and growth hormone (GH), or glycoproteins, such as follicle-stimulating hormone (FSH), luteinizing hormone (LH), and thyroid-stimulating hormone (TSH). Their functions, like those of they hypothalamic hormones, are disparate and cover roughly the same areas of homeostasis and of reproduction.

Although many of the common steroid hormones are synthesized predominantly within the adrenal glands, they are not only synthesized (or interconverted) elsewhere (e.g., the liver, testes, ovaries, placenta, and peripheral body cells) but often extensively so. These steroids are a grab bag set of hormones with a common origin from the cholesterol molecule and two main synthetic pathways that (depending on the specific synthetic branch) part company at the division between pregnenolone and progesterone. One branch is the corticosteroids and the second, more complex branch, the sexual steroids. The corticosteroids (e.g., cortisol) have potent effects on electrolyte levels, glucose metabolism, and immune function. The genetic absence of glucocorticoids, if uncorrected, is fatal. The sexual steroids, including dehydroepiandrosterone (DHEA), are considered reproductive hormones yet have a host of other functions, some probably unknown. Dehydroepiandrosterone, for example, has the highest serum level of circulating steroids (Drucker et al., 1972; Gordon et al., 1999), yet to say that its functions (except as a synthetic intermediary) are poorly defined exaggerates our knowledge. Curiously, this branching point defines an aging difference (Parker, 1999). Aging women have a defect in the δ-5-steroid pathway (to DHEA and its sulfate), but no corresponding defect in the cortisol pathways (Parker et al., 2000).

The thyroid secretes thyroxine (T4) and triiodothyronine (T3), amino acids with bound iodine that control body metabolism. Secretion is initially controlled by the pituitary release of TSH, which is in turn controlled by hypothalamic peptides. Dietary iodine, feedback from circulating free thyroid hormones, and other factors play a role. Too little thyroid results in a progressive hypometabolic state, culminating in myxedema, coma, and death (Bailes, 1999). To much thyroid results in hypermetabolism, putting the elderly at greater risk (from cardiac dysrhythmias, for example) than the young adult.

The anatomic neighbor of the thyroid, the parathyroid gland, excretes calcitonin and parathyroid hormone. These hormones control bone metabolism through their effects on the intakes, metabolism, and renal excretion of calcium, phosphorus, and vitamin D, but have profound (though less often addressed) effects on cardiac, skeletal muscle, and neuronal function.

Clinically, the most common endocrine disease and most common endocrine intervention are the result of pancreatic cell loss. Islets of Langerhans produce insulin; lack of insulin produces diabetes. Despite devastating long-term consequences of diabetes, insulin, a simple polypeptide molecule, is rightfully considered the success story of endocrinology. No other hormone is so remarkable in its rapidity and efficacy as insulin. Without it, patients die in a matter of days, with too much, they can die in a matter of minutes. The extensive morbidity (especially renal, vascular, cardiac, and retinal) attached to the diagnosis of lifelong diabetes is largely the result of our medical inability to maintain appropriate physiological glucose and insulin over the lifetime of diabetics. We are never as smart as a normal pancreas.

Descartes was right in calling the pineal gland the "seat of the soul," as it is at least the seat for melatonin. Melatonin, a tryptophan-derived neurotransmitter, was discovered less than 50 years ago and its functions remain arguable. The clearest role is to synchronize the body to a single diurnal clock, based on environmental light; it also functions as a free radical scavenger (Reiter et al., 1999). Although it has effects on menarche, behavioral arousal, the menstrual cycle, thyroid function, and probably a good many other tissues and organs, it probably plays no fundamental role in determining the rate or progress of aging. Approaches that alter maximal lifespan and aging at a fundamental level, for example, caloric restriction, have no effect on the age-related decline in melatonin normally found in rats (MacGibbon et al., 2001). This implies that melatonin's role in aging, if it has a role, is secondary and not causal. A large and showy body of data claims melatonin affects aging (e.g., Pierpaoli and Regelson, 1995; Pierpaoli and Bulian, 2001), but the more extreme claims are disputed (Reiter et al., 1998) and in disrepute (Fossel, 2001c). Although some evidence suggests that melatonin supplementation may have physiological benefits (at least in mice), including a marginal increase in lifespan, other evidence supports increased tumor incidence (Anisimov et al., 2001).

There is an indefinitely large potpourri of other hormones. Not only are there other commonly known hormones, such as epinephrine (largely from the adrenal) or insulin-like growth factor (IGF; peripheral and hepatic in origin; Arvat et al., 2000), and a few less commonly known hormones, such as relaxin (from the ovary), but a complete list grants trophic factors and growth factors circumscribed status as hormones. Nerve growth factor (NGF), colony-stimulating factor (CSF), lymphokines, cytokines, and literally hundreds of other hormones serve the same basic function that classic hormones do: they communicate between cells and coordinate cell function. In a sense, the entire body is one large endocrine system, with no cell excluded. For brevity and clarity, however, and in keeping with our own venue, clinical aging, we will restrict this chapter to the more common hormones alone.

Aging and Other Pathology

Endocrine aging has, ironically and perennially, been a matter of "always the bride, never the bridesmaid." Since Brown-Sequard first began to use hormones therapeutically more than a century ago (and incidentally failed to prevent his own aging in the experiment), there has been an unfounded and repeatedly disproved belief that hormonal changes cause aging and that replacement causes rejuvenation. Hormones are a prime mover in weddings, but mere uninvited guests as we progress to death do us part.

The earliest attempts to relate aging to hormones tried using testosterone (or testicular extracts) to "rejuvenate" aging males (Morley and Kaiser, 1993). The literature of the past century makes for fascinating sociology, as the use of hormones for rejuvenation waxes and wanes with fashion. Like the phoenix, endocrine therapy for aging is notorious for rising again from its own ashes. Like some doomsday cult on the day after the end of the world, overwhelmingly falsifying data make no difference whatever to the true believers. Grandiose endocrine claims arise almost cyclically, as each generation pins its hopes again on the hypothalamus (Bernardis and Davis, 1996), testosterone (Bagatell and Bremner, 1998; Basaria and Dobs, 1999), estrogen (Martin, 1998), thyroid, melatonin (Reiter et al., 1998; Bulian and Pierpaoli, 2000; Pierpaoli et al., 2000), growth hormone (Bengtsson et al., 1998; Toogood and Shalet, 1998), or its secretagogues (Walker and Bercu, 1998). Although in many cases, investigators have made serious attempts to define the utility of hormonal interventions (O'Connor et al., 1999; Morley, 2001a), the public has shown little interest in the facts. In many cases, negative data and an ironically mocking history are not only uninvited guests at the wedding of charlatan and credulity but are actively bounced at the door.

Contrary to the public understanding, not all hormones decline with age. To the contrary, many hormones don't change significantly or predictably with age (Timiras, 1995a). In several cases, earlier claims for endocrine changes with age have not been supported by more recent data. For example, although several endocrine cell types (those secreting CCK, somatostatin, or serotonin) decline with age in the duodenum (Sandstrom and el-Salhy, 1999a), earlier claims for age-related endocrine changes in the colon have not been borne out by data (Sandstrom and el-Salhy, 1999b). Equally, recent work has questioned earlier claims for a decline in melatonin with age (Kennaway et al., 1999; Zeitzer et al., 1999). In the sympathoadrenal system, there is considerable controversy regarding changes with aging, which species show such changes, and the level at which such changes occur (Young, 2001). Naively (or sardonically) we could wonder if, perhaps we wait long enough, careful data might show that none of our endocrine systems age. Nevertheless, there are clear exceptions to such nihilism; certain age-related endocrine changes are not only accepted but supported by decades of confirmatory data. Estrogen drops dramatically with menopause (Shifren and Schiff, 2000), testosterone falls slowly and linearly with advanced age (Gray et al., 1991; Morley et al., 1997), and other hormones (see below) are accepted as having slow, but inarguable declines (Martin-Du Pan, 1999) (Fig. 12–1).

The changes in hormonal activity that do occur with age can each have various and several causes: diminished secretion, increased clearance, fewer receptors, altered receptor response, and altered intracellular response to the receptor. Nonetheless, most overall changes (to the extent that such hormonal changes are uniform or predictable) result in lower serum levels or in an altered pattern of secretion to normal stimuli. The mean serum level may be "normal" (i.e., the same as in a young adult), but the pattern of secretion, for example, the response to releasing factors (or other hormonal stimulation), may be slower in onset or longer in duration (e.g., corticosteroids), of lower than usual magnitude (e.g., insulin), or occur in an altered temporal pattern (e.g., growth hormone). In addition, aging is marked by a loss of coordination, timeliness of response, and appropriate pattern of response (Roth, 1995; Blackman, 2000) that goes beyond mere changes in mean serum levels and may be the hallmark of endocrine aging (Banks and Morley, 2000).

Although unlikely beneficial, age-related endocrine alterations do not necessarily imply dysfunction. Assumptions that lower serum levels in aging individuals imply failing endocrine systems and replacement will prove beneficial are unwarranted. While this is consistent with what we know of aging endocrine systems, the conclusion demands data, not irrational and enthusiastic inference. The notion that declining hormone

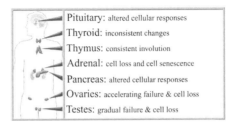

Figure 12–1 Aging endocrine tissue. Among endocrine tissues, the age-related histologic and physiologic changes vary. In the ovary, thymus, and pituitary, these changes are likely to involve multiple inputs and causes. Nonetheless, cell senescence plays a role (even the predominant role) in age-related endocrine change.

levels require replacement is neither logically exclusive nor justifiable without data to support it. Physiology is complex; what we take for a cause of failing health is, a priori, equally likely the body's healthy response to the problem. Consider an analogy in which the error is more apparent. When the body has an infection, a rising white cell count is not the cause of the problem but the body's healthy response. It is a defense, not an offense. It would be foolish to treat an infection by removing the abnormally numerous white cells. Using pheresis to remove them only increases, not decreases, morbidity. In cases such as this, we should not treat the (healthy) response, but the (unhealthy) cause.

Equally, we might imagine an endocrine system whose diminished secretory rate is an appropriate and protective response to aging in other organ systems. This occurs in the hormonal response to dietary restriction, for example (Morley, 2000b). Similarly, decline in a growth factor might be the body's response to an increasing age-related risk of cancer. Were that the case, then attempting to replace the missing growth promoter could be not only foolish but potentially fatal. In the same minatory vein, many have suggested that replacing hormones in the elderly might increase the risk of carcinogenesis (Martin-Du Pan, 1999; Morley, 1999). Although the potential risk of malignancy has been investigated with some vigor for estrogen (Gillum et al., 2000; Van Hoften et al., 2000), data are relatively lacking for other hormones, despite concern. An exception may be the risk of prostate cancer in the face of growth hormone supplementation, with a modicum of suggestive evidence (Colao et al., 1999b) though little firm data (Untergasser et al., 1999). Even without definitive data it remains possible that evolution may have selected for protective lowering of growth hormone levels to increase likelihood of survival, rather than being a primary hormonal deficit requiring replacement.

Similarly, if hormone X was the body's response to osteoporosis, atherosclerosis, or glial cell inflammation, imagine the consequences of naive replacement: aggravation of the underlying problem. The common belief that declines in hormone levels are a problem (rather than the body's solution to more fundamental problems) might be correct, but it is naive to defend generic replacement without evidence of benefit. This issue comes to the fore in discussing the putative benefits of growth hormone in aging. In mice, a genetic absence of growth hormone correlates with longer than normal lifespans (Brown-Borg et al., 1999); transfection with a gene for growth hormone decreases lifespan and decreases the proliferative potential of several cell phenotypes (Pendergrass et al., 1993). This beneficial effect of a genetic absence of growth hormone may be mediated by several specific mechanisms (including fewer cell divisions), but there are broad changes in gene expression (Bartke et al., 2001b). Whatever the mechanism, the contradiction between publicized claims for growth hormone supplementation and available scientific data remains surprisingly complex (Bartke et al., 2001a). As with the segmental lifespan effects of genes in *Caenorhabditis elegans* (Johnson et al., 2001b), the effects of growth hormone may alter markedly, depending on when it acts during the lifespan. It might, for example, be detrimental early in life, but beneficial later (Bartke et al., 20001b). Despite concerns, little is certain. Growth hormone–releasing factor antagonists might even have potential in oncotherapy (Kiaris et al., 1999), again begging the (unanswered) question of the potential cancer risk of secretagogues.

Understanding endocrine function in aging requires thoughtful questions and careful data, rather than rapid and reckless answers. The first question is how hormonal levels and patterns of hormonal response change with age. The second question is the clinical outcomes of proposed therapeutic interventions in endocrine aging. We know too little to accurately answer either question.

Some hormones, such as antidiuretic hormone, have little dispute about outcome (a less concentrated urine) but considerable uncertainty about mechanisms involved (less secretion, diminished renal response, or other factors?). Brain and kidney may become more sluggish and less capable of normal endocrine responses (Timiras, 1995a), but the interaction between these organs remains arguable. Even data are in dispute: opinions range from no change in antidiuretic hormone to severe changes. Judging from the literature, the mechanism of hormonal dysfunction in antidiuretic hormone may be anywhere (if it occurs). Worse, we can't discuss single hormone function in isolation: hormone function is part of an axis, such as the hypothalamic–pituitary–adrenocortical axis, a complex cascade of causes and effects (Timiras, 1995a). It is difficult (perhaps impossible) to tease out isolated effects of aging in such complex systems and attribute them to a particular endocrine organ (Veldhuis et al., 1999).

In discussing thyroid function, for example, metabolism may decrease, but where does the dysfunction lie? We may laugh at the old joke about the frog who jumps progressively less distance with each loud noise as his limbs are amputated one by one, until with no legs he goes deaf, yet this is the logical error we condone if we agree too naively on the cause of thyroid aging. Is age-related thyroid change attributable to a dysfunction in temperature sensors, neurons, the pituitary, the circulation, the thyroid gland, hormone clearance, or the receptor response of the distal cells? Is autoimmune thyroid disorder (Mariotti et al., 1999) a cause or a result of immune system aging? The outcome may be clear—the metabolism no longer "jumps," but to attribute the cause to aging names but fails to explain it. To attribute age-related thyroid dysfunction to a particular portion of the endocrine axis (e.g., the cell receptors are "deaf" to thyroid hormone) requires data. Unfortunately, clinicians may attribute thyroid changes to aging, remaining blind to correctable disease (Bailes, 1999). There are intrinsic, age-related changes in the thyroid axis, including alteration in diurnal variance and reaction to hormonal stimuli (Chakraborti et al., 1999). Normal, nondiseased thyroid glands probably shrink slightly and T4–T3 conversion, secretion, and clearance probably decrease trivially. Serum thyroid levels do not change with age in any widely accepted, predictable way. While there are both changes in patients (Nardi et al., 1999) and an increase in the variance between patients (Maugeri et al., 1999; Ognibene et al., 1999), it is not clear that aging (as opposed to disease, malnutrition, or lack of activity) causes predictable change in circulating thyroid hormones (Timiras, 1995b). The aged show a clear loss of thermoregulatory control and an elevation in heat- and cold-related mortality rates, but scant evidence for uniform and reliable impairment in the thyroid axis to which we might attribute the loss of control or the elevated mortality. Increased heat- and cold-related mortality is at least as attributable to vascular, cardiac, dietary, and other aging changes as it is to thyroid or endocrine aging.

The same general pattern might be expected in any broad review of endocrine aging (Timiras et al., 1995). There are few reliable endocrine changes. Some of the most bruited "facts" of endocrine aging may be erroneous. Growth hormone generally declines with age (Rudman et al., 1981; Veldhuis, 1998; Blackman, 2000), although with variance. Growth hormone levels may decline with age, but also with inactivity, changes in sleep cycles, malnutrition, or disease (von Werder, 1999). The cause of the decline may be a decline in growth hormone–releasing factor (Mulligan et al., 1999b; Russell-Aulet et al., 1999), suggesting a central nervous system basis for the decline, or even an underlying decline in other hormonal systems, such as the thyroid axis (Tagawa et al., 2000). There have been repeated suggestions that declining growth hormone might play a role in age-related diseases, including atherosclerosis, even independently of lipid-related risk factors (O'Connor et al., 1999). This parallels work suggesting that growth hormone supplementation may have beneficial effects on myocardial blood flow (in aging rats) by increasing the capillary density (Khan et al., 2001). Paralleling growth hormone and playing a role in the age-related decline (Span et al., 1999), levels of insulin-like growth factor fall (Savine and Sonksen, 1999), although its relationship to disease (Arvat et al., 2000) or even cell senescence (Sell et al., 1993) is largely unknown. Some decrease is simply attributable to poor nutrition (Hall et al., 1999).

Among the hormones reported to decline with age, melatonin has become a royal favorite. Current literature assumes this decline in serum levels and focuses on the mechanisms (Benot et al., 1999) or associated endocrinological abnormalities (Morales et al., 2000). It may, however, be a case of the emperor's new clothes. Recent data suggest that while melatonin decreases from its peak in adolescence, it may not decrease thereafter in normal, healthy individuals (Kennaway et al., 1999; Zeitzer et al., 1999). During menopause, it may even rise, apparently due to falling estrogen levels (Okatani et al., 2000). Decreasing serum melatonin may be simply a secondary marker of ill health, probably unrelated to aging. In short, a fall in serum melatonin may correlate with advancing years, but the decline may be caused by other factors, not necessarily including age. Moreover, although caloric restriction is one of the only interventions known to affect aging, it has no effect on the normal decline in melatonin seen in aging rats (MacGibbon et al., 2001). A decline in melatonin, if it occurs, may even be protective against malignancy, as melatonin supplementation increases the incidence of murine tumors (Anisimov et al., 2001).

The clearest age-related endocrine change is in sexual steroids. Androgens fall progressively in males, but may reflect a parallel decrease in other hormonal systems rather than independence (Morales et al., 2000). The adrenal glands (a major source of steroid production) change with age, even absent disease. The cortex (particularly the inner zone, the zona reticularis) shrinks, lipofuscin accumulates (Cheng et al., 1999), and a host of other changes occur. Despite this, basal glucocorticoids vary little as aging occurs in humans and other species. Dehydroepiandrosterone and its sulfate (DHEAS), aldosterone, and sex steroids, however, decrease (Timiras, 1995a; Stomati et al., 1999; Kiechl et al., 2000) and each has been speculatively linked (with little data) to the aging process (Harper et al., 1999). These changes are apparently the result of diminished rates of steroidogenesis rather than higher rates of clearance (Romanoff et al., 1961; West et al., 1961).

Within the testes, there is a loss of germ cells and a decrease in the rate of sperm production (Syntin et al., 2001). Whether this is the direct result of aging of the germ cells themselves or aging of the Sertoli cells that support the germ cell development and differentiation is unclear. At least in rats, there are changes in the seminiferous tubules and in the Sertoli cells, but whether this represents primary cellular senescence or is secondary to hormonal or cellular changes elsewhere is unclear (Wright et al., 1993; Zirkin and Chen, 2000). With age, there is gradual depletion of Leydig cells and a consequent decrease in their testosterone production; again, the etiology is unclear. In rats this is probably secondary, due to the effects of trophic or hormonal factors (but not luteinizing hormone) on gene expression in these cells (Luo et al., 1996, 2001; Syntin et al., 2001), rather than to intrinsic Leydig cell aging (Chen et al., 1996). While there is evidence of an increase in free radicals (specifically superoxide) and a decrease in mitochondrial volume in older rat Leydig cells (Chen et al., 2001a), this may be primary or due to changes in gene expression that precede and cause the alteration in metabolic efficiency.

Of sexual steroids, estrogen demonstrates the most apparent and profound temporal changes. Estrogen cycles on a monthly basis, becomes less predictable as menopause approaches, then declines precipitously at menopause. Secondary changes are attributed to this decline because they often parallel its course. These include changes in skin and mucosal membranes, breast characteristics, and risk of osteoporosis, cancer, heart disease, and Alzheimer dementia. Menopause, natural or surgical, is likewise correlated with a decrease in the ability to perform quotidian physical activities (Sowers et al., 2001). Multiple increases in risk occur at menopause. Men show no similar inflection, although risks increase at a more leisurely pace and may be correlated with less striking estrogen (Khosla et al., 1999) or androgen declines. Menopause is not simply related to exhaustion of ovarian follicles (Wise et al., 1994; Wise, 1999) but is a complex failure of communication between ovaries, brain, and pituitary gland. The primary player in this age-related change, variously attributed to each organ, remains uncertain, as does the precise role this change plays in various clinical syndromes likely related to declining serum estrogen levels.

From an interventional perspective, insulin was the first success story and might therefore be the most clinically understood hormone, yet its role in aging remains a complex and fascinating mystery. Given the increased incidence of diabetes in the elderly, one might suppose that serum insulin levels fall with age. However, the increased incidence is predominantly in non–insulin-dependent diabetes and things are a bit more complex than a simple decline in islet cell synthesis. The central issue is not that serum insulin levels fall with age (on the average they rise), but that the response of insulin levels to normal stimuli and cellular response to insulin become erratic and, from a clinical perspective, inappropriate. We might generalize by suggesting that age-related changes in insulin are not quantitative but qualitative: insulin no longer responds appropriately to physiological needs. At a given sampling time, serum insulin may not differ significantly between a centenarian and a 20-year-old. Exposed to an oral glucose load, exercise, infection, or hormonal changes, their responses often diverge markedly. Moreover, even if the insulin responses (rises in serum levels) were perfectly matched, the secondary effects of the insulin rise on cells, organs, and secondary hormonal release may diverge markedly between the old and young. For example, as a primary effect, oral glucose will often induce a slower and less effective rise in serum insulin in the elderly, partially due to a slower insulin clearance (Minaker et al., 1982a). As a secondary effect, even if we control for insulin rise, there will be a much more modest effect on serum norepinephrine release in the elderly than in the young, even though the direct effect of a rise in serum glucose on norepinephrine release is accentuated in the elderly (Minaker et al., 1982b). With age, insulin levels do not so much fall (or rise) as they wander about without regard to need and without inducing the appropriate secondary effects on which normal body function depends.

With regard to insulin, as perhaps in so many other endocrine systems, aging is accompanied by a gradual loss of the tight, responsive coupling that normally occurs between hormonal stimulus and tissue response. If the job of endocrine systems is to provide communication and coordination, aging undermines both. The central problem in communication failure is not volume but fidelity of the message. In endocrine aging the problem is not serum level but appropriateness of the endocrine response. With aging, messages becomes degraded and responses inappropriate, often independently of endocrine levels.

In summary, the aging endocrine systems show fairly well-defined but poorly understood changes (Perry, 1999) that may have profound effects on cell function and cell survival (Lockshin and Zakeri, 1990). These include a loss of reserve capacity to stimulation as well as declines in the baseline of several hormones, including growth hormone, insulin, dehydroepiandrosterone, antidiuretic hormone, and sexual steroids. The clearest age-related endocrine level changes are menopause in women, androgen decline in men, and decreased growth hormone and a major increase in the risk of type 2 diabetes in both sexes (Morley, 2000a). Several age-related diseases are directly (diabetes) or indirectly (cardiovascular disease, bone fractures) attributable to these changes and to the more subtle changes in endocrine communication, independent of serum levels. Potentially, disease risk factors, such as sarcopenia, hyperlipidemia, and osteoporosis, might be attributable to endocrine changes, if indirectly. Although much is known about age-related changes in the endocrine systems, sweeping generalizations about falling hormonal levels are misleading and often simply false. Such changes are complex and involve all endocrine functions, including production, secretion, transport, clearance, temporal regulation, and target tissue response (Bartke and Lane, 2001). The aging endocrine system might best be characterized as having poor homeostasis; its action is characterized by increasingly inappropriate and inadequate temporal characteristics and a clumsy and ineffective physiological response, rather than a simple, linear alteration with age. Endocrine aging is not so much a decline in endocrine levels as it is a decline in endocrine communication leading to a critical degradation of normal endocrine coordination of cellular and tissue functions.

The Role of Cell Senescence

Models of aging based solely on endocrine decline falter on endocrine clocks. If endocrine failure causes (even a significant portion of) aging, then what causes the endocrine failure? As the Romans once asked, in a political system, who guards the guards? Why should serum growth hormone levels decline? What times the fall of testosterone? Why do some hormones, apparently central players in our physiology, diminish with age? In other words, an endocrine theory of aging merely begs the deeper question of what caused endocrine aging in the first place. Here, as elsewhere, is an opportunity to invoke cellular senescence as the prime mover, the final guard from the political analogy.

Until recently, however, while an endocrine theory of aging begged the question, a cell senescence theory of aging begged the data. This was especially true of attempts to apply cell senescence theory to the endocrine system (Kontogeorgos and Kovacs, 1998). The theoretical outline is clear enough. If the role of an aging clock was played by cellular senescence, then we might expect that some cells that synthesize hormones (or cells that physiologically support such synthesizing cells) divide and thereby senesce. Such candidate cells should show shortening telomeres and an altered pattern of gene expression correlating with and underlying the known changes in the aging endocrine system. Ultimately, the hypothesis predicts that resetting such cells should return hormone synthesis, secretion, and serum levels (and, more importantly, tissue function) to those typical of a much younger organism.

The theory is simple, but not the data. The major problem is that we know too little of the origin of the observed changes in the aging endocrine system. We might, for example, attribute changes in the hypothalamic–pituitary axis to glial cell senescence, but not only is there little evidence that glial senescence occurs, there is no agreement that declining hormones levels are attributable to primary CNS changes in the first place. We know far too little about the mechanisms of endocrine changes that occur with age. To the extent that growth hormone levels decline, the "clock" that times this decline might be located within the posterior pituitary or the hypothalamus, but we have insufficient data to support either candidate. In estrogen and menopause, there is good evidence that the hypothalamus orchestrates (in a complex interaction with the ovary and pituitary) the timing and course of menopause (Wise, 1999), but this is not sufficient. If we did have convincing data, what cells time such a decline? There are changes in hypothalamic cells with age (Lloyd et al., 1994; Romero et al., 1994; Bernardis and Davis, 1996), but are these changes the primary "endocrine clock" or secondary to some more fundamental aging clock located elsewhere? The location and mechanism of the prime mover (or movers) in endocrine aging remains at large. It is therefore reasonable to suggest, but unreasonable to assume, that cell senescence functions as the underlying clock. To test the hypothesis, which cells should we look at and why these particular cells?

This problem is especially acute within the female reproductive system. Menopause is fairly well understood, but the complex interrelationship between the ovaries and hypothalamus leaves us uncertain of where the timer lies (Dorland et al., 1998). Is it the geometrically increasing loss of ova that triggers the hypothalamus to shut down the cycles, or is it the hypothalamus that ages and causes the accelerating loss of ova and ends the menses? More likely, neither accurately characterizes the complex timing function that regulates the menses or menopause. Brain and ovaries are menopausal pacemakers (Wise et al., 1996, 1999), but which, if either, contains cells that senesce and time menopause?

The suprachiasmatic nucleus, in which light-induced Fos expression is blunted in middle-aged rats and which may be the synchronizing clock for many endocrine cycles (Harney et al., 1996), is a prime candidate (Cai and Wise, 1996). Some (vasoactive intestinal polypeptide secreting), but not all (arginine vasopressin secreting) cells within the suprachiasmatic nuclei, which play a role in maintaining the cycles on which menses and estrogen secretion depend, show clear changes with age and a loss of cyclicity (Forsling et al., 1998; Krajnak et al., 1998). These cells lose their ability to synchronize the critical neuroendocrine signals on which menstrual cyclicity depends, contributing to the accelerated rate of follicular loss that occurs during middle age. This damping and destabilization of the ultradian, circadian, and infradian neural cycles lead to ovarian failure (Wise et al., 1997). Regarding the issue of cell senescence in the ovary, oocytes do show age-related changes (Kirkwood, 1998). Correspondingly, the little data available show that while oocytes (Wright et al., 1996b) and primordial follicles do not demonstrate telomerase activity, such activity is seen in the granulosa cells of growing follicles (Lavranos et al., 1999).

A similar centrally mediated failure apparently occurs in the gonadotropin-releasing hormone production in men (Mulligan et al., 1999a). Could these neurons fail because of vascular or glial cell senescence (see Chapter 13)? At least in rats, there is an overall change in the pattern of gene expression in relevant hypothalamic neurons (activated gonadotropin-inhibiting hormone neurons, which may explain the falling amplitude of the luteinizing hormone surge that may parallel the mechanisms triggering menopause in humans), but it is unclear if this represents age-related primary changes in neuronal gene expression or primary effects of an altered pattern of neuronal activation with secondary changes in gene expression (Lloyd et al., 1994). Although the ovary does show aging changes and although cell senescence in the ovarian stroma cells may play some role in menopause, the overall mechanism is not one of simple ovarian failure. The mechanism of menopause is not merely neuronal but an interactive one between hypothalamus, pituitary, and ovary, yet triggering events may be predominantly neuronal (Wise, 1994). Though part of this complex system might contain cells whose senescence is responsible for menopause, we have little or no data to support this possibility.

Within the adrenal glands, and relevant to most the aging changes of most other steroidal systems, there is evidence for lifelong cell division. Changes in DNA, RNA, and protein synthesis are consistent with senescence. In rat adrenal gland cortical cells, for example, there are characteristic age-related changes in DNA, RNA, and protein synthesis. Thymidine labeling shows a steady decrease in DNA and RNA synthesis of cells in the medulla and cortex (zona glomerulosa, zona fasciculata, and zona reticularis) as the animal ages. Moreover, human adrenocortical cells show an age-associated loss of telomere length reversible by transfection with hTERT. Normal human adrenocortical cells show a decline in TRFs from 12 kb in fetal donors to 7 kb in the oldest donors, a value consistent with senescence in human fibroblasts. Barring hTERT transfection, adrenocortical cell division occurs slowly over the human lifespan and is associated with a progressive loss of telomere length. This may result in proliferative defects in vivo and explain the age-related changes in the structure and function of the human adrenal cortex (Yang et al., 2001c).

While these latter results might explain the age-related changes in serum steroid hormones, similar changes apparently do not occur in aging Leydig cells in the testes (Nagata et al., 2000). The relevance of this to the lack of senescence in germ (and perhaps Sertoli) cells of the testes (Yashima et al., 1998b) is unknown, as are most mechanisms by which Sertoli cells ensure germ cell survival (Akama et al., 2002), but this begs our interest. Adult spermatozoa do not express telomerase (Wright et al., 1996b). As in estrogen control, discussed above, there is evidence for age-related changes within the hypothalamus and pituitary that may be the basis for adrenal aging. Although there has been speculation that the clock for adrenal aging may reside in the hippocampus (Magri et al., 2000), there is at least good evidence for an age-related decrease in glucocorticoid sensitivity of the pituitary corticotrope cells (Revskoy and Redei, 2000). If cell senescence plays a role in the age-related loss of feedback regulation in the hypothalamic–pituitary–adrenal axis, such senescence might occur at almost any level.

Although perhaps less dramatically, the issues discussed above in several endocrine axes should play out in other axes. Assigning overall causation to cell senescence—

in any endocrine system—is feasible and consistent with known data, but unprovable because of the complexity of the endocrine systems involved and recurrent lacunae in our knowledge of endocrine function within each axis. If the complexity of the endocrine systems is the major obstacle, making it difficult to interpret available data regarding cell senescence in the endocrine system, the minor issue has been the lack of data to interpret.

Exceptions to this pessimism are growing. Data support senescence in specific endocrine cells. Cells within the thyroid and parathyroid tissues show telomere loss, particularly later in life (Kammori et al., 2002b). Initial human results on in vivo adrenocortical cell senescence and in vitro hTERT transfection (Yang et al., 2001c) have not (yet) been used for in vitro human intervention. Recently, however, hTERT was cotransfected (along with SV40 T antigen, neo, and green fluorescent protein) into primary bovine adrenocortical cells. The resulting immortalized clones were then transplanted into immunodeficient (SCID) mice. The recipient animals then successfully survived adrenalectomies. The normal murine corticosterone was replaced by (transplant secreted) bovine cortisol. Transplanted adrenocortical tissue was similar to normal bovine adrenal cortex. These adrenocortical cells had low proliferation rates and no indication of malignant transformation (Thomas et al., 2000a). One cannot help but wonder what will happen when hTERT transformation is attempted in vivo in human trials (and when?).

Models such as this, where immortalized endocrine tissues are observed not for mere normalcy of function but for prolonged normalcy within the aging animal recipient may allow us to experimentally test the hypothesis that cell senescence plays a role in intrinsic aging changes within the endocrine system. Although animal testing will be the most direct test, the prevalence of human endocrine diseases, notably diabetes, prompts considerable investment in endocrinological interventions that have a bearing on the same theoretical issues addressed in animal studies. There are current plans for parallel human interventions, for example, using pancreatic islet cells in insulin-dependent diabetic patients. Given the concern over senescence limiting the utility of transplanted cells, these cells are likely to be transfected with hTERT, undergo telomere lengthening via promoter, or derive from early stem cell sources. In each option, such cells are relatively juvenile (from the standpoint of cell senescence) and offer useful information regarding cell senescence in aging endocrine systems. Although the major concerns are safety and efficacy, the background work for this and long-term outcomes could teach us a good deal.

Intervention

The most popular (and largely ineffective) interventions in aging and age-related disease are endocrinological. Not only are there are clear and glaring exceptions to the general rule that such interventions in age-related diseases lack supportive data (e.g., insulin works reliably and effectively in diabetes), but there are data that hormonal replacement in the aging patient does have some benefits. There are two concerns: (1) there are insufficient data on the cost/benefit ratio, and (2) the public, anticipating benefits, opts for the experimental group without appreciation of the risks. These two observations have been equally true historically for at least the past century, although the current focus has shifted from estrogen and testosterone to melatonin, dehydro-epiandrosterone, and growth hormone.

Although such interventions, such as growth hormone supplementation, might have clinical benefits (perhaps even after balancing the risks; Vance, 1998), this does not imply that endocrine supplementation affects aging. There is no evidence that hormones affect aging. With few exceptions, there is little evidence that hormone replacement affects lifespan or mortality. The most notable exception is insulin replacement, which has profound effects on morbidity and mortality. Type 2 diabetes is linked epidemiologically to advancing age (and independently to obesity and other factors). Although there are data that replacement of other hormones (e.g., thyroid) have clinical benefits, this applies to pathological conditions, independent of aging. Even taking counterbalancing risks into account (and though it does not affect aging), hormonal replacement in aging (even excepting type 2 diabetes) may have net benefits in some well-defined patients (Perry, 1999). Indications include defined hormonal deficits (e.g., hypothyroidism), but emotional thinking and social pressures increase the complexity.

In the elderly, hormonal deficits are often not well defined: we don't know what a healthy normal serum level means in an elderly patient. Equally, we don't know the risks, the efficacy, nor, therefore, the potential net clinical benefit (if any). Not giving hormonal supplements is equivalent to deciding that the optimal dose should be zero— a recommendation nonetheless, and one of ignorance. We are often more comfortable giving nothing and defending such a decision on the (illogical) grounds that we don't know enough (Hermann and Berger, 1999), rather than admitting that any dose recommendation (even the conservative figure of zero) is uncertain and as equally based on ignorance as is the recommendation of replacement therapy. A more honest (but no more useful) appraisal is that we prefer the devil we know (aging with no hormone replacement) to the one we don't (after all, who knows what might happen?). Many patients know aging too well and are willing to take an uncertain risk.

The most common current attempt to intervene in aging is growth hormone. This intervention rests on the observation that growth hormone levels decline in many elderly patients, although this decline, to the extent that it is age related, might be incidental, secondary, or even protective. Most reviews of the literature recommend against the routine use of growth hormone or growth hormone–releasing factors, citing the flawed logic behind their use and specific, legitimate concerns about clinical risks (Welle, 1998; Wolfe, 1998; Morley, 1999; von Werder, 1999; Blackman et al., 2002).

Although many of those spending their money on growth hormone (or its releasing factors) have allowed fashion to consign them to an experimental group of pharmaceutical lemmings, others have been equally unsympathetic toward hormone replacement without fairly considering data. Momentarily ignoring caveats, growth hormone, its releasing factors, or insulin-like growth factor may have potential beneficial effects (Savine and Sonksen, 1999). It has been cited as increasing exercise endurance, bone, and collagen turnover (Wallace et al., 2000); muscle mass, strength, and protein synthesis (Welle, 1998); bone density (Mosekilde et al., 1999) and mood, and perhaps lowering cardiac risk (Colao et al., 1999a; O'Connor et al., 1999). In many cases, the effects may be weak or dependent on additional variables, as in bone density (Christmas et al., 2002). Growth hormone may increase insulin-like growth factor, though not dehydroepiandrosterone sulfate levels (Aimaretti et al., 2000).

The downsides remain (von Werder, 1999): (*1*) growth hormone is given by subcutaneous injection, (*2*) dosage calculation is difficult as elderly patients may show increased sensitivity or be resistant, (*3*) the risk of diabetes may increase, (*4*) it enhances the risk or progression of malignant disease (IGF-I levels correlate with the incidence of prostatic cancer and acromegalic patients have a higher frequency of colonic polyps and gastrointestinal malignancies), and (*5*) the present cost is high and may not be reimbursable (Biller et al., 2000). In Ames dwarf mice, animals genetically deficient in growth hormone live longest, while those mice that overexpress it live the shortest lifespans (Brown-Borg et al., 1999). These data (while not offered as necessarily relevant to humans) scarcely underscore growth hormone as a way to extend lifespan. As with any pharmaceutical, there is unpredictable risk. Cardiac risk versus benefits, for example, may vary widely among individuals (Colao et al., 2001). We might say, with some flippancy but equal insight, that nature has a considerable head start on us in understanding physiology. If more growth hormone were better, then evolution should have selected for it and didn't. Perhaps nature knows something that we should know. Caveat emptor.

Dehydroepiandrosterone and its sulfate have enjoyed a strong public (Hinson and Raven, 1999) interest, but limited scientific or medical support (Huppert et al., 2000), despite some intriguing early data (Schwartz, 1979). The relationship between age and dehydroepiandrosterone has been known for half a century (Pincus et al., 1955; De Neve and Vermeulen, 1965). There have been suggestions that dehydroepiandrosterone or the sulfate might have beneficial clinical effects over about the same period (Kiechl et al., 2000; Tagawa et al., 2000); the field has enjoyed a renewed interest in the past few years. There have been claims that dehydroepiandrosterone might be protective against cardiovascular disease, cancer, immune-modulated diseases, dementia, or aging (Tummala and Svec, 1999; Tagawa et al., 2000). Some suggest that dehydroepiandrosterone might protect against glucocorticoid side effects, including diabetes, amino acid deamination, fattiness, hypertension, immune suppression, myopathy, osteopenia, osteoporosis, and avascular necrosis (Robinzon and Cutolo, 1999). Although some proponents have explored the cell biology (Baulieu, 2000; Williams, 2000)), putative mechanisms are largely ignored in optimistic acceptance of the claims (Dhar, 1999).

Evidence is less spectacular. There is a good correlation between serum dehydroepiandrosterone (or dehydroepiandrosterone sulfate) and vascular diseases, presence of dementia, diabetes mellitus, malignancies, musculoskeletal disorders, and clinical measures of disease, but these correlations may not be causal or predictive (Tilvis et al., 1999). There is growing evidence that it has no protective effect against atherosclerosis (Mazza et al., 1999; Kiechl et al., 2000). With regard to immune function, there is some evidence that it can have beneficial effects (Solerte et al., 1999). There is a correlation between dementia and low serum dehydroepiandrosterone (Hillen et al., 2000; Magri et al., 2000), but no evidence that dehydroepiandrosterone is protective here (Carlson et al., 1999). Despite suggestions that dehydroepiandrosterone might have beneficial effects on mood based on correlational findings (Barrett-Connor et al., 1999; Young, 1999), perhaps via effects on β-endorphin responses (Stomati et al., 1999), interventional studies do not support the suggestion (Huppert et al., 2000). At least in perimenopausal women, there is no demonstrable effect on severity of perimenopausal symptoms, mood, dysphoria, libido, cognition, memory, or well-being (Barnhart et al., 1999). There remains the possibility that it may be effective in preventing osteoporotic bone loss in aging (Gordon et al., 1999). Some interventional studies have shown few results and almost no clinical benefit (Flynn et al., 1999). Other studies (Baulieu et al., 2000) demonstrate some improvement in elderly women in their bone turnover (assessed by the dual-energy X-ray absorptiometry [DEXA] technique), decreased osteoclastic activity, increased libido (in women), and an improvement in skin parameters (hydration, epidermal thickness, sebum production, and pigmentation). The overall evidence that dehydroepiandrosterone has benefit is minimal (Nippoldt and Nair, 1998; Pugh et al., 1999b) and its significance, clinically or to our understanding of endocrine aging, remains speculative.

The upshot is that the endocrine system is, and always has been, an arena for intervention. Over the past century, it has witnessed some clear winners, such as insulin. Despite extensive public interest and usage (and expectation that something dramatic should have been proven), there are surprisingly few data that endocrine supplementation affects aging or age-related diseases (Fisher and Morley, 2002). Hormone use for defined deficit is well grounded. Aging deficits, however, are largely unproven, and data do not support the dramatic effects claimed for supplementation.

Exceptions, where hormone supplementation may have accepted beneficial effects on age-related diseases, are interesting, but annoyingly uncertain. Estrogen supplementation may have indications, previously including atherosclerosis risk (Schwenke, 1998), but it may likewise increase the risk of some cancers (Rodriguez et al., 2001; Stephenson, 2001) and have complex risks and benefits on coagulation (Gottsater et al., 2001) and quality of life (Hlatky et al., 2002; Rexrode and Manson, 2002). Meta-analysis suggests that the risk of ischemic stroke may increase (Gillum et al., 2000), but other data find no increase or decrease in stroke risk (Simon et al., 2001). In this, as in most other aspects of endocrine aging, the complexity of the interactions (Straub et al., 2001) precludes easy generality and encourages contradictory data sets. This is more true of interventions incompletely understood in the first place, such caloric restriction. One of the most commonly accepted interventions in aging, caloric restriction has effects on the endocrine system (Wise, 1995; McShane and Wise, 1996), but the direction of causation and mechanisms involved remain largely guesswork.

Overall, our ability to intervene in endocrine aging has an illusory quality that contradicts the public perception. Endocrine supplementation may not work (and may not affect aging), but it is available. In contrast, cellular or genetic interventions may work, but are unavailable because of the difficult technical issues involved in such interventions and because of our ignorance in the face of endocrine complexity specifically. Experimental transplantation of hTERT transfected cells (Thomas et al., 2000a; Condon et al., 2002) may clarify cell senescence in intrinsic aging of the endocrine system and endocrine-responsive organs. Given the results of human in vitro work (Yang et al., 2001c), human in vivo trials cannot be far behind. Moreover, such transplants are likely to prove immensely effective, although they are not in clinical use. As a result of the enormous impetus for such interventions, it may be that we solve the technical issues and even successfully reverse endocrine aging long before we fully understand how the endocrine systems work, what is responsible for its aging, or even that the system demonstrates primary aging in the first place. It would be ironic if we were to solve the problem before we can all agree that there is one to solve.

CHAPTER 13

Nervous System

Structure and Overview

The human nervous system is ignorant when young, stores a great deal of information as it matures, but has considerable problems with access and processing that information as it grows older. The basis of this failure is known in outline, but the causes of aging and age-related disease in the central nervous system largely escape us. The bulk of our clinical interest lies in the central nervous system, most attributable to two major categories of disease: the dementias and cerebral infarcts.

Even though aging changes in the peripheral nervous system are largely slighted, the peripheral nervous system is important nonetheless and deserves at least parenthetical mention. Although there is evidence for peripheral neuronal aging, many of the clinical changes that we attribute to aging in peripheral neurons are more accurately the result of peripheral vascular disease or reflect diffuse metabolic problems in the elderly, such as chronic hyperglycemia secondary to diabetes. All of our sensory input arrives through the peripheral nervous system. All of our volitional (and much of our autonomic) activities are accomplished by it. The most widely appreciated aging dysfunctions of the sensory system are probably those of retinal degeneration (addressed in Chapter 17) or neural deafness, but the most common is probably a gradual (perhaps we may say, insensible) loss of our dermal receptor input. We no longer feel the world effectively. The most clinically prominent of our motor problems in old age are probably more related to the loss of central dopaminergic motor control (i.e., substantia nigra neuron loss in Parkinson's disease or striatal neuron dysfunction; Roth, 1997) or muscle loss (disuse and idiopathic sarcopenia) than to primary aging changes in our peripheral, secondary motor neurons. Nonetheless, the peripheral nerves do show changes, such as lipofuscin accumulation (Sosunov et al., 1997), whose functional importance (if any) is unknown.

The central nervous system has an estimated 100 billion neurons, but this probably represents only a small percentage (perhaps 10%) of the total number of cells. The majority of the cells making up the brain are glial (from the Greek for *glue*) cells. Neurons are considered the more important active cells, which they are from the electrophysiological perspective, and are considered responsible for all perception, learning, memory, intellectual, and all motor activity. The glial cells, which have historically been given the short shrift with regard to assigned functions and importance (Aschner et al., 1999), have gradually begun to assume a more prominent and less passive role in our limited but growing understanding of brain function (Aschner et al., 1999; Nichols, 1999). Although glial cells provided a physical framework, particularly during neurodevelopment when they act as guides to migrating cortical neurons, their role as insulators and metabolic support units for the intertwining neurons has long been recognized. More recently we have begun to realize that glial cells play some ill-defined role in learning and memory, perhaps by shaping synaptic numbers and location (Ullian et al., 2001), although the limits of such roles remain indistinct and largely unexplored.

Typically the cortex of the human brain comprises layers of distinct neuronal types. Input arrives from peripheral sensory or other neurons, ascends through the subcortical white matter, and is processed by the neurons, and final output descends back into the white matter, bound for other neurons.

The axons, long neuronal arms that carry most neural information (as electrical impulses) away from the neuron, are surrounded by oligodendrocytes whose high lipid content make them good insulators for the rapid electrolyte shifts that the axons depend on for transmitting waves of electrical current to the next neuron. This high lipid content renders the oligodendrocytes whiter than the gray colored (though pink in fresh tissue) neurons, hence dividing the brain into gray (cortex with highs concentration of neurons) and white matter (subcortical axons with high concentrations of oligodendrocytes). Although the oligodendrocytes are numerous and necessary, the brain is replete with astrocytes, microglia, and other cells whose functions have historically attracted less interest.

Astrocytes and oligodendrocytes make up the macroglia. Astrocytes are the largest and most numerous neuroglial cells in the brain and spinal cord. They regulate extracellular ion concentrations, respond to injury, have immune functions (Aschner, 1998), and are capable of releasing (and taking up) some neurotransmitters.

Microglia are inordinately variable in appearance. Having immune functions (Aloisi et al., 2000b), they respond to damage and are capable of phagocytosis, as well as secretion of cytokines and growth factors. Together, the glia comprise the majority of cells in the brain and while most are probably astrocytes, a large percentage of the glial cells (Stoll and Jander, 1999) are microglia.

Electrical impulses travel down axons, often in small but rapid jumps occasioned by a series of nodes between spans of glial insulation, and result in the release of neurotransmitters from the end of the axon. Classically (and to a large degree accurately), each specific neuron releases only a single specific transmitter (e.g., dopamine, acetylcholine, serotonin, and now literally dozens of other transmitter substances) that crosses the synapse separating the axonal button from the dendrite of the next neuron and causes electrical changes: information processing in action. Although the axons are the trunk lines of the brain, it is in the synapses and dendrites that we find the complexity and heart of the processing of information. While the average peripheral neuron may have less than a hundred synapses, the central neurons, the foundation of our ability to think, are more likely to have at least tens of thousands of synapses, resulting in a complexity without intracellular parallel in other systems. In this complexity, somehow, lies our ability to learn, to move, to sense, and to think. And this complexity fails.

Classic teaching was that neurons divided in the fetal organism, but not beyond birth. We learned not by adding or subtracting neurons in this vast web of cells, but by adding or subtracting (or altering the efficacy of) our synapses. In reality, new neurons do form from neural stem ("neural precursor") cells present in all adult mammals, including humans (Shihabuddin et al., 1999; Svendsen et al., 1999; Gage, 2000), and this process is responsive to neural growth factors (Wagner et al., 1999) and probably to environmental stimulation (Nilsson et al., 1999). There are some initial data suggesting that (at least in rat hippocampus) as many as half of all adult neurons are capable of division and proliferation, given the right conditions (Brewer, 1999). Similar though less impressive data are found in human ex vivo cells (Brewer et al., 2001). Nonetheless, in measuring telomere lengths in patients ranging from neonates to centenarians, cortical neurons remain stable in this regard (Takubo et al., 2002). The numbers of neurons generated in adult human cortex, location of such stem cells (Ourednik et al., 2001), mechanisms controlling such stem cells (Groszer et al., 2001), and practical significance of neuron replacement (Kornack and Rakic, 2001), particularly as a mechanism for learning or to a noticeable degree for regeneration after infarction or trauma (Eriksson et al., 1998; Kempermann et al., 1998; Brewer et al., 2001) remain argued and largely unknown. Part of this conclusion lies in our lack of sufficient data, but part is necessarily implied by almost incomprehensible complexity of neural structures and corresponding incomprehensibility of replacing such structures (Horner and Gage, 2000). Consider, for example, the frontal lobe secondary motor neuron just under the skull, whose axon must find its way down into the spinal cord and meet a specific primary motor neuron located within the spine and just below the posterior ribs. The scale is about equivalent to that of a 6-foot-tall man in Los Angeles reaching out one arm, across North America, and shaking hands with a *specific* group of a dozen people located on a *specific* street in New York and then linking hands permanently with only one of them. To a degree, these connections are established prenatally (when the two men are, as it were, standing beside one another in St. Louis). If we lose these neurons in adulthood, how can such incredibly specific connections be reestablished? Even allowing for reprogramming and rerouting (plasticity), it remains unlikely from a theoretical point of view that newly divided neurons play a significant role in adult learning or in adult healing in the central nervous system.

If we assume, conservatively, that neuronal replacement plays no role in the adult nervous system, then what of the glial cells? Do they divide and, in doing so, play some role in learning, repair, or aging? Here too, there are initial problems. The oligodendrocytes that invest and insulate neurons within the central nervous system are themselves (like neurons) complex in morphology and might be thought incapable of division in the adult organism. If they divide, their complexity might run afoul of the same conceptual stumbling block that we impose on neural division: could new cells assume the complexity of shape and function of the cells that they replace? We know that oligodendrocytes can be reprogrammed, becoming multipotential central nervous system cells

(Kondo and Raff, 2000), and such cultured oligodendrocytes apparently do not senesce (Tang et al., 2001). The question is to use these observations clinically.

Glial cells comprise astrocytes and microglia, a different story. Not only are they less complex, and hence easier to envision as replaceable elements, but at least microglia are already known to divide into old age (Schipper et al., 1993). Microglia are small, capable, protean cells that divide readily and are ubiquitous in the nervous system (Streit, 2000). They derive from bone marrow cells (Rezaie and Male, 1999) and at least the perivascular microglia are probably replaced regularly from hematopoetic stem cell lines (Stoll and Jander, 1999), although the issue remains open (Thomas, 1999). Microglia are basically immunocompetent monocytes that reside within and are specific for the central nervous system (Engel and Kohn, 1999; Rezaie and Male, 1999; Aloisi et al., 2000a; Streit, 2002). Although circulating monocytes demonstrate telomerase activity, as least in those under 40 years of age (Iwama et al., 1998), whether microglia demonstrate such activity is unknown. Although having immune functions, microglia have many other nonimmune functions. For example, microglia have hormonal receptors and secondary effects on neighboring neurons through cytokine and growth factor release (Mor et al., 1999). This suggests not only nonimmune regulatory functions for microglia (Rabchevsky and Streit, 1997) but a remarkable complexity and interdependence of their relationship with neurons (Bruce-Keller, 1999; Streit, 2000).

Aging and Other Pathology

If age is a thief, then the greatest treasure we lose is ourselves. Despite social changes over the past century mitigating against home care for elderly, demented relatives, increasing lifespan and consequent increasing incidence of Alzheimer dementia has made it more likely that many of us have parents whom we love and lose—day by day—forever. It is difficult to understand the tragedy until we come face to face with it. Gerard Manley Hopkins (1985), monk and poet, once said that the "mind has mountains; cliffs of fall, Frightful, sheer, no-man-fathomed. Hold them cheap, May who ne'er hung there." More and more of us hang there as we live longer lives, whether poets, parents, or ourselves. The dementias have been variously defined in different studies and incidence depends to a degree on the medical infrastructure of the country in question. In developed nations dementia is rare before age 60, affects 5% of people over age 65, and 20% of those over age 80 (Livingston, 1994). Cognitive impairment in general, and Alzheimer disease in particular, may be unavoidable no matter what the general health of the patient: live long enough and dementia may be the inevitable outcome (McNeal et al., 2001). Moreover, patients with Alzheimer dementia incur additional morbidity and mortality through their increased risk of non-dementia illnesses (Brauner et al., 2000).

The aging central nervous system has two primary pathologies: the loss of its vascular supply—strokes and microinfarct dementias—and loss of neurons without apparent vascular cause—primarily Parkinson and Alzheimer dementias (Fig. 13–1). This age-dependent loss of neurons occurs in other primates as well as in humans (Morris et al., 1999). In addition, there are the less common dementias due to hormonal (e.g., hypothyroidism and, ultimately, myxedematous dementia), infectious (e.g., Lewy body disease), metabolic (e.g., Pick disease), nutritional, or toxic etiologies (e.g., Wernicke-Korsakoff syndrome). The syndrome of cognitive impairment without dementia has been

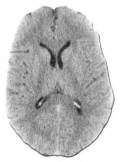
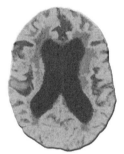

Young brain: Old brain:
53yo Professor   72yo Alzheimer's disease
Speaks 12 languages   Unable to care for self
Perfect GRE scores   Does not recognize family

Figure 13–1 Aging nervous system. Aging brain commonly incurs a gradual loss of brain tissue, often apparent on routine CT scans. Such loss may occur (to a degree) without observable clinical pathology, although the most extreme losses are those in Alzheimer's patients. The patient at the left (with an IQ >180 and three graduate degrees) has barely visible sulci and minimal ventricles; the patient to the right has wide sulci, enormous ventricles, and an obvious loss of brain tissue, correlating with a stunning clinical loss of higher cortical function.

identified in the elderly (Ebly et al., 1995), although further work (Di Carlo et al., 2000) may sort it into one of the above etiologies. In this same context, minimal nutritional deficits have been suggested as playing some role in such cognitive impairment (Calvaresi and Bryan, 2001). When the primary pathology is located within the central nervous system, however, the basic etiology is overwhelmingly vascular or neuronal. Alzheimer disease, for example, is the most common cause of dementia in the elderly (Mayeux and Schofield, 1994), and Parkinson disease affects perhaps 1% of the world's population (de Rijk et al., 1997). By some estimates (Olson, 2000), between 5% and 10% of all individuals over age 60 may have some degree of Parkinson disease. First-degree relatives have a 17% chance of developing Parkinson disease (Marder et al., 1996; Jarman and Wood, 1999).

The pathology of the vascular system is discussed largely in Chapter 9. These diseases fall into three partially overlapping categories: strokes (usually thrombotic), intracranial bleeds (including hemorrhagic stroke), and microinfarct or vascular dementias (Gorelick et al., 1994; Yanagihara, 1999; Erkinjuntti et al., 2000), including Binswanger's disease (Roman, 1999; Ramos-Estebanez et al., 2000; Margolin and Balko, 2001) and a motley collection of other eponyms and abbreviations (Rafalowska, 1999; Loeb, 2000; Thomas et al., 2000b). Vasculitic strokes occur secondary to viral or bacterial infection (Mattila et al., 1998). In all cases, the primary pathology lies within the aging or diseased vessel and risk factors are those of atherosclerotic disease (Gorelick, 1997). In these pathologies, the neuronal loss, while of overwhelming clinical importance, is secondary to the vascular pathology. Nonetheless, vascular changes do occur and there is a large body of data on such changes within the central nervous system. Note that even in disease presentations, such as stroke, that we regard as predominantly vascular in etiology, there is substantial reason to believe that nonvascular factors, such glial cell reactions that change with age, determine the outcome (Kharlamov et al., 2000).

There is a large catalog of changes that occur in the capillary beds and small-caliber arterioles in aging humans (Kalaria, 1996). The composition of connective tissues and arterial smooth muscles alters, there is a thickening of the vascular basement membrane (De Jong et al., 1997), a thinning of the endothelium in some species, and a loss of endothelial mitochondria with an increase in pericytes. Multiple other abnormalities are seen in aging vascular beds within the central nervous system, including unique proteins and membrane lipids and "massive bundles of collagen fibrils" within the blood–brain barrier (De Jong et al., 1997). Although the functional significance (if any) is unknown, age-related changes in the blood–brain barrier (Shah and Mooradian, 1997) might put neurons at risk in some areas, perhaps playing a role in even nonvascular dementias, such as Alzheimer's, in which such changes are more frequent (De Jong et al., 1997). Some authors have suggested that β-amyloid may be the trigger for vascular free radical damage with resultant neuronal damage (Stamler, 1996; Thomas et al., 1996). As the correlation is notable (Goldstein and Reivich, 1991), some have even suggested that Alzheimer's might even be primarily due to an impaired vascular supply (Crawford, 1998; Shi et al., 2000). They suggest that this is consistent with what we know of the association of Alzheimer's with apolipoprotein E4 (Strittmatter et al., 1993; Rosenberg, 2000), effects of drugs (haloperidol, antiinflammatory agents), studies of intellectual function as an independent variable, and pathology (de la Torre, 1997). Moreover, apolipoprotein E4 (apoE4) is underrepresented (Wang et al., 2001c) and E2 is overrepresented in some centenarian populations (Hazzard, 2001). The latter is associated with a lower incidence of Alzheimer and atherosclerotic diseases (Davignon et al., 1988). Alternatively, amyloid deposition might contribute to the decline in vascular function (Kalaria, 1996), although there is no correlation between the stage of Alzheimer disease and degree of capillary abnormalities, suggesting that Alzheimer's does not cause the aberrations (De Jong et al., 1997).

The cells in the vessels and meninges that compose the blood–brain barrier are sources of insulin-like growth factor-1 (IGF-1) for the brain. Although expression of the gene does not change with age, IGF-1 declines (perhaps due to translation or transport defects). Although messenger RNA for corresponding receptors remains constant, receptor count decreases with age (Sonntag et al., 1999a).

Overall, it is clear that vascular abnormalities occur (Mrak et al., 1997), but not what they mean. Such abnormalities correlate clinically with Alzheimer dementia, but the problem of what constitutes the more fundamental cause remains intriguing, yet unanswerable.

In discussing what are (at least superficially) nonvascular pathologies, such as Parkinson's or Alzheimer dementia, we tend to think of them as fundamentally neuronal in etiology: neurons as trigger and target. To a degree, this reflects our current ignorance: we are awash in data, but short on convincing interpretations. Although we know much about the cascade of processes that describe Alzheimer dementia (Selkoe, 1997), we lack an understanding of many issues. Absent postmortem tissue (Fillenbaum et al., 1996; Naslund et al., 2000), and despite encouraging trials (Etcheberrigaray et al., 1998; Mayeux et al., 1999; Friedland et al., 2000; Riemenschneider et al., 2002) and the use of magnetic resonance imaging (MRI; Bartzokis et al., 2000) or positron emission tomography (PET) scans (Rapoport, 1999; Silverman et al., 2001), Alzheimer disease is still not a laboratory or radiologic diagnosis but a clinical one, and even then a diagnosis of exclusion (McCleary et al., 1996) and difficulty (Beck et al., 2000; Knopman et al., 2000; Sternberg et al., 2000). This makes cross-cultural and international epidemiologic studies difficult (Farrer, 2001), although behavioral and lifestyle correlations have maintained support across geographic boundaries (White et al., 1996; Hendrie et al., 2001). In some ways, we know more about what it isn't than what it is. For example, the mechanism of neuronal death is probably apoptotic (Dragunow et al., 1997) and may be stochastic (Lipsitz, 2000). But although we know something of how β-amyloid (Sopher et al., 1996; MacManus et al., 2000) and presenilins (Kim et al., 1997c; Kim and Tanzi, 1997) trigger the apoptotic cascade, and despite an excellent theoretical framework for the overall process (Tanzi et al., 1996; Mattson et al., 1998b; Mattson and Pederson, 1998), there is no consensus on what triggers the amyloid abnormalities. It is a disease in which much is known but little is understood. We have a good grasp of the descriptive pathology at almost all levels. What is not understood is how various etiologies (genetics, viral and bacterial infections, diet, tobacco use, diabetes, vascular disease, toxin exposure, behavior) interact, if some do so (Debanne et al., 2000), to produce Alzheimer disease.

What we do know is profound and represents a large body of knowledge. We know much about the fine pathology, biochemistry, and genetics of this tragic disease. It is a disease of gradual loss of intellectual (Elias et al., 2000) and personal function without clear environmental, hormonal, nutritional, infectious, or vascular etiology (above discussion notwithstanding). It is irreversible and has no current therapy with significant and accepted value.

Histology shows inflammation, neuronal loss (Price et al., 2001), especially of cholinergic neurons (Henderson, 1996), areas of necrosis, neurofibrillary tangles (NFTs) composed of tau proteins, and amyloid plaques throughout affected areas, largely frontal and limbic structures. Curiously, our closest primate relatives, chimpanzees and orangutans, demonstrate β-amyloid deposition, but not the neurofibrillary tangles (Gearing et al., 1994, 1997) and same pattern of substantial neuronal loss (Erwin et al., 2001) common in human central nervous system aging and dementia. Moreover, in fly models, the tau protein and neurodegeneration occur without neurofibrillary tangles, which suggests that such tangles are the outcome, not the cause of the pathology (Wittmann et al., 2001). These and other findings have raised the issue of which effects are primary and which are secondary. More recent work (Gotz et al., 2001; Lewis et al., 2001) suggests an interactive effect between the tau proteins and β-amyloid deposition, in which tau tangles and aggregates are prerequisite to neurogeneration (Lee, 2001). There is an apparent correlation between the level of tau protein expression in oral epithelial cells and incidence of Alzheimer disease; whether this is constitutive or increases during the disease process is unknown (Hattori et al., 2002).

Central to the human pathology is an aberrant metabolism of a protein, β-amyloid (Naslund et al., 2000), whose precursor (Irizarry et al., 1996) is apparently cut inappropriately (Mayeux et al., 1999), aggregates, and becomes insoluble, forming plaques. The mechanisms that control the truncation and aggregation of the precursor protein are debated (Webster and Rogers, 1996; Leveugle et al., 1997; Lin et al., 2000b), although the cleaving enzyme is increased in affected areas (Fukumoto et al., 2002). Whether plaque formation is a primary or merely a secondary event remains arguable (Fowler et al., 1997). Aberrant presenilins (Cook et al., 1996; Kovacs et al., 1996; Page et al.,

1996) correlate with the pathology and genetics (particularly the early-onset familial form) of the disease (Gomez-Isla et al., 1997; Seeger et al., 1997; Athan et al., 2001), although their role is controversial (Xia et al., 1998). Likewise, neurofibrillary tangles play a role (Kim et al., 1997b; Mattson and Guo, 1997; Stege and Bosman, 1999), at least in early-onset familial Alzheimer disease, which accounts for approximately 10% of all cases (Mattson et al., 1998a; McGeer et al., 1998). Interactions between estrogen and presenilins may explain the putative protective effect of estrogen against Alzheimer disease (Mattson et al., 1997b). Although the importance, even correlational validity, of any relationship between presenilins and late-onset Alzheimer disease has been questioned (Romas et al., 2000), the presenilins may play a role in calcium homeostasis (Leissring et al., 2000) and risk of ischemic neuronal damage in early-onset Alzheimer disease (Mattson et al., 2000b).

Although the β-amyloid precursor protein is probably essential and beneficial to normal neuronal and glial function, the altered form found in Alzheimer's disease is not (Mattson, 1997). Some investigators have even argued that the damage that occurs in Alzheimer disease is a product of the decrease in the normally secreted β-amyloid precursor protein and increase in A β-amyloid (Mattson and Pedersen, 1998). There is evidence supporting the benefits of precursor proteins, whose release is activity-dependent. β-Amyloid precursor modulates neurite growth, synaptic plasticity, and neuronal survival and affects glucose and glutamate transport (Mattson et al., 1999b).

The normal precursor is beneficial (and its loss therefore part of the pathology). There are genetic variants of the precursor that are pathologic (Nilsberth et al., 2001) and A β-amyloid protein is cytotoxic (Sopher et al., 1994, 1996), not only in Alzheimer disease but in other diseases, such as Down syndrome (Koudinova et al., 1999), and in other cells, such as melanocytes (Yaar and Gilchrest, 1997; Yaar et al., 1997). This toxicity occurs through several mechanisms, including plasma membrane lipid peroxidation (Joseph, 1992) and other membrane changes (Roth et al., 1995b), impairment of ionmotive ATPases, glutamate uptake, uncoupling of a G protein–linked receptor, impairment of glucose transport, and generation of reactive oxygen species (Mark et al., 1996, 1997; Mattson et al., 1999c). There is evidence (Bence et al., 2001) that the "clumped" form of the protein is taken up by proteosomes, which normally degrade damaged proteins, but the tangled strand then blocks the proteosome, putting it out of commission (Helmuth, 2001). Even a slight degree of down-regulation in amyloid catabolism may play a role in promoting Alzheimer's, and numerous molecular pathways that may play such a role have been explored (Mah et al., 2000; Iwata et al., 2001).

There is a genetic predilection in the 10% of the cases characterized as familial Alzheimer's (Tanzi et al., 1996; Blacker and Tanzi, 1998; Devi et al., 2000), in which three gene abnormalities predominate: the amyloid precursor protein, presenilin 1, and presenilin 2 (Harman, 2000). Expression of the apoE4 allele has been linked to Alzheimer disease (Slooter et al., 1997; Mayeux et al., 1998) and, curiously, the same gene predilection is found in the vascular dementias. Patients who are homozygous for this allele have the highest risk (50% at age 90), heterozygotes have an intermediate risk, while those lacking the allele altogether have a minimal incidence of Alzheimer disease (Henderson et al., 1995). Rate of progression is not strongly correlated with the gene dose (Corder et al., 1995). The lack of full penetrance in the homozygous patient implies that the apoE4 allele is not solely determinant in Alzheimer disease (Zubenko et al., 1996): there are other genetic (Dewj and Singer, 1999; Tang et al., 1998; Devi et al.,

1999), racial (Green et al., 2002), behavioral (Stern et al., 1999; Wilson et al., 2002), toxic (Merchant et al., 1999), physically traumatic, or environmental factors at work (Tang et al., 1996b; Gun et al., 1997; Schofield et al., 1997). ApoE may not be a mere genetic marker, but may play a direct role in the pathology of some forms of Alzheimer's. There is a metabolic link between apoE4 and β-amyloid precursor protein (Kounnas et al., 1995). apoE4 is neurotoxic (Tolar et al., 1999), while apoE2 allele protects against apoptosis induced by the lipid peroxidation product 4-hydroxynonenal (Pedersen et al., 2000). The utility of genetic markers is in flux (Rosenberg, 2002), but they are already in use clinically, with benefits and risks (Tanzi and Blacker, 2000).

Since the mid-1990s (Leveugle et al., 1995; McGeer and McGeer, 1995; Rogers et al., 1996), inflammation in Alzheimer dementia has been brought to center stage (Akiyama et al., 2000a; Halliday et al., 2000) and recent work supports inflammation as being central to the etiology of Alzheimer disease (McGeer and McGeer, 1998b, 1999a; Tan et al., 1999), although with the same caveat regarding the primacy of causation (Eikelenboom et al., 1998). This caveat is undermined by the growing observations on the efficacy of anti-inflammatory compounds in treating or preventing the disease (Broe et al., 2000). Moreover, and despite such caveats, the correlation (with neuronal damage and decreased synapse density) is better for measures of inflammation than it is for β-amyloid deposition or neurofibrillary tangles (Lue et al., 1996), the two classic correlates in Alzheimer pathology. The primary inflammatory cells within the nervous system in general and in Alzheimer disease in particular are the microglial cells (McGeer and McGeer, 1998d; Streit, 2000). Although found predominantly at the periphery of the senile plaques and neurofibrillary tangles (Blain et al., 2000), we do not know if this is because they lead or follow the neuronal damage, although animal studies support the former (Hauss-Wegrzyniak et al., 2002; Jantzen et al., 2002). Curiously, however, inflammation as exemplified by increased microglial expression of interleukins and appears to trigger increased amyloid precursor protein synthesis in astrocytes (Rogers et al., 1999), which suggests that inflammation may be upstream from amyloid deposition in the cascade of Alzheimer pathology.

Microglia are activated by tissue damage, which results in macrophage recruitment and debris clearance (Streit, 1994). Microglia, and to an extent astrocytes (Stege and Bosman, 1999), play an active part in Alzheimer disease (Walker and Beach, 2002) and may be involved in plaque formation (Stoll and Jander, 1999; Streit and Sparks, 1997). But do the microglia cause Alzheimer dementia? Within the central nervous system, damage triggers activation of astrocytes and microglia (Aschner et al., 1999; Streit et al., 1999), and although each may play a central role in the cellular destruction, the core of Alzheimer disease (McGeer and McGeer, 1998c), their roles may not be antagonistic. Perhaps presence of activated glia is merely a reaction (even a beneficial one) to the damage that begins in the neuron (e.g., from advanced glycation end products; Li et al., 1998a) and not in the glial cell. Although either explanation might suffice, data suggest that glia contribute to the pathology (de Vellis, 2002; Walker and Beach, 2002). The same dilemma occurs with regard to HIV dementia (Glass et al., 1995) and central nervous system lesions in simian immunodeficiency virus (Zink et al., 1999a), in which the best correlation with clinical disease and cell damage is not with the presence of viral DNA within the brain but with the presence (and numbers) of macrophages. The recruitment of monocytes, the precursors of macrophages, may be associated with the development of disease (Gartner, 2000), but which is primary, cell destruction or the inflammatory cells?

It remains unclear whether the inflammation is a trigger for the neuronal losses and abnormalities of protein metabolism or whether it is merely a normal, though apparently substantially damaging, response. The possibility remains that the bulk of the damage is attributable to the microglia themselves (Tan et al., 1999), as occurs in other diseases such as multiple sclerosis (Gehrmann et al., 1995; Trapp et al., 1999; Becher et al., 2000). The microglia themselves are an increasing source of inflammatory mediators in older human brains, particularly after exposure to amyloid-β peptide (Lue et al., 2001; Brunden and Frederickson, 2002).

One possible mechanism for microglial damage is suggested by the role of glial cells and particularly astrocytes in clearing glutamate at synapses (Lino et al., 2001; Oliet et al., 2001), whose delayed clearance may play a substantive role in neural damage. Perhaps the pathology is even a ping-pong ball effect in which an underlying neuronal metabolic defect is tolerable until the microglial cells alter (senesce?), triggering inappropriate inflammation, which causes damage, which in turn increases glial activation, etc. In this case, plaque formation may be only a by-product—a marker for but not a cause of pathology (Stege and Bosman, 1999). One function of the microglia (Vekrellis et al., 2000) is degradation of β-amyloid through insulin-degrading enzyme (IDE), a function known to falter in Alzheimer disease (Bertram et al., 2000). This function is, to a degree, shared by the neurons themselves and it remains unclear to what degree this process and other potentially critical and similar microglia functions (Viel et al., 2001) play a causal role in the pathology.

For whatever reasons, the usual reciprocal relationship between neurons and glia is disturbed, contributing to neuronal damage and neurotoxicity (Aschner et al., 1999). Curiously, this same cell lineage—the monocytes—plays a role not only in microglial inflammation in Alzheimer dementia but as foam cells in atherogenesis, and osteoblasts in osteoarthritis. The significance of this is unknown.

Some authors have suggested that, just as free radical damage may play a general role in aging (Harman, 1999), perhaps corresponding to the accumulation of lipofuscin in neurons, so too might free radicals play an equally important role in age-related diseases, such as Alzheimer dementia (Benzi and Moretti, 1995; Lezza et al., 1999; Smith et al., 2000d). This might be attributable not so much to the free radicals themselves as to an age-related metabolic inability to compensate for and respond to such normal free radical production and consequent cellular damage (Perry et al., 2000; Smith et al., 2000b). Circumstantial evidence suggests that free radical damage plays a role (Atwood et al., 1999; Huang et al., 1999a; Castellani et al., 2000), including mitochondrial abnormalities (Smith et al., 2000c), higher than normal oxidized proteins (Smith et al., 1996b; Lyras et al., 1997), and oxidized RNA (Nunomura et al., 1999) and DNA (Mecocci et al., 1994; Lyras et al., 1997). There is a correlational link between free radical damage and β-amyloid deposition (Nunomura et al., 2000) as well as a correlation with the cell cycle (Raina et al., 2000a, 2000b; Zhu et al., 2000b, 2000c). Curiously, there are cell cycle–related proteins (e.g., cyclin-dependent kinases) whose prevalence falls with age but is increased in Alzheimer disease patients compared to that in controls (Zhu et al., 2000d).

Just as aluminum was once believed to play a central role in Alzheimer's disease, many have attempted to resuscitate a similar role for other metal ions, particularly transition metals such as copper or iron (Rottkamp et al., 2000; Smith et al., 2000c). Caloric restriction appears to ameliorate many of the changes (Moore et al., 1995; Forster et al.,

2000), as well as having a protective role for neurons and neural stem cells (Lee et al., 2000b). This effect may be mediated through the corticosteroid stress response (Lee et al., 2000c), although the protection is found in many cell functions (Guo et al., 2000b).

The evidence for lipid peroxidation is less clear (Lovell et al., 1995; Lyras et al., 1997), but growing (Keller and Mattson, 1998). If the overwhelming majority of free radicals derive from faulty mitochondrial respiration, then the putative oxidative cause of Alzheimer's might be mitochondrial damage (Stephenson, 1996; Bonilla et al., 1999; Wallace, 2000), perhaps induced by calcium shifts (Harman, 2000). It is even possible that free radical damage may shorten neuronal telomeres (von Zglinicki et al., 2000a), thereby causing subsequent neuronal changes. Telomeres playing a role or not, there is an increase in mitochondrial DNA (mtDNA) deletions (Lezza et al., 1999) and dysfunction (Mattson et al., 1999c) in neurons from areas of pathology in patients with Alzheimer dementia, lending credence to the role of free radicals (Brewer, 2000; Brewer and Wallimann, 2000). In addition, there is a general association between damaged cytochrome-c oxidase (the key enzyme in mitochondrial respiration) and neurodegeneration (Shapira, 1996) as well as with mtDNA deletions and presbyacusis (Seidman et al., 2000). It has even been suggested that these data fit nicely into the putative role of microglia in releasing free radicals that thereby activate astrocytes and cause the cascade of inflammatory damage in Alzheimer disease (Schubert et al., 1998a, 1998b).

The Role of Cell Senescence

There is no direct evidence that cell senescence plays a role in the causation of Alzheimer dementia. As in the case made for vascular etiologies of Alzheimer disease discussed above, the extant data are consistent with a multiplicity of explanations, while excluding none. Models that use cell senescence as the central player in explaining the pathology of Alzheimer's are consistent, but difficult to support preferentially and difficult to disprove. Although at the other extreme some workers have suggested that cell senescence could not possibly play a role in aging and age-related diseases in the central nervous system (since most neurons are not replaceable by the division of neural precursor cells), this theoretical stance is indefensible and unwarranted.

Inaccuracies require addressing. The criticism that neuronal precursors don't divide in the mature nervous system is factually false but pragmatically true. Although neuronal precursor cells do divide in the adult brain (Cameron and McKay, 1999) and might even have telomerase activity (Prowse, 2002), there is no evidence that neuronal replacement plays enough of a role to cause discernable cell senescence. To the contrary, in vivo measurements of telomeres from adult human donors with ages ranging from 32 to 75 years showed no significant difference ($p = 0.087$) as a function of donor age. This contrasts with a significant ($p = 0.0001$) correlation between telomere length and in vivo aging in mitotically active cells (Allsopp et al., 1995). Neurons (and neuronal precursor stem cells) don't senesce or don't senesce enough to matter. There is, however, some indirect evidence that neurons found in Alzheimer lesions might divide. Many neurons found in regions of Alzheimer disease brain have an increase in a protein related to MORF-4, which may arguably indicate mitotic re-entry (Raina et al., 2001).

Overall, however, the issue of neuronal cell replacement is a straw man and should be disposed of as inadequate for argument against cell senescence in aging nervous systems. No one has argued that neuronal division plays a role in brain aging. No one has ever suggested that neuronal senescence occurs; no one has ever gone on to suggest that neuronal senescence could explain part of aging or central nervous system disease. There have, however, been clearly stated proposals that glial or vascular endothelial cell senescence occurs and can explain aging and age-related neuronal disease (Fossel, 1996). Such models remain unproven but are consistent with existing data and cannot be dismissed absent such falsifying data.

It remains appropriate to clarify a model (neuronal, vascular, glial, or combined) consistent with what we know of aging and central nervous system disease. What is the model and how does it explain the clinical findings? Although (most) adult neurons don't divide, many glial and vascular endothelial cells do. Such cells, whether through inflammatory damage or vascular insufficiency, can logically be tapped as candidates for the primary cause of neuronal pathology. For example, there is correlational evidence that the telomere lengths of circulating monocytes can serve as an independent predictor in at least vascular dementia (von Zglinicki et al., 2000b). mTERT is neuroprotective in the developing murine nervous system and its lack may play a direct role in Alzheimer disease (Fu et al., 2000b; Zhu et al., 2000a). This effect includes specific protection against vulnerability to amyloid-β peptide–induced apoptosis. Curiously, at least in rats, older neurons are more sensitive to the toxic effects of β-amyloid as well as of glutamate and lactic acid (Brewer, 1998), apparently due to an age-related decline in neuroprotective mechanisms (Viel et al., 2001).

One cell senescence model of central nervous system aging might (but need not) rely on vascular aging, another on microglial senescence. Primary endothelial cell aging might reasonably explain atherosclerosis, microinfarct dementia, and chronic ischemic changes within the central nervous system, especially in light of data that demonstrate endothelial senescence in some vascular structures (Chang and Harley, 1995). One could perhaps go further and suggest (as discussed above) that secondary vascular aging underlies Alzheimer dementia. Those who credit a vascular etiology for Alzheimer disease remain distinctly in a minority. Cell senescence could be plugged directly into a theoretical foundation for this vascular rationale. Vascular abnormalities exist in Alzheimer disease and in most age-related neuronal diseases, but to assign cause to correlation is irredeemably naive. Such vascular abnormalities may be merely secondary to the neuronal damage, or vascular and neuronal damage may be secondary to another, yet unspecified, more fundamental process.

Such a more fundamental process could easily involve cell senescence, but in the microglia rather than in endothelial cells. A cell senescence model might explain Alzheimer dementia without primary vascular involvement. Although there is good evidence that glial cells change with age, we must bear in mind two caveats. The first is that the linkage to cell senescence remains merely circumstantial. The second is that there is no evidence that such putative senescence necessarily causes the observed neuronal changes that we wish to explain.

Microglia have been implicated in the inflammation that occurs early in Alzheimer pathology (Lemke et al., 1999), but we have thus far been technically unable to measure glial senescence in vivo, although there are indirect indicators that astrocyte cell division may be accelerated in Alzheimer disease (Schipper et al., 1993). The theory that cell senescence lies at the heart of the pathological cascade of events that results in Alzheimer's is consistent with known data, parallel with what we know of age-related diseases in other tissues, and even elegant but unproven.

Glial cells not only divide but are crucial to neuronal function and indeed to neuronal survival. Glial cells change with age, paralleling their likelihood of accumulated cell divisions and hence of cell senescence. Glial cells mediate normal synaptic remodeling and are involved in the substantial loss of synaptic connections that occurs (Nichols, 1999). Even minor disturbances in the central nervous system homeostasis, particularly neuronal injury, can trigger microglial activation, in which the neuroglial relationship changes dramatically. Activated microglia divide, change in morphology, and alter their cell surface receptor expression and their production of growth factors and cytokines (Streit, 2000). They show a corresponding change in their overall pattern of gene expression (Becher et al., 1996; Matsuo et al., 1996; Williams et al., 1996), becoming central agents in inflammation. That they are players in neuronal damage is no longer arguable, but whether they are the primary cause, simply caught up in the action, or, on balance, a beneficial response team is open to reasoned argument (Stoll et al., 1998). One possibility is that, though initially acting as buffers to neuronal damage, a point comes at which their ability to respond is simply overcome and microglia then "add to neuronal damage by the release of nitric oxide (NO) and by promoting toxic β-amyloid formation" (Schubert et al., 2000).

Secreted or intracellular transcription factors, such as tumor growth factor beta (TGF-β), tumor necrosis factor alpha (TNF-α), activity-dependent neurotrophic factor (ADNF-9), basic fibroblast growth factor (bFGF), transcription factor nuclear factor kappa B (NF-κB), and soluble β-amyloid precursor protein (β-APP) protect neurons against excitotoxic, metabolic, and oxidative insults (Guo and Mattson, 2000b; Mattson et al., 2000a). Microglial senescence, causing or prompted by inflammation, will change gene expression and alter the neuroglial interaction. As these intracellular conditions change, the altered pattern of secretion and altered cellular actions of TGF-β and TNF, coupled with the inappropriate truncation and insolubility of β-amyloid, may lead to neuronal and glial damage, culminating in neurodegenerative disorders (Mattson et al., 1997a).

The incidence of microglia activation correlates with chronologic age, but this does not imply a particular causation. Age-related microglial activation may be merely the secondary result of (increasingly likely) age-related neuronal disease that triggers such activation. It may equally be due to primary intrinsic changes within the glia themselves, such as cell senescence due to cell division and telomere shortening. It is interesting to note that microglial activation is more prominent in patients with known atherosclerosis than in those without disease (Streit and Sparks, 1997).

Other glial cell types, such as astrocytes, activate. Activated astrocytes hypertrophy, surround neurons, and are more likely to express glial fibrillary acidic protein (GFAP). Microglia not only activate but demonstrate increased numbers of specific microglial subsets (e.g., perivascular microglia) likely to be phagocytic and secrete TGF-β1 (Nichols, 1999). Cellular adhesion molecules (selectins, immunoglobulins, and integrins) found on the endothelial cells of brain capillaries change with age, and some of the same changes occur on the adhesion molecules of activated astrocyte and activate microglial cells. Activated microglia secrete low–molecular weight neurotoxins, oxidized lipids, neurotransmitters, and cytokines (Bruce-Keller, 1999; Bacon and Harrison, 2000;

Blain et al., 2000). To a degree, this process parallels that found in multiple sclerosis, in which microglial cells attack neurons (Gilden, 2001), suggesting a parallel to the pathology of Alzheimer dementia (Lee and Benveniste, 1999). A similar involvement of glial cells in the neuronal destruction has been found in AIDS dementia (McArthur et al., 1999; Miller and Meucci, 1999; Zink et al., 1999b).

Alzheimer disease, then, may be a process in which senescing microglial cells become activated and trigger severe inflammatory changes, culminating in neuronal destruction. This model is based largely on the microglial-inflammation work of the McGeers (McGeer and McGeer, 1999a). Microglia attack the plaques and neurofibrillary tangles, but go on to secrete toxins that not only destroy their intended targets—damaged neurons—but healthy cells. The result is a "feed forward" phenomenon, a vicious cycle that irreversibly damages neural tissue (Jones, 2000) and propagates further cell destruction. Theoretically, microglial cell senescence underlies the microglial activation that causes Alzheimer disease. Microglial senescence results from cell division and is probably driven by multiple, unknown factors, including viral infection, toxic damage, genetic predisposition, endocrine changes, and vascular aging. Glial cells divide, senesce, and alter their gene expression into a pattern with profound neuropathological results and severe clinical morbidity.

The activated microglia and astrocytes increasingly synthesize and secrete complement proteins, complement inhibitors, eicosanoids, cytokines (Marx and Blasko, 1999; Luterman et al., 2000), acute-phase reactants, proteases, protease inhibitors (McGeer and McGeer, 1998b), free radicals, nitric oxide, and arachidonic acid derivatives (Fawcett and Asher, 1999). Many components are not only typically found in the cerebral amyloid plaques in Alzheimer dementia but have been suggested as triggers for further β-amyloid synthesis, again initiating further pathology. Equally, microglial cells have been shown to degrade β-amyloid protein (Qiu et al., 1998). Microglial senescence may simply result in the passive accumulation of β-amyloid, without regard for direct microglial inflammatory damage (Marx and Blasko, 1999), for example, by down-regulation of neprilysin (Iwata et al., 2001), which plays a prominent role in amyloid catabolism or effects on the proteosome (Bence et al., 2001). If the degradation is impaired in the putatively senescent glial cells of patients with Alzheimer dementia, this alone might account for the increased susceptibility of older neurons (Brewer, 1998) and, indeed, the human clinical pathology. In short, there are multiple hypotheses—each consistent with what little we know of the pathology—that might account for Alzheimer disease as the outcome of microglial cell senescence. We may rule many out with good data, we cannot rule them out with poor theory.

A curious parallel to Alzheimer disease is seen in Down syndrome (Takashima, 1997; Soliman and Hawkins, 1998a, 1998b; Petronis, 1999). The two diseases share many of the same pathologic features (de la Monte, 1999; Sawa, 1999; van Leeuwen and Hol, 1999), though there are clear differences (Fonseca et al., 1999; Nagy, 1999). From the standpoint of cell senescence, the similarities are remarkable because patients with Down syndrome have accelerated immune senescence (Cuadrado and Barrena, 1996) particularly in lymphocytes, potentially the same cell lineage as microglia. Embryonic development of microglia from patients with Down syndrome is aberrant and microglia show atypical proliferation compared to astrocytes (Wierzba-Bobrowicz et al., 1999). This may explain the correlation between telomere shortening and Alzheimer's status in aging humans (Panossian et al., 2003).

The case for Alzheimer disease as the result of senescing cells is conceptually effortless and a good fit for the pathology; the case for Parkinson disease is a less elegant match. The pathology is not only more anatomically discrete (e.g., neurons of the substantia nigra) but perhaps more discrete in cellular location. The pathology is apparently the result of intracellular processes, although local gliosis does occur. The early-onset form is probably an autosomal mutation; later forms may be due to multiple genetic factors (Martin et al., 2001; Scott et al., 2001; Spillantini and Goedert, 2001). In any case, mutation of the genes for parkin, α-synuclein, or ubiquitin carboxyl-terminal hydrolase result in accumulation of protein inclusions containing α-synuclein and ubiquitin, probably through a common pathway of impaired clearance of glycosylated α-synuclein (Shimura et al., 2001). Cell senescence is not incongruous to this pathology, but Occam's razor might suggest we wait for further evidence of glial involvement before invoking it as an explanation for Parkinson disease.

Cell senescence offers a conceptually broad, clinically enticing, and logically consistent explanation for Alzheimer disease and central nervous system aging. Whether it is true remains unproven. The synopsis of the model is simple. As in other organ systems, multiple factors (e.g., toxins, trauma, infectious agents, genetic risk factors) induce accelerated cell division in a critical cell line, in this case the microglia. As a result, the microglia undergo cell senescence with consequent changes in their pattern of gene expression. This induces direct microglial and indirect neuronal dysfunction that result in neuropathology. The direct changes involve microglial activation with changes in the pattern of neurotrophic secretion, amyloid processing, and inflammation. The indirect changes involve neuronal dysfunction in amyloid processing and an increased likelihood of neuronal apoptosis. These processes result in neuronal destruction, amyloid deposition, and other hallmarks of Alzheimer disease, correlating with clinical outcome.

Intervention

Chief among our fears of aging is the fear of losing ourselves. Our fear of ending our lives with a "brain of feathers and a heart of lead" (Alexander Pope, from Beck, 1968, p 413), has prompted a wide search for therapies, often based more on hope than on knowledge. Not only are the human costs high, but increasingly we have come to realize that there are social and financial costs to Alzheimer dementia (Fillit and Cummings, 2000; Taylor and Sloan, 2000). After neuronal death (as opposed to transient ischemia, inflammatory reactions, and swelling), and despite often impressive behavioral "rewiring," neurologic damage is characterized by its finality. Although we have so far had almost no impact on the course of the disease (Cummings and Cole, 2002) and cannot expect to undo the damage that has already occurred in the brain of a patient with Alzheimer dementia, we can expect to prevent such damage (Mattson, 2000a), particularly by targeting our interventions toward those who are at highest risk, based on genetic and other risk factors (Post, 1999). As might be expected, the usual interventions that affect aging may affect the onset of age-related diseases in the brain. Caloric restriction, for example, is neuroprotective, at least in rats (Bruce-Keller et al., 1999; Guo et al., 2000b; Lee et al., 2000b) and mice (Zhu et al., 1999a). Caloric restriction may be prudent for humans (Mattson, 2000b). Drugs that mimic caloric restriction may likewise have potential clinical value (Mattson, 2000c).

One recurrent and controversial contender for prophylactic (or even therapeutic) intervention for Alzheimer dementia has been estrogen therapy (Fillit et al., 1986; Henderson et al., 1994; Friedrich, 2002b). The original observation was perhaps based on the unremarkable fact that women didn't tend to get Alzheimer disease until after menopause. This was more a prosaic marker of getting old than a cause of age-related disease, but other data supported the possibility that estrogen was no mere correlational bystander in the pathology of dementia. For one thing, women are two to three times as likely to get Alzheimer disease as men (Brinton, 1999). More to the point, women who undergo surgical menopause were likely to demonstrate cognitive dysfunction and this dysfunction responded to estrogen replacement (Henderson et al., 1996b). In twin studies, those who had had a hysterectomy tended to develop Alzheimer disease earlier than did the twin who had not had a hysterectomy (Nee et al., 1999). Intriguingly, the common neuroanatomic sites of Alzheimer pathology matched the sites of estrogen receptors within the brain (Maruyama et al., 2000). There is no significant evidence, however, that a longer reproductive period and later occurrence of natural menopause is protective against Alzheimer dementia (Geerlings et al., 2001).

Assuming (as literature suggests) that estrogen does have a prophylactic (if perhaps not therapeutic) role in Alzheimer disease (Zandi et al., 2002), and despite what we know of estrogen and estrogen receptors (Cyr et al., 2000), its putative mechanism and optimal use (Resnick and Henderson, 2002) are unclear. It has been variously suggested that estrogen is a neuronal growth factor for specific estrogen-responsive neurons, has protective effects on cerebral vasculature, or slows free radical production (Fillit, 1995). It has shown interactional effects with gender (or at least estrogen levels), β-amyloid, and apolipoprotein E (Henderson, 1997; Stone et al., 1997; Bretsky et al., 1999). It may offer protection against the altered glucocorticoid response in aging hippocampal neurons (Sapolsky, 1992; Kudielka et al., 1999; Lupien et al., 1999). Most intriguing, in light of the likely role of microglia in Alzheimer disease, are data confirming the potent effects of estrogens upon cell activation (Bruce-Keller et al., 2000) and their pattern of gene expression (Mor et al., 1999).

Estrogen has a neurotrophic and neuroprotective role (Wise et al., 1999), although it can equally induce apoptosis (Nilsen et al., 2000). Estradiol, for example, has a protective effect in cerebral ischemia (Dubal et al., 1998), apparently decreasing cell death by preventing ischemia-induced down-regulation of *Bcl-2*, a proto-oncogene known to promote cell survival in many tissues (Dubal et al., 1999). In trophic effects, estrogen appears to maintain dendritic spines, help synapse formation, increase the secretion and metabolism of amyloid precursor protein, and protect neurons from toxins (Maruyama et al., 2000). It prevents cognitive and memory losses (perhaps through NGF-responsive cholinergic neurons in the basal forebrain), but the specific role of estrogen in Alzheimer disease is less clear (Thakur, 1999), unless it is mediated via the microglia (Mor et al., 1999).

Initial clinical work suggested that estrogen might be used prophylactically and large-scale studies supported these initial findings (Paganini-Hill and Henderson, 1996; Tang et al., 1996a). Estrogen supplementation even appeared to have some clinical benefits after onset of Alzheimer symptoms (Fillit, 1995; Schneider et al., 1996). This observation suggested that, while the processes underlying Alzheimer disease might be genetic, its disease expression and therefore its therapy might be endocrinological. Recent data have been more equivocal (Mulnard et al., 2000; Zandi et al., 2002); in some cases this may be due to differing patient groups, lack of standardized testing protocols (Doraiswamy et al., 1997), differences in the dose, route, or particular estrogen chosen (Palacios et al., 2000), or other methodological limitations (LeBlanc et al., 2001; Resnick and Henderson, 2002). However, women using estrogen demonstrate increased central atrophy (as measured by an increase in ventricular size seen on MRI) as compared to nonusers (Luoto et al., 2000), paralleling findings in rats (Marriott et al., 2002). The human data might be attributable to vascular disease, rather than pathology due to Alzheimer's, and may additionally represent a selection bias in those who chose to use estrogen for protection in the face of early clinical symptoms, thus biasing the result.

Overall, measures of specific cognitive skills show some improvement in Alzheimer patients who are given supplemental estrogen (Henderson et al., 1996b) and estrogen appears to improve the response to other Alzheimer therapy, such as tacrine (Schneider et al., 1996), perhaps by boosting serum levels (Laine et al., 1999). A placebo-controlled, double-blind pilot study of transdermal estrogen patches (Asthana et al., 1999) found initial improvement in cognitive scores among the treatment (and not the control) group and these benefits diminished when estrogen was withdrawn. Enhancement in verbal memory correlated with plasma estradiol. Subsequent double-blind clinical trials, however, found no short-term benefits from estrogen supplementation for the symptoms of Alzheimer disease (Henderson, 1997; Henderson et al., 2000a) or disease slowing over a 1-year period (Mulnard et al., 2000). Even if confirmed, however, on the one hand these results do not rule out longer-term, higher-dose, or prophylactic effects of such supplementation. On the other hand, such recent double-blind, randomized, placebo-controlled designs do not offer support for estrogen as a therapy.

Generally, Alzheimer disease is a "Humpty Dumpty phenomenon" (Fossel, 1996) in which the impressive complexity of the nervous system is irremediably abrogated and cannot be resurrected by, even theoretical, intervention. Even if this (realistic or pessimistic) evaluation is correct, it does not restrict optimism. There remain the issue of prophylactic therapy and therapies that might effectively slow or stop disease once diagnosed. In short, the probable inability to *reverse* the existing damage of Alzheimer disease does not prevent us from *stopping* further damage.

Studies support the notion that estrogen replacement is effective in stopping progress of Alzheimer disease. Estrogen appears to protect against memory decline and cognitive loss in nondemented women (Resnick et al., 1997). This finding is not only confirmed by neuropsychological tests of figural and verbal memory but by matching findings in the activation of specific brain regions as measured by PET activation (Resnick et al., 1998). These clear effects of estrogen on the altered blood flow in aging patients recall our earlier question of a possible vascular role in Alzheimer disease, but do not allow us an easy answer. Although studies support the efficacy of estrogen supplementation in reducing the prevalence, degree, or progress of Alzheimer disease, they beg the issue of relative risk (Baldereschi et al., 1999). Estrogen is effective because it does have dramatic and widespread effects on gene expression and cell function. Its potency is part of its danger. To the extent that there is consensus that it may decrease the risk of Alzheimer disease and atherosclerosis, there is an equal consensus that it may increase the risk of cancer, particularly ovarian (Rodriguez et al., 2001) and breast (Chen et al., 2002a) cancer.

Although estrogen has been in the therapeutic limelight, there are other interesting therapeutic approaches. These include acetylcholinesterase (or butyrylcholinesterase) inhibitors (Nordberg and Svensson, 1998; Krall et al., 1999), including donepezil, rivastigmine, selegiline, metrifonate, physostigmine, eptastigmine, huperzine (Cheng et al., 1996), tacrine, and galantamine (Medical Letter, 2001b). Many agents, such as galantamine (Rockwood et al., 2001), have shown positive but unremarkable results (e.g., Tariot et al., 2001). This reflects two severe theoretical limitations. Cholinesterase inhibitors and similar interventions attempt to increase the generic effects of the remaining relevant neurotransmitters without regard to fine signaling effects, i.e., they raise the volume of the neural signal without regard for the information content. The second limitation is that such approaches do nothing for the continuing damage, but constitute, at best, a tragic and ineffective holding action, having only modest benefits (Trinh et al., 2003) and not altering progression of the disease (Medical Letter, 2000c; Sramek et al., 2001). Closing the barn door after the horse is gone is the less preferable therapeutic intervention than prevention or intervention in fundamental causes. A compilation of objective reviews (Warner and Butler, 2000) of the efficacy of drugs for Alzheimer dementia suggests that some drugs are effective (donepezil, rivastigmine, and selegiline), while others probably are not (tacrine). Ginkgo biloba has not lived up to early claims that it enhanced memory (Solomon et al., 2002). Melatonin has attracted attention (Pappolla et al., 1998a, 1998b) as a result of early clinical reports (Brusco et al., 1998).

Far more promising is the work with anti-inflammatory agents (Broe et al., 2000), in line with the suggestion that inflammation (Nilsson et al., 1998; Antel and Owens, 1999), particularly microglial activation, underlies the progressive neuronal damage (McGeer and McGeer, 1999b; Halliday et al., 2000). Certain nonsteroidal, specifically anti-inflammatory, agents have shown some degree of efficacy, such as dapsone, ibuprofen, indomethacin, naproxen, and rofecoxib (and other cyclooxygenase-2 [COX-2] inhibitors), perhaps through the COX-2 system known to play a role in the microglial immune response (Aloisi et al., 2000b). Dapsone has been used previously in treating leprosy. Curiously, leprosy patients treated with such drugs had half the incidence of Alzheimer disease of normal patients (McGeer and McGeer, 1999a; Jones, 2000). Initial work with HMG-CoA reductase inhibitors (statins) suggests that these agents may work to reduce the risk of Alzheimer's disease (Jick et al., 2000; Wolozin et al., 2000), probably by modulating immune function (Kwak et al., 2000).

The hypothesis is supported by several studies, although most are relatively small. Indomethacin appears to halt the progressive memory loss seen in Alzheimer's (McGeer and McGeer, 1999a) and at least 20 epidemiological studies suggest that anti-inflammatory drugs may have beneficial effects on the clinical course of Alzheimer disease (McGeer and McGeer, 1998b). Some studies have suggested that aspirin and other drugs that selectively inhibit only the COX-1 arm of the inflammatory process offer little clinical protection despite the association of COX-1 expression with the pathology of Alzheimer disease (Yermakova et al., 1999). Other work, however, suggests that anti-inflammatory medications, including aspirin, offer at least some generic protection even at low doses (Broe et al., 2000).

Cyclooxygenase is expressed in the brain as COX-1 (the constitutive form) and COX-2 (the inducible form), and although there are differences between cells, it remains unclear which cell types express which form (Walker and Beach, 2002). COX-1 inhibitors may interfere with only a portion of the inflammation caused (but not expressed) by microglia and clinical data show them to be ineffective in reducing the formation of senile plaque and neurofibrillary tangles (Blain et al., 2000). There is, however, a reduced risk of Alzheimer disease in patients taking nonsteroidal anti-inflammatory drugs (NSAIDs), which inhibit COX-1 and COX-2 (Blain et al., 2000; Broe et al., 2000). Since COX-2 appears to be the more effective intervention and since the side effects of COX-1 drugs are less acceptable (particularly gastrointestinal bleeding), studies have narrowed in on the newer selective COX-2 inhibiting agents, such as rofecoxib (Vioxx) and celecoxib (Celebrex). This is consistent with the pathology: COX-2 expression is up-regulated within the hippocampus and cortex in Alzheimer disease (Lipsky, 1999) and in the immune response of microglial cells (Aloisi et al., 2000b), and is preferentially expressed in the brain compared to the COX-1 isoform (Medical Letter, 2000a).

The complexity of the immune damage may be a blessing in disguise, as it suggests multiple points of therapeutic intervention, such as the complement system (Webster et al., 1997; McGeer and McGeer, 1998a), microglial activation, cytokine function (Venters et al., 1999), and other components of the inflammatory process in the brain (Nilsson et al., 1998; McGeer and McGeer, 1999a; Akiyama et al., 2000a). Indeed, the complexity of the entire pathology, while daunting, is equally inviting therapeutically. There are a plethora of specific molecular targets including prostate apoptosis response-4 (Par-4; Mattson et al., 1999a) and caspases ("bad guys") and dozens of neurotrophic factors and stress proteins ("good guys") that might provide therapeutic leverage (Mattson et al., 1999c). There is even a separate literature on viral (Dobson and Itzhaki, 1999) or chlamydial infections (Balin et al., 1998) that have periodically been presumed to increase the risk of Alzheimer disease; antibiotics have therefore been suggested as having a direct effect on the cascade of pathology (Howlett et al., 1999) or indirect effects by preventing such infections. Infectious agents may play a role, but data are meager (Renvoize et al., 1987; Nochlin et al., 1999; Gieffers et al., 2000).

To date, however, the attempts to use such trophic factors have been less than promising. Although cortical insulin-like growth factor declines by more than a third with age (Niblock et al., 1998) and is correlated with declines in cortical vascular density (Sonntag et al., 1997), the use of IGF-1 therapeutically in rodents has no effect on loss of sensorimotor function (not Alzheimer disease) that occurs (Markowska et al., 1998).

Other non-estrogen steroids, specifically glucocorticoids, have been considered therapeutic candidates, as they play a role in inflammation and have been used for decades as potent anti-inflammatory agents. They regulate the interactions between glia and neurons and have profound effects on glial gene expression (Tanaka et al., 1997), including GFAP, TGF-β1 (Nichols, 1999), prostaglandins, and nitric oxide (Minghetti et al., 1999). Unfortunately, long-term clinical use of glucocorticoids has overwhelming side effects and increasing morbidity and mortality. If anything, circulating glucocorticoids contribute to, rather than lowering the risk of, the early onset of Alzheimer's disease (Lupien et al., 1999), perhaps especially in the face of estrogen decline (Kudielka et al., 1999). This field has been reviewed extensively and thoroughly by Sapolsky (1992), whose thesis contradicts suggestions that glucocorticoids might be used therapeutically in this venue. On the basis of numerous lines of argument and independent bodies of data, he suggests that the lifetime integral exposure to glucocorticoids may be a cause of age-related neuronal loss (Sapolsky, 1999). Suggestions that glucocorticoids might have a beneficial role are likely naive and at odds with Sapolsky's clear formulation. At least in rats, lower corticosteroids may restore adult production of hippocampal granule neurons, a finding suggesting that the memory problems associated with high corticosteroids result from impaired granule cell replication in the dentate gyrus (Cameron and McKay, 1999).

A different approach altogether has come from the observation that heparin appears to play a role in truncation of the β-amyloid precursor protein (Leveugle et al., 1997). Low–molecular weight heparin has therefore been suggested as a potential therapeutic agent (Leveugle et al., 1998). Similarly, there has been extensive interest in using dietary antioxidants, specifically and especially tocopherols, to delay or prevent Alzheimer dementia (Pitchumoni and Doraiswamy, 1998; Morris et al., 2002c). Although some data implicate a protective effect of antioxidants on some age-related brain changes (den Heijer et al., 2001) and specifically for Alzheimer disease (Engelhart et al., 2002; Morris et al., 2002b), the effects of higher antioxidant levels are not overwhelming clinically (Mendoza-Nunez et al., 1999; Foley and White, 2002) or even in terms of lipid peroxidation levels (Meagher et al., 2001). Our knowledge regarding antioxidant efficacy is minimal. With use of tocopherols at least, side effects are also minimal. While many recommend against tocopherol supplementation (Fitzgerald and Meagher, 2001), clinical recommendation based on judicious assessment of the relative risks, benefits, and efficacy is open to argument.

Cell senescence therapy, while perhaps theoretically offering clinical benefits in preventing Alzheimer disease (Fu et al., 2000b; Mattson, 2000a; Zhu et al., 2000a), remains an unlikely therapy, given our current methods of delivery. Telomerase transfection is feasible in vitro, but Alzheimer disease is a clear example of a complex, interactional, and in vivo disease. In Parkinson disease, where the pathology is slightly more selective anatomically and biochemically than in Alzheimer disease, initial trials of lentiviral vectors to deliver neurotrophic factor to rhesus monkeys suffering from a Parkinson-like disease are promising (Kordower et al., 2000). For the same reasons of relative selectivity, grafting of fetal tissue (Brundin et al., 2000; Friedrich, 2002a) or neuronal stem cells (Kempermann et al., 1998) has more to offer to the Parkinson than to the Alzheimer's patient.

Although it would be interesting to transfect donor microglia from elderly patients in vitro, measuring alterations of gene expression with specific attention to inflammatory patterns, such clinical material (live glial cells from healthy elderly patients who die suddenly or who donate pathology specimens from neurosurgical procedures) is rare. In vivo transfection technology is in its most juvenile phases, no matter what the organ. The brain, enclosed in its bony skull, offers no current practical approach to transfection for the estimated 100 billion cells of the brain at risk in the elderly patient. The only cell senescence approach that might profitably be attempted would be to use a telomerase inducer. None are available.

Nonetheless, there are grounds to suspect that telomerase therapy might have beneficial effects. Given the apparent role of telomerase in protecting against amyloid-β peptide neurotoxicity (Fu et al., 2000b; Zhu et al., 2000a) and the correlation between T-cell telomere length and Alzheimer status (Panossian et al., 2003), there is a clear reason to try such delivery. On theoretical grounds, we might equally posit a beneficial but more indirect effect on microglia, preventing cell senescence and effecting a useful clinical pattern of gene expression. On experimental grounds, we might point out that the apoptosis that occurs in Alzheimer disease might respond handily to telomerization. Elevated telomerase protects pheochromocytoma cells against apoptosis and mitochondrial dysfunction (Fu et al., 1999, 2000b), which may play a role in the etiology of Alzheimer disease (Mattson et al., 1999c).

Therapeutic intervention in Alzheimer disease is at that curious point where there is little to offer but profound and realistic anticipation that new and effective agents will soon be forthcoming. There are promising avenues that deserve clinical trials. Animal (Cummings et al., 1996), or better, experimental animal models of Alzheimer disease (Fisher et al., 1991; Wirak et al., 1991; Tanzi, 1995; Pedersen et al., 1999) and microglial screens for anti-inflammatories (Lombardi et al., 1998) will accelerate understanding and effective testing. Transgenic models may allow better understanding of genetic causes (Price et al., 1998; Guenette and Tanzi, 1999; Gotz et al., 2001; Lewis et al., 2001). Our understanding of secretases and proteases that control amyloid precursor protein offers several potential therapeutic targets (Esler and Wolfe, 2001). Putative vaccines show promise, although ultimate clinical utility is uncertain (Helmuth, 2000). Although we may never have much to offer those who have already suffered the ravages of Alzheimer dementia (Rapoport, 1999), we are likely to have effective prophylactic agents that can retard or prevent the progression of the disease. These agents will have not only medical and even financial benefits (Fillit et al., 1999a, 1999b; Gutterman et al., 1999) but also immeasurable human benefits.

CHAPTER 14

Kidneys

Structure and Overview

The primary function of the kidney is, simplistically, filtration of blood and maintenance of serum electrolyte homeostasis (sodium, potassium, chloride, magnesium, etc). An accurate but insufficient appraisal, the kidneys are also instrumental in modulating blood pressure (via renin secretion and its effects on the renin–angiotensin system), signaling the marrow to increase erythrocyte production (via erythropoetin secretion), activating vitamin D (with consequent effects on calcium and phosphorus metabolism), and filtration of molecules other than the standard electrolytes, such as creatinine, metabolic wastes, endogenous and exogenous toxins, and excess serum glucose.

To grasp the essential importance of renal function, consider the clinical consequences of renal failure. Acutely (within hours to days), the patient suffers from the retention of water (with secondary congestive heart failure, respiratory failure, and general body edema), potassium (with acute secondary risk of fatal cardiac events), and metabolic waste products (urea, creatinine, etc). In chronic renal failure (within weeks to months), even with regular hemodialysis, the red cell count (hematocrit) falls and patients can become critically anemic, although usually the body establishes a new baseline about half to two-thirds of the normal cell count. Risk of infection climbs and patients becomes chronically fatigued, often despite otherwise adequate dialysis.

The kidneys consist of a pair of symmetric organs, each with an arterial supply, a venous drainage system, and a central collecting system that joins in a funnel-shaped "pelvis" that becomes the ureter, draining urine to the bladder. Functionally, the kidney is composed of millions of nephrons, a unit that includes a glomerulus, its associated tubules, and a complex vascular investment. Blood enters the kidney, distributes into smaller arterioles, and enters small vascular tufts (the glomeruli) in which fluid is forced into the collecting tubules, while cells and most proteins are retained. Approximately 20% of fluid volume is removed from the blood entering each glomerulus. This fluid is an ultrafiltrate of plasma, including phosphates, creatinine, uric acid, urea, and some albumin, though seldom larger protein molecules. The filtrate is then passed down and back up a set of parallel tubules that form a counterexchange mechanism that permits reacquisition of most of the fluid (slightly more than 99%, in the normal young kidney) and necessary plasma components, while leaving waste products and excess molecules in the final collected urine. Appropriately, the composition of the urine, and the definition of "excess," depends on the current needs of the body, for it is the actively fluctuating nature of urine composition that permits responsive homeostatic maintenance of molecular concentrations within the blood. Reabsorbed molecules commonly include amino acids, proteins, ascorbic acid, and others that the body can, as a general rule, ill afford to lose and replace. The resultant urine reflects moment-to-moment changes within the blood and integrated physiological needs of the body.

The renal parenchyma comprises a few major cell types, each of which has been subdivided into more specific cell subtypes. The majority of cells are derivatives of vascular endothelial cells or the visceral epithelial cells that form the urinary collecting system. This generalization hides a high degree of specialization, but only a modicum is pertinent to our discussion of age-related changes in the kidney and its function. For example, within the glomeruli, the epithelial cells that line the collecting portion and are in close contact with the vascular epithelial cells have been transmogrified into "podocytes" (Pavenstadt, 2000). These cells resemble cellular octopuses. They have multiple branching and rebranching arms that tangle themselves among similar arms from other podocytes and form (the aquatic analogy fails us) contractile foot processes separated only by tiny (about 250 Å wide) filtration slits. Blood entering the glomerulus flows through successively finer filters: first the endothelial fenestrations and even smaller pores that lie between the vascular endothelial cells, then a charge-selective (Pavenstadt, 1998) basement membrane (the lamina interposed between endothelial cells and podocytes) and, smallest of all, the filtration slits maintained between the smallest podocyte processes (Endlich et al., 2001).

In the context of mechanisms of renal aging, it is critical to recognize that this tissue is dynamic (Bloom and Fawcett, 1975). Renal tissue is in flux, continually turned over, responding to the changing ability of constituent cells to produce and secrete membrane proteins, form processes, and replace lost cells. Basement membrane, for example, is continually renewed in young kidneys. Entrapped particles and molecules (usually those over 100,000 molecular weight) do not long remain within the proteinaceous structure, where collection might potentially impede further filtration or result in dysfunction. This thin (0.1–0.15 μm) membrane is made up of protein filaments within a glycoprotein matrix and is the only continuous layer between the vascular and urinary compartments of the nephron. Several proteins play a role in maintaining the slit diaphragm (Tryggvason and Wartiovaara, 2001) including nephrin, the primary functional protein component in filtration slits (Khoshnoodi and Tryggvason, 2001). Collagen fibers of the membrane are in a macromolecular (rather than fibril) form, perhaps due to its filtration (rather than purely tensile) function.

Synthetically active, podocytes not only produce and maintain the basement membrane (Pavenstadt, 1998) but produce trophic factors, for example vascular endothelial growth factor (VEGF), which modulates endothelial cell growth (Williams, 1998). Just as the podocytes may create the basilar membrane, the mesangial cells may function by removing older, deeper portions of this membrane. Whether the balance between these cells alters in aging or certain diseases is unknown, although podocyte dysfunction has been implicated in some forms of diabetes (Phillips et al., 1999). It is impossible to avoid the conjecture of the potential but unsubstantiated analogy to the loss of balance between osteoblasts and osteoclasts in aging bone. Whatever the (probably multiple) mechanisms, the basal membrane (rather than grosser histological aspects of the glomerulus) is critical in normal renal function and in explaining the loss of filtration that occurs in the aging kidney.

Renal function is most commonly assessed as the glomerular filtration rate (GFR), a measure that shares the dual benefits of clinical practicality and relative validity in assessing overall renal function. As with any clinically useful assessment of physiological function, it integrates the function of several interacting mechanisms. Thus, the glomerular filtration rate integrates renal blood flow, number of functional nephrons, integrity of the glomerular basement membrane, and efficacy of the counter-current mechanism.

Glomerular filtration rate is often estimated using the Cockcroft and Gault (1976) formula:

$$\text{GFR (ml/min)} = \frac{[(140 - \text{age}) \times \text{lean body mass in kg}][\times (0.85 \text{ in females})]}{72 \times \text{serum creatinine in mg/dl}}$$

Alternatively, one of the three more accurate Levey formulas can be employed depending on what additional laboratory data are available:

$$\text{GFR} = 186 \times \text{Cr}^{-1.154} \times \text{age}^{-0.203} [\times 1.212 \text{ if of African ancestry}][\times 0.742 \text{ if female}]$$

or:

$$\text{GFR} = 170 \times \text{Cr}^{-0.999} \times \text{age}^{-0.176} [\times 1.18 \text{ if of African ancestry}][\times 0.762 \text{ if female}] \times \text{BUN}^{-0.017} \times \text{Alb}^{0.318}$$

or:

$$\text{GFR} = 270 \times \text{Cr}^{-1.007} \times \text{age}^{-0.18} [\times 1.178 \text{ if of African ancestry}][\times 0.755 \text{ if female}] \times \text{BUN}^{-0.169}$$

Note that in all cases, the filtration rate is a negative function of age, whether arithmetically (in the first formula) or exponentially (in the other three formulae), an assumption based on population means but is inaccurate as applied to individuals. As with so many age-related measures, aging is correlated less with a decrease in the glomerular filtration rate than with an increase in its variance. While the mean filtration rate falls, the variance rises even more. Not only does the variance increase markedly with age, but in some individuals there is no detectable decrease in renal clearance with age (Lindeman et al., 1985; Timiras, 1994a).

Aging and Other Pathology

Renal anatomic and functional losses have been documented for decades. Anatomically, there is a progressive loss of nephrons and arterial flow (Moore, 1958; Hollenberg et al., 1974). The efficacy of filtration declines, often simply ascribed to "the widespread loss of glomeruli" (Arking, 1998), although it is more complex, involving functional changes within glomeruli (especially the basement membrane) and loops, as well as changes in vascular supply and response (Ungar et al., 2000). The kidney becomes progressively less efficient in filtering the blood (Fig. 14–1), with a mean decline of about 1% per year in its glomerular filtration rate beginning roughly in the fourth decade (Davies and Shock, 1950; Rowe et al., 1976). Serum creatinine levels, responding to a decreasing filtration rate, loss of muscle mass (sarcopenia), and reduced creatinine production (Walser, 1987), change less than might be expected.

No matter how it is assessed, mean renal function declines with age (Rainfray et al., 2000). Although the change in filtration is predictable, the mechanisms underlying this failure are complex (Martins et al., 2001a) and, to an extent, unknown. As mentioned previously, aging changes observed in serum and urine are reflected less in mean values than variance of those values. For example, although hyponatremia and hypokalemia are more common in the elderly, these are closely followed by hypernatremia and hyperkalemia (Adetola et al., 1999; Kugler and Hustead, 2000). It is not so much that electrolyte levels increase or decrease as that they become more labile. As aging occurs, kidney function becomes more variable and less stable. It is less capable of responding to stress and more likely to incur side effects of the usage of drugs such as common loop diuretics (e.g., furosemide), nonsteroidal anti-inflammatory agents (e.g., ibuprofen), and numerous other common clinical agents.

Overall, the increasing lability of renal function results from the loss of compensatory function, stemming from the conjoined decreases in the renal arterial supply, decreasing numbers of several phenotypes of renal cells, and decline in renal cell function, along with the multiplicity of interactive changes throughout the rest of the body that affect renal function, such as blood pressure changes, hypoxia, malnutrition, sarcopenia, and more frequent immune stress. The outcome of this increase in lability is the kidney's inability to respond appropriately to additional metabolic need induced by physical activity, infection, drugs, cardiovascular changes, or a host of changes in demand for renal function. While the young kidney rapidly adjusts to dehydration or water load, the response of the elderly kidney is slow and incomplete (Phillips et al., 1984). The usual clinical approach to renal aging is, therefore, to minimize renal stress by maintaining hydration, optimizing nutrition, minimizing drug use, and monitoring renal function (Martins et al., 2001a).

A number of age-related clinical problems can be ascribed, at least interactively if not solely, to aging renal function. These include hypertension (via the amount of renin secretion, the inappropriate course of the renin response to hemodynamic stimuli, the loss of adequate filtration and resorption capability), renal osteodystrophy (via failure to adequately activate vitamin D), anemia (via inadequate erythropoetin secretion), pro-

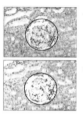

Young kidney
  more nephrons
  better vascularization

Old kidney
  less responsive
  poorer filtration

Figure 14–1 Aging renal tissue. Renal aging is notable for a loss of vascular tissue and simplification of the nephron (circled area). The clinical outcome is both an impaired baseline filtration rate and an impaired response to any alteration in physiological conditions (e.g., changes in arterial pressure, fluid shifts, or electrolyte losses). While renal function may suffice under normal conditions, physiologic stress may expose cryptic, age-related losses in function.

teinuria and nephrotic syndrome (via inadequate protein filtration in the glomerulus), and frank renal failure. The latter is almost always the result of a chronic disease (most commonly diabetes, hypertension, or polycystic kidneys) or a severe acute renal disease (most commonly infectious or autoimmune in origin). In many diseases (Mundel and Shankland, 1999; Pavenstadt, 2000), such as nephrotic syndrome (Smoyer and Mundel, 1998; Deschenes and Martinat, 2000), glomerulonephritis (Schwartz, 2000), glomerulosclerosis (Kriz et al., 1998, 1999; Kriz and Lemley, 1999), and perhaps in aging (Abrass, 2000), the fault is expressed at the level of the podocyte and basement membrane, where filtration fails and results in symptomatic disease. Independent of disease, however, renal aging appears largely a consequence of a loss of cells or a decrement in cell function. The underlying cause of such cell changes, however, remains seldom considered and rarely addressed.

The Role of Cell Senescence

The aging human kidney shows a progressive loss of volume and, specifically, a loss of nephrons (Timiras, 1994a). Not only is there a wholesale loss of cells, but within those cells that remain there are functional changes that have greater implications for the gradual loss of function in the aging kidney. There may be fewer cells in the glomeruli and renal tubules, and those cells are dysfunctional. This is, a fortiori, true of the functional changes in the podocytes and basement membrane of the renal glomeruli. Podocytes may be missing and intact podocytes may be swollen or have a loss of complexity and numbers of processes. Even in apparently intact glomeruli, there is a progressive thickening of the basement membrane. These changes may be attributable to senescing podocytes and endothelial cells.

Unfortunately, there are few data that speak directly to this attribution. There are no published data on podocyte senescence. While vascular endothelial cells show senescence in other organs, there are no published data showing that endothelial cells within the renal vasculature senesce. It is true that telomeres in the human renal cortex shorten (approximately 0.029 kbp, or one-quarter percent per year) with age (Melk et al., 2000), but medullary telomere shortening, by contrast, is less than that found in the cortex and not statistically significant. Renal cortical cells have longer telomeres than those in renal medullary cells and this difference shrinks with age. While there may be some stem cell population within the kidney capable of telomerase expression in response to cytokines or other stimuli, there are no published data supporting this possibility and, at least in the rat, renal cortical cells are negative for telomerase (Golubovskaya et al., 1997).

Nonetheless, whether due to the primary changes of cell senescence or a secondary and adaptive response, there are clear changes in the pattern of gene expression within the renal cortex. In rats, for example, the balance between collagen synthesis and degradation tips in favor of an accumulation of pro-α2(I)collagen (COL-I). These and other changes parallel the consistent histologic changes, such as the increasing renal cortical fibrosis, a hallmark of the aging rat kidney (Gagliano et al., 2000). Overall, however, neither this nor other published evidence has addressed the issue of changes in gene expression due to renal cell senescence. A modicum of evidence suggests that cell senescence plays a role in renal allograft survival, at least in rats (Chkhotua et al., 2002).

While there is little a priori doubt that cell senescence occurs in vivo in the human kidney, there are even fewer a posteriori data supporting this prediction and no direct (as opposed to circumstantial) evidence that cell senescence underlies the increasing clinical dysfunction seen in the aging kidney. Few will be surprised to find that cell senescence plays a role, but the research remains undone.

Intervention

Renal interventions encompass specific therapies aimed at reversible etiologies (such as infections), general therapies aimed at chronic diseases with substantial renal complications (such as diabetes and hypertension), and two expensive and invasive therapies aimed specifically at renal failure, i.e., dialysis (peritoneal and hemodialysis) and renal transplantation. In renal aging, there is little to offer. To many undergoing dialysis or faced with the prospect of renal transplant, and far more so in the elderly, these interventions are insufficient to justify their discomfort, restriction, and cost. No clinician or patient familiar with current renal failure therapy argues against improvement. To the contrary, we can offer little and what we do offer often falls short of ensuring an acceptable quality of life or at an acceptable cost.

Caloric restriction appears to decrease the rate of age-related glomerular loss in rats (Durakovic and Mimica, 1983) and renal epithelial cell senescence in mice (Pendergrass et al., 1995). There is no reason to suspect this does not extend to humans. Equally, however, human studies have not been done. Human patients seldom willingly undergo dietary abnegation to the degree hypothesized to extend renal function, even if proven effective.

More optimistically, proteinuria accompanying impaired renal filtration has prompted research on low-protein diets. High-protein diets can induce glomerular damage and a reduction in dietary protein is protective (Everitt et al., 1982; Timiras, 1994a). This restricted degree of dietary (as opposed to caloric) restriction is not only more attainable but has become a standard dietary recommendation for renal patients worldwide. There are limited data suggesting that dehydroepiandrosterone may induce similar benefits (Pashko et al., 1986; Timiras, 1994a), but neither this nor other endocrine interventions are likely substantive improvements in our clinical armamentarium.

In cell senescence, vascular endothelial cells are already a research target and may improve renal function to the degree to which renal aging can be laid at the doorstep of aging vessels. Realistically, podocytes and cells composing the renal tubules may senesce. Intervention in this process, on the face of it, requires systemic delivery of an hTERT gene (e.g., via a viral carrier) or a promoter. Neither has been attempted in animal or human studies.

CHAPTER 15

Muscle

Structure and Overview

Muscles consist of large numbers of myocytes that join to form visible structures to allow movement. They receive innervation from the motor neurons that control them. Equally, they receive a substantial vascular supply to supply oxygen, glucose, and nutrients, while removing metabolic waste products such as carbon dioxide and lactate. Muscle strength varies histologically with the type of muscle fiber (white or red; type I or II), anatomically with size (diameter) and attachment (leverage), temporally with chronic use (exercise) and acute use (fatigue), and hormonally (testosterone, corticosteroid, thyroid, growth hormone, etc). Finally, and appropriately so, muscle strength varies chronologically with age.

Skeletal muscle makes up most of the visible muscle tissue and is resistant to hypoxic damage. In demonstrating peripheral nerve and motor function, I once gave an hour lecture with a blood pressure cuff clamped off at twice my systolic pressure, preventing all blood flow to my left arm. Despite the transient (and notable) discomfort, not only was I able to continue my entire lecture, in which I discussed peripheral nerve function and vasculature, but my left arm returned to its subjectively normal baseline function almost immediately after I released the pressure. Severe acute ischemic insult may prevent normal function (as it did in this case), but within broad limits has little effect on the survival and long-term functional capacity of skeletal muscle cells. Such muscle cells are capable of surviving outside the normal glycolytic pathway and can build up an oxygen debt by metabolizing glucose to lactate in the relative absence of oxygen. In short, myocytes are tough and sturdy in the face of metabolic insults.

Cardiac muscle, to the contrary, is incapable of functioning and surviving without a ready supply of oxygen. The results of this exquisite dependence is that decreases in coronary artery flow result in corresponding and immediate ischemic dysfunction or permanent infarction of affected cardiac muscle. Cardiac muscle without blood flow not only doesn't function, it dies. This entire pathology, however, is secondary to primary arterial disease, not primary cardiac muscle disease. Myocardial aging has, therefore, already been discussed under the aegis of cardiovascular aging (Chapter 9).

Despite these fatal differences in cardiac and skeletal muscle, the differences between smooth and striated muscle, and the differences between fast and slow, white and red, type I and II muscle fibers, all muscle cells have generic similarities at the cellular level. Muscles comprise fibrous tissue (for strength) and muscle cells in long bundles (for movement). The muscle cells are long, syncytial bundles (although this is not true of cardiac muscle; Bloom and Fawcett, 1975) that include mitochondria, nuclei, and usual cellular components, all of which are overwhelmed by and all but lost among myofibrils, the engines of the human body. Myofibrils are predominantly actin and myosin, two proteins that form bands or stria (hence, striated muscle) and do the work. The thinner actin filaments are pulled relative to the thicker myosin proteins by ATP-dependent stearic changes, causing them to overlap, shorten, and thereby contract. The ionic and metabolic details of this contraction (and subsequent relaxation) are complex and fascinating, but beyond, and largely orthogonal to, the charge of this text.

Aging and Other Pathology

Muscles lose strength and mass with age (Evans, 1995; Hurley, 1995; Visser et al., 2000). While specific muscle diseases occur (Laguno et al., 2002), the primary concern in this venue is age-related loss of strength. The loss of strength is manifold, at a minimum comprising losses of maximal strength, precision control, and ability to maintain contraction (Ranganathan et al., 2001). Although the loss of mass may begin as early as age 25 (Andersen et al., 2000), most muscle loss occurs later; between the second and seventh decades, muscle area declines by 40% and strength by 30% (Rogers and Evans, 1993). By age 80, approximately 50% of muscle mass, mainly as a loss of fibers, is gone (Andersen et al., 2000). Several variables might account for such loss, including diminished use, but circulatory loss and other factors are likely to play a role (Dutta and Hadley, 1995; Hughes et al., 2001). Age-related muscle wasting (loss of mass) is termed *sarcopenia*, a relatively new coinage (Rosenberg, 1989, 1997), but a useful as well as fashionable one. The loss of muscle mass has consequences for motor activity, but other, perhaps more dangerous consequences. Muscle represents protein storage for the body. Sarcopenia decreases the body's ability to mobilize protein in acute needs, thereby indirectly but significantly interfering with antibody and enzyme production for the immune system, the liver, and other organs during infection, trauma, or other stresses. Excepting perhaps intentional weight loss in the obese (Taylor and Ostbye, 2001), weight loss is a predictive risk factor for mortality in the elderly (Newman et al., 2001) and sarcopenia is a major portion of this loss (Metter et al., 2002). In short, sarcopenia prevents adequate response to acute insult and increases the risk of nearly all diseases in the elderly (Roubenoff and Castaneda, 2001), even those with no clear relationship to muscle function.

Sarcopenia is distinguished by an age-related decline in muscle fiber numbers and a decrease in myocyte size, resulting in a composite loss of muscle mass (Evans and Campbell, 1993; Melton et al., 2000) (Fig. 15–1). The concept parallels, in onset and definition, osteoporosis and has been arbitrarily defined as a muscle mass (often appendicular rather than central for ease of measure) less than two standard deviations below mean normal young muscle mass (Baumgartner et al., 1998). Loss of muscle strength with aging is not solely attributable to sarcopenia, but implicates other cellular, neural, or metabolic factors that remain imprecisely defined (Hughes et al., 2001; Metter et al., 2002). To some extent, the specific muscle loss is dependent on fiber type (Moulias et al., 1999) and is probably more prominent in fast fibers (Andersen et al., 2000), although the decline occurs in fast and slow muscle fiber types (Bemben, 1998) and distinction between the two types becomes blurred (Andersen et al., 2000). The deficit can be arguably traced to a decrease in muscle protein synthesis. Specifically, this decline is found in the synthesis rate of myosin heavy chain (MHC) protein (Nair, 2000). Attempts to link this to merely dietary factors, such as increased amino acid requirements in the elderly (Campbell et al., 2001), are insufficient to explain the breadth of cellular changes that define sarcopenia. More recent data (Volpi et al., 2001) have suggested that while the normal anabolic response to specific stimulation declines with age, the basal synthesis, catabolism, and turnover of muscle protein may not, at least in men. Appropriate myogenic stimuli, such as exercise, diet, or hormones, may no longer trigger the normal anabolic increases seen in younger individuals (Roubenoff and Hughes, 2000; Volpi et al., 2000; Roubenoff and Castaneda, 2001).

The blood supply and oxidative enzyme activity decrease, though not necessarily the glycolytic capacity. Overall metabolism decreases, becoming less efficient, a change that has been attributed to significant (Schwarze et al., 1995; Eimon et al., 1996; Arking, 1998) but subtle (Van Zeeland et al., 1999) mitochondrial changes that respond to caloric restriction (Desai et al., 1996; Lee et al., 1998a; Lal et al., 2001). Within the muscles, mitochondrial protein synthesis declines with age (Nair, 2000). Many have assumed that changes in mitochondria, and specifically the mitochondrial genome, may "substantially contribute" to the age-related loss of muscle function (Skorjanc et al., 2001). Consistent with this assumption, the literature reports an

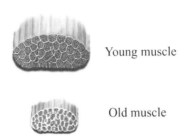

Young muscle

Old muscle

Figure 15–1 Aging muscle tissue. In the aging muscle, the overall gross loss of muscle radius and strength reflects a paralleling histologic sarcopenia. Age-related losses occur at all levels (muscles, muscle fibers, and individual myocytes), although specific patterns of loss vary by muscle, motor fiber type, gender, and pattern of exercise.

increased frequency of mitochondrial DNA damage and mutations in aging myocytes (Lee et al., 1997; Chandwaney et al., 1998; Kowald and Kirkwood, 2000). As is frequently true (but perennially forgotten) of scientific data, a correlation is supported, an inference of causality is not.

Resting capillary flow is less affected by age than is the exercise-induced increase in capillary flow, presumably because of a reduced ability to vasodilate, a reduction in capillary density, and losses to the reserve capillary bed (McCully and Posner, 1995), as well as poorly understood changes in the capillary endothelium (Degens, 1998). The loss of muscle tissue can affect thermoregulation and cardiac work load, perhaps contributing to the risk of congestive heart failure (Kenney and Buskirk, 1995). In addition, the loss of quotidian stress on bony structures (with its impact on osteoporosis; Layne and Nelson, 1999) and decreased muscle strength may interact to increase the risk of falls, with a consequent increase in fracture morbidity and mortality (Marcus, 1995; Dutta, 1997; Melton et al., 2000). Since sufficient exercise results in a return of lost muscle mass and strength (Evans, 1996; McGuigan et al., 2001), it is not clear that sarcopenia is a primary result of intrinsic muscle aging rather than largely secondary to simple disuse (Rogers and Evans, 1993). Nonetheless, weight lifting may simply result in thickening of the remaining fibers but have little or no effect on the progressive loss of individual fibers (Andersen et al., 2000). Such loss may be an outcome of hormonal changes (although probably not growth hormone; Roubenoff et al., 1998), the decrease in neuromuscular innervation (Beaufrere and Boirie, 1998; Proctor et al., 1998; Urbanchek et al., 2001) with its concomitant loss of "neural activation" of the muscle (Lamoureux et al., 2001), or other less defined factors (Moulias et al., 1999).

As muscle function (and mass) are dependent on the contractile proteins, actin and myosin (particularly the MHC), we should not be surprised to find that there is less net muscle protein loss. However, protein synthesis and turnover also decline with age (Nair, 1995; Short and Nair, 1999, 2000).

It is tempting to describe sarcopenia as a simple, generic outcome of aging: another of the myriad outcomes of aging, recalling Emerson's concept of aging as the disease "into which all others run" (Beck, 1968). Perhaps muscles wither because of disuse, as the elderly patient's arthritis inhibits exercise, as angina prohibits it, or as emphysema limits it. Similarly, an ensemble of Alzheimer dementia, infections, social isolation, poor nutrition, and other age-correlated factors might result in disuse atrophy. To what extent, however, does sarcopenia occur as result of what we might term "local" factors, such as cellular changes within myocytes, loss of motoneuron innervation, or loss of microvascular function within the muscle? Even the effects of exercise on ameliorating sarcopenia can be interpreted as implying a surprisingly significant role for vascular factors in sarcopenia (McGuigan et al., 2001). Curiously, at least in rats, regeneration of muscle appears to depend more on the age of the recipient than it does on the age of the organism that donates the aging muscle (Carlson et al., 2001). If specific intracellular changes do play a role, then these cellular changes might include the long-term accumulation of oxidative damage, the result of the high oxygen consumption inherent in this tissue, although there is little clear evidence to support this suggestion (Weindruch, 1995). There is some evidence for alterations in the pattern of gene expression in older myocytes that might explain sarcopenia (Ly et al., 2000), but whether such changes in gene expression are primary or secondary remains unclear.

The Role of Cell Senescence

Conventional wisdom was that "skeletal muscle is a nondividing tissue" (Arking, 1998). If true, muscle cells do not senesce. The mutability of muscle mass remained concordant with this tenet. Hypertrophy, rather than hyperplasia, was considered the basis of muscle enlargement in response to increased use or hormonal stimulation. Nevertheless, more diligent attention to mammalian muscle histology shows that muscle cells do divide (or are replaced) in the mature organism in skeletal (Antonio and Gonyea, 1993) and cardiac (Kajstura et al., 2000) muscles. Replacement myocytes derive not from standard, differentiated muscle cells, however, but rather from a reserve population of satellite stem cells or myoblasts (Anderson, 1998). To an extent, postnatal muscle growth is the result of the proliferation of these satellite cells and their subsequent fusion with existing muscle fibers (Schultz and McCormick, 1994). Muscle mass may be a direct correlative outcome of the proliferative capacity of these cells (Merly et al., 1998) and although we know little of the cell signaling involved (Chambers and McDermott, 1996; Husmann et al., 1996), the mechanisms of development may vary markedly from those of repair (Russell et al., 1992). Part of the normal response to exercise, even in the elderly person with sarcopenia, is an increase in this population of satellite cells (Roth et al., 2001b). The same increase in the population of satellite cells occurs in rats in which muscles are stimulated electrically and, although early studies found an age-related decrement (Schultz and Lipton, 1982; Gibson and Schultz, 1983), this satellite cell response may continue unabated by age (Putnam et al., 2001). Regarding cell senescence in rat skeletal muscle, increases in satellite cells are not accompanied by increases in telomerase activity (Radak et al., 2001). In murine muscle cells, myocyte differentiation is accompanied by a decline in telomerase activity due to a decrease in mTERT mRNA levels and down-regulation of mTERT gene expression (Nozawa et al., 2001).

Although satellite cells are usually located on the fringes of the muscle fibers, i.e., between the mature muscle fiber and its external basement lamina (Anderson, 1998; Yablonka-Reuveni et al., 1999), other far stranger sources have been identified. For example, clonable skeletal myogenic cells have been found in the aortas of mouse embryos. Such findings suggest that a percentage of what we classify as satellite cells, even in mature muscles, might derive from the supplying capillary beds or other vascular origins (De Angelis et al., 1999).

Satellite cells are a small (1%–6%) percentage of muscle cells. As might be expected of dividing cell lines, and specifically stem cell lines, they become slightly less common with age. At least in rats, however, there is no massive depletion of the satellite cell pool. Some investigators have therefore suggested that the diminished regenerative capacity of senile muscle might be due more to changes in microenvironment and satellite cell *response* than to hypothetical attenuation of cellular *capacity* to divide and restore missing myocytes (Nnodim, 2000). While this is consistent with what we do know, next to nothing is known of the details of such putative changes with age. A lack of exercise can reduce the population of satellite cells (Wanek and Snow, 2000). This might support the possibility that even if dysfunctional (or diminished numbers of) satellite cells are the proximate cause of sarcopenia, it might equally be due to the underlying causes already discussed above—diminished use, an altered hormonal milieu, decreased capillary beds, etc.

The division rate of such satellite cells, while not well measured, is probably low and critically dependent on local factors such as muscle damage, inflammation, extracellular matrix, growth factors, and disease (such as muscular dystrophy) (Grounds, 1998; Kajstura et al., 2000). Nonetheless, though the proliferation rate may be low, it is possible that the bulk of muscle tissue regeneration and repair derives not from classic hypertrophy but from satellite cell hyperplasia, i.e., responsive division of satellite cells that supply "fresh" cells to the muscle. Such daughter cells fuse to the extant muscle syncytia and permit the equivalent of hypertrophy through the surreptitious accretion of satellite myoblasts, an interesting example of hyperplasia by proxy. As such satellite cells accumulate divisions with age (and lose telomere length) because of the repeated repair of damaged muscle (Grounds, 1998), they should thereby senesce (Bornemann et al., 1999) and be less capable of rapidly resupplying new cells to the active muscle.

Measurements of telomere lengths in young dystrophic human skeletal (Decary et al., 2000) and rat cardiac muscle (Kajstura et al., 2000) support this suggestion. Telomeres shorten with age and circumstances in a proportion of these myocytes. Although human myoblasts have limited proliferative capacity and skeletal muscle normally has a low rate of replacement, the myoblasts of patients with muscular dystrophy have divided repeatedly and show consequent (and accelerated) telomere shortening at an early age. Although telomere shortening is found in normal aging muscle, the rate of loss is magnified (14-fold) in dystrophic myoblasts (Decary et al., 2000). Whether this is due to replicative aging or to impaired differentiation in the affected myocytes, at least in Duchenne muscular dystrophy, is arguable (Oexle and Kohlschutter, 2001). Moreover, while telomerase transfection into dystrophic human myoblasts results in normal myocyte differentiation, it does not extend the replicative ability of these abnormal cells (Seigneurin-Venin et al., 2000). This finding supports the suggestion that the underlying cause of the dystrophy may (and independently of telomere length) limit cell replication and survival.

The notion that myoblasts senesce and thereby induce age-related changes in functioning myocytes is consistent with the age-related changes in the cellular microenvironment, as seen in patterns of inflammation, growth factors, cell receptors (particularly for FGF-2), and extracellular matrix (Grounds, 1998). Similarly, we see changes in the activation of older satellite cells by insulin-like growth factor I (IGF-1), which can be restored through viral transfection (Barton-Davis et al., 1998). In rats, the satellite cells from older donors are less capable of normal differentiation sequence, marked by myogenin expression and transition to a MyoD+ phenotype. In addition, the response of satellite cells to appropriate growth factors (e.g., fibroblast, but not hepatocyte growth factor) is delayed, although the final proliferation rate is similar. The responses of cells from older donors lag behind those of younger donors (Yablonka-Reuveni et al., 1999). There are changes in gene expression of at least 55 genes in myocytes taken from older donors, compared to younger donors (Lee et al., 1999a). Whether these changes occur because of intrinsic cell senescence of dividing satellite cells or (as may be more likely) the secondary effects of other more distant, dividing (and senescing) cells (such as fibroblasts, endothelial cells, etc) is unknown.

Collectively, such altered responses may imply a gradual but continual loss of muscle fibers without a correspondingly balanced gain of newly differentiated myocytes, with sarcopenia as the outcome. The primary cause of aging-related impairment of muscle function (sarcopenia) is the cumulative failure to repair damage sustained during muscle utilization (Barton-Davis et al., 1998), which in turn is due to cell senescence of the satellite cells as well as the effects of senescence in fibroblasts and vascular structures. In addition, the gradual changes in gene expression result in a decline in myosin synthesis (Nair, 2000), thereby slowing the turnover rate and, pari passu, increasing the percentage of damaged proteins within the cell.

Even if the above model were wrong and satellite cells did not senesce, cell senescence might play a role, albeit indirectly. As we have seen in the heart, cell senescence may be the major single common denominator in myocardial infarction, even if cardiac cells never divide simply because of the ubiquitous and deadly effects of aging cells in the vascular endothelium. In a parallel fashion, the same model may be operating here. As the endothelial cells of the capillary beds and fine arterioles senesce, they have a profound impact on the metabolic function of the end organ: the muscles. That the muscle cells may not divide (enough to cause myocyte senescence) is immaterial. The question is one of cell senescence in the vascular beds. Although it is clear that such beds alter profoundly with age, whether this is due to cell senescence remains unknown. In a similar vein, an age-related decrease in innervation may have a detrimental secondary effect upon satellite cell proliferation (Carlson, 1995). Although uncomfortably circuitous, it is even possible that the rate-limiting step in sarcopenia is not satellite cell senescence but glial or endothelial senescence mediated via a decrease in peripheral motoneuron arborization, resulting in the observed loss of satellite cells (Bornemann et al., 1999).

We are left with two possible (and possibly interacting) venues for cell senescence to play out its effects on sarcopenia: directly through satellite cell senescence or indirectly through vascular or neural changes, themselves putatively the result of cell senescence elsewhere. The model remains consistent with known data, but the data are woefully insufficient.

Intervention

There are myriad possible interventions that might effectively treat age-related sarcopenia. Most clinical trials have focused on exercise, often with an almost religious fervor. Most of this research has used correlational rather than interventional designs, then drawn causal inferences which, though possibly true, are unwarranted on the basis of the merely observational data. More appropriate exercise research suggests that there are benefits not only in muscle strength but in mobility (Westerterp and Meijer, 2001), quality of life (Rejeski and Mihalko, 2001), and other less measurable attributes, though often these latter observations have little hard data.

Morbidity or mortality data, which might confirm the overall clinical value of exercise, are often merely assumed, are difficult to gather, and have, consequently, been slow in coming. Whatever else its value, exercise is an effective determinant of muscle size, regardless of age (Roth et al., 2001a). However, there is now growing evidence that exercise not only increases the lost muscle mass (Evans, 1996; Hagerman et al., 2000; Hikida et al., 2000) and decreases secondary pathology such as atherosclerosis, diabetes, osteoporosis, or fractures (Evans and Campbell, 1993; Layne and Nelson, 1999), but probably, although not certainly (Keysor and Jette, 2001), lowers the outcome frequency of morbidity and mortality (Curl, 2000). Despite problems of correlational data and prevalence of unexamined but a priori dogma that has interfered with objective validation, exercise probably does have objective value in modulating sarcopenia and in altering clinical outcomes.

Although exercise has been the leading idol, even among those who demand bona fide supportive data, other interventions have been considered. Initial research, although tentative, suggests that sarcopenia can be delayed by caloric restriction, at least in some species (Keith et al., 2000). Interventional research on the clinical value of caloric restriction in humans with sarcopenia remains feasible, pending clearer data.

Given the historical enthusiasm among researchers and general public, it is hardly surprising that hormonal intervention has been tried, particularly using testosterone and growth hormone. Although testosterone has been used to affect muscle mass (and for other reasons) since it was first identified in 1849 (Goodman, 1974a), more recent work has been less anecdotal and more predictively valid, yet remains incomplete. There is excellent support for the circumscribed conclusion that, in supraphysiological doses, testosterone increases muscle mass and improves strength in young, eugonadal males (Vermeulen et al., 1999), but beyond this point things become a bit more difficult. Given testosterone, healthy older men demonstrate modest improvements in several parameters (Basaria and Dobs, 1999; Kenny et al., 2001), including muscle mass, strength, and perhaps mood (Seidman and Walsh, 1999), but the incidence of secondary problems and crucial outcomes of morbidity and mortality remain unclear and controversial (Tenover, 1998; Bross et al., 1999). Growth hormone likewise shows effects similar to those of exercise, not only in rats (Mosekilde et al., 1999) but in young athletes (Wallace et al., 2000) and moderately frail old people (Hennessey et al., 2001). Nonetheless, the case for routine clinical use of testosterone or growth hormone in aging patients with sarcopenia is hardly open and shut.

Other interventions have also been considered. Hormone replacement therapy, generally taken to refer specifically to postmenopausal estrogen and/or progesterone supplementation, has conflicting clinical support (Kenny et al., 2003) and no morphological or functional support (Widrick et al., 2003). Data on creatine supplementation are suggestive, particularly in the context of exercise (Brose et al., 2003), but unimpressive.

With an increased understanding that satellite cells may play a central role in not only muscle development and regeneration but in age-related sarcopenia, there has been a corresponding interest in the factors that control satellite cell activation (Anderson and Murray, 1998; Grounds, 1998). Such studies have concentrated largely on local growth factors (Bornemann et al., 1999), neural influences (Carlson, 1995), receptors (Chambers and McDermott, 1996), and oxidative stress (Renault et al., 2002). The older interest in systemic growth factors such as growth hormone, insulin-like growth hormone, and dehydroepiandrosterone, has carried over into this area, but remains equally unexplored (Short and Nair, 1999). While this work qualifies as relevant to questions of intervention, it remains largely experimental and thus premature from the clinical standpoint.

With regard to cell senescence, there is almost a complete void. What data exist may be interpreted to suit the bias of the researcher. There is little known about satellite cell senescence (current information is merely descriptive of a decrease in satellite cell numbers and a change in characteristics with donor age, not cell senescence). There has been no work using myocyte telomerization or reconstituted muscle tissue, with the exception of myometrium. The latter work suggests that uterine smooth muscle cells, immortalized with hTERT, are essentially normal although with the loss of estrogen β receptors (Condon et al., 2002).

There have been suggestions that telomerase gene delivery might be useful in specific muscle diseases, such as Duchenne muscular dystrophy, but there are no interventional studies. To an extent, this absence reflects the conclusion that Duchenne's is not the result of cell senescence but (parallel to HIV) of impaired differentiation, altered cell–cell interactions, and inadequate response to signals for cell replacement. While this explains failure of myoblast transfer experiments to treat Duchenne muscular dystrophy, telomerase gene transfer might be effective nonetheless (Oexle and Kohlschutter, 2001). This potential therapy parallels the use of telomerase to "end-run" the helicase defect in Werner syndrome and induce cell immortalization (Wyllie et al., 2000).

While telomerase induction or transfection has not been used as an experimental intervention in aging muscle, specifically as a treatment for sarcopenia, there is no reason why such an experiment should not be forthcoming in the near future. The primary problem, as in many tissues, is a practical one: targeted and effective delivery to appropriate cells.

CHAPTER 16

Gastrointestinal System

Structure and Overview

The gastrointestinal tract comprises a long tube with associated organs, including the liver and pancreas. Although the tract commonly achieves more interest, the bulk of this chapter will slight the gastrointestinal tract and concern itself with the liver. The gastrointestinal tract will, however, be considered, largely because there is a growing body of research focusing on cell senescence in the esophagus and intestines.

The human liver, a mere 3% of body weight (Goodman, 1974b), is the major chemical factory of the body and largest gland in the body. It receives the entire venous drainage of the gastrointestinal tract, which it detoxifies, modifies, and delivers into the general circulation. Storing (as glycogen) and releasing glucose, it acts as a rapid damper to sudden shifts in serum glucose, tiding the body over until fat stores can serve in the same capacity with a slower time frame. The liver, for example, is drawn upon in sudden strenuous exertions, as during a marathon or tonic-clonic seizure, similar (though not identical) activities from a metabolic perspective. If additional glucose is needed, the liver is capable of producing it from circulating fatty acids (from distant adipocytes), lactate (from muscle activity), or amino acids (from protein breakdown). In this, as in its literally hundreds of other metabolic functions (Robbins, 1974), the liver is the homeostatic organ par excellence. In a sense, it is the body's metabolic banker and money changer, a role essential to the body at every stage of metabolism.

To appreciate its functions, consider the effects of its failure. Acutely, hepatic failure is clinically protean. The most trenchant effects are within the central nervous system: it causes confusion at the earliest stages and coma terminally. More insidious liver failure can initially be subtle, but is ultimately just as fatal. Its effects include increases in circulating estrogens, alterations in glial cell function, changes in the peripheral microvasculature, impaired bilirubin breakdown (from erythrocytic hemoglobin) with resultant jaundice, and secondary failure in other organs (e.g., hepatorenal failure). A full list is nearly interminable, covering almost all aspects of intermediate metabolism: thermal regulation, cholesterol circulation, protein metabolism, clotting efficacy, ammonia accumulation, etc. Curiously, individual hepatic functions can fail with relative independence: clinical liver function tests in human patients frequently show modest impairment of one function without significant impairment of another.

Grossly, the liver appears homogeneous. Although there is a complex vascular and drainage system, the bulk of the liver seems to be a single mass of identical cells. Although it has only the usual single (and unremarkable) venous drainage, the vasculature is anomalous for having two incoming vascular supplies that meet in a complex arrangement. The liver receives not only the portal veins (supplying the bulk of incoming hepatic blood and comprising the entire venous drainage from the intestines) but also the hepatic arteries (supplying a far smaller volume) from the normal arterial circulation. Most of the liver's critical endocrine work is unseen, accomplished by release directly into the venous drainage. The more easily observable exocrine drainage system is less critical and far less subtle: a confluence of bile ducts drain their products into the gall bladder and into the duodenum, allowing digestion of dietary fatty acids.

Microscopically, identical liver cells may form a continuous parenchyma throughout the liver. Cells are arranged like ill-defined orange sections around a central vein and this same arrangement is repeated endlessly within the liver. Each slice of hepatic "orange" defines a liver lobule, in which intestinally derived blood flows from the outer "peel" toward the prominent central vein. Liver cells lie along sinusoid spaces that convey the incoming blood from the outer ring to the hepatic veins, and process the blood as it flows centripetally. A normal arterial blood supply is also available to the hepatocytes, though less subject to the careful filtration and processing that the intestinally derived blood must undergo in traversing the liver.

At the ultrastructural level, there are two main types of hepatic parenchymal cells: endothelial cells and stellate cells. The endothelial cells of the liver are flattened cells with little cytoplasm that line the sinusoidal spaces (Goodman, 1974b; Enzan et al., 1997). Stellate, or "Ito," cells" (Friedman, 1997), in contrast, have a stellate appearance (Friedman, 1999c) and are now known by their shape rather than their eponym. They accumulate retinoids, while the cytoplasm and cytoplasmic variety increase more than flatter endothelial cells. The stellate cells phagocytize erythrocytes and particles of all sorts, are part of the reticuloendothelial system, and may derive from the bone marrow. They are the source of most extracellular matrix in the liver (Lang and Brenner, 1999; Li and Friedman, 1999). Within the lobule, those stellate cells toward the periphery are the more metabolically active, with many large, almost spherical mitochondria; stellate cells toward the center have fewer and thinner mitochondria (Goodman, 1974b). Although simple histologically, the liver is far from simple metabolically. The pathologic reflection of this contrast is equivalent: human hepatic disease is anatomically simple, but clinically complex and occasionally enigmatic.

The topological simplicity of the remainder of the gastrointestinal system is equally misleading. The gastrointestinal tract is a simple layered tube. The inner layer is absorptive, the next layer outward muscular, the outermost layer predominantly vascular. The inner surface epithelium is rough and fractal in its organization. The deepest, proliferative cells, in the crypts of Lieberkühn, are a small population of stem cells from which other epithelial cells continually rederive (Potten et al., 1997a; van den Brink et al., 2001; Yang et al., 2001d). Cell numbers are stringently controlled by balancing the loss and apoptosis of normal or damaged cells against the cell divisions of the stem cell population (Potten and Booth, 1997; Potten et al., 1997b). Stem cells proliferate in response to and are tightly modulated by local cell–cell signals, as occur with the loss of neighboring stem cells (Potten, 1991). The regulation of cell division and survival of the epithelial stem cells of the intestinal crypts are emphatically the responsibility of the vascular endothelial cells. These cells produce at least 20 identified growth factors; their apoptotic loss may be the controlling factor in the gastrointestinal side effects (e.g., the loss of epithelial stem cells in the intestinal crypts) of radiation therapy (Folkman and Camphausen, 2001; Paris et al., 2001).

Grossly, the gastrointestinal tract comprises a small (duodenum, jejunum, and ileum) and a large (cecum, appendix, and colon) intestine. The small intestine averages 7 meters in length and is recoiled upon itself, lying within the outer ring formed by the ascending (right), transverse, and descending (left) portions of the colon. The small intestine processes and absorbs food, while the colon absorbs water and transiently stores feces pending defecation. The histology of the tract reflects these conspicuous functions. The complex inner layer of the small intestine is specialized for the excretion of digestive molecules that break up the available dietary molecules and bind them for easier absorption. The former task is in many ways the more complex and crucial. Many required dietary molecules are not easily absorbed without active alteration by the cells lining the intestines. The activity of the large intestine is different. In the large intestine, specifically the colon, the prolonged storage of unused dietary intake and sloughed cells from the small intestine results in continual exposure to toxins and repeated challenge by colonic bacteria.

In performing these tasks, the gastrointestinal system has, simplistically speaking, three major cell types, each of which can and frequently does go awry. The innermost, mucosal cells are synthetically active, frequently replaced, and subject to considerable chemical and bacterial stress. The intermediate layer consists of muscle cells recurrently active (e.g., in peristalsis or sphincter control) and are required not only for appropriate mechanical function (e.g., directional maintenance and excretion of stool) but for optimal absorption (e.g., through churning motions). The outermost, vascular (and other) cells are critical for not only the same function they have elsewhere in other body tissues (nutrient supply and waste removal) but the absorption of nutrients and their initial (first-pass) delivery to the liver.

Aging and Other Pathology

Gastrointestinal pathology reflects gross and subtle functions, as well as risks implied by these functions. Within the colon, for example, the continual exposure to chemical and bacterial challenges results in its characteristic incidence of disease (e.g., colon cancer, diverticulitis). The acidity of the stomach and anatomic proximity of the lower esophagus and duodenum result in characteristic mucosal risks (e.g., gastric and duodenal ulceration, gastroesophageal reflux disorder). The same is perhaps even more frequently true of the more subtle functions of the gastrointestinal system. Even with a more than adequate oral intake, absent intrinsic factor (IF) secretion by the gastric mucosa, the intestines cannot absorb cyanocobalamin (B_{12}); again, the result is a characteristic clinical outcome (pernicious anemia). Failures of secretion, absorption, motility, and vascular supply all have pathological outcomes and each is channeled by the specific risks and conditions inherent to the tissue involved. Failure at the cellular level likewise accounts for the clinical pathology at the tissue and organismal level, but can only be understood in the context of cell-specific functions within the affected tissue. For example, the failure of endothelial vascular cells in the small intestine results in a different pathology from the same failure of phenotypically identical cells within the coronary arteries. In both, intracellular failure may be identical, including the changes in gene expression incumbent upon cellular senescence (vide infra).

The liver is the site of a large plurality of human disease, partly because hepatic function is so critical, partly because of its subtle effects on so many separate tissues. Liver cancer has been dealt with previously. Although most diseases that affect hepatic function are linked etiologically to (increased risk of) hepatic cancer, they deserve an independent venue. The common clinical hepatic diseases, especially cirrhosis and hepatitis, are far more common than the occasional ominous consequence of cancer. In hepatic disease, fatality often intervenes before malignancy begins.

Liver cirrhosis is the seventh leading cause of death by disease (Rudolph et al., 2000). Although vaguely defined (Robbins, 1974), the pathology is not vague. To the contrary, it is devastating and easy to observe histologically and clinically. Cirrhosis is scarring and necrosis, widely distributed and associated with regenerative hepatocytes. The overwhelming leading cause of cirrhosis in most nations is alcohol hepatitis; the leading cause in many underdeveloped nations is usually the same, but viral hepatitis will occasionally take precedence. Both causes are ubiquitous, plurality varying by country, ethnic group, decade, and chance. Defining alcoholism socially can be as problematic as Wittgenstein's classic attempt to define a chair (Wittgenstein, 1958), varying with fashion and prejudice and often simply encompassing anyone who drinks alcohol "whom you don't like" (Robbins, 1974). The pathologic results, however, are less deconstructionist or subjective and far more tangible. Clinically, alcohol cirrhosis is manifested initially by hepatomegaly and later by liver shrinkage, jaundice, easy bleeding, and ascites. Twenty-five years ago, approximately 80%–90% of all patients diagnosed with alcoholic cirrhosis died within 5 years of initial diagnosis (Robbins, 1974) and current outcome statistics have not improved much.

The anatomic outcomes—fibrous scarring, portal hypertension, gastric bleeding—are widespread regardless of the cause of severe cirrhosis, but fatty deposition is pathognomonic of alcohol. It begins almost immediately upon consumption and occurs independently of other caloric intake (Rubin and Lieber, 1968). Alcohol mobilizes fat from peripheral adipocytes to the liver and blocks its oxidation while it accumulates in hepatocytes, beginning in the centermost cells of the lobules (Goodman, 1974b). The metabolic outcomes of alcohol—an increased $NADH_2/NAD$ ratio, hypoxic hepatocytes, generation of lipid peroxides, eicosanoids, and increased acetaldehyde formation (Hautekeete and Geerts, 1997; Friedman, 1999b)—are usually further complicated by the malnutrition of alcoholics. This can induce secondary pathology such as protein insufficiency (kwashiorkor), thiamine deficiency (Wernicke-Korsakoff syndrome), and a host of other problems. Prominent physiologic changes occur, with an increase in circulating cytokines (Hautekeete and Geerts, 1997) such as transforming growth factor-beta (Bissell,

1998) and interleukin-8, as well as direct induction of plasma endotoxins (a potent inducer of tumor necrosis factor [TNF]-α and interleukin-1; Huang et al., 1999b). The frequency of alcohol cirrhosis increases with age, but probably as a result of accumulated alcohol exposure, rather than because of direct effects of aging. As we shall see, cell senescence may mediate pathology, even if alcohol is the independent variable. Alcohol in cirrhosis may parallel cholesterol in atherosclerosis: cholesterol is important, but cell senescence mediates pathology.

Viral hepatitis has a similar outcome to that of alcohol hepatitis, albeit without fatty accumulation. Histologically, the first sign of infection is hepatic endothelial cell swelling, along with swelling and hyperplasia of stellate cells. This is followed by lymphocytic infiltration, macrophage proliferation, and hepatocyte necrosis. The stellate cells alter, becoming fibrogenic, contractile myofibroblasts (Li and Friedman, 1999). The remaining hepatocytes divide, replacing those that have died, but the balance of these two opposite processes—necrosis and cell division—may achieve a tenuous balance or may go either way and thereby determine the clinical outcome: recovery, chronic infection, or death. In cases in which the immune system can eradicate the active infection, the rate of necrosis slows and, if the rate of hepatocyte division has kept up with the losses, the patient survives and is cured. If the immune system does not eradicate the infection, but the rate of continuous cell division can be maintained and is adequate, the patient survives with chronic infection. If the rate of cell loss falls, acutely or in the long run, behind the rate of cell replacement, the patient dies of hepatic failure.

Descriptions of the transformation from normal to cirrhotic liver can be exceedingly complex (Gressner, 1996), but there are a few clear principles. In the primary forms, alcohol and viral hepatitis, the liver loses functioning hepatocytes and makes some (often heroic) attempt to replace those losses. In both cases there is an inflammatory component and an increase in stellate fibrocytes and fibrous scarring (Li and Friedman, 1999). And in both cases, there is increasing cell division with all that it implies for acceleration of cell senescence.

The intestines themselves have a number of organ-specific diseases, and even the generic pathologies, such as cancer, must be understood in the context of the organs involved. Colon cancer is a frequent cause of death in the elderly and colon has a much higher incidence of cancer than does the small intestine, likely due to the differential exposure to chemical and bacterial stress and duration of those exposures. Beyond these differences in exposure, the cells of the large intestine have a lower frequency of apoptosis (presumably due their expression of the *bcl-2* gene), which may explain some differential risk of malignancy between the two ends of the intestinal tract (Potten, 1998). As in hepatic cancer, a more detailed treatment of gastrointestinal malignancy has already been offered in previous chapters.

Cancer is, of course, not the only age-related pathology of the gastrointestinal tract. Among the preeminent pathology of the body generically and gastrointestinal tract specifically is vascular pathology. Ischemic bowel, for example, may be just as fatal in some patients as ischemic myocardium is in others. Other generic pathologies, such as sarcopenia, have their gastrointestinal counterparts. Although considered a characteristic of appendicular muscles, there is age-related loss of gastrointestinal muscle tone, causing constipation, altered food and water resorption, and increasing risk of diverticular disease and colon cancer. Such changes occur in aging humans as well as other species. Within the murine colon, for example, changes in "age-related colonic dysmotility" may result in subtle changes in the mucosa and intestinal function (Sweet et al., 1996).

Aging in the gastrointestinal tract is subtle yet pervasive (Fig. 16–1). Accurately or not, normal function is ascribed to "redundancy" (Baime et al., 1994). Most functional losses that do occur can be lumped into two classes: inappropriate responses to stress (generic among aging tissues) and inadequate baseline nutritional function (specific to gastrointestinal function). The first implies that baseline function is not so much of a problem as is the inadequate response to altered physiological conditions. Baseline functions may remain unremarkable, but the degree, temporal course, or specificity of physiological responses are measurably impaired.

Although reviews often focus on malnutrition in the elderly (Amarantos et al., 2001; Chernoff, 2001; Wakimoto and Block, 2001), much of this is a simple decline in quantity rather than quality of nutrition (Morley, 2001b), and may be due as much to extrinsic as intrinsic causes. Malnutrition in the elderly may, for example, be due to poverty, physical limitations in getting and preparing meals, depression, loss of appetite, dementia, and a host of etiologies that need not invoke primary gastrointestinal aging. This is not to suggest that primary gastrointestinal aging does not occur, but it must be assessed in a pragmatic context.

Aging in the gastrointestinal system has been categorized and reviewed adequately elsewhere (Baime et al., 1994; Cheskin and Schuster, 1994; Kerr, 1994), although without following such changes down to their intracellular sources. Reviews that consider cellular changes in the aging gastrointestinal system (Arking, 1998; Anantharaju and Feller, 2002) conclude that there are alterations within specific components (or functions) of that system, i.e., connective tissue, muscle cells, and secretory cells. The reader is referred to such sources for competent overviews of our general knowledge of gastrointestinal aging.

That cells of the aging gastrointestinal system divide, show telomere loss, and show resultant changes in gene expression has not been reviewed or considered in detail. What has been considered are the outcomes (moderate changes in function or response) and correlates (specific changes within specific cells) without regard for an underlying cause,

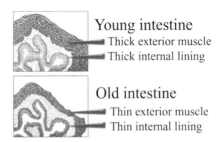

Young intestine
Thick exterior muscle
Thick internal lining

Old intestine
Thin exterior muscle
Thin internal lining

Figure 16–1 Aging gastrointestinal tissue. In the gastrointestinal tract, the most obvious histologic changes are within the external band of muscles and the internal lining. The former reflects smooth muscle cell losses (sarcopenia). The latter reflects both a gradual decrease in stem cell numbers and a slower rate of their division. Without any compensatory decrease in the rate of cell loss within the lumen of the tract, the result is a smaller cell population and, consequently, a thinner lining.

such as cellular senescence. Nevertheless, within the gastrointestinal system, a number of cells divide or are subject to dependence on cells that divide, and this can be expected yield dysfunctional dividends for the gastrointestinal tissues and for the organism.

The Role of Cell Senescence

Cell senescence probably plays a role in several venues within the gastrointestinal system, but will be primarily considered in two manifestations. The first will be an overview of what we know of cell senescence within the mucosal cells of the intestinal wall; the second is a specific overview of cell senescence in hepatic cirrhosis. While a few side issues should and will be raised, the remainder of the chapter will focus on cellular aging within the liver and the link between cellular aging and hepatic cirrhosis. In both cases, the reason for this focus lies in what we know rather than what we might wish to know. While beneficial to consider other aspects of cell senescence in gastrointestinal aging, the field remains wide and data narrow.

Beginning at the top of the tract, there is progressive telomere shortening with age in the esophageal mucosa at the rate of approximately 60 bp per year. The telomeres of older cells are shorter, but exhibit more variance. The relatively slow fall in telomere lengths compared to the rapid turnover in esophageal mucosa suggests the presence of cells with telomerase, i.e., esophageal stem cells (Takubo et al., 1999).

The stomach may contain stem cell populations, but gastric cells show gradual telomere loss notwithstanding. Normal gastric mucosal cells show loss of telomere lengths at a rate of approximately 46 bp per year (Furugori et al., 2000), as do other mucosal cells within the intestines. *Helicobacter pylori*, perhaps responsible for most though not all (Brock et al., 2001; Butler et al., 2001) stomach ulcers, is associated with the risk of stomach cancer (EUROGAST Study Group, 1993). *Helicobacter* infection causes the release of reactive oxygen and nitrogen species, which may trigger hyperplasia among gastric stem cells; these may already be capable of expressing telomerase. *Helicobacter* infection and stem cell division, along with DNA damage and *p53* mutations (found in 30% of intestinal metaplasia), have been cited as part of the cascade of risks underlying gastric cancer (Tahara, 1998).

Although intestinal cells may be less prone to *Helicobacter* infection or acid stress than gastric cells, the large and small intestine mucosal cells nonetheless demonstrate telomere shortening (Hiyama et al., 1996b). Several workers have looked at age-related changes in the stem cells within the crypts of Lieberkühn. In mice, there are age-related alterations in the histology and the apoptotic responses of stem cells to low-dose radiation. The probability of apoptosis increases with exposure to radiation or cytotoxic agents and this is accentuated in older animals, in which there is a twofold increase in the level of apoptosis (Martin et al., 1998b). As a result, older mice exposed to radiation have fewer and smaller surviving crypts than do young mice with equivalent exposures. Regenerative growth responses are delayed in older mice. Surprisingly, however, there are more stem cells per crypt in older mice (Martin et al., 1998a).

The major importance of crypt cells lies in being sources of renewal for the lifelong cell losses. That these stem cells express telomerase is predictable but not assumable. Telomerase-expressing stem cells are found within the intestinal crypts (Bach et al., 2000), but the control of expression is unclear. As elsewhere, such expression should delay telomere loss and cell senescence, responding to cytokines and to the rate of intestinal cell loss. Where telomerase is lacking, we should expect cell senescence to accelerate, resulting in early histological simplification and a loss of intestinal function. This occurs in telomerase knockout mice, which demonstrate atrophy of the small intestine (Herrera et al., 1999b). Stem cells are responsible for long-term intestinal tract function and, likely, telomerase is in turn responsible for long-term stem cell function. Nonetheless, the degree to which telomere loss and cell senescence, held in partial abeyance by telomerase-positive stem cells, directly results in the functional decrements seen in the aging human intestinal tract is unproven.

Close to the far end of the gastrointestinal tract, colon cells show telomere shortening with age (Hastie et al., 1990). Here again, cell turnover is continually occurring in conjunction with cell loss and the result is gradual cell senescence. While telomerase-positive stem cells may be present within the colon and other portions of the large intestine, less is known about this portion of the gastrointestinal tract than about the small intestine. Nonetheless, telomerase activity is found in normal colonic mucosal cells and there are interesting correlations between telomere maintenance and colonic disease. Ulcerative colitis, an inflammatory condition of the large intestine, is associated with increased chromosomal instability, including end-to-end telomere associations (Cottliar et al., 2000). This may be the result of insufficient telomerase expression and telomere shortening (O'Sullivan et al., 2002). Endoscopic biopsies from patients with ulcerative colitis demonstrate deficient telomerase activity in samples from the cecum, transverse colon, sigmoid colon, and rectum. Telomerase activity is highest in colonic cells from patients with cancer, but it is higher in samples from patients with normal colons than in those from patients with ulcerative colitis. Moreover, telomerase activity is low even in normal portions of the colon from patients with ulcerative colitis, "suggesting that telomerase deficiency may contribute to the pathogenesis of the disease" (Usselman et al., 2001). While a number of other diseases, such as diverticulosis and diverticulitis, Crohn's disease, ischemic bowel disease, and mesenteric adenopathy, might have potential relationships to cell senescence or dysfunctional telomere maintenance, data that support or refute such suggestions are lacking.

The most comprehensive evidence for cell senescence within the gastrointestinal system is not in the tract but in one of its major associated organs: the liver. Toxic or infectious insults result in cell necrosis, in turn resulting in cell division. Under normal circumstances, liver cells turn over slowly. Normal human hepatocyte telomeres normally shorten by 55 bp per year, and decelerate in middle age. Although hepatocyte turnover is slower than gastrointestinal mucosal cells turnover, their rates of telomere loss are about equivalent (Takubo et al., 2000), perhaps due to reciprocal differences in telomerase expression. Stimulated hepatocytes are capable of prolonged and stunning regeneration, even replacing the liver. Only days after surgical excision or toxic damage, many animals may regenerate up to 90% of their liver (Goodman, 1974b; Robbins, 1974; Leevy, 1998). This astounding regeneration includes considerable histologic remodeling, resulting in a substantially normal organization and function. Although progress in this area is underway (Martinez-Hernandez and Amenta, 1995), this complex process remains poorly understood.

In cirrhosis, however, this regeneration—by cell division and cell replacement—is insufficient and abnormal. In continual hepatic insult, as in alcoholics, such abnormalities might be attributed solely to cell damage rather than senescence. The literature confirms that cirrhotic cells are dysfunctional, but not why, nor whether cell senescence plays a role.

With this caveat, consider the correlational evidence (Erlitzki and Minuk, 1999). Hepatic cirrhosis includes hepatocyte insult and continuous cell turnover (Pinzani and Gentilini, 1999). A portion occurs in stellate cells (Pinzani et al., 1998; Lang and Brenner, 1999), which become fibrogenic (Gressner, 1998). Accompanying turnover are changes in the extracellular matrix (which stellate cells manufacture) and an accelerated degradation of this matrix (Friedman, 1999b). Cytokine and chemokine production change (Lang and Brenner, 1999) with consequences for their main hepatic target, the stellate cell (Friedman, 1999a; Li and Friedman, 1999). Signaling pathways change (Pinzani et al., 1998) as does cell regulation generally, apoptotic regulation specifically (Gressner, 1998), and protease production and inhibition. Central to this alteration is the stellate cell (Burt, 1999), which divides repeatedly (Friedman, 1999a), activating and transforming from quiescent retinoid-rich cells to fibrogenic and contractile myofibroblasts, devoid of retinoids (Friedman, 1999a; Li and Friedman, 1999).

Cirrhosis is characterized by changes we anticipate in senescing cells, such as expression changes in growth response and other genes (Leevy, 1998), paracrine responses (Friedman, 1999a), matrix production (Friedman, 1999b), cell signaling, and stellate cell activation (Alcolado et al., 1997). Several studies in stellate cells have looked at the transcriptional and post-transcriptional regulation of type I collagen genes, transcription factor nuclear factor kappa B, focal adhesion kinase, and integrin-mediated signal transduction, as well as apoptosis (Lang and Brenner, 1999). There are complex interactive changes in the extracellular matrix, the stellate cells that produce it, and various cytokines in cirrhotic stellate cells. Specific receptors for matrix proteins, many in the integrin family, interact with and activate stellate integrins (such as $\alpha 1 \beta 1$) and are critical to contractility in cirrhosis (Bissell, 1998).

Like many stem cell populations, hepatocytes can express telomerase (Borges and Liew, 1997; Yui et al., 1998; Golubovskaya et al., 1999) at a low level (Burger et al., 1997). This activity increases in hepatic graft rejection (Goto et al., 2000), hepatitis, and cirrhosis (Tahara et al., 1995b), as well as in hepatic regeneration, where there is a generic increase in cytokines, growth response genes, and telomerase activity (Golubovskaya et al., 1997; Leevy, 1998; Inui et al., 2002). Even with telomerase present, most somatic cells senesce, albeit more slowly than otherwise. In rats, telomere erosion may be slower than in other tissues, but senescence is seen in late passaged cells (Golubovskaya et al., 1999), despite stable expression of telomerase with age (Golubovskaya et al., 1997). In keeping with predictions (one division per year, with fibroblasts losing 50–150 bp per year), human hepatocytes lose about 120 bp per year (Aikata et al., 2000), resulting in a mean of 10 kbp in normal 80-year-old hepatocytes. The mean is slightly, but significantly, lower in age-matched patients with chronic hepatitis or cirrhosis (Miura et al., 1997; Aikata et al., 2000). The correlation between telomere loss correlates and degree of pathology. It has been seen as suggesting that fibrotic scarring in cirrhosis might be a consequence of hepatocyte senescence (Gordon, 2000; Wiemann et al., 2002). As in other tissues, the loss of telomere length and senescence may predispose to malignancy (Golubovskaya et al., 1999), but conversely, high telomerase activity serves as a malignant marker (Takaishi et al., 2000).

An absence of telomerase causes cirrhosis and its expression reverses the process. Telomerase knockout mice showed defects in liver regeneration after surgical and toxic hepatic insults and good histological evidence of cirrhosis. Using an adenoviral delivery system, they then restored telomerase activity and telomere function. These mice showed histologic and physiologic reversal of the cirrhosis. This experiment argues for cell senescence in cirrhosis (Rudolph et al., 2000). As a result of damage (over time or acutely), hepatocytes die and the remaining hepatocytes divide and senesce, thereby altering not only their own gene expression but the function of cells that surround them. The resulting dysfunctional changes in physiology and histology define clinical cirrhosis.

Intervention

In at least one venue, diabetes, gastrointestinal interventions have been effective. The advent of injectable insulin transformed an acutely fatal disease into a chronic disease that injures most organs over time. The outcome is horrific. Most clinicians and diabetics pin their hopes on transplanted human β islet cells, a hope tethered to problems with immune rejection and replicative limits in culturing these cells. Although retroviral transfection of the hTERT gene induces telomerase activity, cell senescence cannot yet be prevented (Halvorsen et al., 2000).

Cirrhosis, a significant cause of death worldwide, has no effective treatment. Prevention consists of abstinence from alcohol and, where available, immunization against known viral hepatitides. Despite contemporary and projected advances (Dai and Jiang, 2001), current intervention consists of supportive measures, coupled with antivirals where appropriate.

Several experimental approaches take aim at the fibrotic and inflammatory changes, such as S-adenosylmethionine (in carbon tetrachloride-induced fibrosis), anti-inflammatory compounds, collagen synthesis inhibitors, and antioxidants. In vitro, polyenylphosphatidylcholine can protect against alcohol-induced fibrosis and cirrhosis, attenuate stellate cell transformation, and increase collagen breakdown and is under trial (Lieber, 1999). Agents that alter repair, cytokine mechanisms, stellate cell activation (Bissell, 1998), gluconeogenesis, fatty acid formation (Goodman, 1974b), cell replication, and collagen deposition (Leevy, 1998) are under consideration.

Since accelerated telomere loss has been suggested as a factor in hepatic cirrhosis (Rudolph et al., 2000), telomerase has become a target (Burger et al., 1997). Genetically stable, differentiated, nonmalignant, immortalized hepatocytes "would find broad applications in biomedical research, especially for . . . hepatocyte transplantation" (Cascio, 2001). Experimentally derived telomerase-positive hepatocytes may be morphologically and functionally normal, with microarray patterns similar to those of normal hepatocytes and without evidence of malignant transformation (Schnabl et al., 2002). Adenoviral delivery, as has been used in mice (Rudolph et al., 2000), or other methods deserve consideration in future human trials.

CHAPTER 17

The Eye

Structure and Overview

The eye is a remarkable gestalt—part skin, part muscle, part brain. Like Yeats and his chestnut tree (1963, p 214), it is not "the leaf, the blossom, or the bole," but something more, something critical to our view of the world. For most of us, our eyes create reality.

Scientifically, the eye is just as wondrous. To Charles Darwin (1859, p 133), the notion that "the eye with all its inimitable contrivances for adjusting the focus to different distances, for admitting different amounts of light, and for the correction of spherical and chromatic aberration could have been formed by natural selection, seems . . . absurd in the highest degree." But as Darwin argued at least as well if not as succinctly, biology cannot be understood save in the light of evolution and biology, and so we view the eye.

Each human eye is 24 mm in diameter, comprising a tough external membrane (the cornea and sclera), an intermediate vascular, pigmented layer (the iris, ciliary muscles, and choroid), and an internal layer (the retina), surrounding a central, transparent, relatively protein-free fluid (Gardner et al., 1975).

The cornea, a transparent layer made of keratocytes (fibroblasts), is continuous with the more peripheral sclera. Anterior to the anterior chamber, it is the first cell layer encountered as light enters the eye. Refraction occurs in the cornea, but only to a minor degree compared to the lens, although the cornea has the additional benefit of refraction at the air–tissue interface, which considerably increases its refractive effect upon incoming light. The cornea is avascular (permeation from the limbus serves to supply most nutrients instead), but has transparent, extensive, and exquisitely sensitive free nerve endings throughout. The opaque, white sclera is made of a tough meshwork of collagen and connects to the extraocular muscles that move the eye.

The centripetally deeper, intermediate layer (the uvea) has a more active role in ocular function. This layer contains most of the blood vessels and actively controls the aperture of the eye, the pupil. The ciliary muscles control the shape (and hence focal length) of the lens; the iris, a circular diaphragm of muscles, controls the depth of focus and amount of light that enters the eye via the pupil.

The innermost layer, the retina, is histologically complex, but in essence consists of an external pigment layer and an internal neural layer. In nocturnal animals such as cats, this external pigment layer (the tapetum) is reflective (hence the glow of cats' eyes at night), ensuring that the receptors have a higher rate of photon capture on the rebound and trading off excellent night vision for poorer resolution. In humans, this pigment layer is absorptive, which prevents such reflective scattering, trading off poorer night vision for improved resolution, particularly in the fovea. The fovea, which subtends about 1° of our visual field, is the center of the larger macula, which subtends about 3° of our visual field. This pigment layer is not a passive layer, merely absorbing superfluous photons. Cuboidal cells composing retinal pigment epithelium (RPE) are strategically placed between photoreceptors and the vascular uveal layer. These cells provide phagocytic recycling of photoreceptor membranes, are responsible for vitamin A (retinol) metabolism in the retina, maintain electrolyte homeostasis for normal photoreceptor function, and control all transport between the blood and retina (Schraermeyer and Heimann, 1999). As we shall see, this layer plays a role—one we do not understand—in the etiology of the most prominent age-related ocular diseases, macular degeneration.

The retinal layer lying closest to the center of the globe, the neural layer, consists of two types of photoreceptors. The more sensitive, color-blind, low-light rod receptors (good night vision, poor for fine resolution) are more prominent in the periphery. The color cones come in three types, each with its own characteristic spectral sensitivity. The three types of color-sensitive cones (good for day vision, excellent for resolution) are more prominent in the central macular region (the fovea). The complexity of the neural layer resembles a simpler version of the central cortex and appropriately so. This layer is no mere passive collection of receptors, but an extrusion (embryologically) of the central nervous system into the eye. As such, it extensively processes visual information prior to sending the information onto the brain via the optic nerve.

The optic nerves are among the largest nerve bundles of the body, containing in excess of one million carefully mapped tertiary axons, carrying information on color, contrast, and retinal location to the center of the brain, where the information is further processed in the thalamus before going on to the primary visual cortex and conscious awareness. The eye is capable of transmitting even more visual information than this one million–axon figure might suggest, because raw visual information is processed so heavily before it enters the optic nerve. For example, the brain does not receive information on light energy (brightness), but information on *differences* in light energy (Cornsweet, 1970). Likewise, each optic nerve axon transmits an information composite from several receptors, defining complex visual response fields, rather than single receptor events. The eye is not a passive transducer, taking photons and converting them into neuronal impulses, but a moderately sophisticated visual computer that processes information before "uploading" it to the brain. This complexity makes it vulnerable to damage and lies at the heart of its general pathology and ocular pathology characteristic of aging. It is a complexity value-added within the retina, for we do not see the world, but we create it.

Blake, in "The Everlasting Gospel," called the eyes "life's dim windows of the soul" (Keynes, 1966); but they are not only dim, they are usefully distorted. As Wordsworth wrote at Tintern Abbey, our eyes show us "what they half create and what [they] perceive" (Williams, 1952). This echoes the more banal epistemology of the visual physiologist, for whom our constructed, personal world depends "only indirectly" on incoming light waves, and is by necessity "different in many important ways from the world " (Cornsweet, 1970). We half-see, half-create our visual world. This act of creating makes our world our own, but likewise magnifies the vulnerability and cost of its loss in aging or disease.

Aging and Other Pathology

The poignant fear of blindness is a dread to the elderly: we lose our world, we lose our independence. The most profound aging pathology occurs in the retina and the most profound pathology of the retina is age-related macular degeneration (AMD). Retinal pathology is the primary cause of visual disability in aging (Michaels, 1994). It is predictable (Yoo and Adamis, 1998), can be seen even in the fourth decade (Uchino et al., 2001), and (of all retinal pathology) macular degeneration is the leading cause of blindness in the developed world (Garcia Layana, 1998), especially in patients over 60 years of age (Allikmets, 1999). Not only do we lack effective treatments for macular degeneration (Campochiaro et al., 1999), making it the major focus of geriatric ophthalmology, we do not understand the disease.

Genetic factors, as usual, play a role (Gorin et al., 1999; Zack et al., 1999), but their analysis has been difficult and we have few candidate genes so far (Allikmets, 1999). The few we do have include the *ABCR* gene and a linkage to markers in 1q25–q31. The *ABCR* gene, encoding a retinal rod photoreceptor-specific ATP-binding cassette transporter, may be involved, but is more closely associated with other ocular diseases (e.g., retinitis pigmentosa) than with macular degeneration. *ABCR* gene may increase the risk for macular degeneration even in heterozygous patients (Shroyer et al., 1999). Although there is probably a decrease in the effective capacity of the Na/K ATPase pump in the macula with aging, this is due to the decrease in cell numbers (at least in vitro), not in the number or efficacy of such pumps (Burke and McKay, 1993). In a tantalizing link with genes linked to Alzheimer dementia, the apoE ϵ4 allele has been associated with a reduced risk of macular degeneration (Yates and Moore, 2000).

Behavioral risk factors play a role. Although it is clear that tobacco use (Hawkins et al., 1999) increases the risk of macular degeneration, despite more than two decades of careful research into risk factors for macular degeneration, the role of hypertension, hypercholesterolemia, postmenopausal estrogen, diabetes, and dietary intake of fats and alcohol remain uncertain and (though perhaps likely) largely unproven (Snow and Seddon, 1999). Dietary intake of specific types of fat may be correlated to increased risk (Cho et al., 2001a; Seddon et al., 2001). Obesity, whether due to genetic or behavioral effects, is a risk factor (specifically, the waist-to-hip ratio) for macular degeneration, as well as other age-related ocular diseases (Klein et al., 2001). Photodamage may play a role in macular degeneration, as it does in skin aging (Cruickshanks et al., 2001).

Inadequate vitamin intake (particularly retinoids, hence the name) can cause retinal dysfunction, but the role of other dietary components are disputed. Oxidative damage in macular degeneration is attracting attention (Winkler et al., 1999). Dietary antioxidants (Congdon and West, 1999; Smith, 1999) and other dietary components (Pratt, 1999) have been suggested as having a prominent role in retinal pathology. There have been few data to support or undermine such claims (Cooper et al., 1999). Although larger trials (Age-Related Eye Disease Study Research Group, 2001a) suggest that there may be some protective effect of antioxidant and zinc supplementation (Jampol and Ferris, 2001), other work suggests that zinc has no protective role (Cho et al., 2001b). We remain distressingly far from a clear understanding or an effective intervention. Vascular changes in retrobulbar circulation have been blamed for macular degeneration and glaucoma (Harris et al., 2000), but this may be mere correlation, not cause.

Even though we know next to nothing about the functional etiology of macular degeneration, we do have a good grasp of the descriptive pathology (Fine et al., 2000; Gottlieb, 2002). This includes edema, infarction, exudates, hemorrhage, pigment dispersion, atrophy, and inflammation. It is typically bilateral but asymmetric in onset, with one eye leading the other in its pathology, rarely by more than 4 years (Michaels, 1994). Macular "holes" may occur, whose etiology remains speculative (Ho et al., 1998).

The loss of central vision in macular degeneration occurs because of exudative separation of the pigment epithelium from the photoreceptor layer. Pigment epithelium is protective and fails in this role—although whether primarily or secondarily is unknown—early in its pathology. This protective role is not well understood, but includes defenses against oxidative stress, detoxification of peroxides, the binding of zinc, and lysosomal degradation (Schraermeyer and Heimann, 1999). The uveal layer, just outward from (centrifugal to) the pigment epithelium, plays a role in some forms of macular degeneration. If new vessels invade from the choroid, the result may often be hemorrhage, defeating the presumed physiologic "purpose" of such neovascularization (Green, 1999). Moreover, it results in scarring and further loss of photoreceptors and, hence, vision.

At the fine histologic level, macular degeneration is associated with apoptosis of the retinal ganglion cells, perhaps initiated by ischemia, although other causes have been asserted, including cell senescence of the retinal pigment epithelial cells (Harris et al., 1999a). Vascular defects in the physiologically supportive uveal layer have been identified in nonexudative and exudative macular degeneration. That macular degeneration results in atrophy of the neurons and visual receptors is unfortunate; that it does so at the center of vision—in the macula—is tragic, for it prevents patients from seeing what they are looking at. Patients with macular degeneration typically are unable to recognize friends, watch television, or read. The blind spot is centered in their visual world.

Although macular degeneration may be the most poignant problem of visual aging, it is not the most common. Age-related lens and corneal changes, from simple presbyopia to cataract formation, lead the way in incidence and there are innumerable other visual problems that commonly occur (Fig. 17–1). They might best be categorized and discussed by their anatomic origin within the aging eye, sequentially from the cornea, through the anterior chamber, iris, and lens, until we reach the retina.

The cornea changes in a variety of ways with age (Faragher et al., 1997). These include a decrease in the cell density of keratinocytes (Murphy et al., 1984) by about

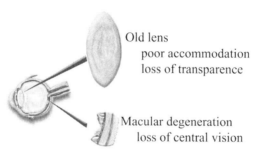

Old lens
poor accommodation
loss of transparence

Macular degeneration
loss of central vision

Figure 17–1 Aging eye tissue. In the aging eye, cell senescence in the lens may well explain presbyopic changes, such as poorer accommodation and altered transmission. Though consistent with current data, a parallel explanation of macular degeneration remains more speculative.

0.6% per year, although the variance increases, making cell density an unreliable biomarker of corneal aging. In addition, there are changes in the shape and optical properties (increasing the odds of astigmatism), an increasing intramolecular and intrafibrillar spacing in the intracellular matrix (possibly as a result of glycation; Malik et al., 1992, 1996), and in increase in the thickness of Descemet's membrane. The normally soluble proteins condense and clump, thereby scattering light (Friedrich, 2001). A catalog of imperfections becomes increasingly and finally overwhelmingly probable, and each of these imperfections can individually impair visual quality. Because the cornea has a high affinity for water (causing an inherent tendency toward cloudiness, i.e., light scattering), the impaired function of the active metabolic pump with age results in decreased visual clarity (Michaels, 1994). In addition, there is a decreased resistance to infection, a failure to regulate inflammation (Hobden et al., 1995), reduced phagocytosis (Hazlett et al., 1990), and changes in cell permeability (Chang and Hu, 1993) and metabolism (Lass et al., 1995). The cornea is slower to recover from hypoxic stress (Polse et al., 1989), probably because of senescent changes in the anterior segments (Faragher et al., 1997b) that normally prevent or limit damage from reactive oxygen species (Green, 1995). Corneal endothelial cells do not normally divide (Mishima, 1982; Treffers, 1982; Schultz et al., 1992) although they are capable of doing so.

The space between the cornea and lens, the anterior chamber, becomes shallower (partly as a result of age-related changes in the shape and size of the lens), increasing the risk and incidence of glaucoma (Michaels, 1994). When the pressure in the anterior chamber rises, as it does in glaucoma (sometimes suddenly), it is often painless, but it can present with progressive pain and cause damage to intraocular cells and the optic nerve and, ultimately, blindness. Risk factors include age, as well as genetic factors, myopia, venous occlusion, diabetes, infection, steroid use, and trauma. Atherosclerosis with secondary ischemia has recently been implicated (Harris et al., 1999a).

The iris changes predictably with age, but has little clinical pathology compared to the rest of the structures discussed here. The muscles of the iris stiffen and can demonstrate sarcopenia. They do not dilate the iris as fully as they do in the younger eye, contributing to poorer night vision and a loss of fine accommodation.

The lens, however, is a different matter and accounts for a large percentage of age-related clinical symptoms, often resulting in surgical excision. An onion-like collection of cells, varying in shape from outer flattened or cuboidal cells to the inner long fiber-like cells, it is serially accreted and continues to grow throughout life. This is a rare example where the body accumulates "dead" cells, not subject to turnover. As a result, the slow racemization of the amino acids can even be used to assess age in some species, such as whales (George et al., 1999), when alternative methods are not practical. The rate of cell division (and accretion) slows with age (Michaels, 1994). The overall mass of the lens triples by age 70 (Arking, 1998) and as it increases, it becomes visually dysfunctional. Specifically, the lens becomes stiffer (making it harder to change focus) and more prone to scatter light (giving poorer resolution at any focus; Beers et al., 1998). The ciliary muscle (which, when it contracts, accentuates the convexity of the lens to achieve a nearer focal length) atrophies, but presbyopia is more the result of lens stiffening (and increasing size) than it is of ciliary sarcopenia. Sclerosis of the lens substance and decreased elasticity of its capsule are the main causes of poorer accommodation.

Worldwide, cataracts are the leading cause of visual impairment as well as causing half of all blindness (Friedrich, 2001). The fine pathology of the aging lens is characteristic: there is degeneration of the epithelium, water clefts, lens fiber fragmentation, and crystal (Ca^{2+} and cholesterol) deposition (Michaels, 1994). At the biochemical level, the lens proteins themselves change. Among the commonest of the lens proteins are the α crystallins, chaperone proteins that putatively protect other lens proteins against oxidative, thermal, and chemical inactivation (Hook and Harding, 1998). Diabetes is a risk factor in cataracts, probably through its hyperglycemic effects on the lens proteins (Bron et al., 1998). Crystallins are normally formed exclusively of L-amino acids, but with age comes progressive racemization. The aspartates at positions 36 and 62 in the αA- and αB-crystallins from the aged human lens become highly racemized (D/L isomer ratios are 0.92 and 0.54, respectively). Strangely, the aspartates at positions 58 and 151 in αA-crystallin become inverted (D/L isomer ratios of 3.1 and 5.7, respectively), which is difficult to attribute to random processes and may therefore be due to active stereo inversion (Fujii et al., 1999). Some process in the cell (and a distinctly chirally biased process at that) putatively induces inversion after the α crystallin is synthesized. Such post-translational changes in α-crystallin properties are probably not unique, and other age-related protein changes, particularly in their chaperone and aggregation properties (Takemoto and Boyle, 1998), have been implicated in cataract formation in particular and age-related lens dysfunction in general. Classic cross-linking and Maillard reactions (Yin, 1996) are common within the lens (Shamsi and Nagaraj, 1999) and while oxidative damage may play a causal role, antioxidant supplementation may not be protective (Age-Related Eye Disease Study Research Group, 2001b; Jampol and Ferris, 2001). All of these factors may underlie the disturbed pattern of fiber-packing causing photon interference (and opacity) in the aging eye (Johnsen, 2000).

Although the retina is most notorious for macular degeneration, it has other age-related pathology, including the same garden-variety vascular pathology found elsewhere in the body. Such pathology is strikingly easier to diagnose and track because of the location. The retina provides a clear view of vascular abnormalities to routine ophthalmoscopy. Diabetic vasculopathy, loss of capillary beds, occlusive vasculopathy (thrombotic or embolic, with or without prior transient ischemia), and hemorrhage all contribute to visual loss in the elderly and can all be followed without invasive tests. Atherosclerosis, hypertension (Schubert, 1998), and diabetes are the major vascular risk factors in the retina as elsewhere, and their histopathologic changes parallel those classically seen in coronary and other critical arterial beds (Michaels, 1994). The retina manifests a plethora of other (at least ostensibly) nonvascular aging changes. It is increasingly likely to detach from its choroid, usually starting peripherally and progressing to central visual loss. Independent of the deficits of iris function, the neural elements of the retina are themselves slower to adapt to the dark, probably because of primary changes in retinal neuron interactions.

It is perhaps surprising then, that many visual functions do not change predictably with age (Enoch et al., 1999). Most age-invariant functions rest upon neural foundations, rather than upon lens, vascular, or fibroblast function. These invariant functions include visual receptor sensitivity to color, motion, and contrast. As in many other systems, it is the tissues with dividing cells that show primary pathology and correlate best with age-related dysfunction. Although many cells, such as retinal neurons, may demonstrate extensive secondary pathology, this is often accurately attributable to vascular (e.g., hypertensive and atherosclerotic), inflammatory, or other secondary etiologies. Nondividing neural cells show little in the way of primary age-related pathology, suggesting a likely role for cell senescence in the pathologies we associate with ocular aging.

The Role of Cell Senescence

The notion that cell senescence may play a role in age-related diseases of the eye is not novel. Indeed, several authors have suggested that cell senescence might play a role in age-related retinal (Eldred, 1993; Silvestri, 1997; Harris et al., 1999a), lens (Tassin et al., 1979; Colitz et al., 1999; Wolf and Pendergrass, 1999a), corneal (Faragher et al., 1997b), or other ocular dysfunction. We might expect such a role to parallel the degree to which cell turnover occurs in particular cell populations of the eye. Corneal epithelial cells divide continuously and turnover is complete within 5 to 7 days of terminal differentiation (LeBlond, 1964; Marshall, 1991). Other cells turn over only in response to stimulation, as in ocular stromal keratocytes (Tuft et al., 1993). Corneal endothelial cells do not demonstrate telomerase activity (Colitz et al., 1999) and seldom turn over, although they are capable of doing so (Mishima, 1982; Treffers, 1982; Schultz et al., 1992). When bovine corneal endothelial cells divide in vitro, they show clear evidence of ongoing telomere loss, correlated with increasing β-galactosidase and p53 expression (Whikehart et al., 2000). Data (Egan et al., 1998) support the conclusion that in vivo corneal endothelial cells do not divide, do not senesce, and are probably not involved in age-related pathology. But whether such cells have senescent characteristics and whether endothelial cell senescence might underlie certain ocular diseases of the elderly is uncertain. For example, the endothelial cells produce excessive amounts of abnormal basement membrane in Fuchs' endothelial dystrophy and this might be such an example of senescent cell changes in gene expression (Bergmanson et al., 1999).

While there is some information about stem cell function within the eye (Colitz et al., 1999), there is considerable uncertainty about it. To the extent that such populations (transiently or otherwise) express telomerase, this has substantial implications for the limits of cell senescence (and hence the pathology) within its intrinsic cell phenotypes. Which cells can divide within the adult human eye is under revision, and this revision extends into the retina. Although traditionally felt to consist largely of terminally differentiated, nondividing cells, some retinal cells are now known to be capable of division. In the adult mouse, for example, pigmented ciliary margin cells can act as stem cells, differentiating into rod photoreceptors, bipolar neurons, and ganglion cells (Tropepe et al., 2000), although again, their ability to express telomerase is unknown.

There is good circumstantial evidence that senescent cells are present in vivo in the older eye. Cultures of keratinocytes from old donors, for example, show an increased fraction of senescent cells (Salla et al., 1996; Faragher et al., 1997b). The same is true of human corneal endothelium, in which there is an age-related increase in senescent cells (Hoppenreijs et al., 1994; Blake et al., 1997; Faragher et al., 1997b). Whether such cells play a role in pathology, however, is a separate issue and needs addressing.

Corneal epithelial cells do not demonstrate telomerase activity (Colitz et al., 1999) and can be expected to senesce more rapidly than might other cells (such as lens epithelial cells) that do have such activity. The overall effect of cell senescence in vitro has been characterized as a catabolic change in cell behavior (Campisi, 1997b) and in fibroblasts is associated with collagen disorganization (Dimri et al., 1995). If this change in collagen metabolism occurs equally in the cornea (Faragher et al., 1997b), it explains the observed loss of collagen organization and appearance of collagen-free spaces (Kanai and Kaufman, 1973; Moller-Pederson, 1997). In a like vein, Faragher et al. (1997b) suggest that the increase in lipofuscin seen in the aging stroma may be the product of senescent cells, similar to the senescence-related accumulation found in retinal pigment epithelial cells (Rawes et al., 1997; Holz et al., 1999). Just as ultraviolet photons have been implicated in telomere shortening in fibroblasts (Kruk et al., 1995; Hande et al., 1997), the constant exposure to near-ultraviolet photons in the structures of the eye, including the retina, may play a role in cell senescence, including changes in gene expression, lipofuscin accumulation, and other markers of retinal pigment cell senescence (Li et al., 1999b).

Clinical findings in patients who demonstrate premature fibroblast senescence, such as those with Hutchinson-Gilford or Werner syndrome (vide supra), provide only limited data. Although anecdotal reports from the parents suggest that progeric children are intolerant of bright light (Fossel, clinical observation), there is no reported increase in macular degeneration and few published reports of ocular problems (e.g., Iordanescu et al., 1995) among progeric children in the literature. In Werner syndrome patients, by contrast, postsurgical healing of the cornea is severely impaired (Jonas et al., 1987). This parallels the clinical observations of a progressive defect in postophthalmic surgery healing in normally aging patients (Waring et al., 1991; Dutt et al., 1994; Chatterjee et al., 1996). An animal model (SAM mice) of accelerated senescence demonstrates early onset of retinal receptor cell and ganglion cell degeneration (Hosokawa and Ueno, 1999), although the degree of relevance to human ocular aging and macular degeneration is arguable.

Ocular photoaging has been offered as a parallel to dermal photoaging and may accelerate ocular senescence. Faragher et al. (1997b) point out that the cornea is saturated in "mutagenic" light, which induces "reactive senescence" in keratinocytes or deeper cell layers. Since turnover is continuous in the corneal epithelium, rapid senescence is expected especially in stem cells. Photoaging may accelerate this.

Within the cornea, a number of changes in function, probably reflecting changes in gene expression, occur and these have been tentatively attributed to cell senescence

(Faragher et al., 1997b). These include changes in cell permeability (Chang and Hu, 1993), changes in integrin subunit function (especially the distribution and continuity of the α6- and β4-subunit components of hemidesmosomes; Trinkaus-Randall et al., 1993), and a reduced ability to up-regulate expression of adhesion molecules (Hobden et al., 1995).

In the lens, ocular keratocytes, like fibroblasts elsewhere, senesce (Tassin et al., 1979; Dropcova et al., 1999), causing many changes in the lens. Some changes are simply morphological, such as the increase in finger-like projections seen in humans and other primates (Boyle and Takemoto, 1998), although morphological change may interfere with normal light transmission. More profound physiological changes occur. These include an increased production of fibronectin, cathepsin D, and hyaluronan, and a decreased synthesis of collagen, chrondroitin sulphate, interkeukin-6, and insulin-like growth factor. There is a general loss of sensitivity to many growth factors and cytokines in such cells (Grey and Norwood, 1995). Most changes described above (decreased metabolism, poorer recovery from hypoxia, increased light scattering secondary to impaired metabolic pumping of water) are attributable to changes in gene expression and to cell senescence.

Rather than being uniform, there are a variety of cells composing the lens that have an equal diversity of mitotic, and hence senescent, potentials (Colitz et al., 1999). The germinative epithelial cells that cover the lens have an unlimited replicative potential, while the older epithelial cells at the core of the lens are considered nonreplicative. Is this distinction correlated with cell senescence or telomerase activity and could it help explain cataract formation? Not simply. Telomerase activity is uniform throughout this cellular spectrum in normal canine, feline, and murine lens tissue. In epithelial cells from lens with cataracts, however, telomerase activity is increased, although it is not clear whether this causes or is the physiological response to cataract formation. Telomerase activity was present in such cells initially, but rapidly disappeared when cultured, a finding suggesting that telomerase activity is not constitutive but dependent on cell milieu and response. In stem cell reserves of the outer epithelial tissue, telomerase expression makes sense in preserving replicative capacity over the lifetime of the lens. In the quiescent, central cells, however, telomerase is more puzzling, perhaps functioning to protect the cell from inappropriate senescent changes induced by the ravages of high oxygen and ultraviolet exposure in this tissue (Colitz et al., 1999). Cell senescence in cataract formation is possible and speculation tempting (Wolf and Pendergrass, 1999), but even the sparse data available are complex and not unambiguously supportive.

Because it is the site of macular degeneration, the retina has received much attention, especially senescence in retinal pigment epithelial cells (Hjelmeland et al., 1999). Senescent retinal pigment epithelial cells have been suggested as playing a central role in age-related maculopathy and age-related macular degeneration (Matsunaga et al., 1999a), but data are sparse and their interpretation ambiguous (Hjelmeland, 1999). Retinal pigment epithelial cells demonstrate the characteristic changes of senescence in vitro, such as β-galactosidase expression as a function of in vivo age (Mishima et al., 1999) and in vitro population doubling and diminution of the mean terminal telomere restriction fragment length (Matsunaga et al., 1999a). But are these relevant to in vivo pathology? Studies of the in vitro kinetics of human retinal pigment epithelial cells parallel in vivo data and might plausibly be used to suggest that such senescence occurs in vivo (Rawes et al., 1997), although only limited in vivo data are available (Hjelmeland et al., 1999). Theoretically, the apoptosis of retinal ganglion cells associated with macular degeneration might be initiated indirectly by ischemia (due to vascular endothelial cell senescence) or directly by cell senescence of the retinal pigment epithelial cells (Harris et al., 1999a). There is good evidence that (at least in vitro) cell senescence of retinal pigment epithelial cells results in characteristic changes in gene expression. Moreover, these changes are characterized by the expression of genes whose products are inflammatory (Shelton et al., 1999) and resemble the pattern found in wound repair (Matsunaga et al., 1999b). This supports the hypothesis that the inflammation found in age-related ocular disease (e.g., macular degeneration) is not secondary to injury but may be primary, as it occurs in vitro in the absence of other cell types and solely as the result of senescence. It is not unreasonable to propose that macular degeneration result from cell senescence alone. Retinal pigment epithelial cells might senesce, become proinflammatory, and trigger the entire cascade of pathology that results in clinical disease. Although simplistic, there is little to contradict such a naive model and much to learn by testing it.

If retinal pigment epithelial cells do senesce in vivo, the consequent changes in gene expression might explain the observed abnormalities of the extracellular matrix, which in turn may promote the choroidal neovascularization that figures so prominently in the gross pathology (Campochiaro et al., 1999). The pattern of gene expression that occurs in senescent retinal pigment epithelial cells in vitro includes the repression of prostaglandin D synthetase, a potential retinoid binding protein, and cellular retinol binding protein-1 (Shelton et al., 1999). These changes, alone or as part of an overall alteration in the pattern of retinal gene expression, might be expected to have profound consequences for the function of the aging human retina in vivo. Other changes have been observed. The cells become altered in their signaling responses, for example, and are unable to respond to express collagen in response to low-serum conditions. Senescent retinal pigment epithelial cells in vivo, like those in vitro, demonstrate increased lipofuscin (Rawes et al., 1997). Such alterations in patterns of gene expression, defective responses to local cell signaling, and lipofuscin accumulation are expected, even predictable, in comprehensive explanations of ocular pathology. Similar parallels between behavior of in vivo and in vitro senescent cells are seen in human corneal cells (Faragher et al., 1997b).

Unfortunately, the cascade of pathology involved in macular degeneration is so complex that a host of hypotheses can be entertained without much fear of (or opportunity for) falsification. The role of apoptosis, rod-cone dependencies, trophic factor requirements, identifying the cells that produce trophic factors, cell–cell contact requirements, and other questions remain unanswered (Adler et al., 1999) and it is in these areas that cell senescence is likely to cause pathology. Our ignorance allows speculation but forbids certainty.

Intervention

The main spur to new interventions, based on cell senescence or not, is the lack of other effective therapeutic interventions for most age-related ocular diseases. Although extant therapies for cataracts (surgery), presbyopia (corrective lenses), and glaucoma (medication) may suffice, the same cannot be said for macular degeneration, for which there is little to offer. Current therapy, such as the destruction of neovascularization (e.g., using verteporfin and 689 nm wavelength light from a nonthermal diode laser), is secondary, not fundamental or preventative. Some age-related ocular pathology can be prevented or ameliorated, at least in lens opacification. Avoidance of ultraviolet exposure is an accepted example; estrogen replacement a more tenuous possibility (Worzala et al., 2001). In macular degeneration, the initial data on dietary supplementation are supportive (Age-Related Eye Disease Study Research Group, 2001a), but their value as a preventive therapeutic intervention remains uncertain (Jampol and Ferris, 2001).

There is a considerable body of data, however, supporting the value of caloric restriction for the aging eye. With regard to cell proliferation in the aging lens, for example, caloric restriction is protective against chronically inflicted oxidative damage in murine epithelial cells (Li et al., 1997, 1998b). Telomere shortening in these same lens cells is slowed (Pendergrass et al., 2001) and replicative potential is maintained longer in restricted mice (Pendergrass et al., 1995; Wolf et al., 1995). Not surprisingly then, cataract formation is delayed in calorically restricted mice (Wolf et al., 2000). Nor is the lens the only site of age-related ocular effects. Caloric restriction delays the changes in the aqueous collecting channels of aging mice, suggesting its potential value in delaying or preventing glaucoma (Li and Wolf, 1997).

Given current interventions, research on ocular pathology (even falsifying the role of cell senescence) would be useful. The possibility that senescence-related changes in gene expression underlies macular dystrophy is testable. In testing the hypothesis, changes in gene expression become ready targets for rationally designed drugs (Campochiaro et al., 1999), even if the overall theory were wrong.

Even if cell senescence were to underlie macular degeneration, genes and gene products, rather than the overall process of cell senescence, might remain the more appropriate and facile therapeutic target. This possibility arises from the recurrent concern over malignant transformation. There is no evidence to support this concern and a considerable absence of evidence in studies looking for such data (Jiang et al., 1999). Admittedly, however, replicative limits are likely to represent one of the cell's bulwarks against malignancy and, as such, deserve a minatory respect. As a result, some workers have expressed concern that inactivating such a mechanism is "intrinsically undesirable" and prefer modification of the results of senescence rather than senescence itself (Faragher et al., 1997b). The initial results of telomerase knock-in mice show the predictable increase in tissue healing and predilection to malignancy (Gonzalez-Suarez et al., 2001; Artandi et al., 2002) that we can expect from constitutive expression. Murine corneal fibroblasts transfected with hTERT and constitutively expressing telomerase, maintain their telomeres over time and demonstrate few of the normal signs of fibroblast senescence (Gendron et al., 2001). Telomerized human retinal pigment epithelial cells express normal proteins, melanize, and remain capable of differentiation (Rambhatla et al., 2002). In either case, cancer or age-related disease, a clearer understanding of the putative role of cell senescence provides testable targets for clinical intervention. Even lacking such understanding, the potential benefits and low risks (Jiang et al., 1999) of retinal cell transfection are clinically attractive.

Besides the possibilities of direct cell telomerization (to prevent senescence) or indirect drug therapy (aimed at the gene products of senescence), there are other avenues by which an understanding of cell senescence may offer clinical benefits. The ability to use stem cells or immortalized, differentiated cells to grow specific organs or tissues is in its infancy but has enormous potential (Lanza et al., 1999a, 1999b; Perry, 2000).

Already, telomerized or otherwise immortalized cells can be used to construct some tissues (Funk et al., 2000) and to replace those damaged by age-related pathology. Although the possibility of doing so for complex cell assemblages such as those of the neural retina is distant, corneal replacements are already feasible. Using recombinant viruses (containing HPV16 genes E6 and E7) or direct transfection (with genes encoding SV40 large T antigen, pSV3neo, and adenovirus E1A 12S), Griffith et al. (1999c) immortalized human corneal cells. They constructed a "human corneal equivalent" comprising all three main layers (epithelium, stroma, and endothelium). Their results suggest that we might be capable of constructing corneal transplants made of viable human cells with low rejection risk. Such immortalized corneas are themselves experiments, allowing us to further assay cell senescence in cataracts, although it is not clear that transformation with E6 and E7 is sufficient for long-term immortalization (Coursen et al., 1997). Although we might reasonably speculate that cataract formation may be dependent on cell senescence (Wolf and Pendergrass, 1999) and might therefore predict that cell immortalization prevents the onset and progression of cataracts, these theories are unproven.

The most tantalizing approach to intervention is direct extension of in vivo ocular cell telomeres. Although this possibility has been discussed privately, the difficulties of transfection or induction of telomerase intraocularly preclude its being among the first intervention that will likely be tried. Intraocular cell senescence therapy remains tempting, however, partly because of the lack of effective therapy, especially for macular degeneration, and partly because of the ease of access compared to other organs that might otherwise be more important clinically (though not necessarily by ophthalmologists or all patients), such as neural or vascular structures. The clinical importance of the eye suggests that interventions will be attempted soon after dermatologic or perhaps endothelial interventions have been tried and found effective.

CHAPTER 18

Towards Therapy

Death is dialog between
The spirit and the dust,
"Dissolve," says death. The spirit, "Sir,
I have another trust."

Emily Dickinson

Interventions

No model of disease has value beyond its ability to improve lives. Despite strident claims, there are no currently effective clinical interventions for human aging. There are interventions that affect a number of biomarkers (e.g., free radicals), superficial cosmetic changes (e.g., retinoic acid), physiological correlates (e.g., hormones), mean lifespan (seatbelts), and age-associated disease mortality (e.g., medications lowering cardiovascular mortality). None of these are clinically effective in altering aging (Butler et al., 2002).

Genetic therapy allows us to affect fundamental and previously inaccessible cellular mechanisms, including those of aging. If changes in gene expression cause cell aging, which underlies age-related disease, then we may be able to alter aging. We can alter gene expression in vitro with beneficial outcomes in multiple human cell phenotypes (e.g., Bodnar et al., 1998; Vaziri, 1998) and in reconstituted human skin (Funk et al., 2000). Resultant cells and tissues have normal physiology, morphology, and function. Extending this work into other tissues and in vivo therapy requires substantial work.

Criticism has been marred by erroneous assumptions, as well as a complex conceptual and historical context (Hirshbein, 2001). Recently, however, many have come to regard aging as "a disease that can be cured" (Guarente and Kenyon, 2000). Aging drives disease and is therefore an appropriate target for clinical research (Osiewacz and Hamann, 1997). To eschew calling aging a disease, despite associated disabilities (Hayflick, 2000b), risks trivializing the loss of health and independence (Kipling and Faragher, 1997; Anderson-Ranberg et al., 2001; Nybo et al., 2001). Aging encroaches upon and circumscribes our lives (Mirowsky, 1997) and, like other diseases, is a state that "places individuals at an increased risk of adverse consequences" (Temple et al., 2001). Aging is the ubiquitous disease.

Moreover, accepting aging as inevitable impedes advances. Popular attempts to laud the virtues of "successful" aging (Rowe and Kahn, 1997, 2000) raise the specter of successfully having Alzheimer disease, heart disease, or arthritis. Curing polio required (and requires; Vastag, 2001a) hard work, not successful fatalism. Microbial disease was accepted in the 1870s. Its basic mechanisms were novel and poorly understood even by medical scientists, who criticized evidence that bacteria caused disease (King, 1991). Medical success is measured in preventions and cures, not conceptual fit (Weng and Hodes, 2000) and certainly not in successful endurance.

Techniques

Resetting gene expression is the most efficient point of aging intervention; relengthening telomeres is the most efficient way to reset gene expression. There are three major approaches involving relengthening of the telomere via hTERT. We can telomerize cells ex vivo, insert an hTERT gene into cells in vivo (Shay and Wright, 2000c; Steinert et al., 2000), or induce native hTERT expression in vivo.

Ex vivo telomerization is technically the simplest. Human cells are removed from the donor, telomerized, and returned. This is easiest for blood-borne cells, such as lymphocytes or circulating stem cells. Absent telomerization, this procedure is already used in bone marrow transplantation, a procedure whose success telomerization might improve, particularly in serial transplantation. The procedure might also be considered for HIV patients, trisomy 21 with immune senescence, or normal immune senescence. Other tissues, such as skin (Funk et al., 2000), could be extracted, telomerized, and replaced. We might reconstitute human skin, myocardial tissue, lenses, and other tissue. Though technically feasible, ex vivo reversal of tissue aging has not been attempted.

Embryonic stem cells have similar potential (Lanza et al., 1999a, 1999b; Perry, 2000). Although raising ethical questions (Lanza et al., 2000a; Juengst and Fossel, 2000), somatic cells might theoretically be used to generate "embryonic" stem cells (Wakayama et al., 2001). Embryonic stem cells are capable of creating any cell phenotype (Thomson et al., 1998) and may express telomerase (Lanzendorf et al., 2001), avoiding subsequent senescence (Amit et al., 2000). Somatic stem cells (Boogaerts et al., 1996) are routinely used to replace marrow-derived cells in cancer (Basser, 1998; Lazarus, 1998), usually after high-dose chemotherapy for malignancy (Territo, 1997; Thomas, 1997; McGuire, 1998). They have been used in autoimmune disorders (Exner et al., 1997; Snowden and Brooks, 1999; Burt et al., 2000), including rheumatoid arthritis (Brooks, 1997), systemic lupus erythematosus, and scleroderma (Tyndall, 1997). Additional uses may include corneal scarring (Kruse and Volcker, 1997; Dua and Azuara-Blanco, 2000), central nervous system diseases (Ourednik et al., 1999; Armstrong and Svendsen, 2000; Bjorklund and Lindvall, 2000), and other diseases (Aubin, 1998). Within poorly understood limits (Slack, 2000; Wagers et al., 2002), specific stem cell lines can be induced to differentiate (or de-differentiate) into replacement cells (Sanchez-Ramos et al., 2000; Theise et al., 2000; Woodbury et al., 2000), including skin (for burn patients), cardiomyocytes (replacing infarcted heart tissue), or insulin-producing β cells (in diabetic patients). Neural stem cells may give rise to myocytes (Galli et al., 2000), muscle satellite cells to hematopoetic cells (Mahmud et al., 2002), and oligodendrocyte precursor cells to generic neural stem cells (Kondo and Raff, 2000), and other cells might likewise be used to replace damaged neural or other tissues (Kaji and Leiden, 2001), although within limits (Castro et al., 2003). While making progress in understanding cell differentiation (Watt and Hogan, 2000; Lumelsky et al., 2001), much remains unknown (Brazelton et al., 2000; Mezey et al., 2000) and obstacles are significant (Weissman, 2000).

Telomerization has the advantage of preventing replicative senescence (Harley, 2000). Telomerized skin grafts, pancreatic islet cells, lymphocyte transplants, chondrocyte joint remodeling, and treatment of osteoporosis via systemically administered osteoblasts all have clinical potential. The functional normality of such tissues is supported by in vitro work and a few studies of hTERT-transfected ex vivo cells, such as adrenocortical cells (Thomas et al., 2000a). Human corneal equivalents have been created, although with virally immortalized (SV40 large T antigens, pSV3neo, and adenovirus E1A 12S) cells that demonstrate random chromosomal breaks, structural rearrangements, and aneuploidy (Griffith et al., 1999c). Telomerized cells lack such damage.

The second approach, in vivo insertion of hTERT gene, poses additional questions that ex vivo approaches can evade: the percentage of cell take, the degree of hTERT expression, and the extent of telomere reset. These are critical to effective use of "telomerase-based gene therapy of age-related diseases" (Samper et al., 2001). Ex vivo approaches permit selection of cells that express telomerase, replicate, and have normal gene expression before reinsertion. Fortunately, cells that are "not completely senescent" can probably be rescued (Steinert et al., 2000), even with critically short telomeres, as in telomerase-deficient mice (Terc−/−). Similarly, HUVEC cells can be reliably rescued at 88/95 (93% of cell lifespan) doublings (Morin, 1999). While rescuing senescent cells is critical, so is functional gene delivery in the first place. One brute-force approach, useful in skin, is a commercially available, high-pressure gene gun. Other approaches include adenovirus (Rudolph et al., 2000), Sendai and other viral vectors, liposomes, dendrimers, and transcatheter application. Targeted introns (Guo et al., 2000a) and similar approaches may improve control of gene expression. Human clinical trials are likely to include syndromes in which telomerase dysfunction is known to underlie pathology: dyskeratosis congenita, Bloom syndrome, Fanconi anemia (Multani et al., 2002), and Hutchinson-Gilford syndrome. In addition, human trials are planned for elderly human patients with diabetic skin ulcers, venous stasis ulcers, and normal aging skin. Trials are planned in 2004.

The third approach induces expression of native hTERT, the most promising target in senescing cells (Santos Ruiz et al., 2000; Fajkus et al., 2002). Although gene insertion of telomerase may be effective (Gonzalez-Suarez et al., 2001) and even safe (Steinert et al., 2000), it is inelegant: hTERT gene is already present in human cells. Moreover, the first two approaches demand gene delivery to all senescing cells; delivering an inducer may be easier and more effective.

Gene induction might allow control of hTERT systemically. Cancer cells unlock hTERT; stem cells turn hTERT on and off predictably. Controlling hTERT, we might emulate natural mechanisms controlling expression. Imagine a dark room (a cell without telomerase). We know that the lights work (telomerase can be expressed), but we don't know where the switches are. The first two approaches are clumsy: we either change the entire room (ex vivo) or import a generator and light bulb (transfection). The third solution (induction) is the more elegant: we find the light switch. The requirements for specific hTERT inducers are daunting. Human chromosomes contain on the order of 10^5 genes. We require a molecule specific for hTERT, with no significant effects on other genes. This informational specificity implies a relatively large, complex molecule, but simultaneously small (or lipophilic) enough to penetrate cell and nuclear membranes and access the chromosome, while being stable and without detrimental effects. On the plus side, the complexity and contextual nature of hTERT regulation (Cong et al., 1999) may offer several possible targets for intervention.

Transcription begins with the enhancer, a short section of DNA with multiple activator binding sites. Activators bind and recruit the RNA polymerase II (Pol II) cascade and other chromatin-modifying proteins that bind the core promoter. Multiple different (and synergistic) activators are possible. This variety and complexity permit enormous adaptability and an ability to integrate information from local cell environment, distant environment within the organism, cell phenotype, and developmental stage of the organism (Struhl, 2001). This may include senescence, i.e., telomeric signaling, through its effects on the pattern of gene expression. Whether telomeric signaling is modular (acting independently of other inputs) or requires specific nonmodular enhancers (acting only if all enhancers are present) to permit and cause cell senescence is unknown.

Information on telomerase regulation and specific promoters has been slowly accumulating, but is accelerating. The hTERT gene is on chromosome 5p (Bryce et al., 2000; Shay and Wright, 2000b); its regulation is under tight control of promoter (Takakura et al., 1999; Koga et al., 2000; Kyo et al., 2000b) and repressor mechanisms (Fujimoto et al., 2000; Kanaya et al., 2000).

The hTERT promoter was first characterized in 1999; considerable interest now focuses on the hTERT 5' gene regulatory region (Poole et al., 2001). The hTERT promoter lacks TATA and CAAT boxes and is in a CpG island (Horikawa et al., 1999) with an E-box (CACGTG) binding site and sites for Sp1 and several for c-Myc (Takakura et al., 1999; Wick et al., 1999; Wu et al., 1999c). hTERT and c-myc are expressed in actively dividing cells, but down-regulated in nondividing cells. Even though their constitutive expression can induce immortalization, c-myc rapidly and directly induces hTERT expression independently of proliferation status (Greenberg et al., 1999b). Myc-induced activation of the hTERT promoter requires an E-box. c-Myc-ER-induced accumulation of hTERT mRNA takes place without de novo protein synthesis (Greenberg et al., 1999b). The hTERT gene is a direct transcriptional target of c-Myc. However, TERT is unable to substitute for c-Myc in transforming rodent fibroblasts, which suggests that c-myc has a role beyond merely inducing telomerase (Greenberg et al., 1999b).

In a series of papers, Kyo's group has clarified the factors influencing the promoter region. The 5' region (containing the E-box) binds Myc/Max and 3' region (containing the GC-box) binds Sp1; both are essential for transactivation. Predictably, mutations of the E-box or GC-box decreased transcription, while Myc/Max or Sp1 overexpression led to activation, with Sp1 required for Myc/Max effects. Fibroblasts show dramatic induction of c-Myc and Sp1 when replicative senescence is overcome via telomerase activation. Apparently, c-Myc and Sp1 are major determinants of hTERT expression (Kyo et al., 2000b). Maximal promoter activity occurs in a 59 bp region (−208 to −150), probably containing the Myc binding site. c-Myc plasmid insertion (Horikawa et al., 1999) or retroviral infection (Falchetti et al., 1999) causes rapid telomerase transcription. hTERT is also transcriptionally regulated by regulatory elements distant from the 5' flanking region, independent of c-Myc and coregulators. (Ducrest et al., 2001).

Specific mechanisms of hTERT repression are gradually becoming understood. There is a 400 bp silencer upstream from the hTERT promoter including multiple binding motifs for myeloid-specific zinc finger protein 2 (MZF-2). Mutation within this region activates TERT transcription. Overexpression of MZF-2 causes down-regulation of hTERT transcription and telomerase activity (Fujimoto et al., 2000). Nor is this the only zinc finger gene associated with senescence or maintenance of the nondividing state: a novel KRAB zinc finger gene, *ZFQR*, is up-regulated in nondividing senescent and quiescent human fibroblasts. Overexpression inhibits cell cycle entry and represses transcription (Ran et al., 2001). The promiscuous p53 can likewise repress telomerase (Kanaya et al., 2000) and play multiple roles (Sharpless and DePinho., 2002). As telomeres shorten and genomic instability increases in telomerase knockout mice, p53 is activated and growth arrest and/or apoptosis ensues. Deleting p53 attenuates these events, but only if deleted early in the cascade (Chin et al., 1999). Several telomerase repressors are on chromosome 3p (Loughran et al., 1997; Horikawa et al., 1998; Mehle et al., 1998; Cuthbert et al., 1999), probably including wnt-5a (Olson et al., 1998; Olson and Gibo, 1998). hTR is located on 3q26.3 (Soder et al., 1997), correlating with "local" telomerase repression (Newbold, 1997). Chromosome 10p also contains a repressor site (Nishimoto et al., 2001). A number of nonspecific agents cause hTERT repression. A demethylating agent, 5-aza-CR, represses transcriptional activity of the hTERT promoter and "the E-box within the core promoter was responsible for this down-regulation." This agent reactivates p16 expression and represses c-Myc expression in some cells (Kitagawa et al., 2000).

Transcriptional switching has been accomplished using a conditional v-Myc-estrogen receptor protein (Falchetti et al., 1999) with resultant estrogen-dependent telomerase activity. Estrogen, specifically, 17β-. Jekyll and Mr. Hyde" molecule with both enormous benefits and unexpected pitfalls (Prescott and Blackburn, 1999). Several predictable risks have been identified. The most obvious is cancer. Not only may we increase cancer incidence merely by extending lifespan, i.e., increasing the denominator—the population at risk (Aragona et al., 2000a), but we may increase the numerator (actual incidence) as well. The latter possibility (caused by obviating limits to cell division) has already been discussed, as well as two potential mitigating factors (increased estradiol, appears to increase hTERT expression (and activity) in cells expressing estrogen receptors (Kyo et al., 1999c). Several proto-oncogenes and tumor suppressor genes play a role in hTERT regulation, including c-Myc, Bcl-2, p21(WAF1), Rb, p53, PKC, Akt/PKB, and protein phosphatase 2A (Liu, 1999). Hsp90-related chaperones (Akalin et al., 2001) play a nontranscriptional regulatory role in telomerase activity, increasing assembly via hsp90 chaperoning.

Several laboratories are currently working on, and may have identified, effective hTERT promoters with molecular characteristics consistent with potential clinical efficacy. None of these compounds have been take to animal trials, let alone phase I human trials. Given the research vector, this work will likely have either borne fruit or proven ineffective prior to publication of this text. A final note on research within the biotech sector is the possibility of using transduced hTERT protein directly in human cells. Originally considered and discounted for technical reasons in the mid-1990s, this possibility has resurfaced (as technical assumptions and limitations shift) and is again being considered using a slightly altered technique (Becker-Hapak et al., 2001; Wadia and Dowdy, 2002). Which of these techniques will prove most effective in giving us clinical control of hTERT expression, activity, and turnover remains to be seen. Putative medical benefits remain still exactly that.

Caveats

Several caveats pertain. The first is that of efficacy. Many conclude that breakthroughs "appear to be just on the horizon" (Hodes et al., 1996a), but "we have not yet determined whether telomere shortening plays a significant role in human aging or in age-related pathology, and it is therefore unclear whether telomere extension or maintenance is likely to modify these processes. These caveats notwithstanding, the mechanisms of telomere length regulation and telomere activity are topics that continue to command considerable interest from the perspective of basic biology and for their possible application to human aging and disease" (Warner and Hodes, 2000).

The second caveat is risk. Historically, risks we can predict are often minor compared to those we cannot. Equally, in our ignorance, we often magnify what prove to be illusory dangers. The best minatory advice is that of Pope's *Essay on Criticism* (Beck, 1969, p 403): "be not the first by whom the new are tried, nor yet the last to lay the old aside." Telomerase may be a Dr. Jekyll and Mr. Hyde molecule with both enormous benefits and unexpected pitfalls (Prescott and Blackburn, 1999). Several predictable risks have been identified. The most obvious is cancer. Not only may we increase cancer incidence merely by extending lifespan, i.e., increasing the denominator, the population at risk (Aragona et al., 2000a), but we may increase the numerator (actual incidence) as well. The latter possibility (caused by obviating limits to cell division) has already been discussed, as well as two potential mitigating factors (increased genomic stability and improved immune surveillance).

Less obvious risks may also be clinically relevant, such as the "Humpty Dumpty phenomena" and functional mismatch (Fossel, 1996). The former, a caveat of omission, occurs when relevant cell populations of a senescent tissue are sufficiently damaged as to preclude rescue via telomerase. Infarcted myocardium, destroyed joint surfaces, and wholesale neuronal losses are examples of such cases, where neither all the king's horses nor any degree of telomerase activation could be expected to offer clinical benefit. The second, a caveat of commission, occurs when beneficial changes in one tissue outstrip the functional capacity of another, on which it is dependent. We might, for example, imagine increasing muscle mass and metabolic activity without sufficient parallel improvement in vascular supply, causing ischemia—a functional mismatch. The degree to which these and other problems have clinical relevance remains to be seen. We might, however, use them to infer other, as yet unpredicted side effects in the clinical use of telomerase for age-related disease.

Obstacles

Remaining obstacles fall into two categories, technical and regulatory, with the former the more compelling. Initial extrapolation predicted prototypic clinical use in about two decades (Fossel, 1996) and while there is little reason to alter this prediction, it remains merely prediction. Clinical use requires not only proof of efficacy (which has been demonstrated in cells and reconstituted tissue) but identification of a lead compound, in vitro demonstration, animal validation, and successful overcoming of routine regulatory hurdles.

Such regulatory hurdles have generally (and on the whole, appropriately) taken the stance that efficacy cannot be aimed at aging but must be aimed at diseases, whether age-related or not. In the United States, this position (on the part of the Food and Drug Administration [FDA]) has two related rationales: the first to force claimants to discuss interventions in a concrete fashion, the second is to permit the use of accepted and definable markers of clinical success. Historically, there have been widespread claims of anti-aging efficacy that rest on two ambiguities: the ambiguity of defining aging and the (consequent) difficulty of proving (or disproving) intervention. By affirmed intent, the FDA stance forces discussions to become concrete and claims to become strictly refutable. The practical outcome in the current context is that any telomerase-based intervention must apply for investigational status in a specific tissue venue. Which tissue is chosen will determine the rapidity and costs of regulatory passage, the acceptability of risks, and the likelihood of success. Initial trials are, for a number of reasons, likely to occur in skin, then progress to arteries and joints. As ever, acceptance for labeled use in one tissue venue does not preclude off-label use in another.

Events controlling progress down this cascade are every bit as complex as those controlling the most arcane biological cascade. Individual beliefs, limitations, and actions determine collective human progress, sometimes slowing, sometimes accelerating its course. Microbes were first described 400 years ago and their role in human disease more than 100 years ago, yet we are only partially capable of clinically arresting microbial disease. The first description of somatic cell mortality versus germ cell immortality was made more than a century ago (Weismann, 1884). Hayflick, who first defined cell senescence, doubts its relevance to human disease or that benefits might accrue from intervention (Hayflick, 1998d). Although we may yet employ our knowledge to ameliorate, even eradicate, the bulk of human disease and suffering, such progress requires not only technical success and regulatory perseverance but also belief, resources, and application. Perhaps, like microbial therapy, success also lies at the mercy of the slow whims of history.

Implications

Clinical implications of cell senescence are unprecedented in breadth and depth of application and in fiscal efficacy. The closest historical analogy, that of curing numerous bacterial infections via knowledge of microbiology and immunity, is suggestive but insufficient. Telomerase therapy promises to break upon us more suddenly and achieve far more than microbial theory. The breadth of application of cell senescence stems from its clinical implications for all age-related disease, regardless of tissue. Its role in basic pathology suggests its depth of efficacy in treatment and prevention. Fiscal efficacy derives from low predicted costs compared to other, currently more expensive and far less effective interventions. In terms of health-care costs alone, we can expect that, again without social precedent, we will see a drop in the percentage of the gross national product spent on medical care, while dramatically improving both medical outcome and, succinctly, human lives. The most profound implication, however, is that such intervention is likely to have the totally unprecedented effect of increasing not merely the mean but the maximum healthy human lifespan. The latter has cultural, social, and economic implications that are impossible to adequately predict and, although likely to generate controversy (Bova, 2000), have yet received only minimal attention. Such implications are likely to be incomparably far-reaching (Fossel, 1996, 1998a, 1998c; Banks and Fossel, 1997), but cannot be adequately or appropriately pursued here.

A number of authors have suggested that not only is aging mutable (Rose and Nusbaum, 1994), but maximum lifespan is likewise (Mueller and Rose, 1996; Banks and Fossel, 1997; Rose, 1999a). Some have criticized suggestions that human lifespan has intrinsic and inevitable limits that cannot be overcome by technical advances not supported by evidence, but only by "ex cathedra pronouncement and mutual citation" (Oeppen and Vaupel, 2002). Not only may technical advances alter aging (Harris, 2000), but an increasing body of current research is specifically "designed to understand and eventually modify the rate of aging" (de Grey et al., 2002). Recent work in cell biology and genetics has suggested that at the most fundamental level, not only are age-related diseases the outcome of cell senescence, but our growing understanding of cell senescence, senescence-associated gene expression, and telomerase biology will soon allow us to prevent, ameliorate, or to some degree even reverse such pathology. This potential includes an effective control of cancer. The dual assumptions that aging is merely the passive accumulation of wear and tear and age-related diseases are merely the outgrowth of such passively accumulated dysfunction are erroneous. Aging occurs as the result of a predictably altered pattern of gene expression specific to cell type and it culminates in dysfunction and disease. In vitro, the process can be prevented or (within predictable limits) reversed. Although many other approaches might be feasible, the most efficient treatment of age-related diseases, cancer, or aging will be the reversible control of native telomerase activity (Steinert et al., 2000) by induction of expression and, in cancer, by telomerase inhibitors. Within technical limits, such intervention is feasible and within the next decade or so (Collins, 2001), we will likely be engaged in trials to extend the human lifespan.

Dorian Gray, in Oscar Wilde's infamous and eponymous novel (Wilde, 1890), said that "we never get back our youth." His book was a portrait of the evil inherent in a grasping for not health, but the outward show of youth at the cost of one's soul. Faustian bargains notwithstanding, health itself has much to offer; the greater evil lies not in bringing health but in doing nothing. Compassion for our fellow creatures needs no defense and is the "firmest and surest guarantee of pure moral conduct" (Schopenhauer, 1965). Until now, we had little to offer those suffering from the diseases of aging, but as this changes, so do our ethical responsibilities. An ethical chasm exists between not helping others because of our inability to intervene and our intentional declining to intervene (Juengst and Fossel, 2000; Fossel, 2003). As we gain the ability to prevent or cure aging diseases, we also gain ethical responsibilities to those who suffer.

The human race has yet to grasp the complex dilemmas of our own natures or to understand what yet remains necessary if we are to attain even a juvenile form of civilization. Chief among obstacles are our ignorance, an inability to think adequately, and a dearth of human kindness. It may, at times, appear impossible that we can ever overcome such problems. It may appear equally impossible that we can ever overcome aging and the abundant human diseases in which aging is manifested. Our limits are not set within our world, nor in any heaven we may conceive. Impossibilities are defined by people, not nature.

References

Abdel-Salam IM, Khaled HM, Gaballah HE, Mansour OM, Kassem HA, Metwaly AM. Telomerase activity in bilharzial bladder cancer. Prognostic implications. *Urol Oncol* 6:149–153, 2001.

Abdenur JE, Brown WT, Friedman S, Smith M, Lifshitz F. Response to nutritional and growth hormone treatment in progeria. *Metabolism* 46:851–856, 1997.

Abdul-Ghani R, Ohana P, Matouk I, Ayesh S, Ayesh B, Laster M, Bibi O, Giladi H, Molnar-Kimber K, Sughayer MA, de Groot N, Hochberg A. Use of transcriptional regulatory sequences of telomerase (hTER and hTERT) for selective killing of cancer cells. *Mol Ther* 2:539–544, 2000.

Abrass CK. The nature of chronic progressive nephropathy in aging rats. *Adv Ren Replace Ther* 7:4–10, 2000.

Adams MR, Kinlay S, Blake GJ, Orford JL, Ganz P, Selwyn AP. Atherogenic lipids and endothelial dysfunction: mechanisms in the genesis of ischemic syndromes. *Annu Rev Med* 51:149–167, 2000.

Adams SP, Hartman TP, Lim KY, Chase MW, Bennett MD, Leitch IJ, Leitch AR. Loss and recovery of Arabidopsis-type telomere repeat sequences 5'-(TTTAGGG)(n)-3' in the evolution of a major radiation of flowering plants. *Proc R Soc Lond B Biol Sci* 268:1541–1546, 2001.

Adelfalk C, Lorenz M, Serra V, von Zglinicki T, Hirsch-Kauffmann M, Schweiger M. Accelerated telomere shortening in Fanconi anemia fibroblasts—a longitudinal study. *FEBS Lett* 506:22–26, 2001.

Adetola A, Pan D, Martins D, Norris KC. Magnitude or acid-base and electrolyte disorders in the elderly. *Ethn Dis* 9:479, 1999.

Adibzadeh M, Mariani E, Bartoloni C, Beckman I, Ligthart G, Remarque E, Shall S, Solana R, Taylor GM, Barnett Y, Pawelec G. Life spans of T lymphocytes. *Mech Ageing Dev* 91:145–154, 1996.

Adibzadeh M, Pohla H, Rehbein A, Pawelec G. Long-term culture of monoclonal human T lymphocytes: models for immunosenescence? *Mech Ageing Dev* 83:171–183, 1995.

Adler R, Curcio C, Hicks D, Price D, Wong F. Cell death in age-related macular degeneration. *Mol Vis* 5:31, 1999.

Afshari CA, Barrett JC, Carman TA. Cellular senescence in telomerase-expressing Syrian hamster embryo cells. *Exp Cell Res* 244:33–42, 1998.

Age-Related Eye Disease Study Research Group. A randomized, placebo-controlled, clinical trial of high-dose supplementation with vitamins C and E, beta carotene, and zinc for age-related macular degeneration and vision loss. AREDS report No. 8. *Arch Ophthalmol* 119:1417–1436, 2001a.

Age-Related Eye Disease Study Research Group. A randomized, placebo-controlled, clinical trial of high-dose supplementation with vitamins C and E, beta carotene, and zinc for age-related cataract and vision loss. AREDS report No. 9. *Arch Ophthalmol* 119:1439–1452, 2001b.

Aggarwal BB, Totpal K, LaPushin R, Chaturvedi MM, Pereira-Smith OM, Smith JR. Diminished responsiveness of senescent normal human fibroblasts to TNF-dependent proliferation and interleukin production is not due to its effect on the receptors or on the activation of a nuclear factor NF-κ B. *Exp Cell Res* 218:381–388, 1995.

Ahmad K, Golic KG. Telomere loss in somatic cells of *Drosophila* causes cell cycle arrest and apoptosis. *Genetics* 151:1041–1051, 1999.

Ahmed A, Tollefsbol T. Telomeres and telomerase: basic science implications for aging. *J Am Geriatr Soc* 49:1105–1109, 2001.

Ahmed S, Alpi A, Hengartner MO, Gartner A. *C. elegans* RAD-5/CLK-2 defines a new DNA damage checkpoint protein. *Curr Biol* 11:1934–1944, 2001.

Ahmed S, Hodgkin J. MRT-2 checkpoint protein is required for germline immortality and telomere replication in *C. elegans*. *Nature* 403:159–164, 2000.

Aigner T, Kurz B, Fukui N, Sandell L. Roles of chondrocytes in the pathogenesis of osteoarthritis. *Curr Opin Rheumatol* 14:578–584, 2002.

Aikata H, Takaishi H, Kawakami Y, Takahashi S, Kitamoto M, Nakanishi T, Nakamura Y, Shimamoto F, Kajiyama G, Ide T. Telomere reduction in human liver tissues with age and chronic inflammation. *Exp Cell Res* 256:578–582, 2000.

Aimaretti G, Baffoni C, Ambrosio MR, Maccario M, Corneli G, Bellone S, Gasperi M, Degli Uberti E, Ghigo E. DHEA-S levels in hypopituitaric patients with severe GH deficiency are strongly reduced across life span. Comparison with IGF-I levels before and during rhGH replacement. *J Endocrinol Invest* 23:5–11, 2000.

Aisner DL, Wright WE, Shay JW. Telomerase regulation: not just flipping the switch. *Curr Opin Genet Dev* 12:80–85, 2002.

Akalin A, Elmore LW, Forsythe HL, Amaker BA, McCollum ED, Nelson PS, Ware JL, Holt SE. A novel mechanism for chaperone-mediated telomerase regulation during prostate cancer progression. *Cancer Res* 61:4791–4796, 2001.

Akama TO, Nakagawa H, Sugihara K, Narisawa S, Ohyama C, Nishimura SI, O'Brien DA, Moremen KW, Millan JL, Fukuda MN. Germ cell survival through carbohydrate-mediated interaction with Sertoli cells. *Science* 295:124–127, 2002.

Akeshima R, Kigawa J, Takahashi M, Oishi T, Kanamori Y, Itamochi H, Shimada M, Kamazawa S, Sato S, Terakawa N. Telomerase activity and p53–dependent apoptosis in ovarian cancer cells. *Br J Cancer* 84:1551–1555, 2001.

Akishita M, Horiuchi M, Yamada H, Zhang L, Shirakami G, Tamura K, Ouchi Y, Dzau VJ. Inflammation influences vascular remodeling through AT2 receptor expression and signaling. *Physiol Genomics* 2:13–20, 2000.

Akiyama H, Barger S, Barnum S, Bradt B, Bauer J, Cole GM, Cooper NR, Eikelenboom P, Emmerling M, Fiebich BL, Finch CE, Frautschy S, Griffin WS, Hampel H, Hull M, Landreth G, Lue L, Mrak R, Mackenzie IR, McGeer PL, O'Banion MK, Pachter J, Pasinetti G, Plata-Salaman C, Rogers J, Rydel R, Shen Y, Streit W, Strohmeyer R, Tooyoma I, Van Muiswinkel FL, Veerhuis R, Walker D, Webster S, Wegrzyniak B, Wenk G, Wyss-Coray T. Inflammation and Alzheimer's disease. *Neurobiol Aging* 21:383–421, 2000a.

Akiyama M, Iwase S, Horiguchi-Yamada J, Saito S, Furukawa Y, Yamada O, Mizoguchi H, Ohno T, Yamada H. Interferon-alpha repressed telomerase along with G1-accumulation of Daudi cells. *Cancer Lett* 142:23–30, 1999.

Akiyama M, Yamada O, Akita S, Urashima M, Horiguchi-Yamada J, Ohno T, Mizoguchi H, Eto Y, Yamada H. Ectopic expression of c-myc fails to overcome downregulation of telomerase activity induced by herbimycin A, but ectopic hTERT expression overcomes it. *Leukemia* 14:1260–1265, 2000b.

Akiyama M, Yamada O, Kanda N, Akita S, Kawano T, Ohno T, Mizoguchi H, Eto Y, Anderson KC, Yamada H. Telomerase overexpression in K562 leukemia cells protects against apoptosis by serum deprivation and double-stranded DNA break inducing agents, but not against DNA synthesis inhibitors. *Cancer Lett* 178:187–197, 2002.

Aladdin H, Von Essen M, Schjerling P, Katzenstein T, Gerstoft J, Skinhoj P, Klarlund Pedersen B, Ullum H. T-cell mean telomere lengths changes in treatment naive HIV-infected patients randomized to G-CSF or placebo simultaneously with initiation of HAART. *Scand J Immunol* 54:301–305, 2001.

Alani RM, Hasskarl J, Grace M, Hernandez MC, Israel MA, Munger K. Immortalization of primary human keratinocytes by the helix-loop-helix protein, Id-1. *Proc Natl Acad Sci USA* 96:9637–9641, 1999.

Alberti P, Ren J, Teulade-Fichou MP, Guittat L, Riou JF, Chaires J, Helene C, Vigneron JP, Lehn JM, Mergny JL. Interaction of an acridine dimer with DNA quadruplex structures. *J Biomol Struct Dyn* 19:505–513, 2001.

Alcolado R, Arthur MJ, Iredale JP. Pathogenesis of liver fibrosis. *Clin Sci (Colch)* 92:103–101, 1997.

Aldous WK. Effects of tamoxifen on telomerase activity in breast cancer. Presented at Telomeres and Telomerase: Implications for Cell Immortality, Cancer, and Age-related Disease. San Francisco, CA, June 1–3, 1998.

Aldous WK, Marean AJ, DeHart MJ, Moore KH. Flourescent detection of telomerase activity. In Double JA, Thompson MJ (eds). *Telomeres and Telomerase: Methods and Protocols.* Humana Press, Totowa, NJ, 2002, pp 137–146.

Alexander F. Neuroblastoma. *Urol Clin North Am* 27:383–392, 2000.

Alexandersen P, Toussaint A, Christiansen C, Devogelaer JP, Roux C, Fechtenbaum J, Gennari C, Reginster JY. Ipriflavone in the treatment of postmenopausal osteoporosis: a randomized controlled trial. *JAMA* 285:1482–1488, 2001.

Alfonso-De Matte MY, Cheng JQ, Kruk PA. Ultraviolet irradiation- and dimethyl sulfoxide–induced telomerase activity in ovarian epithelial cell lines. *Exp Cell Res* 267:13–27, 2001.

Alhasan SA, Aranha O, Sarkar FH. Genistein elicits pleiotropic molecular effects on head and neck cancer cells. *Clin Cancer Res* 7:4174–4181, 2001.

Ali AS, Chopra R, Robertson J, Testa NG. Detection of hTERT protein by flow cytometry. *Leukemia* 14:2176–2181, 2000.

Allen RG, Keogh BP, Gerhard GS, Pignolo R, Horton J, Cristofalo VJ. Expression and regulation of superoxide dismutase activity in human skin fibroblasts from donors of different ages. *J Cell Physiol* 165:576–587, 1995.

Allen RG, Keogh BP, Tresini M, Gerhard GS, Volker C, Pignolo RJ, Horton J, Cristofalo VJ. Development and age-associated differences in electron transport potential and consequences for oxidant generation. *J Biol Chem* 272:24805–24812, 1997.

Allen RG, Tresini M, Keogh BP, Doggett DL, Cristofalo VJ. Differences in electron transport potential, antioxidant defenses, and oxidant generation in young and senescent fetal lung fibroblasts (WI-38). *J Cell Physiol* 180:114–122, 1999.

Allikmets R. Molecular genetics of age-related macular degeneration: current status. *Eur J Ophthalmol* 9:255–265, 1999.

Allison DB, Miller RA, Austad SN, Bouchard C, Leibel R, Klebanov S, Johnson T, Harrison DE. Genetic variability in responses to caloric restriction in animals and in regulation of metabolism and obesity in humans. *J Gerontol A Biol Sci Med Sci* 56A:B55–65, 2001.

Allison JP. Enhancement of anti-tumor immune responses by manipulation of T-cell regulatory signals. Presented at Cancer and Molecular Genetics in the Twenty-first Century, Van Andel Research Institute, Grand Rapids, MI, September 5–9, 2000.

Allison JP, Chambers C, Hurwitz A, Sullivan T, Boitel B, Fournier S, Brunner M, Krummel M. A role for CTLA-4-mediated inhibitory signals in peripheral T cell tolerance? *Novartis Found Symp* 215:92–98, 1998.

Allman RM. Pressure ulcers: using what we know to improve quality of care. *J Am Geriatr Soc* 49:996–997, 2001.

Allshire RC. Elements of chromosome structure and function in fission yeast. *Semin Cell Biol* 6:55–64, 1995.

Allshire RC, Dempster M, Hastie ND. Human telomeres contain at least three types of G-rich repeat distributed non-randomly. *Nucleic Acid Res* 17:4611–4627, 1989.

Allsopp RC. Models of initiation of replicative senescence by loss of telomeric DNA. *Exp Gerontol* 31:235–243, 1996.

Allsopp RC, Chang E, Kashefi-Aazam M, Rogaev EI, Piatyszek MA, Shay JW, Harley CB. Telomere shortening is associated with cell division in vitro and in vivo. *Exp Cell Res* 220:194–200, 1995.

Allsopp RC, Cheshier S, Weissman IL. Telomerase activation and rejuvenation of telomere length in stimulated T cells derived from serially transplanted hematopoietic stem cells. *J Exp Med* 196:1427–1433, 2002.

Allsopp RC, Harley CB. Evidence for a critical telomere length in senescent human fibroblasts. *Exp Cell Res* 219:130–136, 1995.

Allsopp RC, Vaziri H, Patterson C, Goldstein S, Younglai EV, Futcher AB, Greider CW, Harley CB. Telomere length predicts replicative capacity of human fibroblasts. *Proc Natl Acad Sci USA* 89:10114–10118, 1992.

Allsopp RC, Weissman IL. Replicative senescence of hematopoietic stem cells during serial transplantation: does telomere shortening play a role? *Oncogene* 21:3270–3273, 2002.

Aloisi F, Ria F, Adorini L. Regulation of T-cell responses by CNS antigen-presenting cells: different roles for microglia and astrocytes. *Immunol Today* 21:141–147, 2000a.

Aloisi F, Serafini B, Adorini L. Glia–T cell dialogue. *J Neuroimmunol* 107:111–117, 2000b.

Alter BP. Bone marrow failure syndromes in children. *Pediatr Clin North Am* 49:973–988, 2002.

Altkorn D, Vokes T. Treatment of postmenopausal osteoporosis. *JAMA* 285:1415–1418, 2001.

Alvarez Kindelan J, Lopez-Beltran A, Requena Tapia MJ. Molecular biology in bladder cancer [in Spanish]. *Actas Urol Esp* 24:604–625, 2000.

Alves G, Fiedler W, Guenther E, Nascimento P, Campos MM, Ornellas AA. Determination of telomerase activity in squamous cell carcinoma of the penis. *Int J Oncol* 18:67–70, 2001.

Amarantos E, Martinez A, Dwyer J. Nutrition and quality of life in older adults. *J Gerontol A Biol Sci Med Sci* 56:54–64, 2001.

American Cancer Society. The Colon and Rectal *Cancer Res*ource Center. What Are the Key Statistics about Colorectal Cancer? ACS home page. Available at http://www3.cancer.org/cancerinfo/specific.asp. Accessed March 18, 1999. Updated December 20, 1998.

Ames BN, Shigenaga MK, Hagen TM. Oxidants, antioxidants and the degnerative diseases of aging. *Proc Natl Acad Sci USA* 90:7915–7922, 1993.

Amit M, Carpenter MK, Inokuma MS, Chiu CP, Harris CP, Waknitz MA, Itskovitz-Eldor J, Thomson JA. Clonally derived human embryonic stem cell lines maintain pluripotency and proliferative potential for prolonged periods of culture. *Dev Biol* 227:271–278, 2000.

Amoroso G, van Veldhuisen DJ, Tio RA, Mariani M. Pathophysiology of vascular endothelium and circulating platelets: implications for coronary revascularisation and treatment. *Int J Cardiol* 79:265–275, 2001.

Anantharaju A, Feller A, Chedid A. Aging liver. A review. *Gerontology* 48:343–353, 2002.

Ancelin K, Brun C, Gilson E. Role of the telomeric DNA-binding protein TRF2 in the stability of human chromosome ends. *Bioessays* 20:879–883, 1998.

Ancelin K, Brunori M, Bauwens S, Koering CE, Brun C, Ricoul M, Pommier JP, Sabatier L, Gilson E. Targeting assay to study the *cis* functions of human telomeric proteins: evidence for inhibition of telomerase by TRF1 and for activation of telomere degradation by TRF2. *Mol Cell Biol* 22:3474–3487, 2002.

Andersen JL, Schjerling P, Saltin B. Muscle, genes and athletic performance. *Sci Am* 283:49–55, 2000.

Andersen-Ranberg K, Schroll M, Sci M, Jeune B. Healthy centenarians do not exist, but autonomous centenarians do: a population-based study of morbidity among Danish centenarians. *J Am Geriatr Soc* 49:900–908, 2001.

Anderson JE. Murray L. Barr Award Lecture. Studies of the dynamics of skeletal muscle regeneration: the mouse came back! *Biochem Cell Biol* 76:13–26, 1998.

Anderson S, Bankier AT, Barrell BG, de Bruijn MH, Coulson AR, Drouin J, Eperon IC, Nierlich DP, Roe BA, Sanger F, Schreier PH, Smith AJ, Staden R, Young IG. Sequence and organization of the human mitochondrial genome. *Nature* 290:457–465, 1981.

Anderson S, Shera K, Ihle J, Billman L, Goff B, Greer B, Tamimi H, McDougall J, Klingelhutz A. Telomerase activation in cervical cancer. *Am J Pathol* 151:25–31, 1997.

Andrawis N, Jones DS, Abernethy DR. Aging is associated with endothelial dysfunction in the human forearm vasculature. *J Am Geriatr Soc* 48:193–198, 2000.

Andrew D, Aspinall R. Age-associated thymic atrophy is linked to a decline in IL-7 production. *Exp Gerontol* 37:455–463, 2002.

Anglana M, Bacchetti S. Construction of a recombinant adenovirus for efficient delivery of the I-SceI yeast endonuclease to human cells and its application in the in vivo cleavage of chromosomes to expose new potential telomeres. *Nucleic Acids Res* 27:4276–4281, 1999.

Anisimov VN, Zavarzina NY, Zabezhinski MA, Popovich IG, Zimina OA, Shtylick AV, Arutjunyan AV, Oparina TI, Prokopnko VM, Mikhalski AI, Yashin AI. Melatonin increases both life span and tumor incidence in female CBA mice. *J Gerontol A Biol Sci Med Sci* 56:B311–323, 2001.

Anson RM, Bohr VA. Mitochondria, oxidative DNA damage, and aging. *J Am Aging Assoc* 23:199–218, 2001.

Antal M, Boros E, Solymosy F, Kiss T. Analysis of the structure of human telomerase RNA in vivo. *Nucleic Acids Res* 30:912–920, 2002.

Antel JP, Owens T. Immune regulation and CNS autoimmune disease. *J Neuroimmunol* 100:181–189, 1999.

Antonio J, Gonyea WJ. Skeletal muscle fiber hyperplasia. *Med Sci Sports Exerc* 25:1333–1345, 1993.

Anttila T, Saikka P, Koskela P, Bloigu A, Dillner J, Ikaheimo I, Jellum E, Lehtinen M, Lenner P, Hakulinn T, Narvanen A, Pukkala E, Thoresen S, Youngman L, Paavonen J. Serotypes of *Chlamydia trachomatis* and risk for development of cervical squamous cell carcinoma. *JAMA* 285:47–51, 2001.

Aogi K, Woodman A, Urquidi V, Mangham DC, Tarin D, Goodison S. Telomerase activity in soft-tissue and bone sarcomas. *Clin Cancer Res* 6:4776–4781, 2000.

Aoki M, Morishita R, Muraishi A, Moriguchi A, Sugimoto T, Maeda K, Dzau VJ, Kaneda Y, Higaki J, Ogihara T. Efficient in vivo gene transfer into the heart in the rat myocardial infarction model using the HVJ (Hemagglutinating Virus of Japan)—liposome method. *J Mol Cell Cardiol* 29:949–959, 1997.

Aparicio OM, Billington BL, Gottschling DE. Modifiers of position effect are shared between telomeric and silent mating-type loci in *S. cerevisiae*. *Cell* 66:1279–1287, 1991.

Aparicio OM, Gottschling DE. Overcoming telomeric silencing: a trans-activator competes to establish gene expression in a cell cycle-dependent way. *Genes Dev* 8:1133–1146, 1994.

Apfeld J, Kenyon C. Cell nonautonomy of *C. elegans* daf-2 function in the regulation of diapause and life span. *Cell* 95:199–210, 1998.

Apfeld J, Kenyon C. Regulation of lifespan by sensory perception in *Caenorhabditis elegans*. *Nature* 402:804–809, 1999.

Appel A, Horowitz AL, Dorfman A. Cell-free synthesis of hyaluronic acid in Marfan syndrome. *J Biol Chem* 254:12199–12216, 1979.

Aragona M, De Divitiis O, La Torre D, Panetta S, D'Avella D, Pontoriero A, Morelli M, La Torre I, Tomasello F. Immunohistochemical TRF1 expression in human primary intracranial tumors. *Anticancer Res* 21:2135–2139, 2001.

Aragona M, Maisano R, Panetta S, Giudice A, Morelli M, La Torre I, La Torre F. Telomere length maintenance in aging and carcinogenesis. *Int J Oncol* 17:981–989, 2000a.

Aragona M, Panetta S, Rizzotti P, La Torre I, Giudice A, La Torre F. Importance of chemoprevention in oncology [in Italian]. *Minerva Med* 91:169–177, 2000b.

Aragona M, Pontoriero A, Panetta S, La Torre I, La Torre F. The role of telomere-binding proteins in carcinogenesis [in Italian]. *Minerva Med* 91:299–304, 2000c.

Arai J, Yajima T, Yagihashi A, Kobayashi D, Kameshima H, Sasaki M, Tanaka K, Kuwajima K, Miyao N, Tsukamoto T, Watanabe N. Limitations of urinary telomerase activity measurement in urothelial cancer. *Clin Chim Acta* 296:35–44, 2000.

Arai J, Yasukawa M, Ohminami H, Kakimoto M, Hasegawa A, Fujita S. Identification of human telomerase reverse transcriptase-derived peptides that induce HLA-A24-restricted antileukemia cytotoxic T lymphocytes. *Blood* 97:2903–2907, 2001.

Arantes-Oliveira N, Apfeld J, Dillin A, Kenyon C. Regulation of life span by germ-line stem cells in *Caenorhabditis elegans*. *Science* 295:502–505, 2002.

Arbiser JL, Yeung R, Weiss SW, Arbiser ZK, Amin MB, Cohen C, Frank D, Mahajan S, Herron GS, Yang J, Onda H, Zhang HB, Bai X, Uhlmann E, Loehr A, Northrup H, Au P, Davis I, Fisher DE, Gutmann DH. The generation and characterization of a cell line derived from a sporadic renal angiomyolipoma: use of telomerase to obtain stable populations of cells from benign neoplasms. *Am J Pathol* 159:483–491, 2001.

Arbustini E, Morbini P, Bello BD, Prati F, Specchia G. From plaque biology to clinical setting. *Am Heart J* 138:55–60, 1999.

Arias Funez F, Fernandez Fernandez E, Escudero Barrilero A, Moyano Jato A, Caso P, Elaez E. Telomerase activity as marker of superficial tumor of the bladder [in Spanish]. *Arch Esp Urol* 53:231–236, 2000.

Arinaga M, Shimizu S, Gotoh K, Haruki N, Takahashi T, Takahashi T, Mitsudomi T. Expression of human telomerase subunit genes in primary lung cancer and its clinical significance. *Ann Thorac Surg* 70:401–405, 2000.

Arkhipova IR, Morrison HG. Three retrotransposon families in the genome of *Giardia lamblia*: two telomeric, one dead. *Proc Natl Acad Sci USA* 98:14497–14502, 2001.

Arking R. Genetic and environmental determinants of longevity in *Drosophila*. *Basic Life Sci* 42:1–22, 1987a.

Arking R. Genetic and environmental determinants of longevity in *Drosophila*. In Woodhead AD, Thompson KH (eds). *Evolution of Longevity in Animals: A Comparative Approach.* Plenum, New York, 1987b, pp 1–22.

Arking R. Successful selection for increased longevity in *Drosophila*: analysis of the survival data and presentation of a hypothesis on the genetic regulation of longevity. *Exp Gerontol* 22:199–220, 1987c.

Arking R. Genetic analyses of aging processes in *Drosophila*. *Exp Aging Res* 14:125–135, 1988.

Arking R. *Biology of aging.* 2nd ed. Sinauer Associates, Sunderland, MA, 1998.

Arking R, Buck S. Selection for increased longevity in *Drosophila melanogaster*: a reply to Lints. *Gerontology* 41:69–76, 1995.

Arking R, Buck S, Berrios A, Dwyer S, Baker GT 3d. Elevated paraquat resistance can be used as a bioassay for longevity in a genetically based long-lived strain of *Drosophila*. *Dev Genet* 12:362–370, 1991.

Arking R, Buck S, Wells RA, Pretzlaff R. Metabolic rates in genetically based long-lived strains of *Drosophila*. *Exp Gerontol* 23:59–76, 1988.

Arking R, Dudas SP. Review of genetic investigations into the aging processes of *Drosophila*. *J Am Geriatr Soc* 37:757–773, 1989.

Arking R, Dudas SP, Baker GT 3d. Genetic and environmental factors regulating the expression of an extended longevity phenotype in a long-lived strain of *Drosophila*. *Genetica* 91:127–142, 1993.

Arking R, Force AG, Dudas SP, Buck S, Baker GT 3rd. Factors contributing to the plasticity of the extended longevity phenotypes of *Drosophila*. *Exp Gerontol* 31:623–43, 1996.

Arking R, Wells RA. Genetic alteration of normal aging processes is responsible for extended longevity in *Drosophila*. *Dev Genet* 11:141–148, 1990.

Arlett CF, Harcourt SA. Survey of radiosensitivity in a variety of human cell strains. *Cancer Res* 40:926–932, 1980.

Armbruster BN, Banik SS, Guo C, Smith AC, Counter CM. N-terminal domains of the human telomerase catalytic subunit required for enzyme activity in vivo. *Mol Cell Biol* 21:7775–7786, 2001.

Armstrong RJ, Svendsen CN. Neural stem cells: from cell biology to cell replacement. *Cell Transplant* 9:139–152, 2000.

Armstrong SJ, Franklin FC, Jones GH. Nucleolus-associated telomere clustering and pairing precede meiotic chromosome synapsis in *Arabidopsis thaliana*. *J Cell Sci* 114:4207–4217, 2001.

Arnett DK, Boland LL, Evans GW, Riley W, Barnes R, Tyroler HA, Heiss G. Hypertension and arterial stiffness: the Atherosclerosis Risk in Communities study. *Am J Hypertension* 13:317–323, 2000.

Artandi SE. Telomere shortening and cell fates in mouse models of neoplasia. *Trends Mol Med* 8:44–47, 2002.

Artandi SE, Alson S, Tietze MK, Sharpless NE, Ye S, Greenberg RA, Castrillon DH, Horner JW, Weiler SR, Carrasco RD, DePinho RA. Constitutive telomerase expression promotes mammary carcinomas in aging mice. *Proc Natl Acad Sci USA* 99:8191–8196, 2002.

Artandi SE, Chang S, Lee SL, Alson S, Gottlieb GJ, Chin L, DePinho RA. Telomere dysfunction promotes non-reciprocal translocations and epithelial cancers in mice. *Nature* 406:641–645, 2000.

Artandi SE, DePinho RA. A critical role for telomeres in suppressing and facilitating carcinogenesis. *Curr Opin Genet Dev* 10:39–46, 2000a.

Artandi SE, DePinho RA. Mice without telomerase: what can they teach us about human cancer? *Nat Med* 6:852–855, 2000b.

Artlett CM, Black CM, Briggs DC, Stevens CO, Welsh KI. Telomere reduction in scleroderma patients: a possible cause for chromosomal instability. *Br J Rheumatol* 35:732–737, 1996.

Arvat E, Broglio F, Ghigo E. Insulin-like growth factor I: implications in aging. *Drugs Aging* 16:29–40, 2000.

Ascenzioni F, Donini P, Lipps HJ. Mammalian artificial chromosomes—vectors for somatic gene therapy. *Cancer Lett* 118:135–142, 1997.

Aschner M. Astrocytes as mediators of immune and inflammatory responses in the CNS. *Neurotoxicology* 19:269–281, 1998.

Aschner M, Allen JW, Kimelberg HK, LoPachin RM, Streit WJ. Glial cells in neurotoxicity development. *Annu Rev Pharmacol Toxicol* 39:151–173, 1999.

Asfour B, Byrne BJ, Baba HA, Hammel D, Hruban RH, Weyand M, Deng M, Scheld HH. Effective gene transfer in the rat myocardium via adenovirus vectors using a coronary recirculation model. *Thorac Cardiovasc Surg* 47:311–316, 1999.

Ashrafi K, Sinclair D, Gordon JI, Guarente L. Passage through stationary phase advances replicative aging in *Saccharomyces cerevisiae*. *Proc Natl Acad Sci USA* 96:9100–9105, 1999.

Aspnes LE, Lee CM, Weindruch R, Chung SS, Roecker EB, Aiken JM. Caloric restriction reduces fiber loss and mitochondrial abnormalities in aged rat muscle. *FASEB J* 11:573–581, 1997.

Asthana S, Craft S, Baker LD, Raskind MA, Birnbaum RS, Lofgreen CP, Veith RC, Plymate SR. Cognitive and neuroendocrine response to transdermal estrogen in postmenopausal women with Alzheimer's disease: results of a placebo-controlled, double-blind, pilot study. *Psychoneuroendocrinology* 24:657–677, 1999.

Atchley WR, Xu S, Cowley DE. Altering developmental trajectories in mice by restricted index selection. *Genetics* 146:629–640, 1997.

Athan ES, Williamson J, Ciappa A, Santana V, Romas SN, Lee JH, Rondon H, Lantigua RA, Medrano M, Torres M, Arawaka S, Rogaeva E, Song Y-Q, Sato C, Kawarai T, Fafel KC, Boss MA, Seltzer WK, Stern Y, St George-Hyslop P, Tycko B, Mayeux R. A founder mutation in presenilin-1 causing early-onset Alzheimer disease in unrelated Caribbean Hispanic families. *JAMA* 286:2257–2263, 2001.

Atkins L. Progeria: report of a case with post-mortem findings. *N Engl J Med* 250:1065–1069, 1954.

Atwood CS, Huang X, Moir RD, Tanzi RE, Bush AI. Role of free radicals and metal ions in the pathogenesis of Alzheimer's disease. *Met Ions Biol Syst* 36:309–364, 1999.

Aubin JE. Bone stem cells. *J Cell Biochem Suppl* 30–31:73–82, 1998.

Austad SN. Concepts and theories of aging. In Masoro EJ, Austad SN (eds). *Handbook of the Bilogy of Aging, 5th ed.* Academic Press, New York, 2001, pp 3–22.

Autexier C. Telomerase as a possible target for anticancer therapy. *Chem Biol* 6:R299–303, 1999.

Autexier C, Greider CW. Functional reconstitution of wild-type and mutant *Tetrahymena* telomerase. *Genes Dev* 8:563–575, 1994.

Autexier C, Greider CW. Boundary elements of the *Tetrahymena* telomerase RNA template and alignment domains. *Genes Dev* 9:2227–2239, 1995.

Autexier C, Greider CW. Telomerase and cancer: revisiting the telomere hypothesis. *Trends Biochem Sci* 21:387–391, 1996.

Autexier C, Greider CW. Mutational analysis of the *Tetrahymena* telomerase RNA: identification of residues affecting telomerase activity in vitro. *Nucleic Acids Res* 26:787–795, 1998.

Autexier C, Pruzan R, Funk WD, Greider CW. Reconstitution of human telomerase activity and identification of a minimal functional region of the human telomerase RNA. *EMBO J* 15:5928–5935, 1996.

Avilion AA. Human telomerase RNA and telomerase activity in immortal cell lines and tumor tissues. *Cancer Res* 56:645–650, 1996.

Avilion AA, Harrington LA, Greider CW. *Tetrahymena* telomerase RNA levels increase during macronuclear development. *Dev Genet* 13:80–86, 1992.

Avilion AA, Piatyszek MA, Gupta J, Shay JW, Bacchetti S, Greider CW. Human telomerase RNA and telomerase activity in immortal cell lines and tumor tissues. *Cancer Res* 56:645–650, 1996.

Aviv A. Chronology versus biology: telomeres, essential hypertension, and vascular aging. *Hypertension* 40:229–232, 2002a.

Aviv A. Telomeres, sex, reactive oxygen species, and human cardiovascular aging. *J Mol Med* 80:689–695, 2002b.

Aviv A, Aviv H. Telomeres, hidden mosaicism, loss of heterozygosity, and complex genetic traits. *Hum Genet* 103:2–4, 1998.

Aviv A, Aviv H. Telomeres and essential hypertension. *Am J Hypertens* 12(4 Pt 1):427–432, 1999.

Aviv A, Harley CB. How long should telomeres be? *Curr Hypertens Rep* 3:145–151, 2001.

Aviv H, Yusuf Khan M, Skurnick J, Okuda K, Kimura M, Gardner J, Priolo L, Aviv A. Age-dependent aneuploidy and telomere length of the human vascular endothelium. *Atherosclerosis* 159:281–287, 2001.

Bacchetti S. Telomere maintenance in tumour cells. *Cancer Surv* 28:197–216, 1996.

Bach SP, Renehan AG, Potten CS. Stem cells: the intestinal stem cell as a paradigm. *Carcinogenesis* 21:469–476, 2000.

Bachand F, Triki I, Autexier C. Human telomerase RNA–protein interactions. *Nucleic Acids Res* 29:3385–3393, 2001.

Backsch C, Wagenbach N, Nonn M, Leistritz S, Stanbridge E, Schneider A, Durst M. Microcell-mediated transfer of chromosome 4 into HeLa cells suppresses telomerase activity. *Genes Chromosomes Cancer* 31:196–198, 2001.

Bacon KB, Harrison JK. Chemokines and their receptors in neurobiology: perspectives in physiology and homeostasis. *J Neuroimmunol* 104:92–97, 2000.

Badame AJ. Progeria. *Arch Dermatol* 125:540–544, 1989.

Baerlocher GM, Mak J, Tien T, Lansdorp PM. Telomere length measurement by fluorescence in situ hybridization and flow cytometry: tips and pitfalls. *Cytometry* 1;47:89–99, 2002.

Bagatell CJ, Bremner WJ. Androgens in aging men: do men benefit from testosterone replacement? *J Anti-Aging Med* 1:359–364, 1998.

Bagnara GP, Bonsi L, Strippoli P, Bonifazi F, Tonelli R, D'Addato S, Paganelli R, Scala E, Fagiolo U, Monti D, Cossarizza A, Bonafe M, Franceschi C. Hemopoiesis in healthy old people and centenarians: well-maintained responsiveness of CD34+ cells to hematopoetic growth factors and remodeling of cytokine network. *J Gerontol A Biol Sci Med Sci* 55:B61–B66, 2000.

Bailes BK. Hypothyroidism in elderly patients. *AORN J* 69:1026–1030, 1999.

Bailey SM, Cornforth MN, Kurimasa A, Chen DJ, Goodwin EH. Strand-specific postreplicative processing of mammalian telomeres. *Science* 293:2462–2465, 2001.

Bailey SM, Meyne J, Chen DJ, Kurimasa A, Li GC, Lehnert BE, Goodwin EH. DNA double-strand break repair proteins are required to cap the ends of mammalian chromosomes. *Proc Natl Acad Sci USA* 96:14899–14904, 1999.

Baime MJ, Nelson JB, Castell DO. Aging of the gastrointestinal system. In Hazzard WR, Bierman EL, Blass JP, Ettinger WH Jr, Halter JB (eds). *Principles of Medicine and Gerontology*. McGraw-Hill, New York, 1994, pp 665–681.

Baker E, Hinton L, Callen D, Haan E, Dobbie A, Sutherland G. A familial cryptic subtelomeric deletion 12p with variable phenotypic effect. *Clin Genet* 61:198–201, 2002.

Baker PB, Baba N, Boesel CP. Cardiovascular abnormalities in progeria: case report and review of the literature. *Arch Pathol Lab Med* 105:384–386, 1981.

Balajee AS, Machwe A, May A, Gray MD, Oshima J, Martin GM, Nehlin JO, Brosh R, Orren DK, Bohr VA. The Werner syndrome protein is involved in RNA polymerase II transcription. *Mol Biol Cell* 10:2655–2668, 1999.

Balajee AS, Oh HJ, Natarajan AT. Analysis of restriction enzyme-induced chromosome aberrations in the interstitial telomeric repeat sequences of CHO and CHE cells by FISH. *Mutat Res* 307:307–313, 1994.

Balcombe NR, Sinclair A. Ageing: definitions, mechanisms and the magnitude of the problem. *Best Pract Res Clin Gastroenterol* 15:835–849, 2001.

Baldereschi M, Di Carlo A, Lepore V, Bracco L, Maggi S, Grigoletto F, Scarlato G, Amaducci L. Estrogen-replacement therapy and Alzheimer's disease in the Italian Longitudinal Study on Aging. *Neurology* 50:996–1002, 1999.

Baldzhiev V, Khristov Kh, Velev Kh. Incomplete Hutchinson-Gilford syndrome. A patient followed to age 29 [in Bulgarian]. *Vutr Boles* 23:86–90, 1984.

Balin AK, Balin LP, Whittlesey M. *The Life of the Skin*. Bantam Books, New York, 1997.

Balin AK, Goodman DB, Rasmussen H, Cristofalo VJ. The effect of oxygen and vitamin E on the life span of human diploid cells in vitro. *J Cell Biol* 74:58–67, 1977.

Balin BJ, Gerard HC, Arking EJ, Appelt DM, Branigan PJ, Abrams JT, Whittum-Hudson JA, Hudson AP. Identification and localization of *Chlamydia pneumoniae* in the Alzheimer's brain. *Med Microbiol Immunol (Berl)* 187:23–42, 1998.

Bandy B, Davidson AJ. Mitochondrial mutations may increase oxidative stress: implications for carcinogenesis and aging? *Free Radic Biol Med* 8:523–539, 1990.

Bandyopadhyay D, Timchenko N, Suwa T, Hornsby PJ, Campisi J, Medrano EE. The human melanocyte: a model system to study the complexity of cellular aging and transformation in non-fibroblastic cells. *Exp Gerontol* 36:1265–1275, 2001.

Banerjee PP, Banerjee S, Zirkin BR, Brown TR. Lobe-specific telomerase activity in the intact adult Brown Norway rat prostate and its regional distribution within the prostatic ducts. *Endocrinology* 139:513–519, 1998a.

Banerjee PP, Banerjee S, Zirkin BR, Brown TR. Telomerase activity in normal adult Brown Norway rat seminal vesicle: regional distribution and age-dependent changes. *Endocrinology* 139:1075–1081, 1998b.

Banik SS, Guo C, Smith AC, Margolis SS, Richardson DA, Tirado CA, Counter CM. C-terminal regions of the human telomerase catalytic subunit essential for in vivo enzyme activity. *Mol Cell Biol* 22:6234–6246, 2002.

Banks DA, Fossel M. Telomeres, cancer, and aging: altering the human life span. *JAMA* 278:1345–1348, 1997.

Banks WA, Morley JE. Endocrine and metabolic changes in human aging. *J Am Aging Assoc* 23:103–115, 2000.

Barinaga M. The telomerase picture fills in. *Science* 276:528–529, 1997.

Barinaga M. Cancer drugs found to work in new way. *Science* 288:245, 2000.

Barker K, Khayat M, Miller N, Wilson M, Clem LW, Bengten E. Immortal and mortal clonal lymphocyte lines from channel catfish: comparison of telomere length, telomerase activity, tumor suppressor and heat shock protein expression. *Dev Comp Immunol* 26:45–51, 2001.

Barnhart KT, Freeman E, Grisso JA, Rader DJ, Sammel M, Kapoor S, Nestler JE. The effect of dehydroepiandrosterone supplementation to symptomatic perimenopausal women on serum endocrine profiles, lipid parameters, and health-related quality of life. *J Clin Endocrinol Metab* 84:3896–3902, 1999.

Barrett-Connor E, von Muhlen D, Laughlin GA, Kripke A. Endogenous levels of dehydroepiandrosterone sulfate, but not other sex hormones, are associated with depressed mood in older women: the Rancho Bernardo Study. *J Am Geriatr Soc* 47:685–691, 1999.

Bartke A, Brown-Borg H, Kinney B, Mattison J, Wright C, Hauck S, Coschigano K, Kopchick J. Growth hormone and aging. *J Am Aging Assoc* 23:219–225, 2001a.

Bartke A, Coschigano K, Kopchick J, Chandrashekar V, Mattison J, Kinney B, Hauck S. Genes that prolong life: relationships of growth hormone and growth to aging and life span. *J Gerontol A Biol Sci Med Sci* 56:B340–349, 2001b.

Bartke A, Lane M. Endocrine and neuroendocrine regulatory functions. In Masoro EJ, Austad SN (eds). *Handbook of the Biology of Aging, 5th ed.* Academic Press, New York, 2001, pp 297–313.

Barton M. Endothelial dysfunction and atherosclerosis: endothelin receptor antagonists as novel therapeutics. *Curr Hypertens Rep* 2:84–91, 2000.

Barton-Davis ER, Shoturma DI, Musaro A, Rosenthal N, Sweeney HL. Viral mediated expression of insulin-like growth factor I blocks the aging-related loss of skeletal muscle function. *Proc Natl Acad Sci USA* 95:15603–15607, 1998.

Bartzokis G, Sultzer D, Cummings J, Holt LE, Hance DB, Henderson VW, Mintz J. In vivo evaluation of brain iron in Alzheimer disease using magnetic resonance imaging. *Arch Gen Psychiatry* 57:47–53, 2000.

Basaria S, Dobs AS. Risks versus benefits of testosterone therapy in elderly men. *Drugs Aging* 15:131–142, 1999.

Basch PF. *International Health.* Oxford University Press, New York, 1978.

Basser RL. New developments in high-dose chemotherapy for breast cancer. *Recent Results Cancer Res* 152:355–367, 1998.

Bauer JM, Conn JW. Werner's syndrome: a study of adrenocortical and hepatic steroidal metabolism. *Texas State J Med* 49:882–888, 1953.

Baulieu EE. 'New' active steroids and an unforeseen mechanism of action. *CR Acad Sci III* 323:513–518, 2000.

Baulieu EE, Thomas G, Legrain S, Lahlou N, Roger M, Debuire B, Faucounau V, Girard L, Hervy MP, Latour F, Leaud MC, Mokrane A, Pitti-Ferrandi H, Trivalle C, de Lacharriere O, Nouveau S, Rakoto-Arison B, Souberbielle JC, Raison J, Le Bouc Y, Raynaud A, Girerd X, Forette F. Dehydroepiandrosterone (DHEA), DHEA sulfate, and aging: contribution of the DHEAge study to a sociobiomedical issue. *Proc Natl Acad Sci USA* 97:4279–4284, 2000.

Baumann P, Cech TR. Pot1, the putative telomere end-binding protein in fission yeast and humans. *Science* 292:1171–1175, 2001.

Baumgartner RN, Koehler KM, Gallagher D, Romero L, Heymsfield SB, Ross RR, Garry PJ, Lindeman RD. Epidemiology of sarcopenia among the elderly in New Mexico. *Am J Epidemiol* 147:755–763, 1998.

Baur JA, Zou Y, Shay JW, Wright WE. Telomere position effect in human cells. *Science* 292:2075–2077, 2001.

Baylink DJ, Jennings JC. Calcium and bone homeostasis and changes with aging. In Hazzard WR, Bierman EL, Blass JP, Ettinger WH Jr, Halter JB (eds). *Principles of Medicine and Gerontology.* McGraw-Hill, New York, 1994, pp 879–896.

Beach DH. Biology of cellular aging. Presented at Cancer and Molecular Genetics in the Twenty-first Century, Van Andel Research Institute, Grand Rapids, MI, September 5–9, 2000.

Bearss DJ, Hurley LH, Von Hoff DD. Telomere maintenance mechanisms as a target for drug development. *Oncogene* 19:6632–6641, 2000.

Beattie TL, Zhou W, Robinson MO, Harrington L. Polymerization defects within human telomerase are distinct from telomerase RNA and TEP1 binding. *Mol Biol Cell* 11:3329–3340, 2000.

Beaufrere B, Boirie Y. Aging and protein metabolism. *Curr Opin Clin Nutr Metab Care* 1:85–89, 1998.

Becher B, Fedorowicz V, Antel JP. Regulation of CD14 expression on human adult central nervous system–derived microglia. *J Neurosci Res* 45:375–381, 1996.

Becher B, Prat A, Antel JP. Brain-immune connection: immunoregulatory properties of CNS-resident cells. *Glia* 29:293–304, 2000.

Bechter OE, Eisterer W, Dlaska M, Kuhr T, Thaler J. CpG island methylation of the hTERT promoter is associated with lower telomerase activity in B-cell lymphocytic leukemia. *Exp Hematol* 30:26–33, 2002.

Beck C, Cody M, Souder E, Zhang M, Small GW. Dementia diagnostic guidelines: methodologies, results, and implementation costs. *J Am Geriatr Soc* 48:1195–1203, 2000.

Beck EM. *Familiar Quotations by John Bartlett, 14th ed.* Little, Brown and Company, Boston, 1968.

Becker-Hapak M, McAllister SS, Dowdy SF. TAT-mediated protein transduction into mammalian cells. *Methods* 24:247–256, 2001.

Beckman KB, Ames BN. The free radical theory of aging matures. *Physiol Rev* 78:547–581, 1998.

Bednarek A, Budunova I, Slaga TJ, Aldaz CM. Increased telomerase activity in mouse skin premalignant progression. *Cancer Res* 55:4566–4569, 1995.

Beeche M, Bodnar AG, Chang E, Chiu C, Frolkis M, Jiang X, Jimenez G, Kusler B, Sage M, Tlsty TD, Wahl GM. Telomerase expression in human somatic cells does not induce changes associated with a transformed phenotype. *Nat Genet* 21:111–114, 1999.

Beers AP, van der Heijde GL, Dubbelman M. Aging of the crystalline lens and presbyopia [in Dutch]. *Tijdschr Gerontol Geriatr* 29:185–188, 1998.

Beharka AA, Meydani M, Wu D, Leka LS, Meydani A, Meydani SN. Interleukin-6 production does not increase with age. *J Gerontol A Biol Sci Med Sci* 56A:B81–88, 2001a.

Beharka AA, Paiva S, Leka LS, Ribaya-Mercado JD, Russell RM, Meydani SN. Effect of age on the gastrointestinal-associated mucosal immune response of humans. *J Gerontol A Biol Sci Med Sci* 56:218–223, 2001b.

Bekaert S, Koll S, Thas O, Van Oostveldt P. Comparing telomere length of sister chromatids in human lymphocytes using three-dimensional confocal microscopy. *Cytometry* 48:34–44, 2002.

Bell E, Ivarsson B, Merrill C. Production of tissue-like structure by contraction of collagen lattices by human fibroblasts of different proliferative potential in vitro. *Proc Natl Acad Sci USA* 76:1274–1278, 1979.

Bello Y, Phillips TJ. Recent advances in would healing. *JAMA* 283:716–718, 2000.

Bemben MG. Age-related alterations in muscular endurance. *Sports Med* 25:259–269, 1998.

Benard C, McCright B, Zhang Y, Felkai S, Lakowski B, Hekimi S. The *C. elegans* maternal-effect gene *clk-2* is essential for embryonic development, encodes a protein homologous to yeast Tel2p and affects telomere length. *Development* 128:4045–4055, 2001.

Bence NF, Sampat RM, Kopito RR. Impairment of the ubiquitin–proteosome system by protein aggregation. *Science* 292:1552–1555, 2001.

Bender BS, Ulmer JB, DeWitt CM, Cottey R, Taylor SF, Ward AM, Friedman A, Liu MA, Donnelly JJ. Immunogenicity and efficacy of DNA vaccines encoding influenza A proteins in aged mice. *Vaccine* 16:1748–1755, 1998.

Benditt EP, Benditt JM. Evidence for a monoclonal origin of human atherosclerotic plaques. *Proc Natl Acad Sci USA* 70:1753–1756, 1973.

Bengtsson B-A, Johannsson G, Isgaard J. Use of growth hormone for treatment of anatomic and physiologic decrements associated with aging. *J Anti-Aging Med* 1:197–206, 1998.

Bennett DC, Medrano EE. Molecular regulation of melanocyte senescence. *Pigment Cell Res* 15:242–250, 2002.

Bennett SE, Umar A, Oshima J, Monnat RJ Jr, Kunkel TA. Mismatch repair in extracts of Werner syndrome cell lines. *Cancer Res* 57:2956–2960, 1997.

Benot S, Goberna R, Reiter RJ, Garcia-Maurino S, Osuna C, Guerrero JM. Physiological levels of melatonin contribute to the antioxidant capacity of human serum. *J Pineal Res* 27:59–64, 1999.

Benson D, Mitchell N, Dix D. On the role of aging in carcinogenesis. *Mutat Res* 356:209–216, 1996.

Benzacken B, Carbillon L, Dupont C, Siffroi JP, Monier-Gavelle F, Bucourt M, Uzan M, Wolf JP. Lack of submicroscopic rearrangements involving telomeres in reproductive failures. *Hum Reprod* 17:1154–1157, 2002.

Benzi G, Moretti A. Age- and peroxidative stress-related modifications of the cerebral enzymatic activities linked to mitochondria and the glutathione system. *Free Radic Biol Med* 19:77–101, 1995.

Beral V, Banks E, Reeves G, Appleby P. Use of HRT and the subsequent risk of cancer. *J Epidemiol Biostat* 4:191–210; discussion 210–215, 1999.

Bergmanson JP, Sheldon TM, Goosey JD. Fuchs' endothelial dystrophy: a fresh look at an aging disease. *Ophthalmic Physiol Opt* 19:210–222, 1999.

Berlowitz DR, Brandeis GH, Morris JN, Ash AS, Anderson JJ, Kader B, Moskowitz MA. Deriving a risk-adjustment model for pressure ulcer development using the minimum data set. *J Am Geriatr Soc* 49:866–871, 2001.

Bernardis LL, Davis PJ. Aging and the hypothalamus: research perspectives. *Physiol Behav* 59:523–536, 1996.

Bernstein E, Kaye D, Abrutyn E, Gross P, Dorfman M, Murasko DM. Immune response to influenza vaccination in a large healthy elderly population. *Vaccine* 17:82–94, 1999.

Berthold F, Hero B. Neuroblastoma: current drug therapy recommendations as part of the total treatment approach. *Drugs* 59:1261–1277, 2000.

Bertram L, Blacker D, Mullin K, Keeney D, Jones J, Basu S, Yhu S, McInnis MG, Go RCP, Vekrellis K, Selkoe DJ, Saunders AJ, Tanzi RE. Evidence for genetic linkage of Alzheimer's disease to chromosome 10q. *Science* 290:2302–2305, 2000.

Bertram MJ, Berube NG, Hang-Swanson X, Ran Q, Leung JK, Bryce S, Spurgers K, Bick RJ, Baldini A, Ning Y, Clark LJ, Parkinson EK, Barrett JC, Smith JR, Pereira-Smith OM. Identification of a gene that reverses the immortal phenotype of a subset of cells and is a member of a novel family of transcription factor–like genes. *Mol Cell Biol* 19:1479–1485, 1999.

Berube NG, Smith JR, Pereira-Smith OM. The genetics of cellular senescence. *Am J Hum Genet* 62:1015–1019, 1998.

Bestilny LJ, Gill MJ, Mody CH, Riabowol KT. Accelerated replicative senescence of the peripheral immune system induced by HIV infection. *AIDS* 14:771–780, 2000.

Betts D, Bordignon V, Hill J, Winger Q, Westhusin M, Smith L, King W. Reprogramming of telomerase activity and rebuilding of telomere length in cloned cattle. *Proc Natl Acad Sci USA* 98:1077–1082, 2001.

Betts DH, King WA. Telomerase activity and telomere detection during early bovine development. *Dev Genet* 25:397–403, 1999.

Bhawan J, Oh CH, Lew R, Nehal KS, Labadie RR, Tsay A, Gilchrest BA. Histopathologic differences in the photoaging process in facial versus arm skin. *Am J Dermatopathol* 14:224–230, 1992.

Bi X. Domains of gene silencing near the left end of chromosome III in *Saccharomyces cerevisiae*. *Genetics* 160:1401–1407, 2002.

Bialkowska-Hobrzanska H, Bowles L, Bukala B, Joseph MG, Fletcher R, Razvi H. Comparison of human telomerase reverse transcriptase messenger RNA and telomerase activity as urine markers for diagnosis of bladder carcinoma. *Mol Diagn* 5:267–277, 2000.

Bianchi A, de Lange T. Ku binds telomeric DNA in vitro. *J Biol Chem* 274:21223–21227, 1999.

Bianchi A, Stansel RM, Fairall L, Griffith JD, Rhodes D, de Lange T. TRF1 binds a bipartite telomeric site with extreme spatial flexibility. *EMBO J* 18:5735–5744, 1999.

Bibby MC. Introduction to telomeres and telomerase. In Double JA, Thompson MJ (eds). *Telomeres and Telomerase: Methods and Protocols*. Humana Press, Totowa, NJ, 2002, pp 1–12.

Bieche I, Nogues C, Paradis V, Olivi M, Bedossa P, Lidereau R, Vidaud M. Quantitation of hTERT gene expression in sporadic breast tumors with a real-time reverse transcription–polymerase chain reaction assay. *Clin Cancer Res* 6:452–459, 2000.

Bierman EL. The effect of donor age on the in vitro life span of cultured human arterial smooth muscle cells. *In Vitro* 14:951–955, 1978.

Bierman EL. Aging and atherosclerosis. In Hazzard WR, Bierman EL, Blass JP, Ettuger WH Jr, Halter JB (eds). *Principles of Geriatric Medicine and Gerontology, 3rd ed*. McGraw-Hill, New York, 1994, pp 509–516.

Biessmann H, Carter SB, Mason JM. Chromosome ends in *Drosophila* without telomeric sequences. *Proc Nat Acad Sci USA* 87:1758–1761, 1990a.

Biessmann H, Mason JM. Genetics and molecular biology of telomeres. *Adv Genet* 30:185–249, 1992.

Biessmann H, Mason JM, Ferry K, d'Hulst M, Valgeirsdottir K, Traverse KL, Pardue ML. Addition of telomere-associated HeT DNA sequences "heals" broken chromosome ends in *Drosophila*. *Cell* 61:663–673, 1990b.

Biessmann H, Walter MF, Mason JM. *Drosophila* telomere elongation. *Ciba Found Symp* 211:53–67; discussion 67–70, 1997.

Bilaud T, Brun C, Ancelin K, Koering CE, Laroche T, Gilson E. Telomeric localization of TRF2, a novel human telobox protein. *Nat Genet* 17:236–239, 1997.

Biller BM, Vance ML, Kleinberg DL, Cook DM, Gordon T. Clinical and reimbursement issues in growth hormone use in adults. *Am J Manag Care* 6:S817–827, 2000.

Biroccio A, Amodei S, Benassi B, Scarsella M, Cianciulli A, Mottolese M, Del Bufalo D, Leonetti C, Zupi G. Reconstitution of hTERT restores tumorigenicity in melanoma-derived c-Myc low-expressing clones. *Oncogene* 21:3011–3019, 2002.

Bisoffi M, Chakerian AE, Fore ML, Bryant JE, Hernandez JP, Moyzis RK, Griffith JK. Inhibition of human telomerase by a retrovirus expressing telomeric antisense RNA. *Eur J Cancer* 34:1242–1249, 1998.

Bissell DM. Hepatic fibrosis as wound repair: a progress report. *J Gastroenterol* 33:295–302, 1998.

Bjorklund A, Lindvall O. Cell replacement therapies for central nervous system disorders. *Nat Neurosci* 3:537–544, 2000.

Black A, Allison DB, Shapses SA, Tilmont EM, Handy AM, Ingram DK, Roth GS, Lane MA. Calorie restriction and skeletal mass in rhesus monkeys (*Maccaca mulatta*): evidence for an effect mediated through changes in body size. *J Gerontol A Biol Sci Med Sci* 56:B98–107, 2001.

Blackburn E. The telomere and telomerase: how do they interact? *Mt Sinai J Med* 66:292–300, 1999.

Blackburn E, Bhattacharyya A, Gilley D, Kirk K, Krauskopf A, McEachern M, Prescott J, Ware T. The telomere and telomerase: how do they interact? *Ciba Found Symp* 211:2–15, 1997.

Blackburn E, Gilley D, Ware T, Bhattacharyya A, Kirk K, Wang H. Studying the telomerase RNA in *Tetrahymena*. *Methods Cell Biol* 62:417–432, 2000.

Blackburn EH. Telomeres and their synthesis. *Science* 249:489–490, 1990a.

Blackburn EH. Telomeres: structure and synthesis. *J Biol Chem* 265:5919–5921, 1990b.

Blackburn EH. Structure and function of telomeres. *Nature* 350:569–573, 1991.

Blackburn EH. Developmentally programmed healing of chromosomes. In Blackburn EH, Greider CW (eds). *Telomeres*. Cold Spring Harbor Laboratory Press, Cold Spring Harbor, NY, 1995, pp 193–218.

Blackburn EH. The telomere and telomerase: nucleic acid-protein complexes acting in a telomere homeostasis system. A review. *Biochemistry (Mosc)* 62:1196–1201, 1997.

Blackburn EH. Telomere states and cell fates. *Nature* 408:53–56, 2000a.

Blackburn EH. Telomeres and telomerase. *Keio J Med* 49:59–65, 2000b.

Blackburn EH. Telomere capping and cell proliferation. Presented at Cancer and Molecular Genetics in the Twenty-first Century, Van Andel Research Institute, Grand Rapids, MI, September 5–9, 2000c.

Blackburn EH. Switching and signaling at the telomere. *Cell* 106:661–763, 2001.

Blackburn EH, Gall JG. A tandemly repeated sequence at the termini of the extrachromosomal ribosomal RNA genes in *Tetrahymena*. *J Mol Biol* 120:33–53, 1978.

Blackburn EH, Greider CW. *Telomeres*. Cold Spring Harbor Laboratory Press, Cold Spring Harbor, NY, 1995.

Blackburn EH, Szostak JW. The molecular structure of centromeres and telomeres. *Annu Rev Biochem* 53:163–194, 1984.

Blacker D, Tanzi RE. The genetics of Alzheimer disease: current status and future prospects. *Arch Neurol* 55:294–296, 1998.

Blackman MR. Age-related alterations in sleep quality and neuroendocrine function: interrelationships and implications. *JAMA* 284:879–881, 2000.

Blackman MR, Sorkin JD, Munzer T, Bellantoni MF, Busby-Whitehead J, Stevens TE, Jayme J, O'Connor KG, Christmas C, Tobin JD, Stewart KJ, Cottrell E, St. Clair C, Pabst KM, Harman, SM. Growth hormone and sex steroid administration in healthy aged women and men. *JAMA* 288:2282–2292, 2002.

Blagosklonny MV. How carcinogens (or telomere dysfunction) induce genetic instability: associated-selection model. *FEBS Lett* 506:169–172, 2001.

Blain H, Jouzeau JY, Blain A, Terlain B, Trechot P, Touchon J, Netter P, Jeandel C. Non-steroidal anti-inflammatory drugs with selectivity for cyclooxygenase-2 in Alzheimer's disease. Rationale and perspectives [in French]. *Presse Med* 29:267–273, 2000.

Blake DA, Yu H, Young DL, Caldwell DR. Matrix stimulates the proliferation of human corneal endothelial cells in culture. *Invest Ophthalmol Vis Sci* 38:1119–1129, 1997.

Blasco MA. Immunosenescence phenotypes in the telomerase knockout mouse. *Springer Semin Immunopathol* 24:75–85, 2002a.

Blasco MA. Mouse models to study the role of telomeres in cancer, aging and DNA repair. *Eur J Cancer* 38:2222–2228, 2002b.

Blasco MA. Telomerase beyond telomeres. *Nat Rev Cancer* 2:627–633, 2002c.

Blasco MA, DePinho RA, Gottlieb GJ, Greider CW, Horner II JW, Lee H. Essential role of mouse telomerase in highly proliferative organs. *Nature* 392:569–574, 1998.

Blasco MA, DePinho RA, Greider CW, Hande MP, Lansdorp PM, Lee HW, Samper E . Telomere shortening and tumor formation by mouse cells lacking telomerase RNA. *Cell* 91:25–34, 1997a.

Blasco MA, Funk W, Greider CW, Villeponteau B. Functional characterization and developmental regulation of mouse telomerase RNA. *Science* 269:1267–1270 1995.

Blasco MA, Gasser SM, Lingner J. Telomeres and telomerase. *Genes Dev* 13:2353–2359, 1999.

Blasco MA, Lee HW, Rizen M, Hanahan D, DePinho R, Greider CW. Mouse models for the study of telomerase. *Ciba Found Symp* 211:160–170, 1997b.

Blasco MA, Rizen M, Greider CW, Hanahan D. Differential regulation of telomerase activity and telomerase RNA during multi-stage tumorigenesis. *Nat Genet* 12:200–204, 1996.

Blasiak J, Kadlubek M, Kowalik J, Romanowicz-Makowska H, Pertynski T. Inhibition of telomerase activity in endometrial cancer cells by selenium-cisplatin conjugate despite suppression of its DNA-damaging activity by sodium ascorbate. *Teratog Carcinog Mutagen* 22:73–82, 2002.

Blau JN. Cases: Werner's syndrome. *Proc R Soc Med* 55:328, 1962.

Blechner MD, Mandavilli SR, Tsongalis GJ. Measuring telomerase activity for the early detection of cancer. *Conn Med* 65:643–648, 2001.

Bloom W, Fawcett DW. *A Textbook of Histology, 10th ed.* W.B. Saunders Company, Philadelphia, 1975.

Blot WJ, McLaughlin JK. The changing epidemiology of esophageal cancer. *Semin Oncol* 26(5 Suppl 15):2–8, 1999.

Boatwright H, Wheeler CE, Cawley EP. Werner's syndrome. *Arch Intern Med* 90:243–249, 1952.

Bodnar AG, Chiu C, Frolkis M, Harley CB, Holt SE, Lichtsteiner S, Morin GB, Ouellette M, Shay JW, Wright WE. Extension of life span by introduction of telomerase into normal human cells. *Science* 279:349–352, 1998.

Bodnar AG, Kim NW, Effros RB, Chiu CP. Mechanism of telomerase induction during T cell activation. *Exp Cell Res* 228:58–64, 1996.

Boeke JD. A little help for my ends. *Nature* 383:579–581, 1996.

Bohr VA, Anson RM. DNA damage, mutation and fine structure DNA repair in aging. *Mutat Res* 338:25–34, 1995.

Boklan J, Nanjangud G, MacKenzie KL, May C, Sadelain M, Moore MA. Limited proliferation and telomere dysfunction following telomerase inhibition in immortal murine fibroblasts. *Cancer Res* 62:2104–2114, 2002.

Bolli R. Regeneration of the human heart—no chimera? *N Engl J Med* 346:55–56, 2002.

Bolzan AD, Paez GL, Bianchi MS, Bianchi NO. Analysis of telomeric repeats and telomerase activity in human colon carcinoma cells with gene amplification. *Cancer Genet Cytogenet* 120:166–170, 2000.

Bonatz G, Frahm SO, Klapper W, Helfenstein A, Heidorn K, Jonat W, Krupp G, Parwaresch R, Rudolph P. High telomerase activity is associated with cell cycle deregulation and rapid progression in endometrioid adenocarcinoma of the uterus. *Hum Pathol* 32:605–614, 2001.

Bonifacio S, Centrone C, Da Prato L, Scordo MR, Estienne M, Torricelli F. Use of primed in situ labeling (PRINS) for the detection of telomeric deletions associated with mental retardation. *Cytogenet Cell Genet* 93:16–18, 2001.

Bonilla E, Tanji K, Hirano M, Vu TH, DiMauro S, Schon EA. Mitochondrial involvement in Alzheimer's disease. *Biochim Biophys Acta* 1410:171–182, 1999.

Bonin LR, Madden K, Shera K, Ihle J, Matthews C, Aziz S, Perez-Reyes N, McDougall JK, Conroy SC. Generation and characterization of human smooth muscle cell lines derived from atherosclerotic plaque. *Arterioscler Thromb Vasc Biol* 19:575–587, 1999.

Boogaerts MA, Brugger W, Carella AM, Cortes-Funes H, Fibbe WE, Hows J, Khayat D, Linch DC, Link H, Moore MA, Testa NG. Peripheral blood progenitor cell transplantation: where do we stand? Chairman's Summary of the European School of Oncology Task Force Meeting on Peripheral Blood Progenitor Cells held September 29–30, 1995. *Ann Oncol* 7:1–4, 1996.

Booth C, Griffith E, Brady G, Lydall D. Quantitative amplification of single-stranded DNA (QAOS) demonstrates that *cdc13-1* mutants generate ssDNA in a telomere to centromere direction. *Nucleic Acids Res* 29:4414–4422, 2001.

Boral AL, Dessain S, Chabner BA. Clinical evaluation of biologically targeted drugs: obstacles and opportunities. *Cancer Chemother Pharmacol* 42 Suppl:S3–21, 1998.

Borges A, Liew CC. Telomerase activity during cardiac development. *J Mol Cell Cardiol* 29:2717–2724, 1997.

Bornemann A, Maier F, Kuschel R. Satellite cells as players and targets in normal and diseased muscle. *Neuropediatrics* 30:167–175, 1999.

Boroditsky RS. Balancing safety and efficacy focus on endometrial protection. *J Reprod Med* 45(3 Suppl):273–284, 2000.

Bosoy D, Lue NF. Functional analysis of conserved residues in the putative "finger" domain of telomerase reverse transcriptase. *J Biol Chem* 276:46305–46312, 2001.

Bostik P, Brice GT, Greenberg KP, Mayne AE, Villinger F, Lewis MG, Ansari AA. Inverse correlation of telomerase activity/proliferation of CD4+ T lymphocytes and disease progression in simian immunodeficiency virus-infected nonhuman primates. *J Acquir Immune Defic Syndr* 24:89–99, 2000.

Bouchal J, Kolar Z, Mad'arova J, Hlobilkova A, von Angerer E. The effects of natural ligands of hormone receptors and their antagonists on telomerase activity in the androgen sensitive prostatic cancer cell line LNCaP. *Biochem Pharmacol* 63:1177–1181, 2002.

Boucher N, Dufeu-Duchesne T, Vicaut E, Farge D, Effros RB, Schachter F. CD28 expression in T cell aging and human longevity. *Exp Gerontol* 33:267–282, 1998.

Bouffler SD. Involvement of telomeric sequences in chromosomal aberrations. *Mutat Res* 404:199–204, 1998.

Bouffler SD, Blasco MA, Cox R, Smith PJ. Telomeric sequences, radiation sensitivity and genomic instability. *Int J Radiat Biol* 77:995–1005, 2001.

Boukamp P. Ageing mechanisms: the role of telomere loss. *Clin Exp Dermatol* 26:562–565, 2001.

Bourns BD, Alexander MK, Smith AM, Zakian VA. Sir proteins, Rif proteins, and Cdc13p bind *Saccharomyces* telomeres in vivo. *Mol Cell Biol* 18:5600–5608, 1998.

Bova B. Eternal verities, eternal questions. *Nature* 404:439, 2000.

Bowles JT. The evolution of aging: a new approach to an old problem of biology. *Med Hypotheses* 51:179–221, 1998.

Boyd MWJ, Grant AP. Werner's syndrome (progeria of the adult): further pathological and biochemical observations. *BMJ* 2:920–925, 1959.

Boyle DL, Takemoto LJ. Finger-like projections of plasma membrane in the most senescent fiber cells of human lenses. *Curr Eye Res* 17:1118–1123, 1998.

Braekman BP, Houthoofd K, Vanfleteren JR. Patterns of metabolic activity during aging of the wild-type and longevity mutants of *Caenorhabditis elegans*. *J Am Aging Assoc* 23:55–73, 2000.

Brallier JM. *Medical Wit and Wisdom*. Running Press, Philadelphia, 1993.

Brand RM, Iversen PL. Iontophoretic delivery of a telomeric oligonucleotide. *Pharm Res* 13:851–854, 1996.

Branicky R, Benard C, Hekimi S. clk-1, mitochondria, and physiological rates. *Bioessays* 22:48–56, 2000.

Brannan CI, Disteche CM, Park LS, Copeland NG, Jenkins NA. Autosomal telomere exchange results in the rapid amplification and dispersion of *Csf2ra* genes in wild-derived mice. *Mamm Genome* 12:882–886, 2001.

Braun-Dullaeus RC, Mann MJ, Dzau VJ. Cell cycle progression: new therapeutic target for vascular proliferative disease. *Circulation* 98:82–89, 1998.

Braun-Dullaeus RC, Mann MJ, Ziegler A, von der Leyen HE, Dzau VJ. A novel role for the cyclin-dependent kinase inhibitor p27(Kip1) in angiotensin II–stimulated vascular smooth muscle cell hypertrophy. *J Clin Invest* 104:815–823, 1999.

Brauner DJ, Muir JC, Sachs GA. Treating nondementia illnesses in patients with dementia. *JAMA* 283:3230–3235, 2000.

Braunschweig R, Guilleret I, Delacretaz F, Bosman FT, Mihaescu A, Benhattar J. Pitfalls in TRAP assay in routine detection of malignancy in effusions. *Diagn Cytopathol* 25:225–230, 2001a.

Braunschweig R, Yan P, Guilleret I, Delacretaz F, Bosman FT, Mihaescu A, Benhattar J. Detection of malignant effusions: comparison of a telomerase assay and cytologic examination. *Diagn Cytopathol* 24:174–80, 2001b.

Braunstein I, Cohen-Barak O, Shachaf C, Ravel Y, Yalon-Hacohen M, Mills GB, Tzukerman M, Skorecki KL. Human telomerase reverse transcriptase promoter regulation in normal and malignant human ovarian epithelial cells. *Cancer Res* 61:5529–5536, 2001.

Brazelton TR, Rossi FMV, Keshet GI, Blau HM. From marrow to brain: expression of neuronal phenotypes in adult mice. *Science* 290:1775–1779, 2000.

Breitbart E, Wang X, Leka LS, Dallal GE, Meydani SN, Stollar BD. Altered memory B-cell homeostasis in human aging. *J Gerontol A Biol Sci Med Sci* 57A:B304–311, 2002.

Brenneisen P, Gogo J, Bayreuther K. Regulation of DNA synthesis in mitotic and postmitotic WI38 fibroblasts in the fibroblast stem cell system. *J Cell Biochem* 17D:152, 1993.

Brenner S. Introduction: telomeres and telomerase. *Ciba Found Symp* 211:2–15, 1997.

Breslow JL. Mouse models of atherosclerosis. *Science* 272:685–688, 1996.

Breslow RA, Shay JW, Gazdar AF, Srivastava S. Telomerase and early detection of cancer: a National Cancer Institute workshop. *J Natl Cancer Inst* 89:618–623, 1997.

Bretsky PM, Buckwalter JG, Seeman TE, Miller CA, Poirier J, Schellenberg GD, Finch CE, Henderson VW. Evidence for an interaction between apolipoprotein E genotype, gender, and *Alzheimer disease*. *Alzheimer Dis Assoc Disord* 13:216–221, 1999.

Brewer GJ. Age-related toxicity to lactate, glutamate and beta-amyloid in cultured adult neurons. *Neurobiol Aging* 19:561–568, 1998.

Brewer GJ. Regeneration and proliferation of embryonic and adult rat hippocampal neurons in culture. *Exp Neurol* 159:237–247, 1999.

Brewer GJ. Neuronal plasticity and stressor toxicity during aging. *Exp Gerontol* 35:1165–1183, 2000.

Brewer GJ, Espinosa J, McIlhaney MP, Pencek TP, Kesslak JP, Cotman C, Viel J, McManus DC. Culture and regeneration of human neurons after brain surgery. *J Neurosci Methods* 107:15–23, 2001.

Brewer GJ, Wallimann TW. Protective effect of the energy precursor creatine against toxicity of glutamate and beta-amyloid in rat hippocampal neurons. *J Neurochem* 74:1968–1978, 2000.

Briata P, Bellini C, Vignolo M, Gherzi R. Insulin receptor gene expression is reduced in cells from a progeric patient. *Mol Cell Endocrinol* 75:9–14, 1991.

Bridger JM, Bickmore WA. Putting the genome on the map. *Trends Genet* 14:403–409, 1998.

Brinton RD. A women's health issue: Alzheimer's disease and strategies for maintaining cognitive health. *Int J Fertil Womens Med* 44:174–185, 1999.

Britten M, Schachinger V. The role of endothelial function for ischemic manifestations of coronary atherosclerosis [in German]. *Herz* 23:97–105, 1998.

Brittney-Shea H, Pongracz K, Shay JW, Gryaznov SM, Shea-Herbert B. Oligonucleotide N3′→P5′ phosphoramidates as efficient telomerase inhibitors. *Oncogene* 21:638–642, 2002.

Broccoli D, Chong L, Oelmann S, Fernald AA, Marziliano N, van Steensel B, Kipling D, Le Beau MM, de Lange T. Comparison of the human and mouse genes encoding the telomeric protein, TRF1: chromosomal localization, expression and conserved protein domains. *Hum Mol Genet* 6:69–76, 1997.

Broccoli D, Godwin AK. Telomere length changes in human cancer. *Methods Mol Med* 68:271–278, 2002.

Broccoli D, Young JW, de Lange T. Telomerase activity in normal and malignant hematopoietic cells. *Proc Natl Acad Sci USA* 92:9082–9086, 1995.

Brock J, Sauaia A, Ahnen D, Marine W, Schluter W, Stevens BR, Scinto JD, Karp H, Bratzler D. Process of care and outcomes for elderly patients hospitalized with peptic ulcer disease. *JAMA* 286:11985–1993, 2001.

Broe GA, Grayson DA, Creasey HM, Waite LM, Casey BJ, Bennett HP, Brooks WS, Halliday GM. Anti-inflammatory drugs protect against Alzheimer disease at low doses. *Arch Neurol* 57:1586–1591, 2000.

Bron AJ, Brown NA, Harding JJ, Ganea E. The lens and cataract in diabetes. *Int Ophthalmol Clin* 38:37–67, 1998.

Brooke RC, Newbold SA, Telfer NR, Griffiths CE. Discordance between facial wrinkling and the presence of basal cell carcinoma. *Arch Dermatol* 137:751–754, 2001.

Brooks PM. Hematopoietic stem cell transplantation for autoimmune diseases. *J Rheumatol Suppl* 48:19–22, 1997.

Brose A, Parise G, Tarnopolsky MA. Creatine supplementation enhances isometric strength and body composition improvements following strength exercise training in older adults. *J Gerontol A Biol Sci Med Sci* 58:11–19, 2003.

Bross R, Storer T, Bhasin S. Aging and muscle loss. *Trends Endocrinol Metab* 10:194–198, 1999.

Brown AJ, Cormack BP, Gow NA, Kvaal C, Soll DR, Srikantha T. Advances in molecular genetics of *Candida albicans* and *Candida glabrata*. *Med Mycol* 36(Suppl 1):230–237, 1998a.

Brown DF, Gazdar AF, White CL 3rd, Yashima K, Shay JW, Rushing EJ. Human telomerase RNA expression and MIB-1 (Ki-67) proliferation index distinguish hemangioblastomas from metastatic renal cell carcinomas. *J Neuropathol Exp Neurol* 56:1349–1355, 1997a.

Brown FM. Urine cytology: Is it still the gold standard for screening? *Urol Clin North Am* 27:25–37, 2000.

Brown JC, Brown BA 2nd, Li Y, Hardin CC. Construction and characterization of a quadruplex DNA selective single-chain autoantibody from a viable motheaten mouse hybridoma with homology to telomeric DNA binding proteins. *Biochemistry* 37:16338–16348, 1998b.

Brown JP, Wei W, Sedivy JM. Bypass of senescence after disruption of *p21^{CIP1/WAF1}* gene in normal diploid human fibroblasts. *Science* 277:831–834, 1997b.

Brown WR. Progeroid syndromes. In Maddox GL (ed). *The Encyclopedia of Aging, 2nd ed.* Springer Publishing Company, New York, 1995, pp 765–767.

Brown WRA, MacKinnon PH, Villasante A, Spurr N, Buckle VJ, Dobson MJ. Structure and polymorphism of human telomere-associated DNA. *Cell* 63:119–132, 1990.

Brown WT. Progeria: a human-disease model of accelerated aging. *Am J Clin Nutr* 55:1222S–1224S, 1992.

Brown WT, Darlington GJ. Thermolabile enzymes in progeria and Werner syndrome: evidence contrary to the protein error hypothesis. *Am J Hum Genet* 32:614–619, 1980.

Brown WT, Darlington GJ, Arnold A, Fotino M. Detection of HLA antigens on progeria syndrome fibroblasts. *Clin Genet* 17:213–219, 1980a.

Brown WT, Epstein J, Little JB. Progeria cells are stimulated to repair DNA by co-cultivation with normal cells. *Exp Cell Res* 97:291–296, 1976.

Brown WT, Ford JP, Gershey EL. Variation of DNA repair capacity in progenia cells unrelated to growth conditions. *Biochem Biophys Res Commun* 97:347–353, 1980b.

Brown WT, Kieras FJ, Houck GE Jr, Dutkowski R, Jenkins EC. A comparison of adult and childhood progerias: Werner syndrome and Hutchinson-Gilford progeria syndrome. *Adv Exp Med Biol* 190:229–244, 1985.

Brown WT, Little JB, Epstein J, Williams JR. DNA repair defect in progeric cells. *Birth Defects* 14:417–430, 1978.

Brown-Borg HM, Bode AM, Bartke A. Antioxidative mechanisms and plasma growth hormone levels: potential relationship in the aging process. *Endocrine* 11:41–48, 1999.

Bruce-Keller AJ. Microglial–neuronal interactions in synaptic damage and recovery. *J Neurosci Res* 58:191–201, 1999.

Bruce-Keller AJ, Keeling JL, Keller JN, Huang FF, Camondola S, Mattson MP. Antiinflammatory effects of estrogen on microglial activation. *Endocrinology* 141:3646–3656, 2000.

Bruce-Keller AJ, Umberger G, McFall R, Mattson MP. Food restriction reduces brain damage and improves behavioral outcome following excitotoxic and metabolic insults. *Ann Neurol* 45:8–15, 1999.

Bruera E, Sweeney C. Cachexia and asthenia in cancer patients. *Lancet Oncol* 1:138–147, 2000.

Brummendorf TH, Ersoz I, Hartmann U, Bartolovic K, Balabanov S, Wahl A, Paschka P, Kreil S, Lahaye T, Berger U, Gschaidmeier H, Bokemeyer C, Hehlmann R, Dietz K, Lansdorp PM, Kanz L, Hochhaus A. Telomere length in peripheral blood granulocytes reflects response to treatment with imatinib in patients with chronic myeloid leukemia. *Blood* 101:375, 2003.

Brummendorf TH, Holyoake TL, Rufer N, Barnett MJ, Schulzer M, Eaves CJ, Eaves AC, Lansdorp PM. Prognostic implications of differences in telomere length between normal and malignant cells from patients with chronic myeloid leukemia measured by flow cytometry. *Blood* 95:1883–1890, 2000.

Brummendorf TH, Maciejewski JP, Mak J, Young NS, Lansdorp PM. Telomere length in leukocyte subpopulations of patients with aplastic anemia. *Blood* 97:895–900, 2001a.

Brummendorf TH, Mak J, Sabo KM, Baerlocher GM, Dietz K, Abkowitz JL, Lansdorp PM. Longitudinal studies of telomere length in feline blood cells: implications for hematopoietic stem cell turnover in vivo. *Exp Hematol* 30:1147–1152, 2002.

Brummendorf TH, Rufer N, Baerlocher GM, Roosnek E, Lansdorp PM. Limited telomere shortening in hematopoietic stem cells after transplantation. *Ann NY Acad Sci* 938:1–7, 2001b.

Brummendorf TH, Rufer N, Holyoake TL, Maciejewski J, Barnett MJ, Eaves CJ, Eaves AC, Young N, Lansdorp PM. Telomere length dynamics in normal individuals and in patients with hematopoietic stem cell–associated disorders. *Ann NY Acad Sci* 938:293–303, 2001c.

Brunden KR, Frederickson CA. Activated neuroglia in Alzheimer's disease. In de Vellis J (ed). *Neuroglia in the Aging Brain.* Humana Press, Totowa, NJ, 2002, pp 365–374.

Brundin P, Pogarell O, Hagell P, Piccini P, Widner H, Schrag A, Kupsch A, Crabb L, Odin P, Gustavii B, Bjorklund A, Brooks DJ, Marsden CD, Oertel WH, Quinn NP, Rehncrona S, Lindvall O. Bilateral caudate and putamen grafts of embryonic mesencephalic tissue treated with lazaroids in Parkinson's disease. *Brain* 123:1380, 2000.

Brundtland GH. The war against disease: investing in health, investing in our common future. *JAMA* 287:444, 2002.

Brusco LI, Marquez M, Cardinali DP. Monozygotic twins with Alzheimer's disease treated with melatonin: case report. *J Pineal Res* 25:260–263, 1998.

Bruunsgaard H, Jensen MS, Schjerling P, Halkjaer-Kristensen J, Ogawa K, Skinhoj P, Pedersen BK. Exercise induces recruitment of lymphocytes with an activated phenotype and short telomeres in young and elderly humans. *Life Sci* 65:2623–2633, 1999.

Bruunsgaard H, Pedersen BK. The senile immune system [in Danish]. *Ugeskr Laeger* 161:4740–4743, 1999.

Bruunsgaard H, Pedersen BK. The senile immune system [in Danish]. *Tidsskr Nor Laegeforen* 120:29–31, 2000.

Bryan TM, Cech TR. Telomerase and the maintenance of chromosome ends. *Curr Opin Cell Biol* 11:318–324, 1999.

Bryan TM, Englezou A, Dalla-Pozza L, Dunham MA, Reddel RR. Evidence for an alternative mechanism for maintaining telomere length in human tumors and tumor-derived cell lines. *Nat Med* 3:1271–1274, 1997a.

Bryan TM, Englezou A, Dunham MA, Reddel RR. Telomere length dynamics in telomerase-positive immortal human cell populations. *Exp Cell Res* 239:370–378, 1998.

Bryan TM, Engelzou A, Gupta J, Bacchetti S, Reddel RR. Telomere elongation in immortal human cells without detectable telomerase activity. *EMBO J* 14:4240–4248, 1995.

Bryan TM, Marusic L, Bacchetti S, Namba M, Reddel RR. The telomere lengthening mechanism in telomerase-negative immortal human cells does not involve the telomerase RNA subunit. *Hum Mol Genet* 6:921–926, 1997b.

Bryan TM, Reddel RR. Telomere dynamics and telomerase activity in in vitro immortalised human cells. *Eur J Cancer* 33:767–773, 1997.

Bryant JE, Hutchings KG, Moyzis RK, Griffith JK. Measurement of telomeric DNA content in human tissues. *Biotechniques* 23:476–478, 480, 482, passim, 1997.

Bryce LA, Morrison N, Hoare SF, Muir S, Keith WN. Mapping of the gene for the human telomerase reverse transcriptase, hTERT, to chromosome 5p15.33 by fluorescence in situ hybridization. *Neoplasia* 2:197–201, 2000.

Bryce SD, Forsyth NR, Fitzsimmons SA, Clark LJ, Bertram MJ, Cuthbert AP, Newbold RF, Pereira-Smith OM, Parkinson EK. Genetic and functional analyses exclude mortality factor 4 (MORF4) as a keratinocyte senescence gene. *Cancer Res* 59:2038–2040, 1999.

Buchkovich KJ. Telomeres, telomerase, and the cell cycle. *Prog Cell Cycle Res* 2:187–195, 1996.

Buchkovich KJ, Greider CW. Telomerase regulation during entry into the cell cycle in normal human T cells. *Mol Biol Cell* 7:1443–1454, 1996.

Buchler P, Conejo-Garcia JR, Lehmann G, Muller M, Emrich T, Reber HA, Buchler MW, Friess H. Real-time quantitative PCR of telomerase mRNA is useful for the differentiation of benign and malignant pancreatic disorders. *Pancreas* 22:331–340, 2001.

Bucholc M, Park Y, Lustig AJ. Intrachromatid excision of telomeric DNA as a mechanism for telomere size control in *Saccharomyces cerevisiae*. *Mol Cell Biol* 21:6559–6573, 2001.

Buck S, Nicholson M, Dudas S, Wells R, Force A, Baker GT 3d, Arking R. Larval regulation of adult longevity in a genetically selected long-lived strain of *Drosophila*. *Heredity* 71(Pt 1):23–32, 1993a.

Buck S, Vettraino J, Force AG, Arking R. Extended longevity in *Drosophila* is consistently associated with a decrease in developmental viability. *J Gerontol A Biol Sci Med Sci* 55:B292–301, 2000.

Buck S, Wells RA, Dudas SP, Baker GT 3d, Arking R. Chromosomal localization and regulation of the longevity determinant genes in a selected strain of *Drosophila melanogaster*. *Heredity* 71(Pt 1):11–22, 1993b.

Bulian D, Pierpaoli W. The pineal gland and cancer: I. Pinealectomy corrects congenital hormonal dysfunctions and prolongs life of cancer-prone C3H/He mice. *J Neuroimmunol* 108:131–135, 2000.

Burger A. Standard TRAP assay. In Double JA, Thompson MJ (eds). *Telomeres and Telomerase: Methods and Protocols*. Humana Press, Totowa, NJ, 2002, pp 109–124.

Burger AM, Bibby MC, Double JA. Telomerase activity in normal and malignant mammalian tissues: feasibility of telomerase as a target for cancer chemotherapy. *Br J Cancer* 75:516–522, 1997.

Burke EM, Horton WE, Pearson JD, Crow MT, Martin GR. Altered transcriptional regulation of human interstitial collagenase in cultured skin fibroblasts from older donors. *Exp Gerontol* 29:37–53, 1994.

Burke JM, McKay BS. In vitro aging of bovine and human retinal pigment epithelium: number and activity of the Na/K ATPase pump. *Exp Eye Res* 57:51–57, 1993.

Burkle A. Poly(ADP-ribosyl)ation: a posttranslational protein modification linked with genome protection and mammalian longevity. *Biogerontology* 1:41–46, 2000.

Burt AD. Pathobiology of hepatic stellate cells. *J Gastroenterol* 34:299–304, 1999.

Burt RK, Brenner M, Burns W, Courier E, Firestein G, Hahn B, Heslop H, Link C, McFarland H, Roland M, Territo M, Tsokos G, Traynor A. Gene-marked autologous hematopoietic stem cell transplantation of autoimmune disease. *J Clin Immunol* 20:1–9, 2000.

Butler J, Ness R, Speroff T. Improving care for elderly patients with peptic ulcer disease: should the focus be on drugs or bugs? *JAMA* 286:2023–2024, 2001.

Butler MG, Tilburt J, DeVries A, Muralidhar B, Aue G, Hedges L, Atkinson J, Schwartz H. Comparison of chromosome telomere integrity in multiple tissues from subjects at different ages. *Cancer Genet Cytogenet* 105:138–144, 1998.

Butler RN, Fossel M, Harman SM, Heward CB, Olshansky SJ, Perls TT, Rothman DJ, Rothman SM, Warner HR, West MD, Wright WE. Is there an antiaging medicine? *J Gerontol A Biol Sci Med Sci* 57A:B333–338, 2002.

Buys CH. Telomeres, telomerase, and cancer. *N Engl J Med* 342:1282–1283, 2000.

Caddle SD, Counter CC, Eaton EN, Ellisen LW, Haber SD, Meyerson M, Weinberg RA. Telomerase activity is restored in human cells by ectopic expression of hTERT (hEST2), the catalytic subunit of telomerase. *Oncogene* 16:1217–1222, 1998.

Cai A, Wise PM. Age-related changes in light-induced Jun-B and Jun-D expression: effects of transplantation of fetal tissue containing the suprachiasmatic nucleus. *J Biol Rhythms* 11:284–290, 1996.

Cajero-Juarez M, Avila B, Ochoa A, Garrido-Guerrero E, Varela-Echavarria A, Martinez D, Clapp C. Immortalization of bovine umbilical vein endothelial cells: a model for the study of vascular endothelium. *Eur J Cell Biol* 81:1–8, 2002.

Caldarera E, Crooks NH, Muir GH, Pavone-Macaluso M, Carmichael PL. An appraisal of telomerase activity in benign prostatic hyperplasia. *Prostate* 45:267–270, 2000.

Callen E, Ramirez MJ, Creus A, Marcos R, Ortega JJ, Olive T, Badell I, Surralles J. Relationship between chromosome fragility, aneuploidy and severity of the haematological disease in Fanconi anaemia. *Mutat Res* 504:75–83, 2002a.

Callen E, Samper E, Ramirez MJ, Creus A, Marcos R, Ortega JJ, Olive T, Badell I, Blasco MA, Surralles J. Breaks at telomeres and TRF2–independent end fusions in Fanconi anemia. *Hum Mol Genet* 11:439–444, 2002b.

Calvaresi E, Bryan J. B vitamins, cognition, and aging: a review. *J Gerontol A Psychol Sci* 56:P327–339, 2001.

Cameron HA, McKay RD. Restoring production of hippocampal neurons in old age. *Nat Neurosci* 2:894–897, 1999.

Campagnoli C, Ambroggio S, Biglia N, Sismondi P. Conjugated estrogens and breast cancer risk. *Gynecol Endocrinol* 13(Suppl 6):13–19, 1999.

Campbell WW, Trappe TA, Wolfe RR, Evans WJ. The recommended dietary allowance for protein may not be adequate for older people to maintain skeletal muscle. *J Gerontol A Biol Sci Med Sci* 56:M373–380, 2001.

Campisi J. Gene expression in quiescent and senescent fibroblasts. *Ann NY Acad Sci* 663:195–201, 1992a.

Campisi J. Oncogenes, protooncogenes, and tumor suppressor genes: a hitchhiker's guide to senescence? *Exp Gerontol* 27:397–401, 1992b.

Campisi J. Replicative senescence: an old lives' tale? *Cell* 84:497–500, 1996.

Campisi J. Aging and cancer: the double-edged sword of replicative senescence. *J Am Geriatr Soc* 45:482–488, 1997a.

Campisi J. The biology of replicative senescence. *Eur J Cancer* 33:703–709, 1997b.

Campisi J. Cancer and aging: the double edged sword of cell senescence. Abstract presented at Telomeres and Telomerase: Implications for Cell Immortality, Cancer, and Age-related Disease. San Francisco, CA, June 1–3, 1998a.

Campisi J. The role of cellular senescence in skin aging. *J Investig Dermatol Symp Proc* 3:1–5, 1998b.

Campisi J. Aging, chromatin, and food restriction—connecting the dots. *Science* 289:2062–2063, 2000a.

Campisi J. Cancer, aging and cellular senescence. *In Vivo* 14:183–188, 2000b.

Campisi J, Dimri GP, Nehlin JO, Testori A, Yoshimoto K. Coming of age in culture. *Exp Gerontol* 31:7–12, 1996.

Campisi J, Kim SH, Lim CS, Rubio M. Cellular senescence, cancer and aging: the telomere connection. *Exp Gerontol* 36:1619–1637, 2001.

Campochiaro PA, Soloway P, Ryan SJ, Miller JW. The pathogenesis of choroidal neovascularization in patients with age-related macular degeneration. *Mol Vis* 5:34, 1999.

Candore G, Di Lorenzo G, Mansueto P, Melluso M, Frada G, Li Vecchi M, Esposito Pellitteri M, Drago A, Di Salvo A, Caruso C. Prevalence of organ-specific and non-organ-specific autoantibodies in healthy centenarians. *Mech Ageing Dev* 94:183–190, 1997.

Cano MI. Telomere biology of trypanosomatids: more questions than answers. *Trends Parasitol* 17:425–429, 2001.

Cano MI, Dungan JM, Agabian N, Blackburn EH. Telomerase in kinetoplastid parasitic protozoa. *Proc Natl Acad Sci USA* 96:3616–3621, 1999.

Cao Y, Li H, Deb S, Liu JP. TERT regulates cell survival independent of telomerase enzymatic activity. *Oncogene* 21:3130–3138, 2002a.

Cao Y, Li H, Mu FT, Ebisui O, Funder JW, Liu JP. Telomerase activation causes vascular smooth muscle cell proliferation in genetic hypertension. *FASEB J* 16:96–98, 2002b.

Carabello BA. Abnormalities in cardiac contraction: systolic dysfunction. In Hosenpud JD, Greenberg BH (eds). *Congestive Heart Failure.* Lippincott Williams & Wilkins, Philadelphia, 2000, pp 67–82.

Carioto LM, Kruth SA, Betts DH, King WA. Telomerase activity in clinically normal dogs and dogs with malignant lymphoma. *Am J Vet Res* 62:1442–1446, 2001.

Carlin C, Phillips PD, Brooks-Frederich K, Knowles BB, Cristofalo VJ. Cleavage of the epidermal growth factor receptor by a membrane-bound leupeptin-sensitive protease active in nonionic detergent lysates of senescent but not young human diploid fibroblasts. *J Cell Physiol* 160:427–434, 1994.

Carlson BM. Factors influencing the repair and adaptation of muscles in aged individuals: satellite cells and innervation. *J Gerontol A Biol Sci Med Sci* 50(Spec No):96–100, 1995.

Carlson BM, Dedkov EI, Borisov AB, Faulkner JA. Skeletal muscle regeneration in very old rats. *J Gerontol A Biol Sci Med Sci* 56:224–233, 2001.

Carlson LE, Sherwin BB. Relationships among cortisol (CRT), dehydroepiandrosterone-sulfate (DHEAS), and memory in a longitudinal study of healthy elderly men and women. *Neurobiol Aging* 20:315–324, 1999.

Carlton PM, Cande WZ. Telomeres act autonomously in maize to organize the meiotic bouquet from a semipolarized chromosome orientation. *J Cell Biol* 157:231–242, 2002.

Carmeliet P. One cell, two fates. *Nature* 408:43–45, 2000.

Carnero A, Hudson JD, Hannon GJ, Beach DH. Loss-of-function genetics in mammalian cells: the p53 tumor suppressor model. *Nucleic Acids Res* 28:2234–2241, 2000a.

Carnero A, Hudson JD, Price CM, Beach DH. p16INK4A and p19ARF act in overlapping pathways in cellular immortalization. *Nat Cell Biol* 2:148–155, 2000b.

Caron F, Jacq C, Rouviere-Yaniv J. Characterization of a histone-like protein extracted from yeast mitochondria. *Proc Natl Acad Sci USA* 76:4265–4269, 1979.

Carr AM. Piecing together the p53 puzzle. *Science* 287:1765–1766, 2000.

Carr AM. Checking that replication breakdown is not terminal. *Science* 297:557–558, 2002.

Carrel A, Ebeling AH. Age and multiplication of fibroblasts. *J Exp Med* 34:599, 1921.

Carvalho CR, de Paula Pinto Schettino G, Maranhao B, Bethlem EP. Hyperoxia and lung disease. *Curr Opin Pulm Med* 4:300–304, 1998.

Casaregola S, Nguyen HV, Lapathitis G, Kotyk A, Gaillardin C. Analysis of the constitution of the beer yeast genome by PCR, sequencing and subtelomeric sequence hybridization. *Int J Syst Evol Microbiol* 51:1607–1618, 2001.

Casasco A, Casasco M, Zerbinati N, Icaro Cornaglia A, Calligaro A. Cell proliferation and differentiation in a model of human skin equivalent. *Anat Rec* 264:261–272, 2001.

Cascio SM. Novel strategies for immortalization of human hepatocytes. *Artif Organs* 25:529–538, 2001.

Case JP. Old and new drugs used in rheumatoid arthritis: a historical perspective. Part 1: the older drugs. *Am J Ther* 8:123–143, 2001a.

Case JP. Old and new drugs used in rheumatoid arthritis: a historical perspective. Part 2: the newer drugs and drug strategies. *Am J Ther* 8:163–179, 2001b.

Caspary T, Cleary MA, Perlman EJ, Zhang P, Elledge SJ, Tilghman SM. Oppositely imprinted genes *p57(Kip2)* and *igf2* interact in a mouse model for Beckwith-Wiedemann syndrome. *Genes Dev* 13:3115–3124, 1999.

Castellani RJ, Harris PL, Lecroisey A, Izadi-Pruneyre N, Wandersman C, Perry G, Smith MA. Evidence for a novel heme-binding protein, HasAh, in Alzheimer disease. *Antioxid Redox Signal* 2:137–142, 2000.

Castro E, Ogburn CE, Hunt KE, Tilvis R, Louhija J, Penttinen R, Erkkola R, Panduro A, Riestra R, Piussan C, Deeb SS, Wang L, Edland SD, Martin GM, Oshima J. Polymorphisms at the Werner locus: I. Newly identified polymorphisms, ethnic variability of 1367Cy/Arg, and its stability in a population of Finnish centenarians. *Am J Med Genet* 82:399–403, 1999.

Castro RF, Jackson KA, Goodell MA, Robertson CS, Liu H, Shine HD. Failure of bone marrow cells to transdifferentiate into neural cells in vivo. *Science* 297:1299, 2003.

Cawthon RM. Telomere measurement by quantitative PCR. *Nucleic Acids Res* 30:e47, 2002.

Cawthon RM, Smith KR, O'Briend E, Sivatchenkoc A, Kerberc RA. Association between telomere length in blood and mortality in people aged 60 years or older. *Lancet* 361:393–395, 2003.

Cech TR. Life at the end of the chromosome: telomeres and telomerase. *Angew Chem Int Ed Engl* 39:34–43, 2000.

Cech TR, Lingner J. Telomerase and the chromosome end replication problem. *Ciba Found Symp* 211:20–28, 1997.

Cech TR, Nakamura TM, Lingner J. Telomerase is a true reverse transcriptase. A review. *Biochemistry (Mosc)* 62:1202–1205, 1997.

Cefalu WT, Bell-Farrow AD, Wang ZQ, Sonntag WE, Fu MX, Baynes JW, Thorpe SR. Caloric restriction decreases age-dependent accumulation of the glycoxidation products, N ε-(carboxymethyl)lysine and pentosidine, in rat skin collagen. *J Gerontol A Biol Sci Med Sci* 50:B337–B341, 1995.

Cefalu WT, Terry JG, Thomas MJ, Morgan TM, Edwards IJ, Rudel LL, Kemnitz JW, Weindruch R. In vitro oxidation of low-density lipoprotein in two species of nonhuman primates subjected to caloric restriction. *J Gerontol A Biol Sci Med Sci* 55:B355–B361, 2000.

Cefalu WT, Wagner JD, Bell-Farrow AD, Edwards IJ, Terry JG, Weindruch R, Kemnitz JW. Influence of caloric restriction on the development of atherosclerosis in nonhuman primates: progress to date. *Toxicol Sci* 52:49–55, 1999.

Cerimele F, Curreli F, Ely S, Friedman-Kien AE, Cesarman E, Flore O. Kaposi's sarcoma–associated herpesvirus can productively infect primary human keratinocytes and alter their growth properties. *J Virol* 75:2435–4243, 2001.

Cerni C. Telomeres, telomerase, and myc. An update. *Mutat Res* 462:31–47, 2000.

Cerone MA, Londono-Vallejo JA, Bacchetti S. Telomere maintenance by telomerase and by recombination can coexist in human cells. *Hum Mol Genet* 10:1945–1952, 2001.

Cervantes RB, Lundblad V. Mechanisms of chromosome-end protection. *Curr Opin Cell Biol* 14:351–356, 2002.

Chadeneau C, Hay K, Hirte HW, Gallinger S, Bacchetti S. Telomerase activity associated with acquisition of malignancy in human colorectal cancer. *Cancer Res* 55:2533–2536, 1995a.

Chadeneau C, Siegel P, Harley CB, Muller WJ, Bacchetti S. Telomerase activity in normal and malignant murine tissues. *Oncogene* 11:893–898, 1995b.

Chai W, Ford LP, Lenertz L, Wright WE, Shay JW. Human Ku70/80 associates physically with telomerase through interaction with hTERT. *J Biol Chem* 277:47242–47247, 2002.

Chakraborti S, Chakraborti T, Mandal M, Das S, Batabyal SK. Hypothalamic-pituitary-thyroid axis status of humans during development of ageing process. *Clin Chim Acta* 288:137–145, 1999.

Chambers DM, Kipling D, Abbott CM. Isolation of a microsatellite that reveals paralogy between the subtelomeric regions of mouse chromosomes 17 and 19: further evidence for telomere–telomere exchange in the mouse. *Genomics* 53:113–114, 1998.

Chambers RL, McDermott JC. Molecular basis of skeletal muscle regeneration. *Can J Appl Physiol* 21(3):155–184, 1996.

Chan SW, Blackburn EH. New ways not to make ends meet: telomerase, DNA damage proteins and heterochromatin. *Oncogene* 21:553–563, 2002.

Chan SW, Chang J, Prescott J, Blackburn EH. Altering telomere structure allows telomerase to act in yeast lacking ATM kinases. *Curr Biol* 11:1240–1250, 2001.

Chance B, Sies H, Boveris A. Hydroperoxide metabolism in mammalian organs. *Physiol Rev* 59:527–605, 1979.

Chandwaney R, Leichtweis S, Leeuwenburgh C, Ji LL. Oxidative stress and mitochondrial function in skeletal muscle: effects of aging and exercise training. *Age* 21:109–117, 1998.

Chang E, Harley CB. Telomere length and replicative aging in human vascular tissues. *Proc Natl Acad Sci USA* 92:1190–11194, 1995.

Chang JT, Liao CT, Jung SM, Wang TC, See LC, Cheng AJ. Telomerase activity is frequently found in metaplastic and malignant human nasopharyngeal tissues. *Br J Cancer* 82:1946–1951, 2000a.

Chang KW, Sarraj S, Lin SC, Tsai PI, Solt D. P53 expression, p53 and Ha-ras mutation and telomerase activation during nitrosamine-mediated hamster pouch carcinogenesis. *Carcinogenesis* 21:1441–1451, 2000b.

Chang S, Khoo C, DePinho RA. Modeling chromosomal instability and epithelial carcinogenesis in the telomerase-deficient mouse. *Semin Cancer Biol* 11:227–239, 2001.

Chang S, Khoo CM, Naylor ML, Maser RS, DePinho RA. Telomere-based crisis: functional differences between telomerase activation and ALT in tumor progression. *Genes Dev* 17:88–100, 2003.

Chang SW, Hu FR. Changes in corneal autofluorescence and corneal epithelial barrier function with aging. *Cornea* 12:493–499, 1993.

Chao D, Espeland MA, Farmer D, Register TC, Lenchik L, Applegate WB, Ettinger WH. Effect of voluntary weight loss on bone mineral density in older overweight women. *J Am Geriatr Soc* 48:753–759, 2000.

Chapin JW, Kahre J. Progeria and anesthesia. *Anesth Analgesia* 58:424–425, 1979.

Chapman ML, Zaun MR, Gracy RW. Changes in NAD levels in human lymphocytes and fibroblasts during aging and in premature aging syndromes. *Mech Ageing Dev* 21:157–167, 1983.

Chatterjee A, Shah S, Doyle SJ. Effect of age on final refractive outcome for 2342 patients following refractive keratectomy. *Invest Ophthalmol Vis Sci* 37:S57, 1996.

Chatterjee D, Wyche JH, Romero DP, Pantazis P. Telomerase activity, Myc and Bcl-2: possible indicators of effective therapy of prostate cancer with 9-nitrocamptothecin. *Anticancer Res* 20:2885–2889, 2000.

Chaturvedi V, Qin JZ, Denning MF, Choubey D, Diaz MO, Nickoloff BJ. Apoptosis in proliferating, senescent, and immortalized keratinocytes. *J Biol Chem* 274:23358–23367, 1999.

Chatziantoniou VD. Telomerase: biological function and potential role in cancer management. *Pathol Oncol Res* 7:161–170, 2001.

Chen CL, Weiss NS, Newcomb P, Barlow W, White E. Hormone replacement therapy in relation to breast cancer. *JAMA* 287:734–741, 2002a.

Chen G, Upham BL, Sun W, Chang CC, Rothwell EJ, Chen KM, Yamasaki H, Trosko JE. Effect of electromagnetic field exposure on chemically induced differentiation of friend erythroleukemia cells. *Environ Health Perspect* 108:967–972, 2000a.

Chen H, Cangello D, Benson S, Folmer J, Zhu H, Trush MA, Zirkin BR. Age-related increase in mitochondrial superoxide generation in the testosterone-producing cells of Brown Norway rat testes: relationship to reduced steroidogenic function? *Exp Gerontol* 36:1361–1373, 2001a.

Chen H, Huhtaniemi I, Zirkin BR. Depletion and repopulation of Leydig cells in the testes of aging Brown Norway rats. *Endocrinology* 137:3447–3452, 1996.

Chen HJ, Cho CL, Liang CL, Chen L, Chang HW, Lu K, Lee TC. Differential telomerase expression and telomere length in primary intracranial tumors. *Chang Gung Med* J 24:352–360, 2001b.

Chen HJ, Cho CL, Liang CL, Lu K, Lin JW. Implication of telomere length as a proliferation-associated marker in schwannomas. *J Surg Oncol* 81:93–100; discussion 100, 2002b.

Chen HJ, Liang CL, Lu K, Lin JW, Cho CL. Implication of telomerase activity and alternations of telomere length in the histologic characteristics of intracranial meningiomas. *Cancer* 89:2092–2098, 2000b.

Chen JL, Blasco MA, Greider CW. Secondary structure of vertebrate telomerase RNA. *Cell* 100:503–514, 2000c.

Chen JL, Opperman KK, Greider CW. A critical stem-loop structure in the CR4-CR5 domain of mammalian telomerase RNA. *Nucleic Acids Res* 30:592–597, 2002c.

Chen JY, Funk WD, Wright WE, Shay JW, Minna JD. Heterogeneity of transcriptional activity of mutant p53 proteins and p53 DNA target sequences. *Oncogene* 8:2159–2166, 1993.

Chen KY, Chang ZF, Liu AY. Changes of serum-induced ornithine decarboxylase activity and putrescine content during aging of IMR-90 human diploid fibroblasts. *J Cell Physiol* 129:142–146, 1986.

Chen L, Trujillo K, Ramos W, Sung P, Tomkinson AE. Promotion of Dnl4–catalyzed DNA end-joining by the Rad50/Mre11/Xrs2 and Hdf1/Hdf2 complexes. *Mol Cell* 8:1105–1115, 2001c.

Chen LQ, Hu CY, Ghadirian P, Duranceau A. Early detection of esophageal squamous cell carcinoma and its effects on therapy: an overview. *Dis Esophagus* 12:161–167, 1999.

Chen Q, Fischer A, Reagan JD, Yan LJ, Ames BN. Oxidative DNA damage and senescence of human diploid fibroblast cells. *Proc Natl Acad Sci USA* 92:4337–4341, 1995.

Chen QM, Bartholomew JC, Campisi J, Acosta M, Reagan JD, Ames BN. Molecular analysis of H_2O_2-induced senescent-like growth arrest in normal human fibroblasts: p53 and Rb control G1 arrest but not cell replication. *Biochem J* 332:43–50, 1998.

Chen XQ, Bonnefoi H, Pelte MF, Lyautey J, Lederrey C, Movarekhi S, Schaeffer P, Mulcahy HE, Meyer P, Stroun M, Anker P. Telomerase RNA as a detection marker in the serum of breast cancer patients. *Clin Cancer Res* 6:3823–3826, 2000d.

Chen YQ, Mauviel A, Ryynanen J, Sollberg S, Uitto J. Type VII collagen gene expression by human skin fibroblasts and keratinocytes in culture: influence of donor age and cytokine responses. *J Invest Dermatol* 102:205–209, 1994.

Chen Z, Monia BP, Corey DR. Telomerase inhibition, telomere shortening, and decreased cell proliferation by cell permeable 2'-*O*-methoxyethyl oligonucleotides. *J Med Chem* 45:5423–5425, 2002d.

Chen Z, Smith KJ, Skelton HG 3rd, Barrett TL, Greenway HT Jr, Lo SC. Telomerase activity in Kaposi's sarcoma, squamous cell carcinoma, and basal cell carcinoma. *Exp Biol Med (Maywood)* 226:753–757, 2001d.

Cheng B, Hornick TR, Hassan MO, Chou SC, Abraham S, Kowal J. Effects of prolonged ACTH-stimulation on adrenocortical accumulation of lipofuscin granules in aged rats. *Tissue Cell* 31:594–604, 1999.

Cheng CW, Chueh SC, Chern HD. Diagnosis of bladder cancer using telomerase activity in voided urine. *J Formos Med Assoc* 99:920–925, 2000a.

Cheng DH, Ren H, Tang XC. Huperzine A, a novel promising acetylcholinesterase inhibitor. *Neuroreport* 8:97–101, 1996.

Cheng RZ, Shammas MA, Li J, Shmookler Reis RJ. Expression of SV40 large T antigen stimulates reversioin of a chromosomal gene duplication in human cells. *Exp Cell Res* 234:300–312, 1997.

Cheng T, Rodrigues N, Shen H, Yang Y, Dombkowski D, Sykes M, Scadden DT. Hematopoetic stem cell quiescence maintained by p21[cip1/waf1]. *Science* 287:1804–1808, 2000b.

Chernoff R. Nutrition and health promotion in older adults. *J Gerontol A Biol Sci Med Sci* 56:47–53, 2001.

Cherubini A, Zuliani G, Costantini F, Pierdomenico SD, Volpato S, Mezzetti A, Mecocci P, Pezzuto S, Bregnocchi M, Fellin R, Seni U, and the VASA Study Group. High vitamin E plasma levels and low low-density lipoprotein oxidation are associated with the absence of atherosclerosis in octogenarians. *J Am Geriatr Soc* 49:651–654, 2001.

Cheskin LJ, Schuster MM. Colonic disorders. In Hazzard WR, Bierman EL, Blass JP, Ettinger WH Jr, Halter JB (eds). *Principles of Geriatric Medicine and Gerontology, 3rd ed.* McGraw-Hill, New York, 1994, pp 723–732.

Chestnut CH III. Osteoporosis. In Hazzard WR, Bierman EL, Blass JP, Ettinger WH Jr, Halter JB (eds). *Principles of Geriatric Medicine and Gerontology, 3rd ed.* McGraw-Hill, New York, 1994, pp 897–909.

Chestnut CH III. Osteoporosis, an underdiagnosed disease. *JAMA* 286:2865–2866, 2001.

Chiechi LM, Secreto G. Factors of risk for breast cancer influencing post-menopausal long-term hormone replacement therapy. *Tumori* 86:12–16, 2000.

Chikashige Y, Hiraoka Y. Telomere binding of the Rap1 protein is required for meiosis in fission yeast. *Curr Biol* 11:1618–1623, 2001.

Chilton RJ. Recent discoveries in assessment of coronary heart disease: impact of vascular mechanisms on development of atherosclerosis. *J Am Osteopath Assoc* 101:S1–5, 2001.

Chin L, Artandi SE, Shen Q, Tam A, Lee SL, Gottlieb GJ, Greider CW, DePinho RA. p53 deficiency rescues the adverse effects of telomere loss and cooperates with telomere dysfunction to accelerate carcinogenesis. *Cell* 97:527–538, 1999.

Chin L, Merlino G, DePinho RA. Malignant melanoma: modern black plague and genetic black box. *Genes Dev* 12:3467–3481, 1998.

Chiu CP, Dragowska W, Kim NW, Vaziri H, Yui J, Thomas TE, Harley CB, Lansdorp PM. Differential expression of telomerase activity in hematopoietic progenitors from adult human bone marrow. *Stem Cells* 14:239–248, 1996.

Chiu CP, Harley CB. Replicative senescence and cell immortality: the role of telomeres and telomerase. *Proc Soc Exp Biol Med* 214:99–106, 1997.

Chiurillo MA, Sachdeva M, Dole VS, Yepes Y, Miliani E, Vazquez L, Rojas A, Crisante G, Guevara P, Anez N, Madhubala R, Ramirez JL. Detection of *Leishmania* causing visceral leishmaniasis in the Old and New Worlds by a polymerase chain reaction assay based on telomeric sequences. *Am J Trop Med Hyg* 65:573–582, 2001.

Chkhotua A, Shohat M, Tobar A, Magal N, Kaganovski E, Shapira Z, Yussim A. Replicative senescence in organ transplantation—mechanisms and significance. *Transpl Immunol* 9:165–171, 2002.

Cho E, Hung S, Willett WC, Spiegelman D, Rimm EB, Seddon JM, Colditz GA, Hankinson SE. Prospective study of dietary fat and the risk of age-related macular degeneration. *Am J Clin Nutr* 73:209–218, 2001a.

Cho E, Stampfer MJ, Seddon JM, Hung S, Spiegelman D, Rimm EB, Willett WC, Hankinson SE. Prospective study of zinc intake and the risk of age-related macular degeneration. *Ann Epidemiol* 11:328–336, 2001b.

Choe W, Budd M, Imamura O, Hoopes L, Campbell JL. Dynamic localization of an Okazaki fragment processing protein suggests a novel role in telomere replication. *Mol Cell Biol* 22:4202–4217, 2002.

Choi AM, Olsen DR, Cook KG, Deamond SF, Uitto J, Bruce SA. Differential extracellular matrix gene expression of fibroblasts during their proliferative life span in vitro and at senescence. *J Cell Physiol* 151:147–155, 1992.

Choi AM, Pignolo RJ, Rhys CM, Cristofalo VJ, Holbrook NJ. Alterations in the molecular response to DNA damage during cellular aging of cultured fibroblasts: reduced AP-1 activation and collagenase gene expression. *J Cell Physiol* 164:65–73, 1995.

Choi D, Whittier PS, Oshima J, Funk WD. Telomerase expression prevents replicative senescence but does not fully reset mRNA expression patterns in Werner syndrome cell lines. *FASEB J* 15:1014–1020, 2001.

Choi SH, Kang HK, Im EO, Kim YJ, Bae YT, Choi YH, Lee KH, Chung HY, Chang HK, Kim ND. Inhibition of cell growth and telomerase activity of breast cancer cells in vitro by retinoic acids. *Int J Oncol* 17:971–976, 2000.

Chong EYY, Pang JCS, Ko CW, Poon WS, Ng HK. Telomere length and telomerase catalytic subunit expression in non-astrocytic gliomas. *Pathol Res Pract* 196:691–699, 2000.

Chong L, van Steensel B, Broccoli D, Erdjument-Bromage H, Hanish J, Tempst P, de Lange T. A human telomeric protein. *Science* 270:1663–1667, 1995.

Chou WC, Hawkins AL, Barrett JF, Griffin CA, Dang CV. Arsenic inhibition of telomerase transcription leads to genetic instability. *J Clin Invest* 108:1541–1547, 2001.

Choy JC, Granville DJ, Hunt DW, McManus BM. Endothelial cell apoptosis: biochemical characteristics and potential implications for atherosclerosis. *J Mol Cell Cardiol* 33:1673–1690, 2001.

Christiansen M, Kveiborg M, Kassem M, Clark BF, Rattan SI. CBFA1 and topoisomerase I mRNA levels decline during cellular aging of human trabecular osteoblasts. *J Gerontol A Biol Sci Med Sci* 55:B194–200, 2000a.

Christiansen M, Stevnsner T, Bohr VA, Clark BF, Rattan SI. Gene-specific DNA repair of pyrimidine dimers does not decline during cellular aging in vitro. *Exp Cell Res* 256:308–314, 2000b.

Christmas C, O'Connor KG, Harman SM, Tobin JD, Munzer T, Bellantoni MF, St. Clair C, Pabst KM, Sorkin JD, Blackman MR. Growth hormone and sex steroid effects on bone metabolism and bone mineral density in healthy aged women and men. *J Gerontol A Biol Sci Med Sci* 57:M12–M18, 2002.

Christov KT, Shilkaitis AL, Kim ES, Steele VE, Lubet RA. Chemopreventive agents induce a senescence-like phenotype in rat mammary tumours. *Eur J Cancer* 39:230–239, 2003.

Chung SS, Weindruch R, Schwarze SR, McKenzie DI, Aiken JM. Multiple age-associated mitochondrial DNA deletions in skeletal muscle of mice. *Aging (Milano)* 6:193–200, 1994.

Cianciarulo FL, Phillips PD, Cristofalo VJ. Effects of tumor necrosis factor and interferon-beta on proliferation and epidermal growth factor binding in young and senescent WI-38 cells. *In Vitro Cell Dev Biol Anim* 29A:656–660, 1993.

Clancy DJ, Gems D, Harshman LG, Oldham S, Stocker H, Hafen E, Leevers SJ, Partridge L. Extension of life-span by loss of CHICO, a *Drosophila* insulin receptor substrate protein. *Science* 292:104–106, 2001.

Clarfield AM. Commentary on special article, the aging syndrome. The aging syndrome—then and now. *J Am Geriatr Soc* 51:562–563, 2003.

Clark MA, Weiss AS. Elevated levels of glycoprotein gp200 in progeria fibroblasts. *Mol Cell Biochem* 120:51–60, 1993.

Clark MA, Weiss AS. Hutchinson-Gilford progeria types defined by differential binding of lectin DSA. *Biochim Biophys Acta* 1270:142–148, 1995.

Clark WR. *Means to an End: the Biological Basis of Aging and Death.* Oxford University Press, New York, 1999.

Clarkson B, Pavenski K, Dupuis L, Kennedy S, Meyn S, Nezarati MM, Nie G, Weksberg R, Withers S, Quercia N, Teebi AS, Teshima I. Detecting rearrangements in children using subtelomeric FISH and SKY. *Am J Med Genet* 107:267–274, 2002.

Classen S, Ruggles JA, Schultz SC. Crystal structure of the N-terminal domain of oxytricha nova telomere end-binding protein alpha subunit both uncomplexed and complexed with telomeric ssDNA. *J Mol Biol* 314:1113–1125, 2001.

Cockayne EA. Dwarfism with retinal atrophy and deafness. *Arch Dis Child* 11:1–8, 1936.

Cockcroft DW, Gault MH. Prediction of creatinine clearance from serum creatinine. *Nephron* 16:31–41, 1976.

Cockell M, Gasser SM. Nuclear compartments and gene regulation. *Curr Opin Genet Dev* 9:199–205, 1999.

Cockell M, Gotta M, Palladino F, Martin SG, Gasser SM. Targeting Sir proteins to sites of action: a general mechanism for regulated repression. *Cold Spring Harb Symp Quant Biol* 63:401–412, 1998.

Cockell MM, Perrod S, Gasser SM. Analysis of Sir2p domains required for rDNA and telomeric silencing in *Saccharomyces cerevisiae*. *Genetics* 154:1069–1083, 2000.

Cody RJ. Hormonal aterations in heart failure. In Hosenpud JD, Greenberg BH (eds). *Congestive Heart Failure*. Lippincott Williams & Wilkins, 2000, pp 199–212.

Cohen J. Selling the immune system short. *Science* 273:30–31, 1996.

Cohen M, Shelley WB. Ankle ulcer sign of Werner's syndrome. *Arch Dermatol* 87:86–88, 1963.

Colao A, Cuocolo A, Di Somma C, Cerbone G, Della Morte AM, Nicolai E, Lucci R, Salvatore M, Lombardi G. Impaired cardiac performance in elderly patients with growth hormone deficiency. *J Clin Endocrinol Metab* 84:3950–3955, 1999a.

Colao A, Marzullo P, Di Somma C, Lombardi G. Growth hormone and the heart. *Clin Endocrinol (Oxf)* 54:137–154, 2001.

Colao A, Marzullo P, Spiezia S, Ferone D, Giaccio A, Cerbone G, Pivonello R, Di Somma C, Lombardi G. Effect of growth hormone (GH) and insulin-like growth factor I on prostate diseases: an ultrasonographic and endocrine study in acromegaly, GH deficiency, and healthy subjects. *J Clin Endocrinol Metab* 84:1986–1991, 1999b.

Cold S, Jensen NV, Brincker H, Rose C. The influence of chemotherapy on survival after recurrence in breast cancer: a population-based study of patients treated in the 1950's, 1960's, and 1970's. *Eur J Cancer* 29:1146–1152, 1993.

Colgin LM, Reddel RR. Telomere maintenance mechanisms and cellular immortalization. *Curr Opin Genet Dev* 9:97–103, 1999.

Colgin LM, Wilkinson C, Englezou A, Kilian A, Robinson MO, Reddel RR. The hTERTα splice variant is a dominant negative inhibitor of telomerase activity. *Neoplasia* 2:426–432, 2000.

Colige A, Nusgens B, Lapiere CM. Altered response of progeria fibroblasts to epidermal growth factor. *J Cell Sci* 100:649–655, 1991a.

Colige A, Roujeau JC, De la Rocque F, Nusgens B, Lapiere CM. Abnormal gene expression in skin fibroblasts from a Hutchinson-Gilford patient. *Lab Invest* 64:799–806, 1991b.

Colitz CM, Davidson MG, McGahan MC. Telomerase activity in lens epithelial cells of normal and cataractous lenses. *Exp Eye Res* 69:641–649, 1999.

Collins F. Quoted at the European Conference on Pharmaceuticals and the Human Genome, Basel, Switzerland, January 2001.

Collins K, Greider CW. *Tetrahymena* telomerase catalyzes nucleolytic cleavage and nonprocessive elongation. *Genes Dev* 7:1364–1376, 1993.

Collins K, Greider CW. Utilization of ribonucleotides and RNA primers by *Tetrahymena* telomerase. *EMBO J* 14:5422–5432, 1995.

Collins K, Kobayashi R, Greider CW. Purification of *Tetrahymena* telomerase and cloning of genes encoding the two protein components of the enzyme. *Cell* 81:677–686, 1995.

Collins K, Mitchell JR. Telomerase in the human organism. *Oncogene* 21:564–579, 2002.

Colman RJ, Kemnitz JW, Lane MA, Abbott DH, Binkley N. Skeletal effects of aging and menopausal status in female rhesus macaques. *J Clin Endocrinol Metab* 84:4144–4148, 1999a.

Colman RJ, Lane MA, Binkley N, Wegner FH, Kemnitz JW. Skeletal effects of aging in male rhesus monkeys. *Bone* 24:17–23, 1999b.

Colman RJ, Ramsey JJ, Roecker EB, Havighurst T, Hudson JC, Kemnitz JW. Body fat distribution with long-term dietary restriction in adult male rhesus macaques. *J Gerontol A Biol Sci Med Sci* 54:B283–290, 1999c.

Colman RJ, Roecker EB, Ramsey JJ, Kemnitz JW. The effect of dietary restriction on body composition in adult male and female rhesus macaques. *Aging (Milano)* 10:83–92, 1998.

Colucci WS. The sympathetic nervous system in heart failure. In Hosenpud JD, Greenberg BH (eds). *Congestive Heart Failure*. Lippincott Williams & Wilkins, Philadelphia, 2000, pp 189–198.

Comfort A. Werner's syndrome. *Lancet* 2:1152, 1961.

Comfort A. The prospects for living even longer. *Time* August 3, 1970, p 44.

Compton C, Tong T, Trookman N, Zhao H, Roy D. TGF-beta 1 gene expression in cultured human keratinocytes does not decrease with biologic age. *J Invest Dermatol* 103:127–133, 1994.

Compton CC, Tong Y, Trookman N, Zhao H, Roy D, Press W. Transforming growth factor alpha gene expression in cultured human keratinocytes is unaffected by cellular aging. *Arch Dermatol* 131:683–690, 1995.

Condon J, Yin S, Mayhew B, Word RA, Wright WE, Shay JW, Rainey WE. Telomerase immortalization of human myometrial cells. *Biol Reprod* 67:506–514, 2002.

Cong YS, Wen J, Bacchetti S. The human telomerase catalytic subunit hTERT: organization of the gene and characterization of the promoter. *Hum Mol Genet* 8:137–142, 1999.

Cong YS, Wright WE, Shay JW. Human telomerase and its regulation. *Microbiol Mol Biol Rev* 66:407–425, 2002.

Congdon NG, West KP Jr. Nutrition and the eye. *Curr Opin Ophthalmol* 10:464–473, 1999.

Conrad MN, Wright JH, Wolf AJ, Zakian VA. RAP1 protein interacts with yeast telomeres in vivo: overproduction alters telomere structure and decreases chromosome stability. *Cell* 63:739–750, 1990.

Contreras F, Rivera M, Vasquez J, De la Parte MA, Velasco M. Endothelial dysfunction in arterial hypertension. *J Hum Hypertens* 14(Suppl 1):S20–25, 2000.

Conway C, McCulloch R, Ginger ML, Robinson NP, Browitt A, Barry JD. Ku is important for telomere maintenance, but not for differential expression of telomeric VSG genes, in African trypanosomes. *J Biol Chem* 277:21269–21277, 2002.

Conway JE, Rhys CM, Zolotukhin I, Zolotukhin S, Muzyczka N, Hayward GS, Byrne BJ. High-titer recombinant adeno-associated virus production utilizing a recombinant herpes simplex virus type I vector expressing AAV-2 Rep and Cap. *Gene Ther* 6:986–993, 1999.

Cook BD, Dynek JN, Chang W, Shostak G, Smith S. Role for the related poly(ADP-Ribose) polymerases tankyrase 1 and 2 at human telomeres. *Mol Cell Biol* 22:332–342, 2002.

Cook DG, Sung JC, Golde TE, Felsenstein KM, Wojczyk BS, Tanzi RE, Trojanowski JQ, Lee VM, Doms RW. Expression and analysis of presenilin 1 in a human neuronal system: localization in cell bodies and dendrites. *Proc Natl Acad Sci USA* 93:9223–9228, 1996.

Cooke H. Non-programmed and engineered chromosome breakage. In Blackburn and Greider, 1995.

Cooke HJ, Smith BA. Variability at the telomeres of the human X/Y psuedoautosomal region. *Cold Spring Harb Symp Quant Biol* 51:213–219, 1996.

Cooke JP. The endothelium: a new target for therapy. *Vasc Med* 5:49–53, 2000.

Cooke JP, Dzau VJ. Nitric oxide synthase: role in the genesis of vascular disease. *Annu Rev Med* 48:489–509, 1997.

Cooke JV. The rate of growth in progeria, with a report of two cases. *J Pediatr* 42:26–37, 1953.

Cool BL, Sirover MA. Proliferation-dependent regulation of DNA glycosylases in progeroid cells. *Mutat Res* 237:211–220, 1990.

Cooper DA, Eldridge AL, Peters JC. Dietary carotenoids and certain cancers, heart disease, and age-related macular degeneration: a review of recent research. *Nutr Rev* 57:201–214, 1999.

Cooper JP, Nimmo ER, Allshire RC, Cech TR. Regulation of telomere length and function by a Myb-domain protein in fission yeast. *Nature* 385:744–747, 1997.

Cooper LT, Cooke JP, Dzau VJ. The vasculopathy of aging. *J Gerontol* 49:191–196, 1994.

Corcoy R, Aris A, de Leiva A. Fertility in a case of progeria. *Am J Med Sci* 297:383–384, 1989.

Corder EH, Saunders AM, Strittmatter WJ, Schmechel DE, Gaskell PC Jr, Rimmler JB, Locke PA, Conneally PM, Schmader KE, Tanzi RE, et al. Apolipoprotein E, survival in Alzheimer's disease patients, and the competing risks of death and Alzheimer's disease. *Neurology* 45:1323–1328, 1995.

Corey D. Potent inhibition of human telomerase by 2'-*O*-methyl RNA. Presented at Telomeres and Telomerase: Implications for Cell Immortality, Cancer, and Age-related Disease. San Francisco, CA, June 1–3, 1998.

Corey DR. Telomerase inhibition, oligonucleotides, and clinical trials. *Oncogene* 21:631–637, 2002.

Cornforth MN, Meyne J, Littlefield LG, Bailey SM, Moyzis RK. Telomere staining of human chromosomes and the mechanism of radiation-induced dicentric formation. *Radiat Res* 120:205–212, 1989.

Cornsweet TN. *Visual Perception*. Academic Press, New York, 1970.

Corsini J, Cotmore SF, Tattersall P, Winocour E. The left-end and right-end origins of minute virus of mice DNA differ in their capacity to direct episomal amplification and integration in vivo. *Virology* 288:154–163, 2001.

Cortopassi GA, Shibata D, Soong NW, Arnheim N. A pattern of accumulation of a somatic deletion of mitochondrial DNA in aging human tissues. *Proc Natl Acad Sci USA* 89:7370–7374, 1992.

Cosentino F, Luscher TF. Effects of blood pressure and glucose on endothelial function. *Curr Hypertens Rep* 3:79–88, 2001.

Cosgrove AJ, Nieduszynski CA, Donaldson AD. Ku complex controls the replication time of DNA in telomere regions. *Genes Dev* 16:2485–490, 2002.

Cotter PD, Kaffe S, Li L, Gershin IF, Hirschhorn K. Loss of subtelomeric sequence associated with a terminal inversion duplication of the short arm of chromosome 4. *Am J Med Genet* 102:76–80, 2001.

Cottliar A, Fundia A, Boerr L, Sambuelli A, Negreira S, Gil A, Gomez JC, Chopita N, Bernedo A, Slavutsky I. High frequencies of telomeric associations, chromosome aberrations, and sister chromatid exchanges in ulcerative colitis. *Am J Gastroenterol* 95:2301–2307, 2000.

Cottliar AS, Slavutsky IR. Telomeres and telomerase activity: their role in aging and in neoplastic development [in Spanish]. *Medicina (B Aires)* 61:335–342, 2001.

Counter CM. The roles of telomeres and telomerase in cell life span. *Mutat Res* 366:45–63, 1996.

Counter CM, Avilion AA, LeFeuvre CE, Stewart NG, Greider CW, Harley CB, Bacchetti S. Telomere shortening associated with chromosome instability is arrested in immortal cells which express telomerase activity. *EMBO J* 11:1921–1919, 1992.

Counter CM, Botelho FM, Wang P, Harley CB, Bacchetti S. Stabilization of short telomeres and telomerase activity accompany immortalization of Epstein-Barr virus–transformed human B lymphocytes. *J Virol* 68:3410–3414, 1994a.

Counter CM, Gupta J, Harley CB, Leber B, Bacchetti S. Telomerase activity in normal leukocytes and in hematologic malignancies. *Blood* 85:2315–2320, 1995.

Counter CM, Hahn WC, Wei W, Caddle SD, Beijersbergen RL, Lansdorp PM, Sedivy JM, Weinberg RA. Dissociation among in vitro telomerase activity, telomere maintenance, and cellular immortalization. *Proc Natl Acad Sci USA* 95:14723–14728, 1998a.

Counter CM, Hirte HW, Bacchetti S, Harley CB. Telomerase activity in human ovarian carcinoma. *Proc Natl Acad Sci USA* 91:2900–2904, 1994b.

Counter CM, Meyerson M, Eaton EN, Ellisen LW, Caddle SD, Haber DA, Weinberg RA. Telomerase activity is restored in human cells by ectopic expression of hTERT (hEST2), the catalytic subunit of telomerase. *Oncogene* 16:1217–1222, 1998b.

Counter CM, Meyerson M, Eaton EN, Weinberg RA. The catalytic subunit of yeast telomerase. *Proc Natl Acad Sci USA* 94:9202–9207, 1997.

Coursen JD, Bennett WP, Gollahon L, Shay JW, Harris CC. Genomic instability and telomerase activity in human bronchial epithelial cells during immortalization by human papillomavirus-16 E6 and E7 genes. *Exp Cell Res* 235:245–253, 1997.

Coviello-McLaughlin GM, Prowse KR. Telomere length regulation during postnatal development and ageing in Mus spretus. *Nucleic Acids Res* 25:3051–3058, 1997.

Cowell JK. Targeted therapy of human tumors in a mouse model by a 2-5A antisense directed against telomerase RNA. Abstract presented at Telomeres and Telomerase: Implications for Cell Immortality, Cancer, and Age-related Disease. San Francisco, CA, June 1–3, 1998.

Cowell JK. Telomeres and telomerase in ageing and cancer. AGE 22:59–64, 1999.

Crandall CJ. Estrogen replacement therapy and colon cancer: a clinical review. *J Womens Health Gend Based Med* 8:1155–1166, 1999.

Crawford JG. Alzheimer's disease risk factors as related to cerebral blood flow: additional evidence. *Med Hypotheses* 50:25–36, 1998.

Crawshaw A. Carcinoma of the breast and hormone replacement therapy for osteoporosis. *Int J Clin Pract* 54:99–103, 2000.

Cree J, Soskolne CL, Belseck E, Horning J, McElhaney JE, Brant R, Suarez-Almazor M. Mortality and institutionalization following hip fracture. *J Am Geriatr Soc* 48:283–288, 2000.

Cressey TR, Tilby MJ, Newell DR. Decreased telomerase activity is not a reliable indicator of chemosensitivity in testicular cancer cell lines. *Eur J Cancer* 38:586–593, 2002.

Crew MD, Effros RB, Walford RL, Zeller E, Cheroutre H, Brahn E. Transgenic mice expressing a truncated *Peromyscus leucopus* TNF-alpha gene manifest an arthritis resembling ankylosing spondylitis. *J Interferon Cytokine Res* 18:219–225, 1998.

Cristofalo VJ. Cellular biomarkers of aging. *Exp Gerontol* 23:297–307, 1988.

Cristofalo VJ. Ten years later: what have we learned about human aging from studies of cell cultures? *Gerontologist* 36:737–741, 1996.

Cristofalo VJ, Allen RG, Pignolo RJ, Martin BG, Beck JC. Relationship between donor age and the replicative life span of human cells in culture: a reevaluation. *Proc Natl Acad Sci USA* 95:10614–10619, 1998a.

Cristofalo VJ, Gerhard GS, Pignolo RJ. Molecular biology of aging. *Surg Clin North Am* 74:1–21, 1994.

Cristofalo VJ, Parris N, Kritchevsky D. Enzyme activity during the growth and aging of human cells in vitro. *J Cell Physiol* 69:263–271, 1967.

Cristofalo VJ, Phillips PD, Sorger T, Gerhard G. Alterations in the responsiveness of senescent cells to growth factors. *J Gerontol* 44:55–62, 1989.

Cristofalo VJ, Pignolo RJ. Replicative senescence of human fibroblast-like cells in culture. *Physiol Rev* 73:617–638, 1993.

Cristofalo VJ, Pignolo RJ. Molecular markers of senescence in fibroblast-like cultures. *Exp Gerontol* 31:111–123, 1996.

Cristofalo VJ, Pignolo RJ, Cianciarulo FL, DiPaolo BR, Rotenberg MO. Changes in gene expression during senescence in culture. *Exp Gerontol* 27:429–432, 1992a.

Cristofalo VJ, Pignolo RJ, Rotenberg MO. Molecular changes with in vitro cellular senescence. *Ann NY Acad Sci* 663:187–194, 1992b.

Cristofalo VJ, Sharf BB. Cellular senescence and DNA synthesis. *Exp Cell Res* 76:419–427, 1973.

Cristofalo VJ, Tresini M. Defects in signal transduction during replicative senescence of diploid human fibroblasts in vitro. *Aging (Milano)* 10:151–152, 1998.

Cristofalo VJ, Volker C, Francis MK, Tresini M. Age-dependent modifications of gene expression in human fibroblasts. *Crit Rev Eukaryot Gene Expr* 8:43–80, 1998b.

Crocker J. Telomeres and telomerases: intimations of immortality. *Eur J Gastroenterol Hepatol* 13:889–890, 2001.

Croteau DL, Stierum RH, Bohr VA. Mitochondrial DNA repair pathways. *Mutat Res* 434:137–148, 1999.

Crowe DL, Nguyen DC. Rb and E2F-1 regulate telomerase activity in human cancer cells. *Biochim Biophys Acta* 1518:1–6, 2001.

Crowe DL, Nguyen DC, Tsang KJ, Kyo S. E2F-1 represses transcription of the human telomerase reverse transcriptase gene. *Nucleic Acids Res* 29:2789–2794, 2001.

Cruickshanks KJ, Klein R, Klein BE, Nondahl DM. Sunlight and the 5–year incidence of early age-related maculopathy: the Beaver Dam Eye Study. *Arch Ophthalmol* 119:246–250, 2001.

Cryderman DE, Morris EJ, Biessmann H, Elgin SC, Wallrath LL. Silencing at *Drosophila* telomeres: nuclear organization and chromatin structure play critical roles. *EMBO J* 18:3724–3735, 1999.

Cuadrado E, Barrena MJ. Immune dysfunction in Down's syndrome: primary immune deficiency or early senescence of the immune system? *Clin Immunol Immunopathol* 78:209–214, 1996.

Cui Q, Tang C, Huang Y. Effects of lead and selenium on telomere binding protein Rap1p, telomerase and telomeric DNA in *Saccharomyces cerevisiae. Sheng Wu Hua Xue Yu Sheng Wu Wu Li Xue Bao (Shanghai)* 34:240–244, 2002a.

Cui W, Aslam S, Fletcher J, Wylie D, Clinton M, Clark AJ. Stabilization of telomere length and karyotypic stability are directly correlated with the level of hTERT gene expression in primary fibroblasts. *J Biol Chem* 277:38531–38539, 2002b.

Cummings BJ, Head E, Ruehl W, Milgram NW, Cotman CW. The canine as an animal model of human aging and dementia. *Neurobiol Aging* 17:259–268, 1996.

Cummings JL, Cole G. Alzheimer disease. *JAMA* 287:2335–2338, 2002.

Cummings SR, Bauer DC. Do statins prevent both cardiovascular disease *and* fracture? *JAMA* 283:3255–3257, 2000.

Cunado N, Sanchez-Moran E, Barrios J, Santos JL. Searching for telomeric sequences in two *Allium* species. *Genome* 44:640–643, 2001.

Cunningham VJ, Markham N, Shroyer AL, Shroyer KR. Detection of telomerase expression in fine-needle aspirations and fluids. *Diagn Cytopathol* 18:431–436, 1998.

Cure-Cure C, Cure-Ramirez P. Hormone replacement therapy for bone protection in multiparous women: when to initiate it. *Am J Obstet Gynecol* 184:580–583, 2001.

Curl WW. Aging and exercise: are they compatible in women? *Clin Orthop* 372:151–158, 2000.

Curran AJ, Gullane PJ, Irish J, Macmillan C, Freeman J, Kamel-Reid S. Telomerase activity is upregulated in laryngeal squamous cell carcinoma. *Laryngoscope* 110:391–396, 2000.

Curtin VT, Kotzen HF. Progeria: review of the literature with report of a case. *Am J Dis Child* 38:993–1005, 1929.

Curtis HJ. Biological mechanisms underlying the aging process. *Science* 141:686–694, 1963.

Curtsinger JW, Fukui HH, Khazaeli AA, Kirscher A, Pletcher SD, Promislow DE, Tatar M. Genetic variation and aging. *Annu Rev Genet* 29:553–575, 1995.

Cuthbert AP, Bond J, Trott DA, Gill S, Broni J, Marriott A, Khoudoli G, Parkinson EK, Cooper CS, Newbold RF. Telomerase repressor sequences on chromosome 3 and induction of permanent growth arrest in human breast cancer cells. *J Natl Cancer Inst* 91:37–45, 1999.

Cutler RG. Antioxidants and longevity of mammalian species. In Woodhead AD, Blackett AD, Hollaender A (eds). *Molecular Biology of Aging.* Plenum Press, New York, 1985, pp 15–73.

Cypser J, Johnson TE. Hormesis extends the correlation between stress resistance and life span in long-lived mutants of *Caenorhabditis elegans. Belle Newsletter* 9:11–12, 2001.

Cyr M, Calon F, Morissette M, Grandbois M, Di Paolo T, Callier S. Drugs with estrogen-like potency and brain activity: potential therapeutic application for the CNS. *Curr Pharm Des* 6:1287–1312, 2000.

d'Adda di Fagagna F, Hande MP, Tong WM, Lansdorp PM, Wang ZQ, Jackson SP. Functions of poly(ADP-ribose) polymerase in controlling telomere length and chromosomal stability. *Nat Genet* 23:76–80, 1999.

d'Adda di Fagagna F, Hande MP, Tong WM, Roth D, Lansdorp PM, Wang ZQ, Jackson SP. Effects of DNA nonhomologous end-joining factors on telomere length and chromosomal stability in mammalian cells. *Curr Biol* 11:1192–1196, 2001.

Dahse R, Mey J. Telomerase in human tumors: molecular diagnosis and clinical significance. *Expert Rev Mol Diagn* 1:201–210, 2001.

Dai WJ, Jiang HC. Advances in gene therapy of liver cirrhosis: a review. *World J Gastroenterol* 7:1–8, 2001.

Dalla Torre CA, Maciel RM, Pinheiro NA, Andrade JA, De Toledo SR, Villa LL, Cerutti JM. TRAP-silver staining, a highly sensitive assay for measuring telomerase activity in tumor tissue and cell lines. *Braz J Med Biol Res* 35:65–68, 2002.

Damm K, Hemmann U, Garin-Chesa P, Hauel N, Kauffmann I, Priepke H, Niestroj C, Daiber C, Enenkel B, Guilliard B, Lauritsch I, Muller E, Pascolo E, Sauter G, Pantic M, Martens UM, Wenz C, Lingner J, Kraut N, Rettig WJ, Schnapp A. A highly selective telomerase inhibitor limiting human cancer cell proliferation. *EMBO J* 20:6958–6968, 2001.

D'Amours D, Jackson SP. The yeast Xrs2 complex functions in S phase checkpoint regulation. *Genes Dev* 15:2238–2249, 2001.

D'Amours D, Jackson SP. The mre11 complex: at the crossroads of DNA repair and checkpoint signalling. *Nat Rev Mol Cell Biol* 3:317–327, 2002.

Dandjinou AT, Dionne I, Gravel S, LeBel C, Parenteau J, Wellinger RJ. Cytological and functional aspects of telomere maintenance. *Histol Histopathol* 14:517–524, 1999.

Danes BS. Progeria: a cell culture study in aging. *J Clin Invest* 50:2000–2003, 1971.

Danesh J. Smoldering arteries? Low-grade inflammation and coronary heart disease. *JAMA* 282:2169–2171, 1999.

Danis M, Gentilini M. Malaria, a worldwide scourge [in French]. *Rev Prat* 48:254–257, 1998.

Daoudal-Cotterell S, Gallego ME, White CI. The plant Rad50–Mre11 protein complex. *FEBS Lett* 516:164–166, 2002.

Dapic V, Bates PJ, Trent JO, Rodger A, Thomas SD, Miller DM. Antiproliferative activity of G-quartet-forming oligonucleotides with backbone and sugar modifications. *Biochemistry* 41:3676–3685, 2002.

Darimont C, Avanti O, Tromvoukis Y, Vautravers-Leone P, Kurihara N, Roodman GD, Colgin LM, Tullberg-Reinert H, Pfeifer AM, Offord EA, Mace K. SV40 T antigen and telomerase are required to obtain immortalized human adult bone cells without loss of the differentiated phenotype. *Cell Growth Differ* 13:59–67, 2002.

Darlington GJ, Dutkowski R, Brown WT. Sister chromatid exchange frequencies in progeria and Werner syndrome patients. *Am J Hum Genet* 33:762–766, 1981.

Darwin C. *The Origin of Species.* The Modern Library, New York, 1859.

Dasi F, Lledo S, Garcia-Granero E, Ripoll R, Marugan M, Tormo M, Garcia-Conde J, Alino SF. Real-time quantification in plasma of human telomerase reverse transcriptase (hTERT) mRNA: a simple blood test to monitor disease in cancer patients. *Lab Invest* 81:767–769, 2001.

Davidson JM, Zang MC, Zoia O, Giro MG. Regulation of elastin synthesis in pathological states. *Ciba Found Symp* 192:81–94; discussion 94–99, 1995.

Davies D, Shock N. Age changes in glomerular filtration rate, effective renal plasma flow, and tubular excretory capacity in adult males. *J Clin Invest* 29:496–507, 1950.

Davies MJ. Going from immutable to mutable atherosclerotic plaques. *Am J Cardiol* 88(4 Suppl):2F–9F, 2001.

Davignon T, Gregg R, Sing C. Apolipoprotein E polymorphisms and atherosclerosis. *Arteriosclerosis* 8:1–21, 1988.

De Angelis L, Berghella L, Coletta M, Lattanzi L, Zanchi M, Cusella-De Angelis MG, Ponzetto C, Cossu G. Skeletal myogenic progenitors originating from embryonic dorsal aorta coexpress endothelial and myogenic markers and contribute to postnatal muscle growth and regeneration. *J Cell Biol* 147:869–878, 1999.

Debanne SM, Rowland DY, Riedel TM, Cleves MA. Association of Alzheimer's disease and smoking: the case for sibling controls. *J Am Geriatr Soc* 48:800–806, 2000.

De Benedictis G, Carrieri G, Garasto S, Rose G, Varcasia O, Bonafe M, Franceschi C, Jazwinski SM. Does a retrograde response in human aging and longevity exist? *Exp Gerontol* 35:795–801, 2000.

de Boer J, Andressoo JO, de Wit J, Huijmans J, Beems RB, van Steeg H, Weeda G, van der Horst GTJ, van Leeuwen W, Themmen APN, Meradji M, Hoeijmakers JHJ. Premature aging in mice deficient in DNA repair and transcription. *Science* 296:1276–1279, 2002.

de Boer RJ. Mathematical models of human CD4+ T-cell population kinetics. *Neth J Med* 60:17–26; discussion 26, 2002.

DeBusk FL. The Hutchinson-Gilford progeria syndrome. Report of 4 cases and review of the literature. *J Pediatr* 80:697–724, 1972.

DeBusk FL. Progeria. In Vaughn VC, McKay RJ, Berman RE. *Nelson Textbook of Pediatrics. 11th ed.* W.B. Saunders Company, Philadelphia, 1979, pp 1986–1988.

Decary S, Hamida CB, Mouly V, Barbet JP, Hentati F, Butler-Browne GS. Shorter telomeres in dystrophic muscle consistent with extensive regeneration in young children. *Neuromuscul Disord* 10:113–120, 2000.

De Caterina R. Endothelial dysfunctions: common denominators in vascular disease. *Curr Opin Clin Nutr Metab Care* 3:453–467, 2000a.

De Caterina R. Endothelial dysfunctions: common denominators in vascular disease. *Curr Opin Lipidol* 11:9–23, 2000b.

De Divitiis O, La Torre D. Inverse correlation of TRF1 expression and cell proliferation in human primary intracranial tumors. *J Neurosurg Sci* 45:1–6, 2001.

Defossez PA, Park PU, Guarente L. Vicious circles: a mechanism for yeast aging. *Curr Opin Microbiol* 1:707–711, 1998.

Defossez PA, Prusty R, Kaeberlein M, Lin SJ, Ferrigno P, Silver PA, Keil RL, Guarente L. Elimination of replication block protein Fob1 extends the life span of yeast mother cells. *Mol Cell* 3:447–455, 1999.

Degens H. Age-related changes in the microcirculation of skeletal muscle. *Adv Exp Med Biol* 454:343–348, 1998.

de Grey DNJ. A proposed refinement of the mitochondrial free radical theory of aging. *Bioessays* 19:161–166, 1997.

de Grey DNJ. *The Mitochondrial Free Radical Theory of Aging.* RG Landes Co., Austin, TX, 1999.

de Grey DNJ, Gavrilov L, Olshansky SJ, Coles LS, Cutler RG, Fossel MB, Harman SM. Antiaging technology and pseudoscience. *Science* (letters) 296:656, 2002.

De Groot WP, Tafelkruyer J, Woerdean MJ. Familial acrogeria (Gottron). *Br J Dermatol* 103:213–223, 1980.

Dejmek A, Yahata N, Ohyashiki K, Kakihana M, Hirano T, Kawate N, Kato H, Ebihara Y. Correlation between morphology and telomerase activity in cells from exfoliative lung cytologic specimens. *Cancer* 90:117–125, 2000.

De Jong GI, De Vos RA, Steur EN, Luiten PG. Cerebrovascular hypoperfusion: a risk factor for Alzheimer's disease? Animal model and postmortem human studies. *Ann NY Acad Sci* 826:56–74, 1997.

de Kok JB, Ruers TJ, van Muijen GN, van Bokhoven A, Willems HL, Swinkels DW. Real-time quantification of human telomerase reverse transcriptase mRNA in tumors and healthy tissues. *Clin Chem* 46:313–318, 2000.

de la Monte SM. Molecular abnormalities of the brain in Down syndrome: relevance to Alzheimer's neurodegeneration. *J Neural Transm Suppl* 57:1–19, 1999.

de Lange T. Telomere dynamics and genome instability in human cancer. In Blackburn EH, Greider CW (eds). *Telomeres.* Cold Spring Harbor Laboratory Press, Cold Spring Harbor, NY, 1995, pp 265–293.

de Lange T. Telomeres and senescence: ending the debate. *Science* 279:334–335, 1998.

de Lange T. Protection and maintenance of human telomeres. Presentation at Cancer and Molecular Genetics in the Twenty-first Century, Van Andel Research Institute, Grand Rapids, MI, September 5–9, 2000.

de Lange T. Telomere capping—one strand fits all. *Science* 292:1075–1076, 2001.

de Lange T. Protection of mammalian telomeres. *Oncogene* 21:532–540, 2002.

de Lange T, DePinho RA. Unlimited mileage from telomerase? *Science* 283:947–950, 1999.

de Lange T, Shuie L, Myers RM, Cox DR, Naylor SL, Killery AM, Varmus HE. Structure and variability of human chromosome ends. *Mol Cell Biol* 10:518–527, 1990.

de la Torre JC. Cerebromicrovascular pathology in Alzheimer's disease compared to normal aging. *Gerontology* 43:26–43, 1997.

Delhommeau F, Thierry A, Feneux D, Lauret E, Leclercq E, Courtier MH, Sainteny F, Vainchenker W, Bennaceur-Griscelli A. Telomere dysfunction and telomerase reactivation in human leukemia cell lines after telomerase inhibition by the expression of a dominant-negative hTERT mutant. *Oncogene* 21:8262–271, 2002.

Delihas N. Targeting the expression of anti-apoptotic proteins by antisense oligonucleotides. *Curr Drug Targets* 2:167–180, 2001.

Dellambra E, Golisano O, Bondanza S, Siviero E, Lacal P, Molinari M, D'Atri S, De Luca M. Downregulation of 14-3-3σ prevents clonal evolution and leads to immortalization of primary human keratinocytes. *J Cell Biol* 149:1117–1130, 2000.

de Magalhaes JP, Chainiaux F, Remacle J, Toussaint O. Stress-induced premature senescence in BJ and hTERT-BJ1 human foreskin fibroblasts. *FEBS Lett* 523:157–162, 2002.

DeMasi J, Du S, Lennon D, Traktman P. Vaccinia virus telomeres: interaction with the viral I1, I6, and K4 proteins. *J Virol* 75:10090–10105, 2001.

de Maupassant G. *Selected Short Stories*. Penguin Books, London, 1980.

Dempsey AA, Dzau VJ, Liew CC. Cardiovascular genomics: estimating the total number of genes expressed in the human cardiovascular system. *J Mol Cell Cardiol* 33:1879–1886, 2001.

De Neve L, Vermeulen A. The determination of 17-oxosteroid sulphates in human plasma. *J Endocrinol* 32:295–302, 1965.

den Heijer T, Launer LJ, de Groot JC, de Leeuw F-E, Oudkerk M, van Gijn J, Hofman A, Breteler MMB. Serum carotenoids and cerebral white matter lesions: the Rotterdam scan study. *J Am Geriatr Soc* 49:642–646, 2001.

Denisenko O, Bomsztyk K. Yeast hnRNP K-like genes are involved in regulation of the telomeric position effect and telomere length. *Mol Cell Biol* 22:286–297, 2002.

Denke MA. Dietary retinol—a double-edged sword. *JAMA* 287:102–104, 2002.

Denver DR, Morris K, Lynch M, Vassilieva LL, Thomas WK. High direct estimate of the mutation rate in the mitochondrial genome of *Caenorhabditis elegans*. *Science* 289:2342–2344, 2000.

de Pauw ES, Otto SA, Wijnen JT, Vossen JM, van Weel MH, Tanke HJ, Miedema F, Willemze R, Roelofs H, Fibbe WE. Long-term follow-up of recipients of allogeneic bone marrow grafts reveals no progressive telomere shortening and provides no evidence for haematopoietic stem cell exhaustion. *Br J Haematol* 116:491–496, 2002.

de Rijk MC, Tzourio C, Breteler MM, Dartigues JF, Amaducci L, Lopez-Pousa S, Manubens-Bertran JM, Alperovitch A, Rocca WA. Prevalence of parkinsonism and Parkinson's disease in Europe: the EUROPARKINSON Collaborative Study. European Community Concerted Action on the Epidemiology of Parkinson's disease. *J Neurol Neurosurg Psychiatry* 62:10–15, 1997.

De Rubertis F, Kadosh D, Henchoz S, Pauli D, Reuter G, Struhl K, Spierer P. The histone deacetylase RPD3 counteracts genomic silencing in *Drosophila* and yeast. *Nature* 384:589–591, 1996.

Desai VG, Weindruch R, Hart RW, Feuers RJ. Influences of age and dietary restriction on gastrocnemius electron transport system activities in mice. *Arch Biochem Biophys* 333:145–151, 1996.

De Sandre-Giovannoli A, Bernard R, Cau P, Navarro C, Amiel J, Boccaccio I, Lyonnet S, Stewart CL, Munnich A, Le Merrer M, Levy N. Lamin A truncation in Hutchinson-Gilford progeria. *Science* 300:2055, 2003.

Deschenes G, Martinat L. Molecular mechanisms of idiopathic nephrotic syndrome [in French]. *Arch Pediatr* 7:1318–1329, 2000.

Desprez PY, Hara E, Bissell MJ, Campisi J. Suppression of mammary epithelial cell differentiation by the helix-loop-helix protein Id-1. *Mol Cell Biol* 15:3398–3404, 1995.

Dessain SK, Yu H, Reddel RR, Beijersbergen RL, Weinberg RA. Methylation of the human telomerase gene CpG island. *Cancer Res* 60:537–541, 2000.

Deveci M. Telomeres and telomerase and their possible future in plastic surgery. *Plast Reconstr Surg* 104:1588–1589, 1999.

de Vellis J. *Neuroglia in the Aging Brain*. Human Press, Totowa, NJ, 2002.

Devi G, Ottman R, Tang M, Marder K, Stern Y, Tycko B, Mayeux R. Influence of APOE genotype on familial aggregation of AD in an urban population. *Neurology* 53:789–794, 1999.

Devi G, Ottman R, Tang MX, Marder K, Stern Y, Mayeux R. Familial aggregation of Alzheimer disease among whites, African Americans, and Caribbean Hispanics in northern Manhattan. *Arch Neurol* 57:72–77, 2000.

Dewj NN, Singer SJ. Genetic clues to Alzheimer's disease. *Science* 271:159–160, 1996.

Dhaene K, Vancoillie G, Lambert J, Naeyaert JM, Van Marck E. Absence of telomerase activity and telemorase catalytic subunit mRNA in melanocyte cultures. *Br J Cancer* 82:1051–1057, 2000a.

Dhaene K, Van Marck E, Parwaresch R. Telomeres, telomerase and cancer: an update. *Virchows Arch* 437:1–16, 2000b.

Dhar HL. Newer approaches in increasing life span. *Indian J Med Sci* 53:390–392, 1999.

Dhar S, Squire JA, Hande MP, Wellinger RJ, Pandita TK. Inactivation of 14-3-3σ influences telomere behavior and ionizing radiation-induced chromosomal instability. *Mol Cell Biol* 20:7764–7772, 2000.

Di Carlo A, Baldereschi M, Amaducci L, Maggi S, Grigoletto F, Scarlato G, Inzitari D. Cognitive impairment without dementia in older people: prevalence, vascular risk factors, impacto on disability. The Italian Longitudinal Study on Aging. *J Am Geriatr Soc* 48:775–782, 2000.

Dickson MA, Hahn WC, Ino Y, Ronfard V, Wu JY, Weinberg RA, Louis DN, Li FP, Rheinwald JG. Human keratinocytes that express hTERT and also bypass a p16(INK4a)-enforced mechanism that limits life span become immortal yet retain normal growth and differentiation characteristics. *Mol Cell Biol* 20:1436–1447, 2000.

Diede SJ, Gottschling DE. Telomerase-mediated telomere addition in vivo requires DNA primase and DNA polymerases alpha and delta. *Cell* 99:723–733, 1999.

Diede SJ, Gottschling DE. Exonuclease activity is required for sequence addition and Cdc13p loading at a de novo telomere. *Curr Biol* 11:1336–1340, 2001.

Dierick JF, Eliaers F, Remacle J, Raes M, Fey SJ, Larsen PM, Toussaint O. Stress-induced premature senescence and replicative senescence are different phenotypes, proteomic evidence. *Biochem Pharmacol* 64:1011–1017, 2002.

Diet F, Pratt RE, Berry GJ, Momose N, Gibbons GH, Dzau VJ. Increased accumulation of tissue ACE in human atherosclerotic coronary artery disease. *Circulation* 94:2756–2767, 1996.

Dimri GP, Campisi J. Molecular and cell biology of replicative senescence. *Cold Spring Harbor Symp Quant Biol* 54:67–73, 1994a.

Dimri GP, Campisi J. Altered profile of transcription factor–binding activities in senescent human fibroblasts. *Exp Cell Res* 212:132–140, 1994b.

Dimri GP, Hara E, Campisi J. Regulation of two E2F-related genes in presenescent and senescent human fibroblasts. *J Biol Chem* 269:16180–16186, 1994.

Dimri GP, Itahana K, Acosta M, Campisi J. Regulation of a senescence checkpoint response by the E2F1 transcription factor and p14(ARF) tumor suppressor. *Mol Cell Biol* 20:273–285, 2000.

Dimri GP, Lee X, Basile G, Acosta M, Scott G, Roskelley C, Medrano E, Linskens M, Rubelj I, Pereira-Smith O, Peacock M, Campisi J. A biomarker that identifies senescent human cells in culture and in aging skin in vivo. *Proc Natl Acad Sci USA* 92:9363–9367, 1995.

Dimri GP, Testori A, Acosta M, Campisi J. Replicative senescence, aging and growth-regulatory transcription factors. *Biol Signals* 5:154–162, 1996.

DiPaolo BR, Pignolo RJ, Cristofalo VJ. Identification of proteins differentially expressed in quiescent and proliferatively senescent fibroblast cultures. *Exp Cell Res* 220:178–185, 1995.

Dlugosz A, Ciechanowicz A. Telomerase and gastrointestinal cancer [in Polish]. *Pol Merkuriusz Lek* 5:57–59, 1998.

Dluhy RG, Lifton RP. Glucocorticoid-remediable aldosteronism. *J Clin Endocrinol Metab* 84:4341–4344, 1999.

D'Mello NP, Jazwinski SM. Telomere length constancy during aging of *Saccharomyces cerevisiae*. *J Bacteriol* 173:6709–6713, 1991.

Dobson AW, Xu Y, Kelley MR, LeDoux SP, Wilson GL. Enhanced mtDNA repair and cellular survival following oxidative stress by targeting the hOGG repair enzyme to mitochondria. *J Biol Chem* 275:37518–37523, 2000.

Dobson CB, Itzhaki RF. Herpes simplex virus type 1 and Alzheimer's disease. *Neurobiol Aging* 20:457–465, 1999.

Doggett DL, Rotenberg MO, Pignolo RJ, Phillips PD, Cristofalo VJ. Differential gene expression between young and senescent, quiescent WI-38 cells. *Mech Ageing Dev* 65:239–255, 1992.

Dokudovskaya SS, Petrov AV, Dontsova OA, Bogdanov AA. Telomerase is an unusual RNA-containing enzyme. A review. *Biochemistry (Mosc)* 62:1206–1215, 1997.

Dol'nik AV, Luk'ianov DV, Enukashvili NI, Podgornaia OI. Localization of proteins, specifically binding highly repetitive sequences of DNA in human spermatozoids [in Russian]. *Tsitologiia* 43:681–691, 2001.

Domanski M, Mitchel G, Pfeffer M, Neaton JD, Norman J, Svendsen K, Grimm R, Cohen J, Stamler J, for the MRFIT Research Group. Pulse pressure and cardiovascular disease–related mortality: follow-up study of the Multiple Risk Factor Intervention Trial (MRFIT). *JAMA* 287:2677–2683, 2002.

Donaldson L, Fordyce C, Gilliland F, Smith A, Feddersen R, Joste N, Moyzis R, Griffith J. Association between outcome and telomere DNA content in prostate cancer. *J Urol* 162:1788–1792, 1999.

Donati A, Cavallini G, Paradiso C, Vittorini S, Pollera M, Gori Z, Bergamini E. Age-related changes in the regulation of autophagic proteolysis in rat isolated hepatocytes. *J Gerontol A Biol Sci Med Sci* 56:B288–293, 2001.

Doraiswamy PM, Bieber F, Kaiser L, Krishnan KR, Reuning-Scherer J, Gulanski B. The Alzheimer's Disease Assessment Scale: patterns and predictors of baseline cognitive performance in multicenter Alzheimer's disease trials. *Neurology* 48:1511–1517, 1997.

Dorland M, van Kooij RJ, te Velde ER. General ageing and ovarian ageing. *Maturitas* 30:113–118, 1998.

Dorman JB, Albinder B, Shroyer T, Kenyon C. The *age-1* and *daf-2* genes function in a common pathway to control the life span of *Caenorhabditis elegans*. *Genetics* 141:1399–1406, 1995.

Double JA. Telomerase as a therapeutic target: therapeutic potential of telomerase inhibitors. In Double JA, Thompson MJ (eds). *Telomeres and Telomerase: Methods and Protocols*. Humana Press, Totowa, NJ, 2002, pp. 209–216.

Double JA, Thompson MJ. *Telomeres and Telomerase: Methods and Protocols*. Humana Press, Totowa, NJ, 2002.

Dowdy SC, O'Kane DJ, Keeney GL, Boyd J, Podratz KC. Telomerase activity in sex cord–stromal tumors of the ovary. *Gynecol Oncol* 82:257–260, 2001.

Dozmorov I, Bartke A, Miller RA. Array-based expression analysis of mouse liver genes: effect of age and of the longevity mutant Prop1df. *J Gerontol A Biol Sci Med Sci* 56A:B72–80, 2001.

Dragunow M, MacGibbon GA, Lawlor P, Butterworth N, Connor B, Henderson C, Walton M, Woodgate A, Hughes P, Faull RL. Apoptosis, neurotrophic factors and neurodegeneration. *Rev Neurosci* 8:223–265, 1997.

Drissi R, Zindy F, Roussel MF, Cleveland JL. c-Myc mediated regulation of telomerase activity is disabled in immortalized cells. *J Biol Chem* 276:29994–30001, 2001.

Dropcova S, Denyer SP, Lloyd AW, Gard PR, Hanlon GW, Mikhalovsky SV, Sandeman S, Olliff CJ, Faragher RG. A standard strain of human ocular keratocytes. *Ophthalmic Res* 31:33–41, 1999.

Drucker WD, Blumberg JM, Gandy HM, David RR, Verde AL. Biologic activity of dehydro-epiandrosterone sulfate in man. *J Clin Endocrinol Metab* 35:48–54, 1972.

Dua HS, Azuara-Blanco A. Limbal stem cells of the corneal epithelium. *Surv Ophthalmol* 44:415–425, 2000.

Duan J, Zhang Z, Tong T. Senescence delay of human diploid fibroblast induced by anti-sense p16INK4a expression. *J Biol Chem* 276:48325–48331, 2001.

Dubal DB, Kashon ML, Pettigrew LC, Ren JM, Finklestein SP, Rau SW, Wise PM. Estradiol protects against ischemic injury. *J Cereb Blood Flow Metab* 18:1253–1258, 1998.

Dubal DB, Shughrue PJ, Wilson ME, Merchenthaler I, Wise PM. Estradiol modulates bcl-2 in cerebral ischemia: a potential role for estrogen receptors. *J Neurosci* 19:6385–6393, 1999.

Dubrana K, Perrod S, Gasser SM. Turning telomeres off and on. *Curr Opin Cell Biol* 13:281–289, 2001.

Duby F, Cardol P, Matagne RF, Remacle C. Structure of the telomeric ends of mt DNA, transcriptional analysis and complex I assembly in the dum24 mitochondrial mutant of *Chlamydomonas reinhardtii*. *Mol Genet Genomics* 266:109–114, 2001.

Ducrest AL, Amacker M, Mathieu YD, Cuthbert AP, Trott DA, Newbold RF, Nabholz M, Lingner J. Regulation of human telomerase activity: repression by normal chromosome 3 abolishes nuclear telomerase reverse transcriptase transcripts but does not affect c-Myc activity. *Cancer Res* 61:7594–7602, 2001.

Ducy P, Schinke T, Karsenty G. The osteoblast: a sophisticated fibroblast under central surveillance. *Science* 289:1501–1504, 2000.

Dudas SP, Arking R. The expression of the EF1 alpha genes of *Drosophila* is not associated with the extended longevity phenotype in a selected long-lived strain. *Exp Gerontol* 29:645–657, 1994.

Dudas SP, Arking R. A coordinate upregulation of antioxidant gene activities is associated with the delayed onset of senescence in a long-lived strain of *Drosophila*. *J Gerontol A Biol Sci Med Sci* 50:B117–127, 1995.

Duggan BD, Wan M, Yu MC, Roman LD, Muderspach LI, Delgadillo E, Li WZ, Martin SE, Dubeau L. Detection of ovarian cancer cells: comparison of a telomerase assay and cytologic examination. *J Natl Cancer Inst* 90:238–242, 1998.

Dugi KA, Rader DJ. Lipoproteins and the endothelium: insights from clinical research. *Semin Thromb Hemost* 26:513–519, 2000.

Dumont P, Royer V, Pascal T, Dierick JF, Chainiaux F, Frippiat C, de Magalhaes JP, Eliaers F, Remacle J, Toussaint O. Growth kinetics rather than stress accelerate telomere shortening in cultures of human diploid fibroblasts in oxidative stress–induced premature senescence. *FEBS Lett* 502:109–112, 2001.

Duncan EL, Perrem K, Reddel RR. Identification of a novel human mitochondrial D-loop RNA species which exhibits upregulated expression following cellular immortalization. *Biochem Biophys Res Commun* 276:439–446, 2000.

Duncan EL, Reddel RR. Genetic changes associated with immortalization. A review. *Biochemistry (Mosc)* 62:1263–1274, 1997.

Duncan EL, Wadhwa R, Kaul SC. Senescence and immortalization of human cells. *Biogerontology* 1:103–121, 2000.

Dunham MA, Neumann AA, Fasching CL, Reddel RR. Telomere maintenance by recombination in human cells. *Nat Genet* 26:447–450, 2000.

Durakovic Z, Mimica M. Proteinuria in the elderly. *Gerontology* 29:121–124, 1983.

Duthu GS, Braunschweiger KI, Pereira-Smith OM, Norwood TH, Smith JR. A long-lived human diploid fibroblast line for cellular aging studies: applications in cell hybridization. *Mech Ageing Dev* 20:243–252, 1982.

Dutt S, Steinert FR, Raizman MB, Puliafito CA. One-year results of excimer laser photorefractive keratectomy for low to moderate myopia. *Arch Ophthalmol* 112:1427–1436, 1994.

Dutta C. Significance of sarcopenia in the elderly. *J Nutr* 127:992S-993S, 1997.

Dutta C, Hadley EC. The significance of sarcopenia in old age. *J Gerontol A Biol Sci Med Sci* 50 (Spec No):1–4, 1995.

Dyck JD, David TE, Burke B, Webb GD, Henderson MA, Fowler RS. Management of coronary artery disease in Hutchinson-Gilford syndrome. *J Pediatr* 111:407–410, 1987.

Dzau VJ. Cell biology and genetics of angiotensin in cardiovascular disease. *J Hypertens Suppl* 12:S3–10, 1994a.

Dzau VJ. Pathobiology of atherosclerosis and plaque complications. *Am Heart J* 128:1300–1304, 1994b.

Dzau VJ. Mechanism of protective effects of ACE inhibition on coronary artery disease. *Eur Heart J* 19(Suppl J):J2–6, 1998.

Dzau VJ. Theodore Cooper Lecture: tissue angiotensin and pathobiology of vascular disease: a unifying hypothesis. *Hypertension* 37:1047–1052, 2001.

Dzau VJ, Gibbons GH, Kobilka BK, Lawn RM, Pratt RE. Genetic models of human vascular disease. *Circulation* 91:521–531, 1995.

Dzau VJ, Gibbons GH, Mann M, Braun-Dullaeus R. Future horizons in cardiovascular molecular therapeutics. *Am J Cardiol* 80:33I–39I, 1997.

Dzau VJ, Gibbons GH, Morishita R, Pratt RE. New perspectives in hypertension research. Potentials of vascular biology. *Hypertension* 23:1132–1140, 1994.

Dzau VJ, Horiuchi M. In vivo gene transfer and gene modulation in hypertension research. *Hypertension* 28:1132–1137, 1996.

Dzau VJ, Mann MJ, Morishita R, Kaneda Y. Fusigenic viral liposome for gene therapy in cardio-vascular diseases. *Proc Natl Acad Sci USA* 93:11421–11425, 1996.

Eastell R. Risedronate: a new bisphosphonate for the prevention and treatment of osteoporosis. *Clin Geriatr* 9:36–46, 2001.

Ebly EM, Hogan DB, Parhad IM. Cognitive impairment in the nondemented elderly. Results from the Canadian Study of Health and Aging. *Arch Neurol* 52:612–619, 1995.

Edelstein-Keshet L, Israel A, Lansdorp P. Modelling perspectives on aging: can mathematics help us stay young? *J Theor Biol* 213:509–525, 2001.

Edwards IJ, Rudel LL, Terry JG, Kemnitz JW, Weindruch R, Cefalu WT. Caloric restriction in rhesus monkeys reduces low density lipoprotein interaction with arterial proteoglycans. *J Gerontol A Biol Sci Med Sci* 53:B443–448, 1998.

Effros RB. Insights on immunological aging derived from the T lymphocyte cellular senescence model. *Exp Gerontol* 31:21–27, 1996.

Effros RB. Loss of CD28 expression on T lymphocytes: a marker of replicative senescence. *Dev Comp Immunol* 21:471–478, 1997.

Effros RB. Immune senescence—senescence in the immune system. Presented at Telomeres and Telomerase: Implications for Cell Immortality, Cancer, and Age-related Disease. San Francisco, CA, June 1–3, 1998a.

Effros RB. Replicative senescence: impact on T cell immunity in the elderly. *Aging (Milano)* 10:152, 1998b.

Effros RB. Replicative senescence in the immune system: impact of the Hayflick limit on T-cell function in the elderly. *Am J Hum Genet* 62:1003–1007, 1998c.

Effros RB. Costimulatory mechanisms in the elderly. *Vaccine* 18:1661–1665, 2000a.

Effros RB. Long-term immunological memory against viruses. *Mech Ageing Dev* 121:161–171 , 2000b.

Effros RB. Telomeres and HIV disease. *Microbes Infect* 2:69–76 , 2000c.

Effros RB. Ageing and the immune system. *Novartis Found Symp* 235:130–139 and 146–149, 2001a.

Effros RB. Immune system activity. In Masoro EJ, Austad SN (eds). *Handbook of the Biology of Aging, 5th ed.* Academic Press, New York, 2001, pp 324–352.

Effros RB, Allsopp R, Chi CP, Hausner MA, Hirji K, Wang L, Harley CB, Villeponteau B, West MD, Giorgi JV. Shortened telomeres in the expanded CD28-CD8+ cell subset in HIV disease implicate replicative senescence in HIV pathogenesis. *AIDS* 10:F17–22, 1996.

Effros RB, Boucher N, Porter V, Zhu X, Spaulding C, Walford RL, Kronenberg M, Cohen D, Schachter F. Decline in CD28(+) T cells in centenarians and in long-term T cell cultures: a possible cause for both in vivo and in vitro immunosenescence. *Exp Gerontol* 29:601–609, 1994a.

Effros RB, Globerson A. Hematopoietic cells and replicative senescence. *Exp Gerontol* 37:191–196, 2002.

Effros RB, Pawelec G. Replicative senescence of T lymphocytes: does the Hayflick limit lead to immune exhaustion? *Immunol Today* 18:450–454, 1997.

Effros RB, Svoboda K, Walford RL. Influence of age and caloric restriction on macrophage IL-6 and TNF production. *Lymphokine Cytokine Res* 10:347–351, 1991a.

Effros RB, Valenzuela HF. Immunosenescence: analysis and genetic modulation of replicative senescence in T cells. *J Anti-Aging Med* 1:305–313, 1998.

Effros RB, Walford RL, Weindruch R, Mitcheltree C. Influences of dietary restriction on immunity to influenza in aged mice. *J Gerontol A Biol Med Sci* 46B:142–147, 1991b.

Effros RB, Zhu X, Walford RL. Stress response of senescent T lymphocytes: reduced hsp70 is independent of the proliferative block. *J Gerontol* 49:B65–70, 1994b.

Egan CA, Savre-Train I, Shay JW, Wilson SE, Bourne WM. Analysis of telomere lengths in human corneal endothelial cells from donors of different ages. *Invest Ophthalmol Vis Sci* 39:648–53, 1998.

Eggan K, Akutsu H, Loring J, Jackson-Grusby L, Klemm M, Rideout WM 3rd, Yanagimachi R, Jaenisch R. Hybrid vigor, fetal overgrowth, and viability of mice derived by nuclear cloning and tetraploid embryo complementation. *Proc Natl Acad Sci USA* 98:6209–6214, 2001.

Ehsan A, Mann MJ, Dell'Acqua G, Dzau VJ. Long-term stabilization of vein graft wall architecture and prolonged resistance to experimental atherosclerosis after E2F decoy oligonucleotide gene therapy. *J Thorac Cardiovasc Surg* 121:714–722, 2001.

Eickbush TH. Telomerase and retrotransposons: which came first? *Science* 277:911–912, 1997.

Eikelenboom P, Rozemuller JM, van Muiswinkel FL. Inflammation and Alzheimer's disease: relationships between pathogenic mechanisms and clinical expression. *Exp Neurol* 154:89–98, 1998.

Eimon PM, Chung SS, Lee CM, Weindruch R, Aiken JM. Age-associated mitochondrial DNA deletions in mouse skeletal muscle: comparison of different regions of the mitochondrial genome. *Dev Genet* 18:107–113, 1996.

Einhard. *The Life of Charlemagne*. Ann Arbor Paperbacks, The University of Michigan Press, Ann Arbor, 1960.

Elayadi AN, Demieville A, Wancewicz EV, Monia BP, Corey DR. Inhibition of telomerase by 2'-*O*-(2-methoxyethyl) RNA oligomers: effect of length, phosphorothioate substitution and time inside cells. *Nucleic Acids Res* 29:1683–1689, 2001.

Eldred GE. Age pigment structure. *Nature* 364:396, 1993.

Elenbaas B, Spirio L, Koerner F, Fleming MD, Zimonjic DB, Donaher JL, Popescu NC, Hahn WC, Weinberg RA. Human breast cancer cells generated by oncogenic transformation of primary mammary epithelial cells. *Genes Dev* 15:50–65, 2001.

Elias MF, Beiser A, Wolf PA, Au R, White RF, D'Agostino RB. The preclinical phase of alzheimer disease: a 22-year prospective study of the Framingham Cohort. *Arch Neurol* 57:808–813, 2000.

Eller MS, Puri N, Hadshiew IM, Venna SS, Gilchrest BA. Induction of apoptosis by telomere 3' overhang-specific DNA. *Exp Cell Res* 276:185–193, 2002.

Elli R, Petrinelli P, Caporossi D, Nicoletti B, Antonelli A. Cytogenetic investigations on Werner's syndrome, acrogeria, and keratosis palmo-plantaris. *J Genet Hum* 31:211–221, 1983.

Ellis NA, Groden J, Ye TZ, Straughen J, Lennon DJ, Ciocci S, Proytcheva M, German J. The Bloom's syndrome gene product is homologous to RecQ helicases. *Cell* 83:655–666, 1995.

Elmore LW, Holt SE. Telomerase and telomere stability: a new class of tumor suppressor? *Mol Carcinog* 28:1–4, 2000.

Elmore LW, Rehder CW, Di X, McChesney PA, Jackson-Cook CK, Gewirtz DA, Holt SE. Adriamycin-induced senescence in breast tumor cells involves functional p53 and telomere dysfunction. *J Biol Chem* 277:35509–5515, 2002a.

Elmore LW, Turner KC, Gollahon LS, Landon MR, Jackson-Cook CK, Holt SE. Telomerase protects cancer-prone human cells from chromosomal instability and spontaneous immortalization. *Cancer Biol Ther* 1:391–397, 2002b.

Ely SA, Chadburn A, Dayton CM, Cesarman E, Knowles DM. Telomerase activity in B-cell non-Hodgkin lymphoma. *Cancer* 89:445–452, 2000.

Emrich T, Chang SY, Karl G, Panzinger B, Santini C. Quantitative detection of telomerase components by real-time, online RT-PCR analysis with the light cycler. In Double JA, Thompson MJ (eds). *Telomeres and Telomerase: Methods and Protocols*. Humana Press, Totowa, NJ, 2002, pp 99–108.

Emrich T, Karl G. Nonradioactive detection of telomerase activity using a PCR-ELISA-based telomeric repeat amplification protocol. In Double JA, Thompson MJ (eds). *Telomeres and Telomerase: Methods and Protocols*. Humana Press, Totowa, NJ, 2002, pp 147–158.

Endlich K, Kriz W, Witzgall R. Update in podocyte biology. *Curr Opin Nephrol Hypertens* 10:331–340, 2001.

Engel BC, Kohn DB. Stem cell directed gene therapy. *Front Biosci* 4:e26–33, 1999.

Engelhardt M, Kumar R, Albanell J, Pettengell R, Han W, Moore MAS. Telomerase regulation, cell cycle, and telomere stability in primitive hematopoetic cells. *Blood* 90:182–193, 1997.

Engelhardt M, Mackenzie K, Drullinsky P, Silver RT, Moore MA. Telomerase activity and telomere length in acute and chronic leukemia, pre– and post–ex vivo culture. *Cancer Res* 60:610–617, 2000.

Engelhardt M, Martens UM. The implication of telomerase activity and telomere stability for replicative aging and cellular immortality [review]. *Oncol Rep* 5:1043–1052, 1998.

Engelhardt M, Ozkaynak MF, Drullinsky P, Sandoval C, Tugal O, Jayabose S, Moore MAS. Telomerase activity and telomere length in pediatric patients with malignancies undergoing chemotherapy. *Leukemia* 12:13–24, 1998.

Engelhart MJ, Geerlings MI, Ruitenberg A, van Swieten JC, Hofman A, Witteman JCM, Breteler MMB. Dietary intake of antioxidants and risk of Alzheimer disease. *JAMA* 287:3223–3229, 2002.

Enoch JM, Werner JS, Haegerstrom-Portnoy G, Lakshminarayanan V, Rynders M. Forever young: visual functions not affected or minimally affected by aging: a review. *J Gerontol A Biol Sci Med Sci* 54:B336–351, 1999.

Enomoto S, McCune-Zierath PD, Gerami-Nejad M, Sanders MA, Berman J. RLF2, a subunit of yeast chromatin assembly factor-I, is required for telomeric chromatin function in vivo. *Genes Dev* 11:358–370, 1997.

Enzan H, Himeno H, Hiroi M, Kiyoku H, Saibara T, Onishi S. Development of hepatic sinusoidal structure with special reference to the Ito cells. *Microsc Res Tech* 39:336–349, 1997.

Epperly TD, Moore KE. Health issues in men: part I: common genitourinary disorders. *Am Fam Physician* 61:3657–3664, 2000.

Epstein CJ, Martin GM, Motulsky AG. Werner's syndrome; caricature of aging. A genetic model for the study of degenerative diseases. *Trans Assoc Am Physicians* 78:73–81, 1965.

Epstein CJ, Martin GM, Schultz AL, Motulsky A. Werner's syndrome: a review of its symptomatology, natural history, pathologic features, genetics and relationship to the natural aging process. *Medicine* 45:177–221, 1977.

Epstein J, Williams JR, Little JB. Deficient DNA repair in human progeroid cells. *Proc Natl Acad Sci USA* 70:977–981, 1973.

Epstein J, Williams JR, Little JB. Rate of DNA repair in progeric and normal human fibroblasts. *Biochem Biophys Res Commun* 59:850–857, 1974.

Eriksson E. Brown WT, Gordon LB, Glynn MW, Singer J, Scott L, Erdos MR, Robbins CM, Moses MY, Berglund P, Dutra A, Pak E, Durkin S, Csoka AB, Boehnkek M, Glover TW, Collins FS. Recurrent de novo point mutations in lamin A cause Hutchinson-Gilford progeria syndrome. *Nature* 423:293–298, 2003.

Eriksson PS, Perfilieva E, Bjork-Eriksson T, Alborn AM, Nordborg C, Peterson DA, Gage FH. Neurogenesis in the adult human hippocampus. *Nat Med* 4:1313–1317, 1998.

Erkinjuntti T, Inzitari D, Pantoni L, Wallin A, Scheltens P, Rockwood K, Roman GC, Chui H, Desmond DW. Research criteria for subcortical vascular dementia in clinical trials. *J Neural Transm Suppl* 59:23–30, 2000.

Erlitzki R, Minuk GY. Telomeres, telomerase and HCC: the long and the short of it. *J Hepatol* 31:939–945, 1999.

Erwin JM, Nimchinsky EA, Gannon PJ, Perl DP, Hof PR. The study of brain aging in great apes. In Hof PR, Mobbs CV (eds). *Functional Neurobiology of Aging*. Academic Press, New York, 2001, pp 447–456.

Esler WP, Wolfe MS. A portrait of Alzheimer secretases—new features and familiar faces. *Science* 293:1449–1454, 2001.

Espejel S, Blasco MA. Identification of telomere-dependent "senescence-like" arrest in mouse embryonic fibroblasts. *Exp Cell Res* 276:242–248, 2002.

Espejel S, Franco S, Rodriguez-Perales S, Bouffler SD, Cigudosa JC, Blasco MA. Mammalian Ku86 mediates chromosomal fusions and apoptosis caused by critically short telomeres. *EMBO J* 21:2207–2219, 2002a.

Espejel S, Franco S, Sgura A, Gae D, Bailey SM, Taccioli GE, Blasco MA. Functional interaction between DNA-PKcs and telomerase in telomere length maintenance. *EMBO J* 21:6275–6287, 2002b.

Etcheberrigaray R, Hirashima N, Nee L, Prince J, Govoni S, Racchi M, Tanzi RE, Alkon DL. Calcium responses in fibroblasts from asymptomatic members of Alzheimer's disease families. *Neurobiol Dis* 5:37–45, 1998.

Etheridge KT, Banik SS, Armbruster BN, Zhu Y, Terns RM, Terns MP, Counter CM. The nucleolar localization domain of the catalytic subunit of human telomerase. *J Biol Chem* 277:24764–24770, 2002.

EUROGAST Study Group. An international association between *Helicobacter pylori* infection and gastric cancer. *Lancet* 341:1359–1362, 1993.

Evans SK, Bertuch AA, Lundblad V. Telomeres and telomerase: at the end, it all comes together. *Trends Cell Biol* 9:329–331, 1999.

Evans WJ. What is sarcopenia? *J Gerontol A Biol Sci Med Sci* 50(Spec No):5–8, 1995.

Evans WJ. Reversing sarcopenia: how weight training can build strength and vitality. *Geriatrics* 51:46–47, 1996.

Evans WJ, Campbell WW. Sarcopenia and age-related changes in body composition and functional capacity. *J Nutr* 123:465–468, 1993.

Everitt AV, Porter BD, Wyndham JR. Effects of caloric intake and dietary composition on the development of proteinuria, age-associated renal disease, and longevity in the male rat. *Gerontology* 28:168–175, 1982.

Ewbank JJ, Barnes TM, Lakowski B, Lussier M, Bussey H, Hekimi S. Structural and functional conservation of the *Caenorhabditis elegans* timing gene *clk-1*. *Science* 275:980–983, 1997.

Exner BG, Groninger JH, Ildstad ST. Bone marrow transplantation for therapy in autoimmune disease. *Stem Cells* 15:171–175; discussion 175–176, 1997.

Fairall L, Chapman L, Moss H, de Lange T, Rhodes D. Structure of the TRFH dimerization domain of the human telomeric proteins TRF1 and TRF2. *Mol Cell* 8:351–361, 2001.

Fairfield KM, Fletcher RH. Vitamins for chronic disease prevention: scientific review. *JAMA* 287:3116–3126, 2002.

Faivre L, Van Kien PK, Madinier-Chappat N, Nivelon-Chevallier A, Beer F, LeMerrer M. Can Hutchinson-Gilford progeria syndrome be a neonatal condition? *Am J Med Genet* 87:450–452, 1999.

Fajkus J, Simickova M, Malaska J. Tiptoeing to chromosome tips: facts, promises and perils of today's human telomere biology. *Philos Trans R Soc Lond B Biol Sci* 357:545–562, 2002.

Falchetti ML, Falcone G, D'Ambrosio E, Verna R, Alema S, Levi A. Induction of telomerase activity in v-myc-transformed avian cells. *Oncogene* 18:1515–1519, 1999.

Fang DC, Yang SM, Zhou XD, Wang DX, Luo YH. Telomere erosion is independent of microsatellite instability but related to loss of heterozygosity in gastric cancer. *World J Gastroenterol* 7:522–526, 2001.

Fang G, Cech TR. Telomere proteins. In Blackburn EH, Greider CW (eds). *Telomeres*. Cold Spring Harbor Press, Cold Spring Harbor, NY, 1995, pp 69–105.

Fanti L, Giovinazzo G, Berloco M, Pimpinelli S. The heterochromatin protein 1 prevents telomere fusions in *Drosophila*. *Mol Cell* 2:527–38, 1998.

Faragher RG. Cell senescence and human aging: where's the link? *Biochem Soc Trans* 28:221–226, 2000.

Faragher RG, Hardy SP, Davis T, Dropcova S, Allen MC. Cycling Werner's syndrome fibroblasts display calcium-dependent potassium currents. *Exp Cell Res* 231:119–122, 1997a.

Faragher RG, Jones CJ, Kipling D. Telomerase and cellular lifespan: ending the debate? *Nat Biotechnol* 16:701–702, 1998.

Faragher RG, Kill IR, Hunter JA, Pope FM, Tannock C, Shall S. The gene responsible for Werner syndrome may be a cell division "counting" gene. *Proc Natl Acad Sci USA* 90:12030–12034, 1993.

Faragher RG, Kipling D. How might replicative senescence contribute to human ageing? *Bioessays* 20:985–991, 1998.

Faragher RG, Mulholland B, Tuft SJ, Sandeman S, Khaw PT. Aging and the cornea. *Br J Ophthalmol* 81:814–817, 1997b.

Faraoni I, Graziani G. Telomerase as a potential anticancer target: growth inhibition and genomic instability. *Drug Resist Update* 3:3–6, 2000.

Faraoni I, Graziani G, Turriziani M, Masci G, Mezzetti M, Testori A, Veronesi U, Bonmassar E. Suppression of telomerase activity as an indicator of drug-induced cytotoxicity against cancer cells: in vitro studies with fresh human tumor samples. *Lab Invest* 79:993–1005, 1999.

Faraoni I, Turriziani M, Masci G, De Vecchis L, Shay JW, Bonmassar E, Graziani G. Decline in telomerase activity as a measure of tumor cell killing by antineoplastic agents in vitro. *Clin Cancer Res* 3:579–585, 1997.

Faravelli M, Azzalin CM, Bertoni L, Chernova O, Attolini C, Mondello C, Giulotto E. Molecular organization of internal telomeric sequences in Chinese hamster chromosomes. *Gene* 283:11–16, 2002.

Farrer LA. Intercontinental epidemiology of Alzheimer disease: a global approach to bad gene hunting. *JAMA* 285:796–798, 2001.

Farwell DG, Shera KA, Koop JI, Bonnet GA, Matthews CP, Reuther GW, Coltrera MD, McDougall JK, Klingelhutz AJ. Genetic and epigenetic changes in human epithelial cells immortalized by telomerase. *Am J Pathol* 156:1537–1547, 2000.

Fawcett JW, Asher RA. The glial scar and central nervous system repair. *Brain Res Bull* 49:377–391, 1999.

Fearon DT, Manders P, Wagner SD. Arrested differentiation, the self-renewing memory lymphocyte, and vaccination. *Science* 293:248–250, 2001.

Feinberg RN, Beebe DC. Hyaluronate in vasculogenesis. *Science* 220:1177–1179, 1983.

Feist H, Zeidler R, Skrebsky T, Schmatloch S, Kreipe H. Induction of telomerase activity in stimulated human lymphocytes precedes expression of topoisomerase II alpha. *Ann Hematol* 76:111–115, 1998.

Felkai S, Ewbank JJ, Lemieux J, Labbe JC, Brown GG, Hekimi S. CLK-1 controls respiration, behavior and aging in the nematode *Caenorhabditis elegans*. *EMBO J* 18:1783–1792, 1999.

Feng J, Funk WD, Wang SS, Weinrich SL, Avilion AA, Chiu CP, Adams RR, Chang E, Allsopp RC, Yu J Le S, West MD, Harley CB, Andrews WE, Greider CW, Villeponteau B. The RNA component of human telomerase. *Science* 269:1236–1241, 1995.

Ferber A, Chang C, Sell C, Ptasznik A, Cristofalo VJ, Hubbard K, Ozer HL, Adamo M, Roberts CT Jr, LeRoith D, et al. Failure of senescent human fibroblasts to express the insulin-like growth factor-1 gene. *J Biol Chem* 268:17883–17888, 1993.

Ferbeyre G, Lowe SW. The price of tumour suppression? *Nature* 415:26–27, 2002.

Ferguson BM, Brewer BJ, Fangman WL. Temporal control of DNA replication in yeast. *Cold Spring Harb Symp Quant Biol* 56:293–302, 1991.

Fernandez-Palazzi F, McLaren AT, Slowie DF. Report on a case of Hutchinson-Gilford progeria, with special reference to orthopedic problems. *Eur J Pediatr Surg* 2:378–382, 1992.

Feskanich D, Singh V, Willett WC, Colditz GA. Vitamin A intake and hip fractures among postmenopausal women. *JAMA* 287: 47–54, 2002.

Feuers RJ, Weindruch R, Hart RW. Caloric restriction, aging, and antioxidant enzymes. *Mutat Res* 295:191–200, 1993.

Fichtlscherer S, Zeiher AM. Endothelial dysfunction in acute coronary syndromes: association with elevated C-reactive protein levels. *Ann Med* 32:515–518, 2000.

Figueiredo LM, Freitas-Junior LH, Bottius E, Olivo-Marin JC, Scherf A. A central role for *Plasmodium falciparum* subtelomeric regions in spatial positioning and telomere length regulation. *EMBO J* 21:815–824, 2002.

Figueroa R, Lindenmaier H, Hergenhahn M, Nielsen KV, Boukamp P. Telomere erosion varies during in vitro aging of normal human fibroblasts from young and adult donors. *Cancer Res* 60:2770–2774, 2000.

Filatov L, Golubovskaya V, Hurt JC, Byrd LL, Phillips JM, Kaufmann WK. Chromosomal instability is correlated with telomere erosion and inactivation of G2 checkpoint function in human fibroblasts expressing human papillomavirus type 16 E6 oncoprotein. *Oncogene* 16:1825–1838, 1998.

Fillenbaum GG, Huber MS, Beekly D, Henderson VW, Mortimer J, Morris JC, Harrell LE. The Consortium to Establish a Registry for Alzheimer's Disease (CERAD). Part XIII. Obtaining autopsy in Alzheimer's disease. *Neurology* 46:142–145, 1996.

Fillit H. Future therapeutic developments of estrogen use. *J Clin Pharmacol* 35:25S–28S, 1995.

Fillit H, Cummings J. Practice guidelines for the diagnosis and treatment of Alzheimer's disease in a managed care setting: Part II—Pharmacologic therapy. Alzheimer's Disease (AD) Managed Care Advisory Council. *Manag Care Interface* 13:51–56, 2000.

Fillit H, Gutterman EM, Lewis B. Donepezil use in managed Medicare: effect on health care costs and utilization. *Clin Ther* 21:2173–2185, 1999a.

Fillit H, Knopman D, Cummings J, Appel F. Opportunities for improving managed care for individuals with dementia: Part 1—The issues. *Am J Manag Care* 5(3):309–315, 1999b.

Fillit H, Weinreb H, Cholst I, Luine V, McEwen B, Amador R, Zabriskie J. Observations in a preliminary open trial of estradiol therapy for senile dementia, Alzheimer's type. *Psychoneuroendocrinology* 11:337–345, 1986.

Finch CE. *Longevity, Senescence, and the Genome.* University of Chicago Press, Chicago, 1990.

Finch CE, Tanzi RE. Genetics of aging. *Science* 278:407–411, 1997.

Fine SL, Berger JW, Maguire MG, Ho AC. Age-related macular degeneration. *N Engl J Med* 342:483–492, 2000.

Finkel E. The mitochondrion: is it central to apoptosis? *Science* 292:624–625, 2001.

Finkel T, Holbrook NJ. Oxidants, oxidative stress and the biology of ageing. *Nature* 408:239–247, 2000.

Finnon P, Silver AR, Bouffler SD. Upregulation of telomerase activity by X-irradiation in mouse leukaemia cells is independent of Tert, Terc, Tnks and Myc transcription. *Carcinogenesis* 21:573–578, 2000.

Finnon P, Wong HP, Silver AR, Slijepcevic P, Bouffler SD. Long but dysfunctional telomeres correlate with chromosomal radiosensitivity in a mouse AML cell line. *Int J Radiat Biol* 77:1151–1162, 2001.

Fisher A, Morley JE. Antiaging medicine: the good, the bad, and the ugly. *J Gerontol A Biol Sci Med Sci* 57:636–639, 2002.

Fisher S, Gearhart JD, Oster-Granite ML. Expression of the amyloid precursor protein gene in mouse oocytes and embryos. *Proc Natl Acad Sci USA* 88:1779–1782, 1991.

Fitzgerald GA, Meagher E. Vitamin E supplementation in healthy persons: reply in Letters to the Editor. *JAMA* 285:2450, 2001.

Fleming JE, Spicer GS, Garrison RC, Rose MR. Two-dimensional protein electrophoretic analysis of postponed aging in *Drosophila*. *Genetica* 91:183–198, 1993.

Flescher E, Tripoli H, Salnikow K, Burns FJ. Oxidative stress suppresses transcription factor activities in stimulated lymphocytes. *Clin Exp Immunol* 112:242–247, 1998.

Fletcher RH, Fairfield KM. Vitamins for chronic disease prevention: clinical applications. *JAMA* 287:3127–3129, 2002.

Fletcher SW, Colditz GA. Failure of estrogen plus progestin therapy for prevention. *JAMA* 288:366–367, 2002.

Flynn MA, Weaver-Osterholtz D, Sharpe-Timms KL, Allen S, Krause G. Dehydroepiandrosterone replacement in aging humans. *J Clin Endocrinol Metab* 84:1527–1533, 1999.

Foddis R, De Rienzo A, Broccoli D, Bocchetta M, Stekala E, Rizzo P, Tosolini A, Grobelny JV, Jhanwar SC, Pass HI, Testa JR, Carbone M. SV40 infection induces telomerase activity in human mesothelial cells. *Oncogene* 21:1434–1442, 2002.

Foley DJ, White LR. Dietary intake of antioxidants and risk of Alzheimer disease. *JAMA* 287:3261–3263, 2002.

Folini M, Colella G, Villa R, Lualdi S, Daidone MG, Zaffaroni N. Inhibition of telomerase activity by a hammerhead ribozyme targeting the RNA component of telomerase in human melanoma cells. *J Invest Dermatol* 114:259–267, 2000.

Folkman J, Camphausen K. What does radiotherapy do to endothelial cells? *Science* 293:227–228, 2001.

Fonseca MI, Head E, Velazquez P, Cotman CW, Tenner AJ. The presence of isoaspartic acid in beta-amyloid plaques indicates plaque age. *Exp Neurol* 157:277–288, 1999.

Fontaine KR, Redden DT, Wang C, Westfall AO, Allison DB. Years of life lost due to obesity. *JAMA* 289:187–193, 2003.

Force AG, Staples T, Soliman S, Arking R. Comparative biochemical and stress analysis of genetically selected *Drosophila* strains with different longevities. *Dev Genet* 17:340–351, 1995.

Ford LP, Shay JW, Wright WE. The La antigen associates with the human telomerase ribonucleoprotein and influences telomere length in vivo. *RNA* 7:1068–1075, 2001.

Ford LP, Wright WE, Shay JW. A model for heterogeneous nuclear ribonucleoproteins in telomere and telomerase regulation. *Oncogene* 21:580–583, 2002.

Fordyce CA, Heaphy CM, Griffith JK. Chemiluminescent measurement of telomere DNA content in biopsies. *Biotechniques* 33:144–146, 148, 2002.

Forejt J, Saam JR, Gregorova S, Tilghman SM. Monoallelic expression of reactivated imprinted genes in embryonal carcinoma cell hybrids. *Exp Cell Res* 252:416–422, 1999.

Forgione MA, Leopold JA, Loscalzo J. Roles of endothelial dysfunction in coronary artery disease. *Curr Opin Cardiol* 15:409–415, 2000.

Forsling ML, Montgomery H, Halpin D, Windle RJ, Treacher DF. Daily patterns of secretion of neurohypophysial hormones in man: effect of age. *Exp Physiol* 83:409–418, 1998.

Forstemann K, Hoss M, Lingner J. Telomerase-dependent repeat divergence at the 3' ends of yeast telomeres. *Nucleic Acids Res* 28:2690–2694, 2000.

Forstemann K, Lingner J. Molecular basis for telomere repeat divergence in budding yeast. *Mol Cell Biol* 21:7277–7286, 2001.

Forster MJ, Sohal BH, Sohal RS. Reversible effects of long-term caloric restriction on protein oxidative damage. *J Gerontol A Biol Sci Med Sci* 55:B522–529, 2000.

Forsyth NR, Wright WE, Shay JW. Telomerase and differentiation in multicellular organisms: turn it off, turn it on, and turn it off again. *Differentiation* 69:188–197, 2002.

Forsythe HL, Elmore LW, Jensen KO, Landon MR, Holt SE. Retroviral-mediated expression of telomerase in normal human cells provides a selective growth advantage. *Int J Oncol* 20:1137–1143, 2002.

Forsythe HL, Jarvis JL, Turner JW, Elmore LW, Holt SE. Stable association of hsp90 and p23, but Not hsp70, with active human telomerase. *J Biol Chem* 276:15571–15574, 2001.

Fossel M. *Reversing Human Aging.* William Morrow and Company, New York, 1996.

Fossel M. Implications of recent work in telomeres and cell senescence. *J Anti-Aging Med* 1:39–43, 1998a.

Fossel M. Telomerase and aging health. Presented at Telomeres and Telomerase: Implications for Cell Immortality, Cancer, and Age-related Disease. San Francisco, CA, June 1–3, 1998b.

Fossel M. Telomerase and the aging cell: implications for human health. *JAMA* 279:1732–1735, 1998c.

Fossel M. Cell senescence and human aging: a review of the theory. *In Vivo* 14:29–34, 2000a.

Fossel M. E-mails to the editor. The function of mitochondrial dysfunction in aging. *J Anti-Aging Med* 3:103–104, 2000b.

Fossel M. Human aging and progeria. *J Pediatr Endosc Metab* 13:1477–1481, 2000c.

Fossel M. The role of cell senescence in human aging. *J Anti-Aging Med* 3:91–98, 2000d.

Fossel M. *Science* by fiat. *J Anti-Aging Med* 4:183–184, 2001a.

Fossel M. The role of telomerase in age-related degenerative disease and cancer. In Mattson MP (ed). *Interorganellar Signaling in Age-Related Disease.* Elsevier *Science*, Amsterdam, 2001b, pp 163–204.

Fossel M. Why we publish. *J Anti-Aging Med* 4:1–2, 2001c.

Fossel M. The ethics of longevity: should we extend the healthy maximum lifespan? In Cutler R, Rodriguez H, (eds). *Critical Reviews in Oxidative Stress and Aging: Advances in Basic Science, Diagnostics and Intervention.* World Scientific Publishing, 2003, pp 1503–1513.

Foster RS, Nichols CR. Testicular cancer: what's new in staging, prognosis, and therapy. *Oncology (Huntingt)* 13:1689–1694, 1999.

Fouladi B, Sabatier L, Miller D, Pottier G, Murnane JP. The relationship between spontaneous telomere loss and chromosome instability in a human tumor cell line. *Neoplasia* 2:540–554, 2000.

Fowler CJ, Cowburn RF, Joseph JA. Alzheimer's, ageing and amyloid: an absurd allegory? *Gerontology* 43:132–142, 1997.

Fraccaro M, Bott MG, Calvert HT. Chromosomes in Werner's syndrome. *Lancet* 1:536, 1962.

Frame PS. Routine screening for lung cancer? Maybe someday, but not yet. *JAMA* 284:1980–1983, 2000.

Franceschi C, Bonafe M, Valensin S. Human immunosenescence: the prevailing of innate immunity, the failing of clonotypic immunity, and the filling of immunological space. *Vaccine* 18:1717–1720, 2000.

Franceschi C, Valensin S, Fagnoni F, Barbi C, Bonafe M. Biomarkers of immunosenescence within an evolutionary perspective: the challenge of heterogeneity and the role of antigenic load. *Exp Gerontol* 34:911–921, 1999.

Francis SC, Raizada MK, Mangi AA, Melo LG, Dzau VJ, Vale PR, Isner JM, Losordo DW, Chao J, Katovich MJ, Berecek KH. Genetic targeting for cardiovascular therapeutics: are we near the summit or just beginning the climb? *Physiol Genomics* 7:79–94, 2001.

Franco S, Alsheimer M, Herrera E, Benavente R, Blasco MA. Mammalian meiotic telomeres: composition and ultrastructure in telomerase-deficient mice. *Eur J Cell Biol* 81:335–340, 2002a.

Franco S, MacKenzie KL, Dias S, Alvarez S, Rafii S, Moore MA. Clonal variation in phenotype and life span of human embryonic fibroblasts (MRC-5) transduced with the catalytic component of telomerase (hTERT). *Exp Cell Res* 268:14–25, 2001.

Franco S, Segura I, Riese HH, Blasco MA. Decreased B16F10 melanoma growth and impaired vascularization in telomerase-deficient mice with critically short telomeres. *Cancer Res* 62:552–559, 2002b.

Francon P, Maiorano D, Mechali M. Initiation of DNA replication in eukaryotes: questioning the origin. *FEBS Lett* 452:87–91, 1999.

Frazier AL, Colditz GA, Fuchs CS, Kuntz KM. Cost-effectiveness of screening for colorectal cancer in the general population. *JAMA* 284:1954–1961, 2000.

Freedman RS, Tomasovic B, Templin S, Atkinson EN, Kudelka A, Edwards CL, Platsoucas CD. Large-scale expansion in interleukin-2 of tumor-infiltrating lymphocytes from patients with ovarian carcinoma for adoptive immunotherapy. *J Immunol Methods* 167:145–160, 1994.

Freitag L, Litterst P, Obertrifter B, Velehorschi V, Kemmer HP, Linder A, Brightman I. Telomerase in lung cancer. Testing the activity of the "immortaligy enzyme" bronchial biopsies increases the diagnostic yield in cases of suspected peripheral bronchogenic carcinomas [in German]. *Pneumologie* 54:480–485, 2000.

Freitas-Junior LH, Bottius E, Pirrit LA, Deitsch KW, Scheidig C, Guinet F, Nehrbass U, Wellems TE, Scherf A. Frequent ectopic recombination of virulence factor genes in telomeric chromosome clusters of *P. falciparum. Nature* 407:1018–1022, 2001.

Frenck RJ, Blackburn EH, Shannon KM. The rate of telomere sequence loss in human leukocytes varies with age. *Proc Nat Acad Sci USA* 95:5607–5610, 1998.

Freud S. *Beyond the Pleasure Principle.* Standard Edition, translated by J. Strachey. W.W. Norton & Company, London, 1961.

Friedland RP, Shi J, Lamanna JC, Smith MA, Perry G. Prospects for noninvasive imaging of brain amyloid beta in Alzheimer's disease. *Ann NY Acad Sci* 903:123–128, 2000.

Friedman SL. Molecular mechanisms of hepatic fibrosis and principles of therapy. *J Gastroenterol* 32:424–430, 1997.

Friedman SL. Cytokines and fibrogenesis. *Semin Liver Dis* 19:129–140, 1999a.

Friedman SL. Stellate cell activation in alcoholic fibrosis—an overview. *Alcohol Clin Exp Res* 23:904–910, 1999b.

Friedman SL. The virtuosity of hepatic stellate cells. *Gastroenterology* 1117:1244–1246, 1999c.

Friedrich MJ. Insight into opacity: clues to cataract formation. *JAMA* 286:1705, 2001.

Friedrich MJ. Research yields clues to improving cell therapy for Parkinson disease. *JAMA* 287:175–176, 2002a.

Friedrich MJ. Teasing out effects of estrogen on the brain. *JAMA* 287:29–30, 2002b.

Fu J, Li C, Yang X, Li X. IL-4 gene transfer induces the differentiation of cells and inhibits the activity of telomerase in hepatoblastoma cells [in Chinese]. *Chung Hua I Hsueh I Chuan Hsueh Tsa Chih* 17:87–90, 2000a.

Fu W, Begley JG, Killen MW, Mattson MP. Anti-apoptotic role of telomerase in pheochromocytoma cells. *J Biol Chem* 274:7264–7271, 1999.

Fu W, Killen M, Culmsee C, Dhar S, Pandita TK, Mattson MP. The catalytic subunit of telomerase is expressed in developing brain neurons and serves a cell survival–promoting function. *J Mol Neurosci* 14:3–15, 2000b.

Fuchs E, Segre JA. Stem cells: a new lease on life. *Cell* 100:143–155, 2000.

Fujii N, Momose Y, Ishii N, Takita M, Akaboshi M, Kodama M. The mechanisms of simultaneous stereoinversion, racemization, and isomerization at specific aspartyl residues of aged lens proteins. *Mech Ageing Dev* 107:347–358 1999.

Fujimoto K, Kyo S, Takakura M, Kanaya T, Kitagawa Y, Itoh H, Takahashi M, Inoue M. Identification and characterization of negative regulatory elements of the human telomerase catalytic subunit (hTERT) gene promoter: possible role of MZF-2 in transcriptional repression of hTERT. *Nucleic Acids Res* 28:2557–2562, 2000.

Fujimoto K, Takahashi M. Telomerase activity in human leukemic cell lines is inhibited by antisense pentadecadeoxynucleotides targeted against c-myc mRNA. *Biochem Biophys Res Commun* 241:775–781, 1997.

Fujimoto R, Kamata N, Yokoyama K, Ueda N, Satomura K, Hayashi E, Nagayama M. Expression of telomerase components in oral keratinocytes and squamous cell carcinomas. *Oral Oncol* 37:132–140, 2001.

Fujiwara M, Okayasu I, Takemura T, Tanaka I, Masuda R, Furuhata Y, Noji M, Oritsu M, Kato M, Oshimura M. Telomerase activity significantly correlates with chromosome alterations, cell differentiation, and proliferation in lung adenocarcinomas. *Mod Pathol* 13:723–729, 2000.

Fujiwara Y, Higashikawa T, Tatsumi M. A retarded rate of DNA replication and normal level of DNA repair in Werner's syndrome fibroblasts in culture. *J Cell Physiol* 92:365–374, 1977.

Fukuchi K, Martin GM, Monnat RJ Jr. Mutator phenotype of Werner syndrome is characterized by extensive deletions. *Proc Natl Acad Sci USA* 86:5893–5897, 1989.

Fukumoto H, Cheung BS, Hyman BT, Irizarry MC. β-Secretase protein and activity are increased in the neocortex in Alzheimer disease. *Arch Neurol* 59:1381–1389, 2002.

Fukushima T, Yoshino A, Katayama Y, Watanabe T, Kusama K, Moro I. Prediction of clinical course of diffusely infiltrating astrocytomas from telomerase expression and quantitated activity level. *Cancer Lett* 187:191–198, 2002.

Fukutomi M, Enjoji M, Iguchi H, Yokota M, Iwamoto H, Nakamuta M, Sakai H, Nawata H. Telomerase activity is repressed during differentiation along the hepatocytic and biliary epithelial lineages: verification on immortal cell lines from the same origin. *Cell Biochem Funct* 19:65–68, 2001.

Funk W. The senescent cell phenotype and its relation to age-related pathologies. Presented at Telomeres and Telomerase: Implications for Cell Immortality, Cancer, and Age-related Disease. San Francisco, CA, June 1–3, 1998.

Funk WD, Wang CK, Shelton DN, Harley CB, Pagon GD, Hoeffler WK. Telomerase expression restores dermal integrity to in vitro–aged fibroblasts in a reconstituted skin model. *Exp Cell Res* 258:270–278, 2000.

Furth JJ, Allen RG, Tresini M, Keogh B, Cristofalo VJ. Abundance of alpha 1(I) and alpha 1(III) procollagen and p21 mRNAs in fibroblasts cultured from fetal and postnatal dermis. *Mech Ageing Dev* 97:131–142, 1997.

Furugori E, Hirayama R, Nakamura KI, Kammori M, Esaki Y, Takubo K. Telomere shortening in gastric carcinoma with aging despite telomerase activation. *J Cancer Res Clin Oncol* 126:481–485, 2000.

Furumoto K, Inoue E, Nagao N, Hiyama E, Miwa N. Age-dependent telomere shortening is slowed down by enrichment of intracellular vitamin C via suppression of oxidative stress. *Life Sci* 63:935–948, 1998.

Fuxe J, Akusjarvi G, Goike HM, Roos G, Collins VP, Pettersson RF. Adenovirus-mediated overexpression of p15INK4B inhibits human glioma cell growth, induces replicative senescence, and inhibits telomerase activity similarly to p16INK4A. *Cell Growth Differ* 11:373–384, 2000.

Fyfe G. Clinical development of an antibody to vascular endothelial growth factor. Presented at Cancer and Molecular Genetics in the Twenty-first Century, Van Andel Research Institute, Grand Rapids, MI, September 5–9, 2000.

Gabb M, Hashem N, Hashem M, Fahmi A, Safouh M. Progeria, a pathologic study. *J Pediatr* 57:70–77, 1960.

Gabr M. Progeria: review of the literature with report of a case. *Arch Pediatr* 71:35–46, 1954.

Gabr M, Hashem N, Hashem M. Progeria, a pathologic study. *J Pediatr* 57:70–77, 1960.

Gabriel SE, Coyle D, Moreland LW. A clinical and economic review of disease-modifying antirheumatic drugs. *Pharmacoeconomics* 19:715–728 , 2001.

Gadaleta MN, Rainaldi G, Lezza AM, Milella F, Fracasso F, Cantatore P. Mitochondrial DNA copy number and mitochondrial DNA deletion in adult and senescent rats. *Mutat Res* 275:181–193, 1992.

Gafni A. Protein structure and turnover. In Masoro EJ, Austad SN (eds). *Handbook of the Biology of Aging, 5th ed.* Academic Press, New York, 2001, pp 59–83.

Gage FH. Mammalian neural stem cells. *Science* 287:1433–1438, 2000.

Gagliano N, Arosio B, Santambrogio D, Balestrieri MR, Padoani G, Tagliabue J, Masson S, Vergani C, Annoni G. Age-dependent expression of fibrosis-related genes and collagen deposition in rat kidney cortex. *J Gerontol A Biol Sci Med Sci* 55:B365–372, 2000.

Gahan PB, Middleton J. Euploidization of human hepatocytes from donors of different ages and both sexes compared with those from cases of Werner's syndrome and progeria. *Exp Gerontol* 19:355–358, 1984.

Gall JG. Beginning of the end: origins of the telomere concept. In Blackburn EH, Greider LW (eds). *Telomeres.* Cold Spring harbor Laboratory Press, Cold Spring Harbor, NY, 1995, pp 1–10.

Gallant JA, Prothero J. Testing models of error propagation. *J Theor Biol* 83:561–578, 1980.

Galli R, Borello U, Gritti A, Minasi MG, Bjornson C, Coletta M, Mora M, De Angelis MG, Fiocco R, Cossu G, Vescovi AL. Skeletal myogenic potential of human and mouse neural stem cells. *Nat Neurosci* 3:986–991, 2000.

Gamble JG. Hip disease in Hutchinson-Gilford progeria syndrome. *J Pediatr Orthop* 4:585–589, 1984.

Gan Y, Engelke KJ, Brown CA, Au JL. Telomere amount and length assay. *Pharm Res* 18:1655–1659, 2001a.

Gan Y, Lu J, Johnson A, Wientjes MG, Schuller DE, Au JL. A quantitative assay of telomerase activity. *Pharm Res* 18:488–493, 2001b.

Gan Y, Mo Y, Johnston J, Lu J, Wientjes MG, Au JL. Telomere maintenance in telomerase-positive human ovarian SKOV-3 cells cannot be retarded by complete inhibition of telomerase. *FEBS Lett* 527:10–14, 2002.

Gapstur SM, Gann P. Is pancreatic cancer a preventable disease? *JAMA* 286:967–968, 2001.

Garcia-Cao M, Gonzalo S, Dean D, Blasco MA. A role for the Rb family of proteins in controlling telomere length. *Nat Genet* 32:415–419, 2002.

Garcia Layana A. Age-related macular degeneration [in Spanish]. *Rev Med Univ Navarra* 42:42–48, 1998.

Gardner E, Gray DJ, O'Rahilly R. *Anatomy: A Regional Study of Human Structure, 4th ed.* W.B. Saunders Company, Philadelphia, 1975.

Gardner ID. The effect of aging on susceptibility to infection. *Rev Infect Dis* 2:801–810, 1980.

Garfinkel S, Hu X, McMahon GA, Kapnik EM, McDowell SD, Maciag T. FGF-1 dependent proliferative and migratory responses are impaired in senescent human umbilical vein endothelial cells and correlate with the inability to signal tyrosine phosphorylation of fibroblast growth factor receptor-1 substrates. *J Cell Biol* 134:783–791, 1996.

Garmyn M, Degreef H, Gilchrest BA. The effect of acute and chronic photodamage on gene expression in human keratinocytes. *Dermatology* 190:305–308, 1995.

Garmyn M, Yaar M, Boileau N, Backendorf C, Gilchrest BA. Effect of aging and habitual sun exposure on the genetic response of cultured human keratinocytes to solar-simulated irradiation. *J Invest Dermatol* 99:743–748, 1992.

Gartner S. HIV infection and dementia. *Science* 287:602–604, 2000.

Gasser SM. A sense of the end. *Science* 288:1377–1379, 2000.

Gasser SM, Gotta M, Renauld H, Laroche T, Cockell M. Nuclear organization and silencing: trafficking of Sir proteins. *Novartis Found Symp* 214:114–126; discussion 126–132, 1998.

Gauthier LR, Granotier C, Soria JC, Faivre S, Boige V, Raymond E, Boussin FD. Detection of circulating carcinoma cells by telomerase activity. *Br J Cancer* 84:631–635, 2001.

Gavory G, Farrow M, Balasubramanian S. Minimum length requirement of the alignment domain of human telomerase RNA to sustain catalytic activity in vitro. *Nucleic Acids Res* 30:4470–4480, 2002.

Gazdar AF, Kurvari V, Virmani A, Gollahon L, Sakaguchi M, Westerfield M, Kodagoda D, Stasny V, Cunningham HT, Wistuba II, Tomlinson G, Tonk V, Ashfaq R, Leitch AM, Minna JD, Shay JW. Characterization of paired tumor and non-tumor cell lines established from patients with breast cancer. *Int J Cancer* 78:766–774, 1998.

Gearing M, Rebeck G, Hyman BT, Tigges J, Mirra SS. Neuropathology and apolipoprotein E profile of aged chimpanzees: implications for Alzheimer's disease. *Proc Natl Acad Sci USA* 91:9382–9386, 1994.

Gearing M, Tigges J, Mori H, Mirra SS. Beta-amyloid (Aβ)deposition in the brains of aged orangutans. *Neurobiol Aging* 18:139–146, 1997.

Geba GP, Weaver AL, Polis AB, Dixon ME, Schnitzer TJ, for the VACT Group. Efficacy of rofecoxib, celecoxib, and acetaminophen in osteoarthritis of the knee. A randomized trial. *JAMA* 287:64–71, 2002.

Gebhart E, Bauer R, Raub U, Schinzel M, Ruprecht KW, Jonas JB. Spontaneous and induced chromosomal instability in Werner syndrome. *Hum Genet* 80:135–139, 1988.

Geerlings MI, Ruitenberg A, Witteman JCM, van Swieten JC, Hofman A, van Duijn CM, Breteler MB, Launer LJ. Reproductive period and risk of dementia in postmenopausal women. *JAMA* 285:1475–1488, 2001.

Gehrmann J, Banati RB, Cuzner ML, Kreutzberg GW, Newcombe J. Amyloid precursor protein (APP) expression in multiple sclerosis lesions. *Glia* 15:141–151, 1995.

Gelmini S, Crisci A, Salvadori B, Pazzagli M, Selli C, Orlando C. Comparison of telomerase activity in bladder carcinoma and exfoliated cells collected in urine and bladder washings, using a quantitative assay. *Clin Cancer Res* 6:2771–2776, 2000.

Gems D. Nematode ageing: putting metabolic theories to the test. *Curr Biol* 9:R614–616, 1999.

Gems D, Sutton AJ, Sundermeyer ML, Albert PS, King KV, Edgley ML, Larsen PL, Riddle DL. Two pleiotropic classes of *daf-2* mutation affect larval arrest, adult behavior, reproduction and longevity in *Caenorhabditis elegans*. *Genetics* 150:129–155, 1998.

Genazzani AR, Gambacciani M. Hormone replacement therapy: the perspectives for the 21st century. *Maturitas* 32:11–17, 1999.

Gendron RL, Liu CY, Paradis H, Adams LC, Kao WW. MK/T-1, an immortalized fibroblast cell line derived using cultures of mouse corneal stroma. *Mol Vis* 7:107–113, 2001.

George JC, Bada J, Zeh J, Scott L, Brown SE, O'Hara T, Suydam R. Age and growth estimates of bowhead whales (*Balaena mysticetus*) via aspartic acid racemization. *Can J Zool* 77:571–580, 1999.

Gerland LM, Ffrench M, Magaud JP. Cyclin-dependent kinase inhibitors and replicative senescence [in French]. *Pathol Biol (Paris)* 49:830–839, 2001.

Gerstein AD, Phillips TJ, Rogers GS, Gilchrest BA. Wound healing and aging. *Dermatol Clin* 11:749–757, 1993.

Gertler R, Rosenberg R, Stricker D, Werner M, Lassmann S, Ulm K, Nekarda H, Siewert JR. Prognostic potential of the telomerase subunit human telomerase reverse transcriptase in tumor tissue and nontumorous mucosa from patients with colorectal carcinoma. *Cancer* 95:2103–2111, 2002.

Gewin L, Galloway DA. E box–dependent activation of telomerase by human papillomavirus type 16 E6 does not require induction of c-myc. *J Virol* 75:7198–7201, 2001.

Giacomoni PU, Rein G. Factors of skin ageing share common mechanisms. *Biogerontology* 2:219–229, 2001.

Gibbons GH, Dzau VJ. The emerging concept of vascular remodeling. *N Engl J Med* 330:1431–1438, 1994.

Gibbons GH, Dzau VJ. Molecular therapies for vascular diseases. *Science* 272:689–693, 1996.

Gibson MC, Schultz E. Age-related differences in absolute numbers of skeletal muscle satellite cells. *Muscle Nerve* 6:574–580, 1983.

Gieffers J, Reusche E, Solbach W, Maass M. Failure to detect *Chlamydia pneumoniae* in brain sections of Alzheimer's disease patients. *J Clin Microbiol* 38:881–882, 2000.

Gilchrest BA. Relationship between actinic damage and chronologic aging in keratinocyte cultures of human skin. *J Invest Dermatol* 72:219–223, 1979.

Gilchrest BA. In vitro assessment of keratinocyte aging. *J Invest Dermatol* 81(1 Suppl):184s–189s, 1983a.

Gilchrest BA. Relationship between actinic damage and chronologic aging in keratinocyte cultures in human skin. *J Invest Dermatol* 81:184s–189s, 1983b.

Gilchrest BA. Skin aging and photoaging. *Dermatol Nurs* 2:79–82, 1990.

Gilchrest BA. A review of skin ageing and its medical therapy. *Br J Dermatol* 135:867–875, 1996.

Gilchrest BA. Treatment of photodamage with topical tretinoin: an overview. *J Am Acad Dermatol* 36:S27–S36, 1997.

Gilchrest BA, Bohr VA. Aging processes, DNA damage, and repair. *FASEB J* 11:322–330, 1997.

Gilchrest BA, Garmyn M, Yaar M. Aging and photoaging affect gene expression in cultured human keratinocytes. *Arch Dermatol* 130:82–86, 1994.

Gilchrest BA, Szabo G, Flynn E, Goldwyn RM. Chronologic and actinically induced aging in human facial skin. *J Invest Dermatol* 80(Suppl):81s–85s, 1983.

Gilchrest BA, Yaar M. Ageing and photoageing of the skin: observations at the cellular and molecular level. *Br J Dermatol* 127(Suppl 41):25–30, 1992.

Gilden DH. Viruses and multiple sclerosis. *JAMA* 286:3127–3129, 2001.

Gilford H. On a condition of mixed premature and immature development. *Medicochir Trans* 80:17–45, 1897.

Gilford H. Progeria: a form of senilism. *Practitioner* 73:188, 1904.

Gilford H. Progeria and ateleiosis. *Lancet* 1:412–413, 1913.

Gilkes JJH, Sharvill DE, Wells RS. The premature ageing syndromes: report of eight new cases and description of a new entity named metageria. *Br J Dermatol* 91:243–262, 1974.

Gillar PJ, Kaye CI, McCourt JW. Progressive early dermatologic changes in Hutchinson-Gilford progeria syndrome. *Pediatr Dermatol* 8:199–206, 1991.

Gilley D, Blackburn EH. The telomerase RNA pseudoknot is critical for the stable assembly of a catalytically active ribonucleoprotein. *Proc Natl Acad Sci USA* 96:6621–6625, 1999.

Gilley D, Tanaka H, Hande MP, Kurimasa A, Li GC, Oshimura M, Chen DJ. DNA-PKcs is critical for telomere capping. *Proc Natl Acad Sci USA* 98:15084–15088, 2001.

Gillum LA, Mamidipudi SK, Johnston SC. Ischemic stroke risk with oral contraceptives. *JAMA* 284:72–78, 2000.

Gimbrone MA Jr, Topper JN, Nagel T, Anderson KR, Garcia-Cardena G. Endothelial dysfunction, hemodynamic forces, and atherogenesis. *Ann NY Acad Sci* 902:230–239, 2000.

Ginaldi L, De Martinis M, D'Ostilio A, Marini L, Loreto MF, Martorelli V, Quaglino D. The immune system in the elderly: II. Specific cellular immunity. *Immunol Res* 20:109–115, 1999a.

Ginaldi L, De Martinis M, D'Ostilio A, Marini L, Loreto MF, Quaglino D. The immune system in the elderly: III. Innate immunity. *Immunol Res* 20:117–126, 1999b.

Giro M, Davidson JM. Familial co-segregation of the elastin phenotype in skin fibroblasts from Hutchinson-Gilford progeria. *Mech Ageing Dev* 70:163–36, 1993.

Gisselsson D, Jonson T, Petersen A, Strombeck B, Dal Cin P, Hoglund M, Mitelman F, Mertens F, Mandahl N. Telomere dysfunction triggers extensive DNA fragmentation and evolution of complex chromosome abnormalities in human malignant tumors. *Proc Natl Acad Sci USA* 98:12683–12688, 2001.

Gisselsson D, Jonson T, Yu C, Martins C, Mandahl N, Wiegant J, Jin Y, Mertens F, Jin C. Centrosomal abnormalities, multipolar mitoses, and chromosomal instability in head and neck tumours with dysfunctional telomeres. *Br J Cancer* 87:202–207, 2002.

Glaessl A, Bosserhoff AK, Buettner R, Hohenleutner U, Landthaler M, Stolz W. Increase in telomerase activity during progression of melanocytic cells from melanocytic naevi to malignant melanomas. *Arch Dermatol Res* 291:81–87, 1999.

Glass J, Fedor H, Wesselingh S, McArthur J. Immunocytochemical quantitation of human immunodeficiency virus in the brain: correlations with dementia. *Ann Neurol* 38:755–762, 1995.

Glasser SP. On arterial physiology, pathophysiology of vascular compliance, and cardiovascular disease. *Heart Dis* 2:375–379, 2000.

Globerson A. Hematopoietic stem cells and aging. *Exp Gerontol* 34:137–146, 1999.

Globerson A, Effros RB. Ageing of lymphocytes and lymphocytes in the aged. *Immunol Today* 21:515–521, 2000.

Go AS, Hylek EM, Phillips KA, Chang YC, Henault LE, Selby JV, Singer DE. Prevalence of diagnosed atrial fibrillation in adults. *JAMA* 285:2370–2375, 2001.

Goldberg AL, Elledge SJ, Harper JW. The cellular chamber of doom. *Sci Am* 284:68–73, 2000.

Goldie SJ, Kuhn L, Denny L, Pollack A, Wright TC. Policy analysis of cervical cancer screening strategies in low-resource settings. *JAMA* 285:3107–3115, 2001.

Goldstein S. Lifespan of cultured cells in progeria. *Lancet* 1:424, 1969.

Goldstein S. The biology of aging. *N Engl J Med* 285:1120–1129, 1971a.

Goldstein S. The role of DNA repair in aging of cultured fibroblasts from xeroderma pigmentosum and normals. *Proc Soc Exp Med* 137:730–734, 1971b.

Goldstein S. Replicative senescence: the human fibroblast comes of age. *Science* 249:1129–1130, 1990.

Goldstein S, Ballantyne SR, Robson AL, Moerman EJ. Energy metabolism in cultured human fibroblasts during aging in vitro. *J Cell Physiol* 112:419–424, 1982.

Goldstein S, Harley CB. In vitro studies of age-associated diseases. *FASEB J* 38:1862–1867, 1979.

Goldstein S, Harley CB, Moerman EJ. Some aspects of cellular aging. *J Chron Dis* 36:103–116, 1983.

Goldstein S, Korczack LB. Status of mitochondria in living human fibroblasts during growth and senescence in vitro: use of the laser dye rhodamine 123. *J Cell Biol* 91:392–398, 1981.

Goldstein S, Lin CC. Rescue of senescent human fibroblasts by hybridization with hamster cells in vitro. *Exp Cell Res* 70:436–439, 1972.

Goldstein S, Moerman EJ. Heat-labile enzymes in circulating erythrocytes of a progeria family. *Am J Hum Genet* 30:167–173, 1978.

Goldstein S, Moerman EJ, Porter K. High-voltage electron microscopy of human diploid fibroblasts during ageing in vitro. Morphometric analysis of mitochondria. *Exp Cell Res* 154:101–111, 1984.

Goldstein S, Niewiarowski S, Singal DP. Pathological implications of cell aging in vitro. *Fed Proc* 34:56–63, 1975.

Goldstein S, Reivich M. Cerebral blood flow and metabolism in aging and dementia. *Clin Neuropharmacol* 14(Suppl 1):S34–44, 1991.

Goldstein S, Singal DP. Alteration of fibroblast gene products in vitro from a subject with Werner's syndrome. *Nature* 251:719–721, 1974.

Goldstein S, Wojtyk RI, Harley CB, Pollard JW, Chamberlain JW, Stanners CP. Protein synthetic fidelity in aging human fibroblasts. *Adv Exp Med Biol* 190:495–508, 1985.

Goletz TJ, Hensler PJ, Ning Y, Adami GR, Pereira-Smith OM. Evidence for a genetic basis for the model system of cellular senescence. *J Am Geriatr Soc* 41:1255–1258, 1993.

Goletz TJ, Robetorye S, Pereira-Smith OM. Genetic analysis of indefinite division in human cells: evidence for a common immortalizing mechanism in T and B lymphoid cell lines. *Exp Cell Res* 215:82–89, 1994a.

Goletz TJ, Smith JR, Pereira-Smith OM. Molecular genetic approaches to the study of cellular senescence. *Cold Spring Harb Symp Quant Biol* 59:59–66, 1994b.

Gollahon LS, Holt SE. Alternative methods of extracting telomerase activity from human tumor samples. *Cancer Lett* 159:141–149, 2000.

Gollahon LS, Kraus E, Wu TA, Yim SO, Strong LC, Shay JW, Tainsky MA. Telomerase activity during spontaneous immortalization of Li-Fraumeni syndrome skin fibroblasts. *Oncogene* 17:709–717, 1998.

Gollahon LS, Shay JW. Immortalization of human mammary epithelial cells transfected with mutant p53 (273his). *Oncogene* 12:715–725, 1996.

Golubev AG. The natural history of telomeres [in Russian]. *Adv Gerontol* 7:95–104, 2001.

Golubovskaya VM, Filatov LV, Behe CI, Presnell SC, Hooth MJ, Smith GJ, Kaufmann WK. Telomere shortening, telomerase expression, and chromosome instability in rat hepatic epithelial stem-like cells. *Mol Carcinog* 24:209–217, 1999.

Golubovskaya VM, Presnell SC, Hooth MJ, Smith GJ, Kaufmann WK. Expression of telomerase in normal and malignant rat hepatic epithelia. *Oncogene* 15:1233–1240, 1997.

Gomez D, Mergny JL, Riou JF. Detection of telomerase inhibitors based on G-quadruplex ligands by a modified telomeric repeat amplification protocol assay. *Cancer Res* 62:3365–3368, 2002.

Gomez-Isla T, Wasco W, Pettingell WP, Gurubhagavatula S, Schmidt SD, Jondro PD, McNamara M, Rodes LA, DiBlasi T, Growdon WB, Seubert P, Schenk D, Growdon JH, Hyman BT,

Tanzi RE. A novel presenilin-1 mutation: increased beta-amyloid and neurofibrillary changes. *Ann Neurol* 41:809–813, 1997.

Gonos ES, Dervenzi A, Kveiborg M, Agiostratidou G, Kassem M, Clark BF, Jat PS, Rattan SI. Cloning and identification of genes that associate with mammalian replicative senescence. *Exp Cell Res* 240:66–74, 1998.

Gonzalez-Suarez E, Samper E, Flores JM, Blasco MA. Telomerase-deficient mice with short telomeres are resistant to skin tumorigenesis. *Nat Genet* 26:114–117, 2000.

Gonzalez-Suarez E, Samper E, Ramirez A, Flores JM, Martin-Caballero J, Jorcano JL, Blasco MA. Increased epidermal tumors and increased skin wound healing in transgenic mice overexpressing the catalytic subunit of telomerase, mTERT, in basal keratinocytes. *EMBO J* 20:2619–2630, 2001.

Good L, Dimri GP, Campisi J, Chen KY. Regulation of dihydrofolate reductase gene expression and E2F components in human diploid fibroblasts during growth and senescence. *J Cell Physiol* 168:580–588, 1996.

Goodman HM. Reproduction. In Mountcastle VB. *Medical Physiology, 13th ed.* C.V. Mosby Company, St. Louis, 1974a, pp 1741–1775.

Goodman HM. The pancreas and regulation of metabolism. In Mountcastle VB. *Medical Physiology, 13th ed.* C.V. Mosby Company, St. Louis, 1974b, pp 1776–1807.

Goodwin AT, Yacoub MH. Role of endogenous endothelin on coronary flow in health and disease. *Coron Artery Dis* 12:517–525, 2001.

Goodwin EC, DiMaio D. Induced senescence in HeLa cervical carcinoma cells containing elevated telomerase activity and extended telomeres. *Cell Growth Differ* 12:525–534, 2001.

Goodwin EC, Yang E, Lee CJ, Lee HW, DiMaio D, Hwang ES. Rapid induction of senescence in human cervical carcinoma cells. *Proc Natl Acad Sci USA* 97:10978–10983, 2000.

Gorbunova V, Seluanov A, Pereira-Smith OM. Expression of human telomerase (hTERT) does not prevent stress-induced senescence in normal human fibroblasts but protects the cells from stress-induced apoptosis and necrosis. *J Biol Chem* 277:38540–549, 2002.

Gorbunova V, Seluanov A, Pereira-Smith OM. Evidence that high telomerase activity may induce a senescent-like growth arrest in human fibroblasts. *J Biol Chem* 279:7692–7698, 2003.

Gordon CM, Glowacki J, LeBoff MS. DHEA and the skeleton (through the ages). *Endocrine* 11:1–11, 1999.

Gordon D. Telomere deficiency worsens liver disease. *Gastroenterology* 118:818, 2000.

Gorelick PB. Status of risk factors for dementia associated with stroke. *Stroke* 28:459–463, 1997.

Gorelick PB, Roman G, Mangone CA. Vascular dementia. In Gorelick PB, Alter MA (eds). *Handbook of Neuroepidemiology.* Marcel Dekker, New York, 1994, pp 197–214.

Gorham H, Yoshida K, Sugino T, Marsh G, Manek S, Charnock M, Tarin D, Goodison S. Telomerase activity in human gynaecological malignancies. *J Clin Pathol* 50:501–504, 1997.

Gorin MB, Breitner JC, De Jong PT, Hageman GS, Klaver CC, Kuehn MH, Seddon JM. The genetics of age-related macular degeneration. *Mol Vis* 5:29, 1999.

Gorman SD, Cristofalo VJ. Analysis of the G1 arrest position of senescent WI38 cells by quinacrine dihydrochloride nuclear fluorescence. *Exp Cell Res* 167:87–94, 1981.

Gorman SD, Hoffman E, Nichols WW, Cristofalo VJ. Spontaneous transformation of a cloned cell line of normal diploid bovine vascular endothelial cells. *In Vitro* 20:339–345, 1984.

Goshi K, Uchida T, Lezhava A, Yamasaki M, Hiratsu K, Shinkawa H, Kinashi H. Cloning and analysis of the telomere and terminal inverted repeat of the linear chromosome of *Streptomyces griseus.* *J Bacteriol* 184:3411–3415, 2002.

Goto M, Horiuchi Y, Okumura K, Tada T. Immunological abnormalities of aging: an analysis of T lymphocyte subpopulations of Werner's syndrom. *J Clin Invest* 64:695–699, 1979.

Goto M, Rubinstein M, Weber J, Woods, K, Drayna D. Genetic linkage of Werner's syndrome to five markers on chromosome 8. *Nature* 355:735–738, 1992.

Goto M, Tanimoto K, Aotsuka S, Okawa M, Yokohari R. Age-related changes in auto- and natural antibody in the Werner syndrome. *Am J Med* 72:607–613, 1982.

Goto S, Lin YC, Lai CY, Lee CM, Pan TL, Lord R, Chiang KC, Tseng HP, Lin CL, Cheng YF, Yokoyama H, Kitano S, Chen CL. Telomerase activity in rat liver allografts. *Transplantation* 69:1013–1015, 2000.

Gotta M, Cockell M. Telomeres, not the end of the story. *Bioessays* 19:367–370, 1997.

Gottesman S, Maurizi MR. Surviving starvation. *Science* 293:614–615, 2001.

Gottlieb JL. Age-related macular degeneration. *JAMA* 288:2233–2236, 2002.

Gottsater A, Rendell M, Hulthen UL, Berntorp E, Mattiasson I. Hormone replacement therapy in healthy postmenopausal women: a randomized, placebo-controlled study of effects on coagulation and fibrinolytic factors. *J Intern Med* 249:237–246, 2001.

Gottschling DE. Telomere-proximal DNA in *Saccharomyces cerevisiae* is refractory to methyltransferase activity in vivo. *Proc Natl Acad Sci USA* 89:4062–4065, 1992.

Gottschling DE, Aparicio OM, Billington BL, Zakian VA. Position effect at *S. cerevisiae* telomeres: reversible repression of Pol II transcription. *Cell* 63:751–762, 1990.

Gottschling DE, Cech TR. Chromatin structure of the molecular ends of Oxytricha macronuclear DNA: phased nucleosomes and a telomeric complex. *Cell* 38:501–510, 1984.

Gottschling DE, Stoddard B. Telomeres: structure of a chromosome's aglet. *Curr Biol* 9:R164–167, 1999.

Gottschling DE, Zakian VA. Telomere proteins: specific recognition and protection of the natural termini of Oxytricha macronuclear DNA. *Cell* 47:195–205, 1986.

Gotz J, Chen F, van Dorpe J, Nitsch RM. Formation of neurofibrillary tangels in P301L tau transgenic mice induced by Aβ42 fibrils. *Science* 293:1491–1495, 2001.

Goukassian D, Sanz-Gonzalez SM, Perez-Roger I, Font de Mora J, Urena J, Andres V. Inhibition of the cyclin D1/E2F pathway by PCA-4230, a potent repressor of cellular proliferation. *Br J Pharmacol* 132:1597–1605, 2001.

Gourdeau H, Speevak MD, Jette L, Chevrette M. Whole-cell and microcell fusion for the identification of natural regulators of telomerase. In Double JA, Thompson MJ (eds). *Telomeres and Telomerase: Methods and Protocols*. Humana Press, Totowa, NJ, 2002, pp 173–196.

Gowan SM, Harrison JR, Patterson L, Valenti M, Read MA, Neidle S, Kelland LR. A G-quadruplex-interactive potent small-molecule inhibitor of telomerase exhibiting in vitro and in vivo antitumor activity. *Mol Pharmacol* 61:1154–1162, 2002.

Gowan SM, Heald R, Stevens MF, Kelland LR. Potent inhibition of telomerase by small-molecule pentacyclic acridines capable of interacting with G-quadruplexes. *Mol Pharmacol* 60:981–988, 2001.

Goyns MH. Genes, telomeres and mammalian ageing. *Mech Ageing Dev* 123:791–799, 2002.

Goyns MH, Charlton MA, Dunford JE, Lavery WL, Merry BJ, Salehi M, Simoes DC. Differential display analysis of gene expression indicates that age-related changes are restricted to a small cohort of genes. *Mech Ageing Dev* 101:73–90, 1998.

Goyns MH, Lavery WL. Telomerase and mammalian ageing: a critical appraisal. *Mech Ageing Dev* 114:69–77, 2000.

Goytisolo FA, Blasco MA. Many ways to telomere dysfunction: in vivo studies using mouse models. *Oncogene* 21:584–591, 2002.

Graat JM, Schouten EG, Kok FJ. Effect of daily vitamin E and multivitamin–mineral supplementation on acute respiratory tract infections in elderly persons: a randomized controlled trial. *JAMA* 288:715–721, 2002.

Grady D, Cummings SR. Postmenopausal hormone therapy for prevention of fractures. *JAMA* 285:2909–2910, 2001.

Grady D, Herrington D, Bittner V, Blumenthal R, Davidson M, Hlatky M, Hsia J, Hulley S, Herd A, Khan S, Newby LK, Waters D, Vittinghoff E, Wenger N, for the HERS Research Group. Cardiovascular disease outcomes during 6.8 years of hormone therapy. *JAMA* 288:49–57, 2002.

Grady D, Rubin SM, Petitti DB, Fox CS, Black D, Ettinger B, Ernster VL, Cummings SR. Hormone therapy to prevent disease and prolong life in postmenopausal women. *Ann Intern Med* 117:1016–1037, 1992.

Graham DY. *Helicobacter pylori* infection is the primary cause of gastric cancer. *J Gastroenterol* 35(Suppl 12):90–97, 2000.

Grand CL, Han H, Munoz RM, Weitman S, Von Hoff DD, Hurley LH, Bearss DJ. The cationic porphyrin TMPyP4 down-regulates c-MYC and human telomerase reverse transcriptase expression and inhibits tumor growth in vivo. *Mol Cancer Ther* 1:565–573, 2002.

Grandin N, Damon C, Charbonneau M. Cdc13 prevents telomere uncapping and Rad50-dependent homologous recombination. *EMBO J* 20:6127–6139, 2001.

Granger MP, Wright WE, Shay JW. Telomerase in cancer and aging. *Crit Rev Oncol Hematol* 41:29–40, 2002.

Grant JD, Broccoli D, Muquit M, Manion FJ, Tisdall J, Ochs MF. Telometric: a tool providing simplified, reproducible measurements of telomeric DNA from constant field agarose gels. *Biotechniques* 31:1314–1316, 1318, 2001.

Gravel S, Wellinger RJ. Maintenance of double-stranded telomeric repeats as the critical determinant for cell viability in yeast cells lacking Ku. *Mol Cell Biol* 22:2182–2193, 2002.

Gray A, Berlin JA, McKinlay JB, Longcope C. An examination of research design effects on the association of testosterone and male aging: results of a meta-analysis. *J Clin Epidemiol* 44:671–684, 1991.

Gray JT, Celander DW. Cloning and expression of genes for the Oxytrica telomere-binding protein: specific subunit interactions in the telomeric complex. *Cell* 67:807–814, 1991.

Gray MD, Shen JC, Kamath-Loeb AS, Blank A, Sopher BL, Martin GM, Oshima J, Loeb LA. The Werner syndrome protein is a DNA helicase. *Nat Genet* 17:100–103, 1997.

Gray MD, Wang L, Youssoufian H, Martin GM, Oshima J. Werner helicase is localized to transcriptionally active nucleoli of cycling cells. *Exp Cell Res* 242:487–494, 1998.

Greally JM, Boone LY, Lenkey SG, Wenger SL, Steele MW. Acrometageria: a spectrum of "premature aging" syndromes. *Am J Med Genet* 44:334–339, 1992.

Green K. Free radicals and ageing of anterior segment tissues of the eye: a hypothesis. *Ophthalmic Res* 27(Suppl):143–149, 1995.

Green LN. Progeria with carotid artery aneurysms: report of a case. *Arch Neurol* 38:659–661, 1981.

Green RC, Cupples LA, Go R, Benke KS, Edeki T, Griffith PA, Williams M, Hipps Y, Graff-Radford N, Bachman D, Farrer LA, for the MIRAGE Study Group. Risk of dementia among white and African American relatives of patients with Alzheimer disease. *JAMA* 287:329–336, 2002.

Green WR. Histopathology of age-related macular degeneration. *Mol Vis* 5:27, 1999.

Greenberg RA, Allsopp RC, Chin L, Morin GB, DePinho RA. Expression of mouse telomerase reverse transcriptase during development, differentiation and proliferation. *Oncogene* 16:1723–1730, 1998.

Greenberg RA, Chin L, Femino A, Lee KH, Gottlieb GJ, Singer RH, Greider CW, DePinho RA. Short dysfunctional telomeres impair tumorigenesis in the INK4a(delta2/3) cancer-prone mouse. *Cell* 97:515–525, 1999a.

Greenberg RA, O'Hagan RC, Deng H, Xiao Q, Hann SR, Adams RR, Lichtsteiner S, Chin L, Morin GB, DePinho RA. Telomerase reverse transcriptase gene is a direct target of c-Myc but is not functionally equivalent in cellular transformation. *Oncogene* 18:1219–1226, 1999b.

Greener M. Telomerase: the search for a universal cancer vaccine. *Mol Med Today* 6:257, 2000.

Greenwell PW, Kronmal SL, Porter SE, Gassenhuber J, Obermaier B, Petes TD. *TEL1*, a gene involved in controlling telomere length in *S. cerevisiae*, is homologous to the human ataxia telangectasia gene. *Cell* 82:823–829, 1985.

Greider CW. Telomeres, telomerase and senescence. *Bioessays* 12:363–369, 1990.

Greider CW. Chromosome first aid. *Cell* 67:645–647, 1991a.

Greider CW. Telomerase is processive. *Mol Cell Biol* 11:4572–4580, 1991b.

Greider CW. Telomeres. *Curr Opin Cell Biol* 3:444–451 , 1991c.

Greider CW. Telomerase and telomere-length regulation: lessons from small eukaryotes to mammals. *Cold Spring Harb Symp Quant Biol* 58:719–723, 1993.

Greider CW. Mammalian telomere dynamics: healing, fragmentation shortening and stabilization. *Curr Opin Genet Dev* 4:203–211, 1994.

Greider CW. Telomerase biochemistry and regulation. In Blackburn EH, Greider CW (eds). *Telomeres*. Cold Harbor Laboratory Press, Cold Spring Harbor, NY, 1995, pp 35–68.

Greider CW. Telomere length regulation. *Annu Rev Biochem* 65:337–365, 1996.

Greider CW. Telomerase activity, cell proliferation, and cancer. *Proc Natl Acad Sci USA* 95:90–92, 1998a.

Greider CW. Telomeres and senescence: the history, the experiment, the future. *Curr Biol* 8:R178–181, 1998b.

Greider CW. Telomerase activation. One step on the road to cancer? *Trends Genet* 15:109–112, 1999a.

Greider CW. Telomeres do D-loop-T-loop. *Cell* 97:419–422, 1999b.

Greider CW, Blackburn EH. Identification of a specific telomere terminal transferase activity in *Tetrahymena* extracts. *Cell* 43:405–413, 1985.

Greider CW, Blackburn EH. Telomeres, telomerase and cancer. *Sci Am* 274:92–97, 1996.

Gressner AM. Transdifferentiation of hepatic stellate cells (Ito cells) to myofibroblasts: a key event in hepatic fibrogenesis. *Kidney Int Suppl* 54:S39–45, 1996.

Gressner AM. The cell biology of liver fibrogenesis—an imbalance of proliferation, growth arrest and apoptosis of myofibroblasts. *Cell Tissue Res* 292:447–452, 1998.

Grey MD, Norwood TH. Cellular aging in vitro. *Rev Clin Gerontol* 5:369–381, 1995.

Griffith JD, Bianchi A, de Lange T. TRF1 promotes parallel pairing of telomeric tracts in vitro. *J Mol Biol* 278:79–88, 1998.

Griffith JD, Comeau L, Rosenfield S, Stansel RM, Bianchi A, Moss H, de Lange T. Mammalian telomeres end in a large duplex loop. *Cell* 97:503–514, 1999a.

Griffith JK, Bryant JE, Fordyce CA, Gilliland FD, Joste NE, Moyzis RK. Reduced telomere DNA content is correlated with genomic instability and metastasis in invasive human breast carcinoma. *Breast Cancer Res Treat* 54:59–64, 1999b.

Griffith M, Osborne R, Munger R, Xiong X, Doillon CJ, Laycock NLC, Hakin M, Song Y, Watsky MA. Functional human corneal equivalents constructed from cell lines. *Science* 286:2169–2172, 1999c.

Griffiths CE. Drug treatment of photoaged skin. *Drugs Aging* 14:289–301, 1999.

Grimes B, Cooke H. Engineering mammalian chromosomes. *Hum Mol Genet* 7:1635–1640, 1998.

Grimes BR, Warburton PE, Farr CJ. Chromosome engineering: prospects for gene therapy. *Gene Ther* 9:713–718, 2002.

Grobelny JV, Godwin AK, Broccoli D. ALT-associated PML bodies are present in viable cells and are enriched in cells in the G(2)/M phase of the cell cycle. *J Cell Sci* 113:4577–4585, 2000.

Grobelny JV, Kulp-McEliece M, Broccoli D. Effects of reconstitution of telomerase activity on telomere maintenance by the alternative lengthening of telomeres (ALT) pathway. *Hum Mol Genet* 10:1953–1961, 2001.

Grodstein F, Newcomb PA, Stampfer MJ. Postmenopausal hormone therapy and the risk of colorectal cancer: a review and meta-analysis. *Am J Med* 106:574–582, 1999.

Grossi S, Bianchi A, Damay P, Shore D. Telomere formation by rap1p binding site arrays reveals end-specific length regulation requirements and active telomeric recombination. *Mol Cell Biol* 21:8117–8128, 2001.

Grossman L, Wei Q. DNA repair and epidemiology of basal cell carcinoma. *Clin Chem* 41:1854–1863, 1995.

Grossmann A, Maggio-Price L, Jinneman JC, Wolf NS, Rabinovitch PS. The effect of long-term caloric restriction on function of T-cell subsets in old mice. *Cell Immunol* 31:191–204, 1990.

Groszer M, Erickson R, Scripture-Adams DD, Lesche R, Trumpp A, Zack JA, Kornblum HI, Liu X, Wu H. Negative regulation of neural stem/progenitor cell proliferationby the *Pten* tumor suppressor gene in vivo. *Science* 294:2186–2189, 2001.

Grounds MD. Age-associated changes in the response of skeletal muscle cells to exercise and regeneration. *Ann NY Acad Sci* 854:78–91, 1998.

Grundy SM. Early detection of high cholesterol levels in young adults. *JAMA* 284:365–367, 2000.

Grune T, Davies KJA. Oxidative processes in aging. In Masoro EJ, Austad SN (eds). *Handbook of the Biology of Aging, 5th ed.* Academic Press, New York, 2001, pp 25–58.

Grune T, Shringarpure R, Sitte N, Davies K. Age-related changes in protein oxidation and proteolysis in mammalian cells. *J Gerontol A Biol Sci Med Sci* 56:B459–467, 2001.

Grune T, Sommerburg O, Siems WG. Oxidative stress in anemia. *Clin Nephrol* 53(1 Suppl):S18–22, 2000.

Grunstein M. Molecular model for telomeric heterochromatin in yeast. *Curr Opin Cell Biol* 9:383–387, 1997.

Gu J, Kagawa S, Takakura M, Kyo S, Inoue M, Roth JA, Fang B. Tumor-specific transgene expression from the human telomerase reverse transcriptase promoter enables targeting of the therapeutic effects of the *Bax* gene to cancers. *Cancer Res* 60:5359–5364, 2000.

Guarente L. Do changes in chromosomes cause aging? *Cell* 86:9–12, 1996.

Guarente L. Chromatin and ageing in yeast and in mammals. *Ciba Found Symp* 211:104–107; discussion 107–111, 1997a.

Guarente L. Link between aging and the nucleolus. *Genes Dev* 11:2449–2455, 1997b.

Guarente L. Diverse and dynamic functions of the Sir silencing complex. *Nat Genet* 23:281–285, 1999.

Guarente L, Kenyon C. Genetic pathways that regulate ageing in model organisms. *Nature* 408:255–262, 2000.

Guarente L, Ruvkun G, Amasino R. Aging, life span, and senescence. *Proc Natl Acad Sci USA* 95:11034–11036, 1998.

Guenette SY, Tanzi RE. Progress toward valid transgenic mouse models for Alzheimer's disease. *Neurobiol Aging* 20:201–211, 1999.

Guertl B, Noehammer C, Hoefler G. Metabolic cardiomyopathies. *Int J Exp Pathol* 81:349–372, 2000.

Guilleret I, Yan P, Grange F, Braunschweig R, Bosman FT, Benhattar J. Hypermethylation of the human telomerase catalytic subunit (hTERT) gene correlates with telomerase activity. *Int J Cancer* 101:335–341, 2002a.

Guilleret I, Yan P, Guillou L, Braunschweig R, Coindre JM, Benhattar J. The human telomerase RNA gene (hTERC) is regulated during carcinogenesis but is not dependent on DNA methylation. *Carcinogenesis* 23:2025–2030, 2002b.

Gum PA, Thamilarasan M, Watanabe J, Blackstone EH, Lauer MS. Aspirin use and all-cause mortality among patients being evaluated for known or suspected coronary artery disease. *JAMA* 286:1187–1194, 2001.

Gun RT, Korten AE, Jorm AF, Henderson AS, Broe GA, Creasey H, McCusker E, Mylvaganam A. Occupational risk factors for Alzheimer disease: a case–control study. *Alzheimer Dis Assoc Disord* 11:21–27, 1997.

Gunes C, Lichtsteiner S, Vasserot AP, Englert C. Expression of the hTERT gene is regulated at the level of transcriptional initiation and repressed by Mad1. *Cancer Res* 60:2116–2121, 2000.

Guo H, Karberg M, Long M, Jones JP III, Sullenger B, Lambowitz AM. Group II introns designed to insert into therapeutically relevant DNA target sites in human cells. *Science* 289:452–457, 2000a.

Guo Q, Lu M, Kallenbach NR. Adenine affects the structure and stability of telomeric sequences. *J Biol Chem* 267:15293–15300, 1992.

Guo W, Kang MK, Kim HJ, Park NH. Immortalization of human oral keratinocytes is associated with elevation of telomerase activity and shortening of telomere length. *Oncol Rep* 5:799–804, 1998.

Guo W, Okamoto M, Park NH, Lee YM, Park NH. Cloning and expression of hamster telomerase catalytic subunit cDNA. *Int J Mol Med* 8:73–78, 2001.

Guo Z, Ersoz A, Butterfield DA, Mattson MP. Beneficial effects of dietary restriction on cerebral cortical synaptic terminals: preservation of glucose and glutamate transport and mitochondrial function after exposure to amyloid beta-peptide, iron, and 3-nitropropionic acid. *J Neurochem* 75:314–320, 2000b.

Guo ZH, Mattson MP. In vivo 2-deoxyglucose administration preserves glucose and glutamate transport and mitochondrial function in cortical synaptic terminals after exposure to amyloid beta-peptide and iron: evidence for a stress response. *Exp Neurol* 166:173–179, 2000a.

Guo ZH, Mattson MP. Neurotrophic factors protect cortical synaptic terminals against amyloid and oxidative stress–induced impairment of glucose transport, glutamate transport and mitochondrial function. *Cereb Cortex* 10:50–57, 2000b.

Gupta J, Han LP, Wang P, Gallie BL, Bacchetti S. Development of retinoblastoma in the absence of telomerase activity. *J Natl Cancer Inst* 88:1152–1157, 1996.

Gupta M, Shogreen MR, Braden GA, White WL, Sane DC. Prevalence of telomerase in coronary artery atherosclerosis. *J Anti-Aging Med* 3:15–24, 2000.

Gupta RD, Fuchs E. Multiple roles for activated LEF/TCF transcription complexes during hair follicle development and differentiation. *Development* 126:4557–4568, 1999.

Gupte S. Progeria with Marcus-Gunn phenomenon. *Indian Pediatr* 20:694–695, 1983.

Gutterman EM, Markowitz JS, Lewis B, Fillit H. Cost of Alzheimer's disease and related dementia in managed-Medicare. *J Am Geriatr Soc* 47:1065–1071, 1999.

Ha JW, Shim WH, Chung NS. Cardiovascular findings of Hutchinson-Gilford syndrome—a Doppler and two-dimensional echocardiographic study. *Yonsei Med* J 34:352–355, 1993.

Haber DA. Clinical implications of basic research: telomeres, cancer, and immortality. *N Engl J Med* 332:955–956, 1995.

Hackett JA, Feldser DM, Greider CW. Telomere dysfunction increases mutation rate and genomic instability. *Cell* 106:275–286, 2001.

Hackett JA, Greider CW. Balancing instability: dual roles for telomerase and telomere dysfunction in tumorigenesis. *Oncogene* 21:619–626, 2002.

Haddad MM, Xu W, Schwahn DJ, Liao F, Medrano EE. Activation of a cAMP pathway and induction of melanogenesis correlate with association of p16(INK4) and p27(KIP1) to CDKs, loss of E2F-binding activity, and premature senescence of human melanocytes. *Exp Cell Res* 253:561–572, 1999.

Hadley EC, Dutta C, Finkelstein J, Harris TB, Lane MA, Roth GS, Sherman SS, Starke-Reed PE. Human implications of caloric restriction's effects on aging in laboratory animals: an overview of opportunities for research. *J Gerontol A Biol Sci Med Sci* 56A:B5–6, 2001.

Hadshiew IM, Eller MS, Gilchrest BA. Age-associated decreases in human DNA repair capacity: implications for the skin. *AGE* 22:45–58, 1999.

Hagberg JM, Zmuda JM, McCole SD, Rodgers KS, Ferrell RE, Wilund KR, Moore GE. Moderate physical activity is associated with higher bone mineral density in postmenopausal women. *J Am Geriatr Soc* 49:1411–1417, 2001.

Hagen TM, Liu J, Lykkesfeldt J, Wehr CM, Ingersoll RT, Vinarsky V, Bartholomew JC, Ames BN. Feeding acetyl-L-carnitine and lipoic acid to old rats significantly improves metabolic function while decreasing oxidative stress. *Proc Natl Acad Sci USA* 99: 1870–1875, 2002.

Hagerman, FC, Walsh SJ, Staron RS, Hikida RS, Gilders RM, Murray TF, Toma K, Ragg KE. Effects of high-intensity resistance training on untrained older men. I. Strength, cardiovascular, and metabolic responses. *J Gerontol A Biol Sci Med Sci* 55:B336–B346, 2000.

Hagman M. Arthritis: a gene for smooth-running joints. *Science* 289:225–226, 2000.

Haguenauer D, Welch V, Shea B, Tugwell P. Anabolic agents to treat osteoporosis in older people: is there still place for fluoride? *J Am Geriatr Soc* 49:1387–1389, 2001.

Hahn WC, Counter CM, Lundberg AS, Beijersbergen RL, Brooks MW, Weinberg RA. Creation of human tumour cells with defined genetic elements. *Nature* 400:464–468, 1999a.

Hahn WC, Meyerson M. Telomerase activation, cellular immortalization and cancer. *Ann Med* 33:123–129, 2001.

Hahn WC, Stewart SA, Brooks MW, York SG, Eaton E, Kurachi A, Beijersbergen RL, Knoll JH, Meyerson M, Weinberg RA. Inhibition of telomerase limits the growth of human cancer cells. *Nat Med* 5:1164–1170, 1999b.

Hall DM, Oberley TD, Moseley PM, Buettner GR, Oberley LW, Weindruch R, Kregel KC. Caloric restriction improves thermotolerance and reduces hyperthermia-induced cellular damage in old rats. *FASEB J* 14:78–86, 2000.

Hall DM, Sattler GL, Sattler CA, Zhang HJ, Oberley LW, Pitot HC, Kregel KC. Aging lowers steady-state antioxidant enzyme and stress protein expression in primary hepatocytes. *J Gerontol A Biol Sci Med Sci* 56:B259–267, 2001.

Hall K, Hilding A, Thoren M. Determinants of circulating insulin-like growth factor-I. *J Endocrinol Invest* 22(5 Suppl):48–57, 1999.

Halliday G, Robinson SR, Shepherd C, Kril J. Alzheimer's disease and inflammation: a review of cellular and therapeutic mechanisms. *Clin Exp Pharmacol Physiol* 27:1–8, 2000.

Halvorsen TL, Beattie GM, Lopez AD, Hayek A, Levine F. Accelerated telomere shortening and senescence in human pancreatic islet cells stimulated to divide in vitro. *J Endocrinol* 166:103–109, 2000.

Hamilton E. *Mythology. Timeless Tales of Gods and Heroes.* Mentor Books, New York, 1940.

Hamilton SE, Pitts AE, Katipally RR, Jia X, Rutter JP, Davies BA, Shay JW, Wright WE, Corey DR. Identification of determinants for inhibitor binding within the RNA active site of human telomerase using PNA scanning. *Biochemistry* 36:11873–11880, 1997.

Han H, Hurley LH. G-quadruplex DNA: a potential target for anti-cancer drug design. *Trends Pharmacol Sci* 21:136–142, 2000.

Hanaoka S, Nagadoi A, Yoshimura S, Aimoto S, Li B, de Lange T, Nishimura Y. NMR structure of the hRap1 Myb motif reveals a canonical three-helix bundle lacking the positive surface charge typical of Myb DNA-binding domains. *J Mol Biol* 312:167–175, 2001.

Hande MP, Balajee AS, Natarajan AT. Induction of telomerase activity by UV-irradiation in Chinese hamster cells. *Oncogene* 15:1747–1752, 1997.

Hande MP, Balajee AS, Tchirkov A, Wynshaw-Boris A, Lansdorp PM. Extra-chromosomal telomeric DNA in cells from Atm(–/–) mice and patients with ataxia-telangiectasia. *Hum Mol Genet* 10:519–528, 2001.

Hande MP, Samper E, Lansdorp P, Blasco MA. Telomere length dynamics and chromosomal instability in cells derived from telomerase null mice. *J Cell Biol* 144:589–601, 1999a.

Hande P, Slijepcevic P, Silver A, Bouffler S, van Buul P, Bryant P, Lansdorp P. Elongated telomeres in *scid* mice. *Genomics* 56:221–223, 1999b.

Hannan EL, Magaziner J, Wang JJ, Eastwood EA, Silberzweig SB, Gilbert M, Morrison RS, McLaughlin MA, Orosz GM, Siu AL. Mortality and locomotion 6 months after hospitalization for hip fracture. *JAMA* 285:2736–2742, 2001.

Hanson H, Mathew CG, Docherty Z, Mackie Ogilvie C. Telomere shortening in Fanconi anaemia demonstrated by a direct FISH approach. *Cytogenet Cell Genet* 93:203–206, 2001.

Hao YH, Tan Z. Telomeres at the chromosome X(p) might be critical in limiting the proliferative potential of human cells. *Exp Gerontol* 36:1639–1647, 2001.

Hao YH, Tan Z. The generation of long telomere overhangs in human cells: a model and its implication. *Bioinformatics* 18:666–671, 2002.

Hara E, Uzman JA, Dimri GP, Nehlin JO, Testori A, Campisi J. The helix-loop-helix protein Id-1 and a retinoblastoma protein binding mutant of SV40 T antigen synergize to reactivate DNA synthesis in senescent human fibroblasts. *Dev Genet* 18:161–172, 1996.

Hara E, Yamaguchi T, Nojima H, Ide T, Campisi J, Okayama H, Oda K. Id-related genes encoding helix-loop-helix proteins are required for G1 progression and are repressed in senescent human fibroblasts. *J Biol Chem* 269:2139–2145, 1994.

Hara M, Ono K, Hwang MW, Iwasaki A, Okada M, Nakatani K, Sasayama S, Matsumori A. Evidence for a role of mast cells in the evolution to congestive heart failure. *J Exp Med* 195:375–381, 2002.

Hara T, Noma T, Yamashiro Y, Naito K, Nakazawa A. Quantitative analysis of telomerase activity and telomerase reverse transcriptase expression in renal cell carcinoma. *Urol Res* 29:1–6, 2001a.

Hara Y, Iwase H, Toyama T, Yamashita H, Omoto Y, Fujii Y, Kobayashi S. Telomerase activity levels for evaluating the surgical margin in breast-conserving surgery. *Surg Today* 31:289–294, 2001b.

Harada K, Yasoshima M, Ozaki S, Sanzen T, Nakanuma Y. PCR and in situ hybridization studies of telomerase subunits in human non-neoplastic livers. *J Pathol* 193:210–217, 2001.

Hardy JD, Bard P. Body temperature regulation. In Mountcastle VB (ed). *Medical Physiology, 13th ed.* C.V. Mosby Company, St. Louis, 1974, pp 1305–1342.

Hari R, Burde V, Arking R. Immunological confirmation of elevated levels of CuZn superoxide dismutase protein in an artificially selected long-lived strain of *Drosophila melanogaster*. *Exp Gerontol* 33:227–237, 1998.

Harjacek M, Batinic D, Sarnavka V, Uzarevic B, Mardesic D, Marusic M. Immunological aspects of progeria (Hutchinson-Gilford syndrome) in a 15-month-old child. *Eur J Pediatr* 150:40–42, 1990.

Hark AT, Schoenherr CJ, Katz DJ, Ingram RS, Levorse JM, Tilghman SM. CTCF mediates methylation-sensitive enhancer-blocking activity at the H19/Igf2 locus. *Nature* 405:486–489, 2000.

Harle-Bachor C, Boukamp P. Telomerase activity in the regenerative basal layer of the epidermis in human skin and in immortal and carcinoma-derived skin keratinocytes. *Proc Natl Acad Sci USA* 93:6476–6481, 1996.

Harley C. Telomerase and cell immortality in humans. Program and Abstracts of the 89th Annual Meeting of the American Association for Cancer Research, March 28–April 1, 1998, New Orleans, LA, 1998a.

Harley CB. Biology and evolution of aging: implications for basic gerontological health research. *Can J Aging* 7:100–113, 1988.

Harley CB. Telomere loss: mitotic clock or genetic time bomb? *Mutat Res* 256:271–282, 1991.

Harley CB. Telomerases. *Pathol Biol (Paris)* 42:342–345, 1994.

Harley CB. Human ageing and telomeres. *Ciba Found Symp* 211:129–139; discussion 139–144, 1997.

Harley CB. The story of the end, and its future. Presented at Telomeres and Telomerase: Implications for Cell Immortality, Cancer, and Age-related Disease. San Francisco, CA, June 1–3, 1998b.

Harley CB. Cloning: techniques and applications in human health. *Generations* 24:65–71, 2000.

Harley CB. Telomerase is not an oncogene. *Oncogene* 21:494–502, 2002.

Harley CB, Futcher AB, Greider CW. Telomeres shorten during aging of human fibroblasts. *Nature* 345:458–460, 1990.

Harley CB, Goldstein S. Retesting the commitment theory of cellular aging. *Science* 207:191–193, 1980.

Harley CB, Goldstein S, Posner BI, Guyda H. Decreased sensitivity of old and progeric human fibroblasts to a preparation of factors with insulinlike activity. *J Clin Invest* 68:988–994, 1981.

Harley CB, Kim NW. Telomerase and cancer. *Important Adv Oncol* 57–67, 1996.

Harley CB, Kim NW, Prowse KR, Weinrich SL, Hirsch KS, West MD, Bacchetti S, Hirte HW, Counter CM, Greider CW, et al. Telomerase, cell immortality, and cancer. *Cold Spring Harb Symp Quant Biol* 59:307–315, 1994.

Harley CB, Pollard JW, Chamberlain JW, Stanners CP, Goldstein S. Protein synthetic errors do not increase during aging of cultured human fibroblasts. *Proc Natl Acad Sci USA* 77:1885–1889, 1980.

Harley CB, Sherwood SW. Aging of cultured human skin fibroblasts. *Methods Mol Biol* 75:23–30, 1997a.

Harley CB, Sherwood SW. Telomerase, checkpoints and cancer. *Cancer Surv* 29:263–284, 1997b.

Harley CB, Shmookler Reis RJ, Goldstein S. Loss of repetitious DNA in proliferating somatic cells may be due to unequal recombination. *J Theor Biol* 94:1–12, 1982.

Harley CB, Vaziri H, Counter CM, Allsopp RC. The telomere hypothesis of cellular aging. *Exp Gerontol* 27:375–382, 1992.

Harley CB, Villeponteau B. Telomeres and telomerase in aging and cancer. *Curr Opin Genet Dev* 5:249–255, 1995.

Harman D. Aging: a theory based on free redial and radiation chemistry. *J Gerontol* 11:298–300, 1956.

Harman D. Free radical theory of aging: increasing the average life expectancy at birth and the maximum life span. *J Anti-Aging Med* 2:199–208, 1999.

Harman D. Alzheimer's disease: a hypothesis on pathogenesis. *J Am Aging Assoc* 23:147–161, 2000.

Harms W, Rothamel T, Miller K, Harste G, Grassmann M, Heim A. Characterization of human myocardial fibroblasts immortalized by HPV16 E6–E7 genes. *Exp Cell Res* 268:252–261, 2001.

Harney JP, Scarbrough K, Rosewell KL, Wise PM. In vivo antisense antagonism of vasoactive intestinal peptide in the suprachiasmatic nuclei causes aging-like changes in the estradiol-induced luteinizing hormone and prolactin surges. *Endocrinology* 137:3696–3701, 1996.

Harper AJ, Buster JE, Casson PR. Changes in adrenocortical function with aging and therapeutic implications. *Semin Reprod Endocrinol* 17:327–338, 1999.

Harper ME, Monemdjou S, Ramsey JJ, Weindruch R. Age-related increase in mitochondrial proton leak and decrease in ATP turnover reactions in mouse hepatocytes. *Am J Physiol* 275(2 Pt 1):E197–206, 1998.

Harrington L, McPhail T, Mar V, Zhou W, Oulten R, Amgen EST program, Bass MB, Arruda I, Robinson MO. A mammalian telomerase-associated protein. *Science* 275:973–976, 1997a.

Harrington L, Robinson MO. Telomere dysfunction: multiple paths to the same end. *Oncogene* 21:592–597, 2002.

Harrington L, Zhou W, McPhail T, Oultion R, Yeung DS, Mar D, Bass MD, Robinson MD. Human telomerase contains evolutionarily conserved catalytic and structural subunits. *Genes Dev* 11:3109–3115, 1997b.

Harrington LA, Greider CW. Telomerase primer specificity and chromosome healing. *Nature* 353:451–454 , 1991.

Harris A, Chung HS, Ciulla TA, Kagemann L. Progress in measurement of ocular blood flow and relevance to our understanding of glaucoma and age-related macular degeneration. *Prog Retin Eye Res* 18:669–687, 1999a.

Harris A, Harris M, Biller J, Garzozi H, Zarfty D, Ciulla TA, Martin B. Aging affects the retrobulbar circulation differently in women and men. *Arch Ophthalmol* 118:1076–1080, 2000.

Harris J. Intimations of immortality. *Science* 288:59, 2000.

Harris ST, Watts NB, Genant HK, McKeever CD, Hangartner T, Keller M, Chesnut CH, Brown J, Eriksen EF, Hoseyni MS, Axelrod DW, Miller PD. Effects of risedronate treatment on vertebral and nonvertebral fractures in women with postmenopausal osteoporosis. A randomized controlled trial. *JAMA* 282:1344–1352, 1999b.

Harrison DE. Potential misinterpretations using models of accelerated aging. *J Gerontol Biol Sci* 49:B245, 1994.

Hartwell LH, Kastan MB. Cell cycle control and cancer. *Science* 266:1821–1828, 1994.

Hasle H, Clemmensen IH, Mikkelsen M. Incidence of cancer in individuals with Down syndrome [in Danish]. *Tidsskr Nor Laegeforen* 120:2878–2881, 2000.

Hass BS, Lewis SM, Duffy PH, Ershler W, Feuers RJ, Good RA, Ingram DK, Lane MA, Leakey JE, Lipschitz D, Poehlman ET, Roth GS, Sprott RL, Sullivan DH, Turturro A, Verdery RB, Walford RL, Weindruch R, Yu BP, Hart RW. Dietary restriction in humans: report on the Little Rock Conference on the value, feasibility, and parameters of a proposed study. *Mech Ageing Dev* 91:79–94, 1996.

Hasselgren PO, Wray C, Mammen J. Molecular regulation of muscle cachexia: it may be more than the proteasome. *Biochem Biophys Res Commun* 290:1–10, 2002.

Hastie ND, Dempster M, Dunlop M, Thompson AM, Green DK, Allshire RC. Telomere reduction in human colorectal carcinoma and with ageing. *Nature* 346:866–868, 1990.

Hasty P, Vijg J. Genomic priorities in aging. *Science* 296:1250–1251, 2002.

Hathcock KS, Hemann MT, Opperman KK, Strong MA, Greider CW, Hodes RJ. Haploinsufficiency of mTR results in defects in telomere elongation. *Proc Natl Acad Sci USA* 99:3591–3596, 2002.

Hathcock KS, Kaech SM, Ahmed R, Hodes RJ. Induction of telomerase activity and maintenance of telomere length in virus-specific effector and memory CD8+ T cells. *J Immunol* 170:147–152, 2003.

Hattori H, Matsumoto M, Iwai K, Tsuchiya H, Miyauchi E, Takasaki M, Kamino K, Munehira J, Kimura Y, Kawanishi K, Hoshino T, Murai H, Ogata H, Maruyama H, Yoshida H. The τ protein of oral epithelium increases in Alzheimer disease. *J Gerontol A Biol Sci Med Sci* 57:M64–70, 2002.

Hattori K, Tanaka M, Sugiyama S, Obayashi T, Ito T, Satake T, Hanaki Y, Asai J, Nagano M, Ozawa T. Age-dependent increase in deleted mitochondrial DNA in the human heart: possible contributory factor to presbycardia. *Am Heart J* 121:1735–1742, 1991.

Haussmann MF, Winkler DW, O'Reilly KM, Huntington CE, Vleck CM. Can an old bird be taught new tricks? Telomere length increases with age in a long-lived bird. Presented at the Annual Meeting of the American Aging Association, San Diego, June 7–11, 2002.

Hauss-Wegrzyniak B, Lynch MA, Vraniak PD, Wenk GL. Chronic brain inflammation results in cell loss in the entorhinal cortex and impaired LTP in perforant path-granule cell synapses. *Exp Neurol* 176:336–341, 2002.

Hautekeete ML, Geerts A. The hepatic stellate (Ito) cell: its role in human liver disease. *Virchows Arch* 430:195–207, 1997.

Haw R, Yarragudi AD, Uemura H. Isolation of a *Candida glabrata* homologue of RAP1, a regulator of transcription and telomere function in *Saccharomyces cerevisiae*. *Yeast* 18:1277–1284, 2001.

Hawkins BS, Bird A, Klein R, West SK. Epidemiology of age-related macular degeneration. *Mol Vis* 5:26, 1999.

Hawley RS. Unresolvable endings: defective telomeres and failed separation. *Science* 275:1441–1443, 1997.

Hayashi T, Ito I, Kano H, Endo, H, Iguchi A. Estriol (E3) replacement improves endothelial function and bone mineral density in very elderly women. *J Gerontol A Biol Sci Med Sci* 55:B183–190, 2000.

Hayflick L. The limited in vitro lifetime of human diploid cell strains. *Exp Cell Res* 37:614–636, 1965.

Hayflick L. *Oncogene*sis in vitro. *Natl Cancer Inst Monogr* 26:355–385, 1967.

Hayflick L. Human cells and aging. *Sci Am* 218:32–37, 1968.

Hayflick L. Aging under glass. *Exp Gerontol* 5:291–303, 1970.

Hayflick L. The cell biology of human aging. *N Engl J Med* 295:1302–1308, 1976.

Hayflick L. The cell biology of aging. *J Invest Dermatol* 73:8–14, 1979.

Hayflick L. Cell aging. In Eisdorfer C (ed). *Annual Review of Gerontology and Geriatrics, Volume 1*. Springer Publishing, New York, 1980, pp 26–67.

Hayflick L. Intracellular determinants of cell aging. *Mech Ageing Dev* 28:177–185, 1984a.

Hayflick L. When does aging begin? *Res Aging* 6:99–103, 1984b.

Hayflick L. The cell biology of aging. *Clin Geriatr Med* 1:15–27, 1985.

Hayflick L. Antecedents of cell aging research. *Exp Gerontol* 24:355–365, 1989.

Hayflick L. Aging under glass. *Mutat Res* 256:69–80, 1991.

Hayflick L. Aging, longevity, and immortality in vitro. *Exp Gerontol* 27:363–368, 1992.

Hayflick L. *How and Why We Age*. Ballantine Books, New York, 1994.

Hayflick L. Mortality and immortality at the cellular level. A review. *Biochemistry (Mosc)* 62:1180–1190, 1997a.

Hayflick L. SV40 and human cancer. *Science* 276:337–338, 1997b.

Hayflick L. A brief history of cell mortality and immortality. Presented at Telomeres and Telomerase: Implications for Cell Immortality, Cancer, and Age-related Disease. San Francisco, CA, June 1–3, 1998a.

Hayflick L. A brief history of the mortality and immortality of cultured cells. *Keio J Med* 47:174–182, 1998b.

Hayflick L. Aging is not a disease. *Aging (Milano)* 10:146, 1998c.

Hayflick L. How and why we age. *Exp Gerontol* 33:639–653, 1998d.

Hayflick L. A brief overview of the discovery of cell mortality and immortality and of its influence on concepts about aging and cancer [in French]. *Pathol Biol (Paris)* 47:1094–1104, 1999.

Hayflick L. New approaches to old age. *Nature* 403:365, 2000a.

Hayflick L. The future of aging. *Nature* 408:267–269, 2000b.

Hayflick L. The illusion of cell immortality. *Br J Cancer* 83:841–846, 2000c.

Hayflick L. Hormesis, aging, and longevity determination. *Belle Newsletter* 9:8–9, 2001.

Hayflick L, Moorhead PS. The serial cultivation of human diploid strains. *Exp Cell Res* 25:585–621, 1961.

Hazlett LD, Kreindler FB, Berk RS, Barrett R. Aging alters the phagocytic capability of inflammatory cells induced into cornea. *Curr Eye Res* 9:129–138, 1990.

Hazzard WR. What heterogeneity among centenarians can teach us about genetics, aging, and longevity. *J Am Geriatr Soc* 49:1568–1569, 2001.

Hazzard WR, Bierman EL, Blass JP, Ettinger WH Jr, Halter JB. *Principles of Geriatric Medicine and Gerontology, 3rd ed.* McGraw-Hill, New York, 1994.

Heath EI, Limburg PJ, Hawk ET, Forastiere AA. Adenocarcinoma of the esophagus: risk factors and prevention. *Oncology (Huntingt)* 14:507–514; discussion 518–520, 522–523, 2000.

Hecht A, Strahl-Bolsinger S, Grunstein M. Spreading of transcriptional repressor SIR3 from telomeric heterochromatin. *Nature* 383:92–96, 1996.

Heinlein RA. *Methuselah's Children*. Signet, New York, 1958.

Heiser A, Dahm P, Yancey DR, Maurice MA, Boczkowski D, Nair SK, Gilboa E, Vieweg J. Human dendritic cells transfected with RNA encoding prostate-specific antigen stimulate prostate-specific CTL responses in vitro. *J Immunol* 164:5508–5514, 2000.

Heiser A, Maurice MA, Yancey DR, Coleman DM, Dahm P, Vieweg J. Human dendritic cells transfected with renal tumor RNA stimulate polyclonal T-cell responses against antigens expressed by primary and metastatic tumors. *Cancer Res* 61:3388–3393, 2001a.

Heiser A, Maurice MA, Yancey DR, Wu NZ, Dahm P, Pruitt SK, Boczkowski D, Nair SK, Ballo MS, Gilboa E, Vieweg J. Induction of polyclonal prostate cancer–specific CTL using dendritic cells transfected with amplified tumor RNA. *J Immunol* 166:2953–2960, 2001b.

Heiss NS, Bachner D, Salowsky R, Kolb A, Kioschis P, Poustka A. Gene structure and expression of the mouse dyskeratosis congenita gene, *dkc1*. *Genomics* 67:153–163, 2000.

Heiss NS, Megarbane A, Klauck SM, Kreuz FR, Makhoul E, Majewski F, Poustka A. One novel and two recurrent missense *DKC1* mutations in patients with dyskeratosis congenita (DKC). *Genet Couns* 12:129–136, 2001.

Hekimi S, Burgess J, Bussiere F, Meng Y, Benard C. Genetics of life span in *C. elegans*: molecular diversity, physiological complexity, mechanistic simplicity. *Trends Genet* 17:712–718, 2001.

Hekimi S, Lakowski B, Barnes TM, Ewbank JJ. Molecular genetics of life span in *C. elegans*: how much does it teach us? *Trends Genet* 14:14–20, 1998.

Helder MN, Jong S, Vries EG, Zee AG. Telomerase targeting in cancer treatment: new developments. *Drug Resist Updat* 2:104–115, 1999.

Helder MN, Wisman GB, van der Zee GJ. Telomerase and telomeres: from basic biology to cancer treatment. *Cancer Invest* 20:82–101, 2002.

Helenius M, Hanninen M, Lehtinen SK, Salminen A. Aging-induced up-regulation of nuclear binding activities of oxidative stress responsive NF-κB transcription factor in mouse cardiac muscle. *J Mol Cell Cardiol* 28:487–498, 1996.

Helmuth L. Further progress on a β-amyloid vaccine. *Science* 289:375, 2000.

Helmuth L. Detangling Alzheimer's disease. *Sci aging knowledge environ.* 2001 Oct 3; 2001(1):oa2.

Hemann MT, Greider CW. G-strand overhangs on telomeres in telomerase-deficient mouse cells. *Nucleic Acids Res* 27:3964–3969, 1999.

Hemann MT, Strong MA, Hao LY, Greider CW. The shortest telomere, not average telomere length, is critical for cell viability and chromosome stability. *Cell* 2001;17:67–77, 2001.

Henderson AS, Easteal S, Jorm AF, Mackinnon AJ, Korten AE, Christensen H, Croft L, Jacomb PA. Apolipoprotein E allele epsilon 4, dementia, and cognitive decline in a population sample. *Lancet* 346:1387–1390, 1995.

Henderson E. Telomere DNA structure. In Blackburn EH, Greider, CW. *Telomeres.* Cold Spring Harbor Laboratory Press, Cold Spring Harbor, NY, 1995, pp 11–34.

Henderson ER, Moore M, Malcolm BA. Telomere G-strand structure and function analyzed by chemical protection base analogue substitution and utilization by telomerase in vitro. *Biochemistry* 29:732–737, 1990.

Henderson S, Allsopp R, Spector D, Wang SS, Harley C. In situ analysis of changes in telomere size during replicative aging and cell transformation. *J Cell Biol* 134:1–12, 1996a.

Henderson VW. The epidemiology of estrogen replacement therapy and Alzheimer's disease. *Neurology* 48:S27–35, 1997.

Henderson VW, Paganini-Hill A, Emanuel CK, Dunn ME, Buckwalter JG. Estrogen replacement therapy in older women. *Arch Neurol* 51:896–900, 1994.

Henderson VW, Paganini-Hill A, Miller BL, Elble RJ, Reyes PF, Shoupe D, McCleary CA, Klein RA, Hake AM, Farlow MR. Estrogen for Alzheimer's disease in women: randomized, double-blind, placebo-controlled trial. *Neurology* 54:295–301, 2000a.

Henderson VW, Watt L, Buckwalter JG. Cognitive skills associated with estrogen replacement in women with Alzheimer's disease. *Psychoneuroendocrinology* 21:421–430, 1996b.

Henderson YC, Breau RL, Liu TJ, Clayman GL. Telomerase activity in head and neck tumors after introduction of wild-type p53, p21, p16, and E2F-1 genes by means of recombinant adenovirus. *Head Neck* 22:347–354, 2000b.

Henderson Z. Responses of basal forebrain cholinergic neurons to damage in the adult brain. *Prog Neurobiol* 48:219–254, 1996.

Hendrie HC, Ogunniyi A, Hall KS, Baiyewu O, Unverzagt FW, Gureje O, Gao S, Evans RM, Ogunseyinde AO, Adeyinka AO, Musick B, Hui SL. Incidence of dementia and Alzheimer disease in 2 communities: Yoruba residing in Ibadan, Nigeria, and African Americans residing in Indianopolis, Indiana. *JAMA* 285:739–747, 2001.

Hennessey JV, Chromiak JA, Ventura SD, Reinert SE, Puhl J, Kiel DP, Rosen CJ, Vandenburgh H, MacLean DB. Growth hormone administration and exercise effects on muscle fiber type and diameter in moderately frail older people. *J Am Geriatr Soc* 49:852–858, 2001.

Hennessy S, Strom BL. Statins and fracture risk. *JAMA* 285:1888–1889, 2001.

Henschke CI, McCauley DI, Yankelevitz DF, Naidich DP, McGuinness G, Miettinen OS, Libby DM, Pasmantier, Koizumi J, Altorki NK, Smith JP. Early lung cancer action project: overall design and findings from baseline screening. *Lancet* 354:99–105, 1999.

Hensler PJ, Annab LA, Barrett JC, Pereira-Smith OM. A gene involved in control of human cellular senescence on human chromosome 1q. *Mol Cell Biol* 14:2291–2297, 1994.

Henson JD, Neumann AA, Yeager TR, Reddel RR. Alternative lengthening of telomeres in mammalian cells. *Oncogene* 21:598–610, 2002.

Herbert B, Pitts AE, Baker SI, Hamilton SE, Wright WE, Shay JW, Corey DR. Inhibition of human telomerase in immortal human cells leads to progressive telomere shortening and cell death. *Proc Natl Acad Sci USA* 96:14276–14281, 1999.

Herbert BS, Wright AC, Passons CM, Wright WE, Ali IU, Kopelovich L, Shay JW. Effects of chemopreventive and antitelomerase agents on the spontaneous immortalization of breast epithelial cells. *J Natl Cancer Inst* 93:39–45, 2001a.

Herbert BS, Wright WE, Shay JW. Telomerase and breast cancer. *Breast Cancer Res* 3:146–149, 2001b.

Hermann M, Berger P. Hormone replacement in the aging male? *Exp Gerontol* 34:923–933, 1999.

Herrera E, Martinez-A C, Blasco MA. Impaired germinal center reaction in mice with short telomeres. *EMBO J* 19:472–481, 2000.

Herrera E, Samper E, Blasco MA. Telomere shortening in mTR–/– embryos is associated with failure to close the neural tube. *EMBO J* 18:1172–1181, 1999a.

Herrera E, Samper E, Martin-Caballero J, Flores JM, Lee HW, Blasco MA. Disease states associated with telomerase deficiency appear earlier in mice with short telomeres. *EMBO J* 18:2950–2960, 1999b.

Herrero A, Barja G. Effect of aging on mitochondrial and nuclear DNA oxidative damage in the heart and brain throughout the life-span of the rat. *J Am Aging Assoc* 24:45–50, 2001.

Herrington DM, Reboussin DM, Brosnihan KB, Sharp PC, Shumaker SA, Snyder TE, Furberg CD, Kowalchuk GJ, Stuckey TD, Rogers WJ, Givens DH, Waters D. Effects of estrogen replacement on the progression of coronary-artery disease. *N Engl J Med* 343:522–529, 2000.

Herron GS. Vascular aneurysms: a side-splitting affair. *Cardiovasc Res* 31:224–230, 1996.

Herron GS, Unemori E, Wong M, Rapp JH, Hibbs MH, Stoney RJ. Connective tissue proteinases and inhibitors in abdominal aortic aneurysms. Involvement of the vasa vasorum in the pathogenesis of aortic aneurysms. *Arterioscler Thromb* 11:1667–1677, 1991.

Herrmann J, Lerman A. The endothelium: dysfunction and beyond. *J Nucl Cardiol* 8:197–206, 2001.

Herstone ST, Bower J. Werner's syndrome. *AJR Am J Roentgenol* 51:639–643, 1944.

Herzberg AJ, Dinehart SM. Chronologic aging in black skin. *Am J Dermatopathol* 11:319–328, 1989.

Hess JL, Highsmith WE Jr. Telomerase detection in body fluids. *Clin Chem* 48:18–24, 2002.

Higami Y, Shimokawa I, Okimoto T, Ikeda T. Vulnerability to oxygen radicals is more important than impaired repair in hepatocytic deoxyribonucleic acid damage in aging. *Lab Invest* 71:650–656, 1994.

Higashi T, Nouso K, Tsuji T. Usefulness of telomerase activity in the diagnosis of small hepato-cellular carcinoma [in Japanese]. *Nippon Rinsho* 56:1248–1252, 1998.

Hikida RS, Staron RS, Hagerman FC, Walsh S, Kaiser E, Shell S, Hervey S. Effects of high-intensity resistance training on untrained older men. II. Muscle fiber characteristics and nucleo-cytoplasmic relationships. *J Gerontol A Biol Sci Med Sci* 55:B347–B354, 2000.

Hillen T, Lun A, Reischies FM, Borchelt M, Steinhagen-Thiessen E, Schaub RT. DHEA-S plasma levels and incidence of Alzheimer's disease. *Biol Psychiatry* 47:161–163, 2000.

Hinkley CS, Blasco MA, Funk WD, Feng J, Villeponteau B, Greider CW, Herr W. The mouse telomerase RNA 5'-end lies just upstream of the telomerase template sequence. *Nucleic Acids Res* 26:532–536, 1998.

Hinnebusch J, Barbour AG. Linear plasmids of *Borrelia burgdorferi* have a telomeric structure and sequence similar to those of a eukaryotic virus. *J Bacteriol* 173:7233–7239, 1991.

Hinson JP, Raven PW. DHEA deficiency syndrome: a new term for old age? *J Endocrinol* 163: 1–5, 1999.

Hirai H. Relationship of telomere sequence and constitutive heterochromatin in the human and apes as detected by PRINS. *Methods Cell Sci* 23:29–35, 2001.

Hirao A, Kong YY, Matsuoka S, Wakeham A, Ruland J, Yoshida H, Liu D, Elledge SJ, Mak TW. DNA damage-induced activation of p53 by the checkpoint kinase Chk2. *Science* 287:1824–1827, 2000.

Hiraoka Y. Meiotic telomeres: a matchmaker for homologous chromosomes. *Genes Cells* 3:405–413, 1998.

Hirashima T, Komiya T, Nitta T, Takada Y, Kobayashi M, Masuda N, Matui K, Takada M, Kikui M, Yasumitu T, Ohno A, Nakagawa K, Fukuoka M, Kawase I. Prognostic significance of telomeric repeat length alterations in pathological stage I-IIIA non-small cell lung cancer. *Anticancer Res* 20:2181–2187, 2000.

Hirose M. A new method for the detection and the measurement of telomerase activity. Presented at Telomeres and Telomerase: Implications for Cell Immortality, Cancer, and Age-related Disease. San Francisco, CA, June 1–3, 1998.

Hirose M, Abe-Hashimoto J, Ogura K, Tahara H, Ide T, Yoshimura T. A rapid, useful and quantitative method to measure telomerase activity by hybridization protection assay connected with a telomeric repeat amplification protocol. *J Cancer Res Clin Oncol* 123:337–344, 1997.

Hirshbein LD. Popular views of old age in America, 1900–1950. *J Am Geriatr Soc* 49:1555–1560, 2001.

Hirsch AT, Criqui MH, Treat-Johnson D, Regensteiner JG, Creager MA, Olin JW, Krook SH, Hunninghake DB, Camerota AJ, Walsh ME, McDermott MM, Hiatt HR. Peripheral arterial disease detection, awareness, and treatment in primary care. *JAMA* 286:1317–1324, 2001.

Hisama FM, Chen YH, Meyn MS, Oshima J, Weissman SM. WRN or telomerase constructs reverse 4-nitroquinoline 1-oxide sensitivity in transformed Werner syndrome fibroblasts. *Cancer Res* 60:2372–2376, 2000.

Hisatomi H, Nagao K, Kanamaru T, Endo H, Tomimatsu M, Hikiji K. Levels of telomerase catalytic subunit mRNA as a predictor of potential malignancy. *Int J Oncol* 14:727–732, 1999.

Hiyama E, Gollahon L, Kataoka T, Kuroi K, Yokoyama T, Gazdar AF, Hiyama K, Piatyszek MA, Shay JW. Telomerase activity in human breast tumors. *J Natl Cancer Inst* 88:116–122, 1996a.

Hiyama E, Hiyama K, Ohtsu K, Yamaoka H, Ichikawa T, Shay JW, Yokoyama T. Telomerase activity in neuroblastoma: is it a prognostic indicator of clinical behaviour? *Eur J Cancer* 33:1932–1936, 1997a.

Hiyama E, Hiyama K, Tatsumoto N, Kodama T, Shay JW, Yokoyama T. Telomerase activity in human intestine. *Int J Oncol* 9:453–458, 1996b.

Hiyama E, Hiyama K, Yokoyama T, Fukuba I, Yamaoka H, Shay JW, Matsuura Y. Rapid detection of *MYCN* gene amplification and telomerase expression in neuroblastoma. *Clin Cancer Res* 5:601–609, 1999.

Hiyama E, Hiyama K, Yokoyama T, Ichikawa T, Matsuura Y. Length of telomeric repeats in neuroblastoma: correlation with prognosis and other biological characteristics. *Jpn J Cancer Res* 83:159–164, 1992.

Hiyama E, Hiyama K, Yokoyama T, Matsuura Y, Piatyszek MA, Shay JW. Correlating telomerase activity levels with human neuroblastoma outcomes. *Nat Med* 1:249–255, 1995a.

Hiyama E, Hiyama K, Yokoyama T, Shay JW. Immunohistochemical detection of telomerase (hTERT) protein in human cancer tissues and a subset of cells in normal tissues. *Neoplasia* 3:17–26, 2001.

Hiyama E, Kodama T, Shinbara K, Iwao T, Itoh M, Hiyama K, Shay JW, Matsuura Y, Yokoyama T. Telomerase activity is detected in pancreatic cancer but not in benign tumors. *Cancer Res* 57:326–331, 1997b.

Hiyama E, Saeki T, Hiyama K, Takashima S, Shay JW, Matsuura Y, Yokoyama T. Telomerase activity as a marker of breast carcinoma in fine-needle aspirated samples. *Cancer* 90:235–238, 2000a.

Hiyama E, Yokoyama T, Hiyama K, Matsuura Y. Relationship between telomere length and clinical and biological characteristics of the cancers with telomerase reactivation [in Japanese]. *Nippon Rinsho* 56:1139–1145, 1998a.

Hiyama E, Yokoyama T, Hiyama K, Yamakido M, Santo T, Kodama T, Ichikawa T, Matsuura Y. Alteration of telomeric repeat length in adult and childhood solid neoplasia. *Int J Oncol* 6:13–16 1995b.

Hiyama E, Yokoyama T, Hiyama K, Yamaoka H, Matsuura Y, Nishimura Si, Ueda K.Multifocal neuroblastoma: biologic behavior and surgical aspects. *Cancer* 88:1955–1963, 2000a.

Hiyama E, Yokoyama T, Tatsumoto N, Hiyama K, Imamura Y, Murakami Y, Kodama T, Piatyszek MA, Shay JW, Matsuura Y. Telomerase activity in gastric cancer. *Cancer Res* 55:3258–3262, 1995c.

Hiyama K, Hiyama E. Telomere and telomerase in lung cancer [in Japanese]. *Nippon Rinsho* 60:737–742, 2002.

Hiyama K, Hirai Y, Kyoizumi S, Akiyama M, Hiyama E, Piatyszek MA, Shay JW, Ishioka S, Yamakido M. Activation of telomerase in human lymphocytes and hematopoietic progenitor cells. *J Immunol* 155:3711–3715, 1995d.

Hiyama K, Hiyama E, Ishioka S, Yamakido M. Lung cancer: progress in diagnosis and treatment. IV. Related topics: 1. Telomere and telomerase, new targets for diagnosis and treatment of lung cancer [in Japanese]. *Nippon Naika Gakkai Zasshi* 86:95–99, 1997c.

Hiyama K, Hiyama E, Ishioka S, Yamakido M. Telomere and telomerase in human cancer [in Japanese]. *Gan To Kagaku Ryoho* 24:196–201, 1997d.

Hiyama K, Hiyama E, Ishioka S, Yamakido M, Inai K, Gazdar AF, Piatyszek MA, Shay JW. Telomerase activity in small-cell and non-small-cell lung cancers. *J Natl Cancer Inst* 87:895–902, 1995e.

Hiyama K, Ishioka S, Hiyama E, Yamakido M. Advance of research on telomerase [in Japanese]. *Gan To Kagaku Ryoho* 25:1105–1110, 1998b.

Hiyama K, Ishioka S, Hiyama E, Yamakido M. Telomerase activity as a novel marker of lung cancer [in Japanese]. *Nippon Rinsho* 56:1253–1257, 1998c.

Hiyama K, Ishioka S, Shay JW, Taooka Y, Maeda A, Isobe T, Hiyama E, Maeda H, Yamakido M. Telomerase activity as a novel marker of lung cancer and immune-associated lung diseases. *Int J Mol Med* 1:545–549, 1998d.

Hiyama K, Ishioka S, Shirotani Y, Inai K, Hiyama E, Murakami I, Isobe T, Inamizu T, Yamakido M. Alterations in telomeric repeat length in lung cancer are associated with loss of heterozygosity in p53 and Rb. *Oncogene* 10:937–944, 1995f.

Hjelmeland LM. Senescence of the retinal pigmented epithelium. *Invest Ophthalmol Vis Sci* 40:1–2, 1999.

Hjelmeland LM, Cristofolo VJ, Funk W, Rakoczy E, Katz ML. Senescence of the retinal pigment epithelium. *Mol Vis* 5:33, 1999.

Hlatky MA, Boothroyd D, Vittinghoff E, Sharp P, Whooley MA, for the HERS Group. Quality-of-life and depressive symptoms in postmenopausal women after receiving hormone therapy. Results from the Heart and Estrogen/Progestin Replacement Study (HERS) Trial. *JAMA* 287:591–597, 2002.

Ho AC, Guyer DR, Fine SL. Macular hole. *Surv Ophthalmol* 42:393–416, 1998.

Ho AM, Johnson MD, Kingsley DM. Role of the mouse *ank* gene in control of tissue calcification and arthritis. *Science* 289:265–270, 2000.

Hoare SF, Bryce LA, Wisman GB, Burns S, Going JJ, van der Zee AG, Keith WN. Lack of telomerase RNA gene hTERC expression in alternative lengthening of telomeres cells is associated with methylation of the hTERC promoter. *Cancer Res* 61:27–32, 2001.

Hobden JA, Masinick SA, Barrett RP, Hazlett LD. Aged mice fail to upregulate ICAM-1 after *Pseudomonas aeruginosa* corneal infection. *Invest Ophthalmol Vis Sci* 36:1107–1114, 1995.

Hodes RJ. Aging and the immune system. *Immunol Rev* 160:5–8, 1997.

Hodes RJ. Telomere length, aging, and somatic cell turnover. *J Exp Med* 190:153–156, 1999.

Hodes RJ. Molecular targeting of cancer: telomeres as targets. *Proc Natl Acad Sci USA* 98:7649–7651, 2001.

Hodes RJ, Cahan V, Pruzan M. The National Institute on Aging at its twentieth anniversary: achievements and promise of research on aging. *J Am Geriatr Soc* 44:204–206, 1996a.

Hodes RJ, Hathcock KS, Weng NP. Telomeres in T and B cells. *Nat Rev Immunol* 2:699–706, 2002.

Hodes RJ, McCormick AM, Pruzan M. Longevity assurance genes: how do they influence aging and life span? *J Am Geriatr Soc* 44:988–991, 1996b.

Hoeg JM. Can genes prevent atherosclerosis? *JAMA* 276:989–992, 1996.

Hoeijmakers JH. Genome maintenance mechanisms for preventing cancer. *Nature* 411:366–374, 2001.

Hollenberg NK, Adams DF, Solomon HS, Rashid A, Abrams HL, Merrill JP. Senescence and the renal vasculature in normal man. *Circ Res* 34:309–316, 1974.

Holliday R. Neoplastic transformation: the contrasting stability of human and mouse cells. *Cancer Surv* 28:103–115, 1996.

Holliday R, Huschtscha LI, Tarrant GM, Kirkwood TBL. Testing the commitment theory of cellular aging. *Science* 198:366–372, 1977.

Holliday R, Porterfield JS, Gibbs DD. Premature ageing and occurrence of altered enzyme in Werner's syndrome fibroblasts. *Nature* 248:762–763, 1974.

Holloszy JO. The biology of aging. *Mayo Clin Proc* 75(Suppl):S3–8; discussion S8–9, 2000.

Holt SE, Aisner DL, Baur J, Tesmer VM, Dy M, Ouellette M, Trager JB, Morin GB, Toft DO, Shay JW, Wright WE, White MA. Functional requirement of p23 and Hsp90 in telomerase complexes. *Genes Dev* 13:817–826, 1999a.

Holt SE, Aisner DL, Shay JW, Wright WE. Lack of cell cycle regulation of telomerase activity in human cells. *Proc Natl Acad Sci USA* 94:10687–10692, 1997a.

Holt SE, Glinsky VV, Ivanova AB, Glinsky GV. Resistance to apoptosis in human cells conferred by telomerase function and telomere stability. *Mol Carcinog* 25:241–248, 1999b.

Holt SE, Shay JW. Role of telomerase in cellular proliferation and cancer. *J Cell Physiol* 180:10–18, 1999.

Holt SE, Shay JW, Wright WE. Refining the telomere-telomerase hypothesis of aging and cancer. *Nat Biotechnol* 14:836–839, 1996a.

Holt SE, Wright WE, Shay JW. Regulation of telomerase activity in immortal cell lines. *Mol Cell Biol* 16:2932–2939, 1996b.

Holt SE, Wright WE, Shay JW. Multiple pathways for the regulation of telomerase activity. *Eur J Cancer* 33:761–766, 1997b.

Holyoake TL, Jiang X, Drummond MW, Eaves AC, Eaves CJ. Elucidating critical mechanisms of deregulated stem cell turnover in the chronic phase of chronic myeloid leukemia. *Leukemia* 16:549–558, 2002.

Holz FG, Schutt F, Kopitz J, Volcker HE. Introduction of the lipofuscin-fluorophor A2E into the lysosomal compartment of human retinal pigment epithelial cells by coupling to LDL particles. An in vitro model of retinal pigment epithelium cell aging [in German]. *Ophthalmologe* 96:781–785, 1999.

The Homocysteine Studies Collaboration. Homocysteine and risk of ischemic heart disease and stroke. *JAMA* 288:2015–2022, 2002.

Honda S, Hjelmeland LM, Handa JT. Oxidative stress–induced single-strand breaks in chromosomal telomeres of human retinal pigment epithelial cells in vitro. *Invest Ophthalmol Vis Sci* 42:2139–2144, 2001.

Honda T, Sadamori N, Oshimura M, Horikawa I, Omura H, Komatsu K, Watanabe M. Spontaneous immortalization of cultured skin fibroblasts obtained from a high-dose atomic bomb survivor. *Mutat Res* 354:15–26, 1996.

Honda Y, Honda S. The *daf-2* gene network for longevity regulates oxidative stress resistance and Mn-superoxide dismutase gene expression in *Caenorhabditis elegans*. *FASEB J* 13:1385–1393, 1999.

Hood JD, Bednarski M, Frausto R, Guccione S, Reisfeld RA, Xiang R, Cheresh DA. Tumor regression by targeted gene delivery to the neovasculature. *Science* 287:2404–2407, 2003.

Hoogendoorn D. Observations on the current status concerning the epidemic of acute myocardial infarction [in Dutch]. *Ned Tijdschr Geneeskd* 134:592–595, 1990.

Hooijberg E, Ruizendaal JJ, Snijders PJ, Kueter EW, Walboomers JM, Spits H. Immortalization of human CD8+ T cell clones by ectopic expression of telomerase reverse transcriptase. *J Immunol* 165:4239–4245, 2000.

Hook DW, Harding JJ. Protection of enzymes by alpha-crystallin acting as a molecular chaperone. *Int J Biol Macromol* 22:295–306, 1998.

Hopkins GM. *Poems and Prose*. Penguin Books, London, 1985.

Hoppenreijs VPT, Pels E, Vrensen GFJM, Treffers WF. Effects of platelet-derived growth factor on endothelial wound healing of human corneas. *Invest Ophthalmol Vis Sci* 35:150–161, 1994.

Horikawa I, Cable PL, Afshari C, Barrett JC. Cloning and characterization of the promoter region of human telomerase reverse transcriptase gene. *Cancer Res* 59:826–830, 1999.

Horikawa I, Oshimura M, Barrett JC. Repression of the telomerase catalytic subunit by a gene on human chromosome 3 that induces cellular senescence. *Mol Carcinog* 22:65–72, 1998.

Horiuchi M, Akishita M, Dzau VJ. Molecular and cellular mechanism of angiotensin II–mediated apoptosis. *Endocr Res* 24:307–314, 1998.

Horner PJ, Gage FH. Regenerating the damaged central nervous system. *Nature* 407:963–970, 2000.

Hornsby PJ. Cloning of animals from senescent cell nuclei—what are the implications for aging research? *Mech Ageing Dev* 115:123–126, 2000.

Hornsby PJ. Cell proliferation in mammalian aging. In Masoro EJ, Austad SN (eds). *Handbook of the Biology of Aging, 5th ed*. Academic Press, New York, 2001, pp 207–245.

Hornsby PJ. Cellular senescence and tissue aging in vivo. *J Gerontol A Biol Sci Med Sci* 57A:B251–256, 2002.

Hosenpud JD, Greenberg BH. *Congestive Heart Failure*. Lippincott Williams & Wilkins, Philadelphia, 2000.

Hosokawa M, Ueno M. Aging of blood–brain barrier and neuronal cells of eye and ear in SAM mice. *Neurobiol Aging* 20:117–123, 1999.

Howard BH. Replicative senescence: considerations relating to the stability of heterochromatin domains. *Exp Gerontol* 31:281–293, 1996.

Howlett DR, George AR, Owen DE, Ward RV, Markwell RE. Common structural features determine the effectiveness of carvedilol, daunomycin and rolitetracycline as inhibitors of Alzheimer beta-amyloid fibril formation. *Biochem J* 343:419–423, 1999.

Hrabko RP, Milgrom H, Schwartz RA. Werner's syndrome with associated malignant neoplasms. *Arch Dermatol* 118:106–108, 1982.

Hsieh HF, Harn HJ, Chiu SC, Liu YC, Lui WY, Ho LI. Telomerase activity correlates with cell cycle regulators in human hepatocellular carcinoma. *Liver* 20:143–151, 2000.

Hsin H, Kenyon C. Signals from the reproductive system regulate the life span of *C. elegans*. *Nature* 399:362–366, 1999.

Hsu HL, Gilley D, Blackburn EH, Chen DJ. Ku is associated with the telomere in mammals. *Proc Natl Acad Sci USA* 96:12454–12458, 1999.

Hsueh WA, Law RE. PPAR-γ and atherosclerosis: effects on cell growth and movement. *Arterioscler Thromb Vasc Biol* 21:1891–1895, 2001.

Hu Y, Lam KY, Wan TS, Fang W, Ma ES, Chan LC, Srivastava G. Establishment and characterization of HKESC-1, a new cancer cell line from human esophageal squamous cell carcinoma. *Cancer Genet Cytogenet* 118:112–120, 2000.

Huang HS, Hwang JM, Jen YM, Lin JJ, Lee KY, Shi CH, Hsu HC. Studies on anthracenes. 1. Human telomerase inhibition and lipid peroxidation of 9-acyloxy 1,5-dichloroanthracene derivatives. *Chem Pharm Bull (Tokyo)* 49:969–973, 2001.

Huang JJ, Lin MC, Bai YX, Jing da D, Wong BC, Han SW, Lin J, Xu B, Huang CF, Kung HF. Ectopic expression of a COOH-terminal fragment of the human telomerase reverse transcriptase leads to telomere dysfunction and reduction of growth and tumorigenicity in HeLa cells. *Cancer Res* 62:3226–3232, 2002.

Huang S, Li B, Gray MD, Oshima J, Mian IS, Campisi J. The premature ageing syndrome protein, WRN, is a 3'→5' exonuclease. *Nat Genet* 20:114–116, 1998.

Huang TT, Carlson EJ, Gillespie AM, Shi Y, Epstein CJ. Ubiquitous overexpression of CuZn superoxide dismutase does not extend life span in mice. *J Gerontol A Biol Sci Med Sci* 55:B5–9, 2000.

Huang X, Atwood CS, Hartshorn MA, Multhaup G, Goldstein LE, Scarpa RC, Cuajungco MP, Gray DN, Lim J, Moir RD, Tanzi RE, Bush AI. The A beta peptide of Alzheimer's disease directly produces hydrogen peroxide through metal ion reduction. *Biochemistry* 38:7609–7616, 1999a.

Huang YS, Wu JC, Chang FY, Lee SD. Interleukin-8 and alcoholic liver disease. *Chung Hua I Hsueh Tsa Chih (Taipei)* 62:418–424, 1999b.

Hubbard K, Ozer HL. Senescence and immortalization of human cells. In Studzinski GP (ed). *Cell Growth and Apoptosis: A Practical Approach.* IRL Press, Oxford, 1995, pp 229–249.

Hubbard K, Ozer HL. Mechanisms of immortalization. AGE 22:65–70, 2000.

Hudson JD, Shoaibi MA, Maestro R, Carnero A, Hannon GJ, Beach DH. A proinflammatory cytokine inhibits p53 tumor suppressor activity. *J Exp Med* 190:1375–1382, 1999.

Huemer RP, Lee KD, Reeves AE, Bickert C. Mitochondrial studies in senescent mice — II. Specific activity, bouyant density, and turnover of mitchondrial DNA. *Exp Gerontol* 6:327–334, 1971.

Huffman KE, Levene SD, Tesmer VM, Shay JW, Wright WE. Telomere shortening is proportional to the size of the G-rich telomeric 3'-overhang. *J Biol Chem* 275:19719–19722, 2000.

Hughes TR, Morris DK, Salinger A, Walcott N, Nugent CI, Lundblad V. The role of the EST genes in yeast telomere replication. *Ciba Found Symp* 211:41–47; discussion 47–52, 71–75, 1997.

Hughes VA, Frontera WR, Wood M, Evans WJ, Dallal GE, Roubenoff R, Singh MAF. Longitudinal muscle strength changes in older adults: influence of muscle mass, physical activity, and health. *J Gerontol A Biol Sci Med Sci* 56:209–217, 2001.

Hultdin M, Gronlund E, Norrback KF, Just T, Taneja K, Roos G. Replication timing of human telomeric DNA and other repetitive sequences analyzed by fluorescence in situ hybridization and flow cytometry. *Exp Cell Res* 271:223–229, 2001.

Hulley S, Furberg C, Barrett-Connor E, Cauley J, Grady D, Haskell W, Knopp R, Lowery M, Satterfield S, Schrott H, Vittinghoff E, Hunninghake D, for the HERS Research Group. Noncardiovascular disease outcomes during 6.8 years of hormone therapy. *JAMA* 288:58–66, 2002.

Hulley S, Grady D, Bush T, Furberg C, Herrington D, Riggs B, Vittinghoff E. Randomized trial of estrogen plus progestin for secondary prevention of coronary heart disease in postmenopausal women. *JAMA* 280:605–613, 1998.

Humphreys D, Eggan K, Akutsu H, Hochedlinger K, Rideout WMIII, Biniszkiewicz D, Yanagimachi R, Jaenisch R. Epigenetic instability in ES cells and cloned mice. *Science* 293:95–97, 2001.

Hunt BJ. The endothelium in atherogenesis. *Lupus* 9:189–193, 2000.

Huo Y, Ley K. Adhesion molecules and atherogenesis. *Acta Physiol Scand* 173:35–43, 2001.

Huppert FA, Van Niekerk JK, Herbert J. Dehydroepiandrosterone (DHEA) supplementation for cognition and well-being. *Cochrane Database Syst Rev* 2:CD000304, 2000.

Hur K, Gazdar AF, Rathi A, Jang JJ, Choi JH, Kim DY. Overexpression of human telomerase RNA in *Helicobacter pylori*–infected human gastric mucosa. *Jpn J Cancer Res* 91:1148–1153, 2000.

Hurley BF. Age, gender, and muscular strength. *J Gerontol A Biol Sci Med Sci* 50(Spec No):41–44, 1995.

Hurwitz AA, Foster BA, Kwon ED, Truong T, Choi EM, Greenberg NM, Burg MB, Allison JP. Combination immunotherapy of primary prostate cancer in a transgenic mouse model using CTLA-4 blockade. *Cancer Res* 60:2444–2448, 2000.

Huschtscha LI, Reddel RR. p16(INK4a) and the control of cellular proliferative life span. *Carcinogenesis* 20:921–926, 1999.

Husmann I, Soulet L, Gautron J, Martelly I, Barritault D. Growth factors in skeletal muscle regeneration. *Cytokine Growth Factor Rev* 7:249–258, 1996.

Hutchinson EW, Rose MR. Quantitative genetics of postponed aging in *Drosophila melanogaster*. I. Analysis of outbred populations. *Genetics* 127:719–727, 1991.

Hutchinson EW, Shaw AJ, Rose MR Quantitative genetics of postponed aging in *Drosophila melanogaster*. II. Analysis of selected lines. *Genetics* 127:729–737, 1991.

Hutchinson J. Congenital absence of hair and mammary glands, with atrophic condition of the skin and its appendages in a boy. *Medicochir Trans* 69:473–477, 1886.

Hutter E, Unterluggauer H, Uberall F, Schramek H, Jansen-Durr P. Replicative senescence of human fibroblasts: the role of Ras-dependent signaling and oxidative stress. *Exp Gerontol* 37:1165–1174, 2002.

Hwang ES. Replicative senescence and senescence-like state induced in cancer-derived cells. *Mech Ageing Dev* 123:1681–1694, 2002.

Hwang JJ, Dzau VJ, Liew CC. Genomics and the pathophysiology of heart failure. *Curr Cardiol Rep* 3:198–207, 2001a.

Hwang MG, Chung IK, Kang BG, Cho MH. Sequence-specific binding property of *Arabidopsis thaliana* telomeric DNA binding protein 1 (AtTBP1). *FEBS Lett* 503:35–40, 2001b.

Hytiroglou P, Kotoula V, Thung SN, Tsokos M, Fiel MI, Papadimitriou CS. Telomerase activity in precancerous hepatic nodules. *Cancer* 82:1831–1838, 1998.

Ichimiya S, Nakagawara A, Sakuma Y, Kimura S, Ikeda T, Satoh M, Takahashi N, Sato N, Mori M. p73: structure and function. *Pathol Int* 50:589–593, 2000.

Ide T, Tahara H. Telomerase [in Japanese]. *Gan To Kagaku Ryoho* 23:247–256, 1996.

Ide T, Tahara H, Nakashio R, Kitamoto M, Nakanishi T, Kajiyama G. Telomerase in hepatocellular carcinogenesis. *Hum Cell* 9:283–286, 1996.

Idei T, Sakamoto H, Yamamoto T. Terminal restriction fragments of telomere are detectable in plasma and their length correlates with clinical status of ovarian cancer patients. *J Intern Med Res* 30:244–250, 2002.

Iida A, Yamaguchi A, Hirose K. Telomerase activity in colorectal cancer and its relationship to bcl-2 expression. *J Surg Oncol* 73:219–223, 2000.

Iki K, Tsujiuchi T, Majima T, Sakitani H, Tsutsumi M, Takahama M, Yoshimoto M, Nakae D, Tsunoda T, Konishi Y. Increased telomerase activity in intrahepatic cholangiocellular carcinomas induced by *N*-nitrosobis(2-oxopropyl)amine in hamsters. *Cancer Lett* 131:185–190, 1998.

Imai S, Armstrong CM, Kaeberlein M, Guarente L. Transcriptional silencing and longevity protein Sir2 is an NAD-dependent histone deacetylase. *Nature* 403:795–800, 2000.

Imai S, Kitano H. Heterochromatin islands and their dynamic reorganization: a hypothesis for three distinctive features of cellular aging. *Exp Gerontol* 33:555–570, 1998.

Ingram DK, Cutler RG, Weindruch R, Renquist DM, Knapka JJ, April M, Belcher CT, Clark MA, Hatcherson CD, Marriott BM, et al. Dietary restriction and aging: the initiation of a primate study. *J Gerontol* 45:B148–163, 1990.

Ingram DK, Lane MA, Cutler RG, Roth GS. Longitudinal study of aging in monkeys: effects of diet restriction. *Neurobiol Aging* 14:687–688, 1993.

Ingvarsson T, Stefansson SE, Gulcher JR, Jonsson HH, Jonsson H, Frigge ML, Palsdottir E, Olafsdottir G, Jonsdottir T, Walters GB, Lohmander LS, Stefansson K. A large Icelandic family with early osteoarthritis of the hip associated with a susceptibility locus on chromosome 16p. *Arthritis Rheum* 44:2548–2555, 2001.

Inoue H, Tsuchida A, Kawasaki Y, Fujimoto Y, Yamasaki S, Kajiyama G. Preoperative diagnosis of intraductal papillary-mucinous tumors of the pancreas with attention to telomerase activity. *Cancer* 91:35–41, 2001.

Inoue K, Wen R, Rehg JE, Adachi M, Cleveland JL, Roussel MF, Sherr CJ. Disruption of the ARF transcriptional activator DMP1 facilitates cell immortalization, Ras transformation, and tumorigenesis. *Genes Dev* 14:1797–1809, 2000.

Inui A. Cancer anorexia-cachexia syndrome: current issues in research and management. *CA Cancer J Clin* 52:72–91, 2002.

Inui T, Shinomiya N, Fukasawa M, Kobayashi M, Kuranaga N, Ohkura S, Seki S. Growth-related signaling regulates activation of telomerase in regenerating hepatocytes. *Exp Cell Res* 273:147–156, 2002.

Iordanescu C, Denislam D, Avram E, Chiru A, Busuioc M, Cioabla D. Ocular manifestations in progeria [in Romanian]. *Oftalmologia* 39:56–57, 1995.

Irizarry MC, Kim TW, McNamara M, Tanzi RE, George JM, Clayton DF, Hyman BT. Characterization of the precursor protein of the non-A beta component of senile plaques (NACP) in the human central nervous system. *J Neuropathol Exp Neurol* 55:889–895, 1996.

Irving J, Feng J, Wistrom C, Pikaart M, Villeponteau B. An altered repertoire of fos/jun (AP-1) at the onset of replicative senescence. *Exp Cell Res* 202:161–166, 1992.

Ishibe N, Prieto D, Hosack DA, Lempicki RA, Goldin LR, Raffeld M, Marti GE, Caporaso NE. Telomere length and heavy-chain mutation status in familial chronic lymphocytic leukemia. *Leuk Res* 26:791–794, 2002.

Ishii K, Yang WL, Cvijic ME, Kikuchi Y, Nagata I, Chin KV. Telomere shortening by cisplatin in yeast nucleotide excision repair mutant. *Exp Cell Res* 255:95–101, 2000.

Ishii T. Progeria: autopsy report of one case, with a review of pathologic findings reported in the literature. *J Am Geriatr Soc* 24:193–202, 1976.

Ishii T, Hosoda Y. Werner's syndrome: autopsy report of one case, with a review of pathologic findings reported in the literature. *J Am Geriatr Soc* 23:145–154, 1975.

Ishii Y, Tsuyama N, Maeda S, Tahara H, Ide T. Telomerase activity in hybrids between telomerase-negative and telomerase-positive immortal human cells is repressed in the different complementation groups but not in the same complementation group of immortality. *Mech Ageing Dev* 110:175–193, 1999.

Ishikawa F. Regulation mechanisms of mammalian telomerase. A review. *Biochemistry (Mosc)* 62:1332–1337, 1997.

Ishikawa F. Aging clock: the watchmaker's masterpiece. *Cell Mol Life Sci* 57:698–704, 2000a.

Ishikawa F. Cellular senescence and chromosome telomeres [in Japanese]. *Nippon Ronen Igakkai Zasshi* 37:19–25, 2000b.

Ishikawa F, Naito T. Why do we have linear chromosomes? A matter of Adam and Eve. *Mutat Res* 434:99–107, 1999.

Itahana K, Zou Y, Itahana Y, Martinez JL, Beausejour C, Jacobs JJ, Van Lohuizen M, Band V, Campisi J, Dimri GP. Control of the replicative life span of human fibroblasts by p16 and the polycomb protein Bmi-1. *Mol Cell Biol* 23:389–401, 2003.

Ito H, Kyo S, Kanaya T, Takakura M, Inoue M, Namiki M. Expression of human telomerase subunits and correlation with telomerase activity in urothelial cancer. *Clin Cancer Res* 4:1603–1608, 1998a.

Ito H, Kyo S, Kanaya T, Takakura M, Koshida K, Namiki M, Inoue M. Detection of human telomerase reverse transcriptase messenger RNA in voided urine samples as a useful diagnostic tool for bladder cancer. *Clin Cancer Res* 4:2807–2810, 1998b.

Itoi T, Ohyashiki K, Yahata N, Shinohara Y, Takei K, Takeda K, Nagao K, Hisatomi H, Ebihara Y, Shay JW, Saito T. Detection of telomerase activity in exfoliated cancer cells obtained from bile. *Int J Oncol* 15:1061–1067, 1999.

Itoi T, Shinohara Y, Takeda K, Takei K, Ohno H, Ohyashiki K, Yahata N, Ebihara Y, Saito T. Detection of telomerase activity in biopsy specimens for diagnosis of biliary tract cancers. *Gastrointest Endosc* 52:380–386, 2000.

Ivessa AS, Zhou JQ, Zakian VA. The *Saccharomyces* Pif1p DNA helicase and the highly related Rrm3p have opposite effects on replication fork progression in ribosomal DNA. *Cell* 100:479–489, 2000.

Iwama H, Ohyashiki K, Ohyashiki JH, Hayashi S, Kawakubo K, Shay JW, Toyama K. The relationship between telomere length and therapy-associated cytogenetic responses in patients with chronic myeloid leukemia. *Cancer* 79:1552–1560, 1997.

Iwama H, Ohyashiki K, Ohyashiki JH, Hayashi S, Yahata N, Ando K, Toyama K, Hoshika A, Takasaki M, Mori M, Shay JW. Telomeric length and telomerase activity vary with age in peripheral blood cells obtained from normal individuals. *Hum Genet* 102:397–402, 1998.

Iwao T, Hiyama E, Yokoyama T, Tsuchida A, Hiyama K, Murakami Y, Shimamoto F, Shay JW, Kajiyama G. Telomerase activity for the preoperative diagnosis of pancreatic cancer. *J Natl Cancer Inst* 89:1621–1623, 1997.

Iwao T, Tsuchida A, Hiyama E, Kajiyama G. Telomerase activity in pancreatic juice for the preoperative diagnosis of pancreatic cancer [in Japanese]. *Nippon Rinsho* 56:1229–1233, 1998.

Iwasaka T, Zheng PS, Yokoyama M, Fukuda K, Nakao Y, Sugimori H. Telomerase activation in cervical neoplasia. *Obstet Gynecol* 91:260–262, 1998.

Iwata N, Tsubuki S, Takaki Y, Shirotani K, Lu B, Gerard NP, Gerard C, Hama E, Lee H-J, Saido TC. Metabolic regulation of brain Aβ by neprilysin. *Science* 292:1550–1552, 2001.

Izbicka E, Barnes LD, Robinson AK, Davidson KK, Lawrence RA, Hannibal GT. Alterations in DNA repair and telomere maintenance mechanism affect response to porphyrins in yeast. *Anticancer Res* 21:1899–1903, 2001.

Izbicka E, Sommer E, Skopinska-Rozewska E, Davidson K, Wu RS, Orlowski T, Pastewka K. Tetracationic porphyrins inhibit angiogenesis induced by human tumor cells in vivo. *Anticancer Res* 20:3205–3210, 2000.

Izumi H, Hara T, Oga A, Matsuda K, Sato Y, Naito K, Sasaki K. High telomerase activity correlates with the stabilities of genome and DNA ploidy in renal cell carcinoma. *Neoplasia* 4:103–111, 2002.

Jacks T, Weinberg RA. Cell-cycle control and its watchman. *Nature* 381:643–644, 1996.

Jacob NK, Skopp R, Price CM. G-overhang dynamics at *Tetrahymena* telomeres. *EMBO J* 20:4299–4308, 2001.

Jacobs JJ, Kieboom K, Marino S, DePinho RA, van Lohuizen M. The oncogene and Polycomb-group gene *bmi-1* regulates cell proliferation and senescence through the ink4a locus. *Nature* 397:164–168, 1999.

Jacobson HG, Rifkin H, Zucker-Franklin D. Werner's syndrome: a clinical-roentgen entity. *Radiology* 74:373–385, 1960.

Jaeger V, Schneider-Stock R, Gerresheim F, Epplen JT, Serra M, Lippert H, Roessner A. Myxoid liposarcoma with transition to round-cell lesion-cell cycle regulator genes and telomerase activity characterizing tumor progression: a case report. *Hum Pathol* 30:1515–1519, 1999.

James SE, Faragher RG, Burke JF, Shall S, Mayne LV. Werner's syndrome T lymphocytes display a normal in vitro life span. *Mech Ageing Dev* 121:139–149, 2001.

Jampol LM, Ferris FL, Antioxidants and zinc to prevent progression of age-related macular degeneration. *JAMA* 286:2466–2468, 2001.

Janeway CA, Travers P. *The Immune System in Health and Disease*. Garland Publishing, New York, 1997.

Jansen-Durr P. The making and the breaking of senescence: changes of gene expression during cellular aging and immortalization. *Exp Gerontol* 33:291–301, 1998.

Jantzen PT, Connor KE, DiCarlo G, Wenk GL, Wallace JL, Rojiani AM, Coppola D, Morgan D, Gordon MN. Microglial activation and beta-amyloid deposit reduction caused by a nitric oxide-releasing nonsteroidal anti-inflammatory drug in amyloid precursor protein plus presenilin-1 transgenic mice. *J Neurosci* 22:2246–2254, 2002.

Jarman P, Wood N. Parkinson's disease genetics comes of age. *BMJ* 318:1641–1642, 1999.

Jazwinski SM. Longevity, genes, and aging. *Science* 273:54–59, 1996.

Jazwinski SM. Aging and longevity genes. *Acta Biochim Pol* 47:269–279, 2000a.

Jazwinski SM. Coordination of metabolic activity and stress resistance in yeast longevity. *Results Probl Cell Differ* 9:21–44, 2000b.

Jazwinski SM. Metabolic control and ageing. *Trends Genet* 16:506–511, 2000c.

Jazwinski SM. Metabolic control and gene dysregulation in yeast aging. *Ann NY Acad Sci* 908:21–30, 2000d.

Jazwinski SM. Metabolic mechanisms of yeast ageing. *Exp Gerontol* 35:671–676, 2000e.

Jazwinski SM. Commentary on "applying hormesis in aging research and therapy". *Belle Newsletter* 9:10, 2001.

Jazwinski SM, Howard BH, Nayak RK. Cell cycle progression, aging, and cell death. *J Gerontol A Biol Sci Med Sci* 50A:B1–8, 1995.

Jeanclos E, Schork NJ, Kyvik KO, Kimura M, Skurnick JH, Aviv A. Telomere length inversely correlates with pulse pressure and is highly familial. *Hypertension* 36:195–200, 2000.

Jeanson L, Mouscadet JF. Ku represses the HIV-1 transcription: identification of a putative Ku binding site homologous to the MMTV NRE1 sequence in the HIV-1 LTR. *J Biol Chem* 277:4918–4924, 2002.

Jee SH, Suh I, Kim IS, Appel, LJ. Smoking and atherosclerotic cardiovascular disease in men with low levels of serum cholesterol. The Korea Medical Insurance Corporation Study. *JAMA* 282:2149–2155, 1999.

Jenkins TC. Targeting multi-stranded DNA structures. *Curr Med Chem* 7:99–115, 2000.

Jentsch S, Tobler H, Muller F. New telomere formation during the process of chromatin diminution in *Ascaris suum*. *Int J Dev Biol* 46:143–148, 2002.

Jenuwein T, Allis CD. Translating the histone code. *Science* 293:1074–1080, 2001.

Jha KK, Banga S, Palejwala V, Ozer HL. SV40-mediated immortalization. *Exp Cell Res* 245:1–7, 1998.

Jiang D, Fei RG, Pendergrass WR, Wolf NS. An age-related reduction in the replicative capacity of two murine hematopoietic stroma cell types. *Exp Hematol* 20:1216–1222, 1992.

Jiang JC, Jaruga E, Repnevskaya MV, Jazwinski SM. An intervention resembling caloric restriction prolongs life span and retards aging in yeast. *FASEB J* 14:2135–2137, 2000.

Jiang XR, Jimenez G, Chang E, Frolkis M, Kusler B, Sage M, Beeche M, Bodnar AG, Wahl GM, Tlsty TD, Chiu CP. Telomerase expression in human somatic cells does not induce changes associated with a transformed phenotype. *Nat Genet* 21:111–114, 1999.

Jick H, Zornberg GL, Jick SS, Seshadri S, Drachman DA. Statins and the risk of dementia. *Lancet* 356:1627–1631, 2000.

Jin S, Zhang W, Teng M. Clinical implications of telomerase activity in breast cancer fine-needle aspirates [in Chinese]. *Zhonghua Zhong Liu Za Zhi* 22:132–134, 2000.

Jin S, Zhang W, Teng M, Zhang Z, Liu Y, Li M, Qu P, Wang S, Jin Y, Wang H, Pan Q, Liu S. Significance of telomerase activity detection by fine-needle aspiration in patients with breast cancer [in Chinese]. *Zhonghua Bing Li Xue Za Zhi* 28:334–336, 1999.

Joaquin AM, Gollapudi S. Functional decline in aging and disease: a role for apoptosis. *J Am Geriatr Soc* 49:1234–1240, 2001.

Joenje H. Genetic toxicology of oxygen. *Mutat Res* 219:193–208, 1989.

Johnsen S. Transparent animals. *Sci Am* 282:80–89, 2000.

Johnson FB, Marciniak RA, Guarente L. Telomeres, the nucleolus and aging. *Curr Opin Cell Biol* 10:332–338, 1998.

Johnson FB, Marciniak RA, McVey M, Stewart SA, Hahn WC, Guarente L. The *Saccharomyces cerevisiae* WRN homolog Sgs1p participates in telomere maintenance in cells lacking telomerase. *EMBO J* 20:905–913, 2001a.

Johnson M, Dimitrov D, Vojta PJ, Barrett JC, Noda A, Pereira-Smith OM, Smith JR. Evidence for a p53-independent pathway for upregulation of SDI1/CIP1/WAF1/p21 RNA in human cells. *Mol Carcinog* 11:59–64, 1994.

Johnson TE. Aging can be genetically dissected into component processes using long lived lines of *Caenorhabditis elegans*. *Proc Natl Acad Sci USA* 84:3777–3781, 1987.

Johnson TE. Genetic influences on aging. *Exp Gerontol* 32:11–22, 1997.

Johnson TE, Wu D, Tedesco P, Dames S, Vaupel JW. Age-specific demographic profiles of longevity mutants in *Caenorhabditis elegans* show segmental effects. *J Gerontol A Biol Sci Med Sci* 56:B331–339, 2001b.

Johnston CC Jr, Bjarnason NH, Cohen FJ, Shah A, Lindsay R, Mitlak BH, Huster W, Draper MW, Harper KD, Heath H 3rd, Gennari C, Christiansen C, Arnaud CD, Delmas PD. Long-term effects of raloxifene on bone mineral density, bone turnover, and serum lipid levels in early postmenopausal women: three-year data from 2 double-blind, randomized, placebo-controlled trials. *Arch Intern Med* 160:3444–3450, 2000a.

Johnston MV, Trescher WH, Ishida A, Nakajima W. Novel treatments after experimental brain injury. *Semin Neonatol* 5:75–86, 2000b.

Johnston S, Stebbing J. Breast cancer: metastatic. *Clin Evidence* 3:846–862, 2000.

Jonas JB, Ruprecht KW, Schmitz-Valckenberg P, Brambring D, Platt D, Gebhart E, Schacht-schabel DO, Naumann GO. Ophthalmic surgical complications in Werner's syndrome: report of 18 eyes of nine patients. *Ophthalmic Surg* 18:760–764, 1987.

Jones CJ, Soley A, Skinner JW, Gupta J, Haughton MF, Wyllie FS, Schlumberger M, Bacchetti S, Wynford-Thomas D. Dissociation of telomere dynamics from telomerase activity in human thyroid cancer cells. *Exp Cell Res* 240:333–339, 1998.

Jones KL, Smith DW, Harvey MA, Hall BD, Quan L. Older paternal age and fresh gene mutation: data on additional disorders. *J Pediatr* 86:84–88, 1975.

Jones N. Soothing the brain [news and analysis]. *Sci Am* 282:24, 2000.

Jones SJ, Riddle DL, Pouzyrev AT, Velculescu VE, Hillier L, Eddy SR, Stricklin SL, Baillie DL, Waterston R, Marra MA. Changes in gene expression associated with developmental arrest and longevity in *Caenorhabditis elegans*. *Genome Res* 11:1346–1352, 2001.

Jorgensen HG, Holyoake TL. A comparison of normal and leukemic stem cell biology in chronic myeloid leukemia. *Hematol Oncol* 19:89–106, 2001.

Joseph JA. The putative role of free radicals in the loss of neuronal functioning in senescence. *Integr Physiol Behav Sci* 27:216–227, 1992.

Joshi VV, Tsongalis GJ. Correlation between morphologic and nonmorphologic prognostic markers of neuroblastoma. *Ann NY Acad Sci* 824:71–83, 1997.

Joyce CA, Dennis NR, Cooper S, Browne CE. Subtelomeric rearrangements: results from a study of selected and unselected probands with idiopathic mental retardation and control individuals by using high-resolution G-banding and FISH. *Hum Genet* 109:440–451, 2001.

Juengst E, Fossel M. The ethics of embryonic stem cells: now and forever, cells without end. *JAMA* 284:3180–3184, 2000.

Jung D, Neron S, Lemieux R, Roy A, Richard M. Telomere-independent reduction of human B lymphocyte: proliferation during long-term culture. *Immunol Invest* 30:157–168, 2001.

Jyoti V, Gadekar HA, Harchandani K. Progeria. *Indian Pediatr* 18:827–828, 1981.

Kadar A, Glasz T. Development of atherosclerosis and plaque biology. *Cardiovasc Surg* 9:109–121, 2001.

Kadenbach B, Bender E, Reith A, Becker A, Hammershmidt S, Lee I, Arnold S, Huttemann M. Possible influence of metabolic activity on aging. *J Anti-Aging Med* 2:255–264, 1999.

Kado DM, Browner WS, Palermo L, Nevitt MC, Genant HK, Cummings SR. Vertebral fractures and mortality in older women: a prospective study. *Arch Intern Med* 159:1215–1220, 1999.

Kaeberlein M, McVey M, Guarente L. The SIR2/3/4 complex and SIR2 alone promote longevity in *Saccharomyces cerevisiae* by two different mechanisms. *Genes Dev* 13:2570–2580, 1999.

Kagawa Y, Cha SH, Hasegawa K, Hamamoto T, Endo H. Regulation of energy metabolism in human cells in aging and diabetes: FoF(1), mtDNA, UCP, and ROS. *Biochem Biophys Res Commun* 266:662–676, 1999.

Kaji EJ, Leiden JM. Gene and stem cell therapies. *JAMA* 285: 545–550, 2001.

Kajstura J, Pertoldi B, Leri A, Beltrami CA, Deptala A, Darzynkiewicz Z, Anversa P. Telomere shortening is an in vivo marker of myocyte replication and aging. *Am J Pathol* 156:813–819, 2000.

Kakeji Y, Maehara Y, Koga T, Shibahara K, Kabashima A, Tokunaga E, Sugimachi K. Gastric cancer with high telomerase activity shows rapid development and invasiveness. *Oncol Rep* 8:107–110, 2001.

Kakizoe T. Asian studies of cancer chemoprevention: latest clinical results. *Eur J Cancer* 36:1303–1309, 2000.

Kakuo S, Asaoka K, Ide T. Human is a unique species among primates in terms of telomere length. *Biochem Biophys Res Commun* 263:308–314, 1999.

Kala DN, Orhii PB, Chen C, Lee DY, Hubbard GB, Lee S, Olatunji-Bello Y. Aged-rodent models of long-term growth hormone therapy: lack of deleterious effect on longevity. *J Gerontol A Biol Sci Med Sci.* 53:452–463, 1998.

Kalaria RN. Cerebral vessels in ageing and Alzheimer's disease. *Pharmacol Ther* 72:193–214, 1996.

Kalidas M, Kantarjian H, Talpaz M. Chronic myelogenous leukemia. *JAMA* 286:895–898, 2001.

Kallassy M, Martel N, Damour O, Yamasaki H, Nakazawa H. Growth arrest of immortalized human keratinocytes and suppression of telomerase activity by *p21WAF1* gene expression. *Mol Carcinog* 21:26–36, 1998.

Kalous M, Drahota Z. The role of mitochondria in aging. *Physiol Res* 45:351–359, 1996.

Kameshima H, Yagihashi A, Yajima T, Kobayashi D, Denno R, Hirata K, Watanabe N. *Helicobacter pylori* infection: augmentation of telomerase activity in cancer and noncancerous tissues. *World J Surg* 24:1243–1249, 2000.

Kameshima H, Yagihashi A, Yajima T, Kobayashi D, Hirata K, Watanabe N. Expression of telomerase-associated genes: reflection of telomerase activity in gastric cancer? *World J Surg* 25:285–289, iv, 2001.

Kaminer MS, Gilchrest BA. Aging of the skin. In Hazzard WR, Bierman EL, Blass JP, Ettinger WH Jr, Halter JB. *Principles of Geriatric Medicine and Gerontology, 3rd ed.* McGraw-Hill, New York, 1994, 411–429.

Kamma H, Fujimoto M, Fujiwara M, Matsui M, Horiguchi H, Hamasaki M, Satoh H. Interaction of hnRNP A2/B1 isoforms with telomeric ssDNA and the in vitro function. *Biochem Biophys Res Commun* 280:625–360, 2001.

Kammori M, Nakamura K, Kanauchi H, Obara T, Kawahara M, Mimura Y, Kaminishi M, Takubo K. Consistent decrease in telomere length in parathyroid tumors but alteration in telomerase activity limited to malignancies: preliminary report. *World J Surg* 26:1083–1087, 2002a.

Kammori M, Nakamura K, Kawahara M, Mimura Y, Kaminishi M, Takubo K. Telomere shortening with aging in human thyroid and parathyroid tissue. *Exp Gerontol* 37:513–521, 2002b.

Kamnert I, Lopez CC, Rosen M, Edstrom JE. Telomeres terminating with long complex tandem repeats. *Hereditas* 127:175–180, 1997.

Kamohara Y, Kanematsu T. Treatment of liver cancer: current status and future prospectives [in Japanese]. *Gan To Kagaku Ryoho* 27:987–992, 2000.

Kanai A, Kaufman HE. Electron microscopic studies of corneal stroma: aging changes of collagen fibers. *Ann Ophthalmol* 5:285–292, 1973.

Kanamaru T, Morita Y, Itoh T, Yamamoto M, Kuroda Y, Hisatomi H. Surgical significance of telomerase activity in noncancerous liver tissue from patients with hepatocellular carcinoma. *Jpn J Cancer Res* 89:727–732, 1998.

Kanamaru T, Yamamoto M, Morita Y, Itoh T, Kuroda Y, Hisatomi H. Clinical implications of telomerase activity in resected hepatocellular carcinoma. *Int J Mol Med* 4:267–271, 1999.

Kanaya T, Kyo S, Hamada K, Takakura M, Kitagawa Y, Harada H, Inoue M. Adenoviral expression of p53 represses telomerase activity through down-regulation of human telomerase reverse transcriptase transcription. *Clin Cancer Res* 6:1239–1247, 2000.

Kanaya T, Kyo S, Takakura M, Ito H, Namiki M, Inoue M. hTERT is a critical determinant of telomerase activity in renal-cell carcinoma. *Int J Cancer* 78:539–543, 1998.

Kanazawa Y, Ohkawa K, Ueda K, Mita E, Takehara T, Sasaki Y, Kasahara A, Hayashi N. Hammerhead ribozyme-mediated inhibition of telomerase activity in extracts of human hepatocellular carcinoma cells. *Biochem Biophys Res Commun* 225:570–576, 1996.

Kaneda Y, Morishita R, Dzau VJ. Prevention of restenosis by gene therapy. *Ann NY Acad Sci* 811:299–308; discussion 308–310, 1997.

Kaneko H, Morimoto W, Fukao T, Kasahara K, Kondo N. Telomerase activity in cell lines and lymphoma originating from Bloom syndrome. *Leuk Lymphoma* 42:757–760, 2001.

Kaneko T, Tahara S, Matsuo M. Non-linear accumulation of 8'-hydroxy-2'-deoxyguanosine, a marker of oxidized DNA damage, during aging. *Mutat Res* 316:277–285, 1996.

Kaneko Y, Knudson AG. Mechanism and relevance of ploidy in neuroblastoma. *Genes Chromosomes Cancer* 29:89–95, 2000.

Kang HK, Kim MS, Kim ND, Yoo MA, Kim KW, Kim J, Ikeno Y, Yu BP, Chung HY. Down-regulation of telomerase in rat during the aging process. *Mol Cells* 9:286–291, 1999.

Kang MK, Guo W, Park NH. Replicative senescence of normal human oral keratinocytes is associated with the loss of telomerase activity without shortening of telomeres. *Cell Growth Differ* 9:85–95, 1998.

Kang MK, Park NH. Conversion of normal to malignant phenotype: telomere shortening, telomerase activation, and genomic instability during immortalization of human oral keratinocytes. *Crit Rev Oral Biol Med* 12:38–54, 2001.

Kang MK, Swee J, Kim RH, Baluda MA, Park NH. The telomeric length and heterogeneity decrease with age in normal human oral keratinocytes. *Mech Ageing Dev* 123:585–592, 2002.

Kanzaki Y, Onoue F, Ishikawa F, Ide T. Telomerase rescues the expression levels of keratinocyte growth factor and insulin-like growth factor-II in senescent human fibroblasts. *Exp Cell Res* 279:321–329, 2002.

Kapahi P, Boulton ME, Kirkwood TB. Positive correlation between mammalian life span and cellular resistance to stress. *Free Radic Biol Med* 26:495–500, 1999.

Karlseder J, Broccoli D, Dai Y, Hardy S, de Lange T. p53- and ATM-dependent apoptosis induced by telomeres lacking TRF2. *Science* 283:1321–1325, 1999.

Karlseder J, Smogorzewska A, de Lange T. Senescence induced by altered telomere state, not telomere loss. *Science* 295:2446–2449, 2002.

Karow JK, Chakraverty RK, Hickson ID. The Bloom's syndrome gene product is a 3'-5' DNA helicase. *J Biol Chem* 272:30611–30614, 1997.

Kass-Eisler A, Greider CW. Recombination in telomere-length maintenance. *Trends Biochem Sci* 25:200–204, 2000.

Kassem M, Ankersen L, Eriksen EF, Clark BF, Rattan SI. Demonstration of cellular aging and senescence in serially passaged long-term cultures of human trabecular osteoblasts. *Osteoporos Int* 7:514–524, 1997.

Kassem M, Kveiborg M, Eriksen EF. Production and action of transforming growth factor-beta in human osteoblast cultures: dependence on cell differentiation and modulation by calcitriol. *Eur J Clin Invest* 30:429–437, 2000.

Katakura Y, Yamamoto K, Miyake O, Yasuda T, Uehara N, Nakata E, Kawamoto S, Shirahata S. Bidirectional regulation of telomerase activity in a subline derived from human lung adenocarcinoma. *Biochem Biophys Res Commun* 237:313–317, 1997.

Katayama S, Kitamura K, Lehmann A, Nikaido O, Toda T. Fission yeast F-box protein Pof3 is required for genome integrity and telomere function. *Mol Biol Cell* 13:211–224, 2002.

Katz MS: Geriatrics grand rounds: Eve's rib, or a revisionist view of osteoporosis in men. *J Gerontol A Biol Sci Med Sci* 55:M560–569, 2000.

Kaul SC, Wadhwa R, Matsuda Y, Hensler PJ, Pereira-Smith OM, Komatsu Y, Mitsui Y. Mouse and human chromosomal assignments of mortalin, a novel member of the murine hsp70 family of proteins. *FEBS Lett* 361:269–272, 1995.

Kaur H, Richardson E, Murty L. Preparation of monoclonal antibodies against human telomerase. *Hybridoma* 20:183–188, 2001.

Kawai K, Yaginuma Y, Tsuruoka H, Griffin M, Hayashi H, Ishikawa M. Telomerase activity and human papillomavirus (HPV) infection in human uterine cervical cancers and cervical smears. *Eur J Cancer* 34:2082–2086, 1998.

Kazimirchuk EV, Egorov EE, Karachentsev DN, Zelenin AV. Effect of azidothymidine on reactivation of DNA synthesis in macrophage nuclei contained in heterokaryons [in Russian]. *Mol Biol (Mosk)* 35:908–911, 2001.

Keaney JF Jr. Atherosclerosis: from lesion formation to plaque activation and endothelial dysfunction. *Mol Aspects Med* 21:99–166, 2000.

Keating JT, Ince T, Crum CP. Surrogate biomarkers of HPV infection in cervical neoplasia screening and diagnosis. *Adv Anat Pathol* 8:83–92, 2001.

Keith N, Bronson RT, Lipman RD, Ding W, Lamont L, Cosmas AC, Manfredi TG. Diet restriction and age alters skeletal muscle capillarity in B6C3F1 mice. *J Am Aging Assoc* 23:141–146, 2000.

Keith WN, Sarvesvaran J, Downey M. Analysis of telomerase RNA gene expression by in situ hybridization. In Double JA, Thompson MJ. *Telomeres and Telomerase: Methods and Protocols.* Humana Press, Totowa, NJ, 2002, pp 65–83.

Kelland LR. Telomerase inhibitors: targeting the vulnerable end of cancer? *Anticancer Drugs* 11:503–513, 2000.

Kelland LR. Telomerase: biology and phase I trials. *Lancet Oncol* 2:95–102, 2001.

Keller JN, Mattson MP. Roles of lipid peroxidation in modulation of cellular signaling pathways, cell dysfunction, and death in the nervous system. *Rev Neurosci* 9:105–116, 1998.

Kemnitz JW, Roecker EB, Weindruch R, Elson DF, Baum ST, Bergman RN. Dietary restriction increases insulin sensitivity and lowers blood glucose in rhesus monkeys. *Am J Physiol* 266:E540–547, 1994.

Kempermann G, Kuhn HG, Winkler J, Gage FH. New nerve cells for the adult brain. Adult neurogenesis and stem cell concepts in neurologic research [in German]. *Nervenarzt* 69:851–857, 1998.

Kennaway DJ, Lushington K, Dawson D, Lack L, van den Heuvel C, Rogers N. Urinary 6-sulfatoxymelatonin excretion and aging: new results and a critical review of the literature. *J Pineal Res* 27:210–220, 1999.

Kenney WL, Buskirk ER. Functional consequences of sarcopenia: effects on thermoregulation. *J Gerontol A Biol Sci Med Sci* 50(Spec No):78–85, 1995.

Kenny AM, Dawson L, Kleppinger A, Iannuzzi-Sucich M, Judge JO. Prevalence of sarcopenia and predictors of skeletal muscle mass in nonobese women who are long-term users of estrogen-replacement therapy. *J Gerontol A Biol Sci Med Sci* 58:436–440, 2003.

Kenny AM, Prestwood KM, Gruman CA, Marcello KM, Raisz LG. Effects of transdermal testosterone on bone and muscle in older men with low bioavailable testosterone levels. *J Gerontol A Biol Sci Med Sci* 56:266–272, 2001.

Kenny AM, Prestwood KM, Marcello KM, Raisz LG. Determinants of bone density in healthy older men with low testosterone levels. *J Gerontol A Biol Sci Med Sci* 55:M492–497, 2000.

Kenyon C. Ponce d'elegans: genetic quest for the fountain of youth. *Cell* 84:501–504, 1996.

Kenyon C, Chang J, Gensch E, Rudner A, Tabtiang R. A *C. elegans* mutant that lives twice as long as wild type. *Nature* 366(6454):461–464, 1993.

Keogh BP, Allen RG, Pignolo R, Horton J, Tresini M, Cristofalo VJ. Expression of hydrogen peroxide and glutathione metabolizing enzymes in human skin fibroblasts derived from donors of different ages. *J Cell Physiol* 167:512–522, 1996a.

Keogh BP, Tresini M, Cristofalo VJ, Allen RG. Effects of cellular aging on the induction of c-fos by antioxidant treatments. *Mech Ageing Dev* 86:151–160, 1996b.

Kermici M, Pruche F, Roguet R, Prunieras M. Evidence for an age-correlated change in glutathione metabolism enzyme activities in human hair follicle. *Mech Ageing Dev* 53:73–84, 1990.

Kerr RM. Disorders of the stomach and duodenum. In Hazzard WR, Bierman EL, Blass JP, Ettinger WH Jr, Halter JB. *Principles of Geriatric Medicine and Gerontology, 3rd ed.* McGraw-Hill, New York, 1994, pp 693–705.

Kerwin SM. G-Quadruplex DNA as a target for drug design. *Curr Pharm Des* 6:441–478, 2000.

Kessler PD, Byrne BJ. Myoblast cell grafting into heart muscle: cellular biology and potential applications. *Annu Rev Physiol* 61:219–242, 1999.

Kettani A, Gorin A, Majumdar A, Hermann T, Skripkin E, Zhao H, Jones R, Patel DJ. A dimeric DNA interface stabilized by stacked A(GGGG)A hexads and coordinated monovalent cations. *J Mol Biol* 297:627–644, 2000.

Keynes G. *Blake: Complete Writings.* Oxford University Press, London, 1966.

Keysor JJ, Jette AM. Have we oversold the benefit of late-life exercise? *J Gerontol A Biol Sci Med Sci* 56:A412–423, 2001.

Khalifa MM. Hutchinson-Gilford progeria syndrome: report of a Libyan family and evidence of autosomal recessive inheritance. *Clin Genet* 35:125–132, 1989.

Khalil Z, Merhi M. Effects of aging on neurogenic vasodilator responses evoked by transcutaneous electrical nerve stimulation: relevance to would healing. *J Gerontol A Biol Sci Med Sci* 55:B257–263, 2000.

Khan AS, Lynch CD, Sane DC, Willingham MC, Sonntag WE. Growth hormone increases regional coronary blood flow and capillary density in aged rats. *J Gerontol A Biol Sci Med Sci* 56A:B364–371, 2001.

Kharbanda S, Kumar V, Dhar S, Pandey P, Chen C, Majumder P, Yuan ZM, Whang Y, Strauss W, Pandita TK, Weaver D, Kufe D. Regulation of the hTERT telomerase catalytic subunit by the c-Abl tyrosine kinase. *Curr Biol* 10:568–575, 2000.

Kharlamov A, Kharlamov E, Armstrong DM. Age-dependent increase in infarct volume following photochemically induced cerebral infarction: putative role of astroglia. *J Gerontol A Biol Sci Med Sci* 55:B135–B141, 2000.

Khaw PT, Doyle JW, Sherwood MB, Grierson I, Schultz G, McGorray S. Prolonged localized tissue effects from 5–minute exposures to fluorouracil and mitomycin. *C Arch Ophthalmol* 111:263–267, 1993.

Khoshnoodi J, Tryggvason K. Unraveling the molecular make-up of the glomerular podocyte slit diaphragm. *Exp Nephrol* 9:355–359, 2001.

Khosla S, Melton LJ 3rd, Riggs BL. Osteoporosis: gender differences and similarities. *Lupus* 8:393–396, 1999.

Kiaris H, Schally AV. Decrease in telomerase activity in U-87MG human glioblastomas after treatment with an antagonist of growth hormone-releasing hormone. *Proc Natl Acad Sci USA* 96:226–231, 1999.

Kiberstis P, Smith O, Norman C. Bone health in the balance. *Science* 289:1497, 2000.

Kiechl S, Willeit J, Bonora E, Schwarz S, Xu Q. No association between dehydroepiandrosterone sulfate and development of atherosclerosis in a prospective population study (Bruneck Study). *Arterioscler Thromb Vasc Biol* 20:1094–1100, 2000.

Kieras FJ, Brown WT, Houck GE Jr, Zebrower M. Elevation of urinary hyaluronic acid in Werner's syndrome and progeria. *Biochem Med Metab Biol* 36:276–282, 1986.

Kiger AA, Jones DL, Schulz C, Rogers MB, Fuller MT. Stem cell self-renewal specified by JAK-STAT activation in response to a support cell cue. *Science* 294:2542–2545, 2002.

Kiger AA, White-Cooper H, Fuller MT. Somatic support cells restrict germline stem cell self-renewal and promote differentiation. *Nature* 407:750–754, 2000.

Kikuchi Y. The mechanism of cisplatin-resistance in ovarian cancer [in Japanese]. *Hum Cell* 14:115–133, 2001.

Kilian A, Bowtell DD, Abud HE, Hime GR, Venter DJ, Keese PK, Duncan EL, Reddel RR, Jefferson RA. Isolation of a candidate human telomerase catalytic subunit gene which reveals complex splicing patterns in different cell types. *Hum Mol Genet* 6:2011–2019, 1997.

Kilian A, Stiff C, Kleinhofs A. Barley telomeres shorten during differentiation but grow in callus culture. *Proc Natl Acad Sci USA* 92:9555–9559, 1995.

Kill IR, Faragher RG, Lawrence K, Shall S. The expression of proliferation-dependent antigens during the life span of normal and progeroid human fibroblasts in culture. *J Cell Sci* 107:571–579, 1994.

Kill IR, Shall S. Senescent human diploid fibroblasts are able to support DNA synthesis and to express markers associated with proliferation. *J Cell Sci* 97:473–478, 1990.

Kim H, Farris J, Christman SA, Kong BW, Foster LK, O'Grady SM, Foster DN. Events in the immortalizing process of primary human mammary epithelial cells by the catalytic subunit of human telomerase. *Biochem J* 365:765–772, 2002a.

Kim H, You S, Farris J, Kong BW, Christman SA, Foster LK, Foster DN. Expression profiles of p53-, p16(INK4a)-, and telomere-regulating genes in replicative senescent primary human, mouse, and chicken fibroblast cells. *Exp Cell Res* 272:199–208, 2002b.

Kim H, You S, Kim IJ, Foster LK, Farris J, Ambady S, Ponce de Leon FA, Foster DN. Alterations in p53 and E2F-1 function common to immortalized chicken embryo fibroblasts. *Oncogene* 20:2671–2682, 2001a.

Kim HR, Kim YJ, Kim HJ, Kim SK, Lee JH. Change of telomerase activity in rectal cancer with chemoradiation therapy. *J Korean Med Sci* 15:167–172, 2000.

Kim HR, Kim YJ, Kim HJ, Kim SK, Lee JH. Telomere length changes in colorectal cancers and polyps. *J Korean Med Sci* 17:360–365, 2002c.

Kim JD, McCarter RJ, Yu BP. Influence of age, exercise, and dietary restriction on oxidative stress in rats. *Aging (Milano)* 8:123–129, 1996.

Kim JH, Lee GE, Kim JC, Lee JH, Chung IK. A novel telomere elongation in an adriamycin-resistant stomach cancer cell line with decreased telomerase activity. *Mol Cells* 13:228–236, 2002d.

Kim JH, Skates SJ, Uede T, Wong KK, Schorge JO, Feltmate CM, Berkowitz RS, Cramer DW, Mok SC. Osteopontin as a potential diagnostic biomarker for ovarian cancer. *JAMA* 287:1671–1679, 2002e.

Kim JW, Baek BS, Kim YK, Herlihy JT, Ikeno Y, Yu BP, Chung HY. Gene expression of cyclooxygenase in the aging heart. *J Gerontol A Biol Sci Med Sci* 56A:B350–355, 2001b.

Kim MJ, Aiken JM, Havighurst T, Hollander J, Ripple MO, Weindruch R. Adult-onset energy restriction of rhesus monkeys attenuates oxidative stress-induced cytokine expression by peripheral blood mononuclear cells. *J Nutr* 127:2293–2301, 1997a.

Kim MM, Rivera MA, Botchkina IL, Shalaby R, Thor AD, Blackburn EH. From the cover: a low threshold level of expression of mutant-template telomerase RNA inhibits human tumor cell proliferation. *Proc Natl Acad Sci USA* 98:7982–7987, 2001c.

Kim NW. Telomere and cell replication. Presented at Telomeres and Telomerase: Implications for Cell Immortality, Cancer, and Age-related Disease. San Francisco, CA, June 1–3, 1998.

Kim NW, Hruszkewycz AM. Telomerase activity modulation in the prevention of prostate cancer. *Urology* 57:148–153, 2001.

Kim NW, Pietyszek MA, Prowse KR, Harley CB, West MD, Ho PLC Coviello GM, Wright WE, Weinrich SL, Shay JW. Specific association of human telomerase activity with immortal cells and cancer. *Science* 266:2011–2015, 1994.

Kim SH, Kaminker P, Campisi J. TIN2, a new regulator of telomere length in human cells. *Nat Genet* 123:405–412, 1999.

Kim SH, Kaminker P, Campisi J. Telomeres, aging and cancer: in search of a happy ending. *Oncogene* 21:503–511, 2002f.

Kim TW, Pettingell WH, Hallmark OG, Moir RD, Wasco W, Tanzi RE. Endoproteolytic cleavage and proteasomal degradation of presenilin 2 in transfected cells. *J Biol Chem* 272:11006–11010, 1997b.

Kim TW, Pettingell WH, Jung YK, Kovacs DM, Tanzi RE. Alternative cleavage of Alzheimer-associated presenilins during apoptosis by a caspase-3 family protease. *Science* 277:373–376, 1997c.

Kim TW, Tanzi RE. Presenilins and Alzheimer's disease. *Curr Opin Neurobiol* 7:683–688, 1997.

Kimura KD, Tissenbaum HA, Liu Y, Ruvkun G. daf-2, an insulin receptor–like gene that regulates longevity and diapause in *Caenorhabditis elegans*. *Science* 277:942–946, 1997.

Kimura Y, Matsumoto M, Den YB, Iwai K, Munehira J, Hattori H, Hoshino T, Yamada K, Kawanishi K, Tsuchiya H. Impaired endothelial function in hypertensive elderly patients evaluated by high-resolution ultrasonography. *Can J Cardiol* 15:563–568, 1999.

King CR, Lemmer J, Campbell JR, Atkins AR. Osteosarcoma in a patient with Hutchinson-Gilford progeria. *J Med Genet* 15:481–484, 1978.

King HC, Sinha AA. Gene expression profile analysis: promise and pitfalls. *JAMA* 286:2280–2288, 2001.

King LM, Song J, Wojcinski ZW, Baker KW, Walker RM. Absence of correlation between telomerase activity and hepatic neoplasia in B6C3F1 mice. *Toxicol Lett* 106:247–254, 1999.

King LS. *Transformations in American Medicine*. Johns Hopkins University Press, Baltimore, 1991.

Kinlay S, Libby P, Ganz P. Endothelial function and coronary artery disease. *Curr Opin Lipidol* 12:383–389, 2001.

Kipling D. Telomerase: immortality enzyme or oncogene? *Nat Genet* 9:104–106, 1995a.

Kipling D. *The Telomere*. Oxford University Press, New York, 1995b.

Kipling D. Mammalian telomerase: catalytic subunit and knockout mice. *Hum Mol Genet* 6:1999–2004, 1997a.

Kipling D. Telomere structure and telomerase expression during mouse development and tumorigenesis. *Eur J Cancer* 33:792–800, 1997b.

Kipling D, Ackford HE, Taylor BA, Cooke HJ. Mouse minor satellite DNA genetically maps to the centromere and is physically linked to the proximal telomere. *Genomics* 11:235–241, 1991.

Kipling D, Cooke HJ. Hypervariable ultra-long telomeres in mice. *Nature* 347:400–402, 1990.

Kipling D, Cooke HJ. Beginning or end? Telomere structure, genetics and biology. *Hum Mol Genet* 1:3–6, 1992.

Kipling D, Faragher RG. Progeroid syndromes: probing the molecular basis of aging? *Mol Pathol* 50:234–241, 1997.

Kipling D, Faragher RG. Telomeres. Ageing hard or hardly ageing? *Nature* 398:191, 193, 1999.

Kipling D, Wilson HE, Mitchell AR, Taylor BA, Cooke HJ. Mouse centromere mapping using oligonucleotide probes that detect variants of the minor satellite. *Chromosoma* 103:46–55, 1994.

Kipling D, Wilson HE, Thomson EJ, Cooke HJ. YAC cloning *Mus musculus* telomeric DNA: physical, genetic, in situ and STS markers for the distal telomere of chromosome 10. *Hum Mol Genet* 4:1007–1014, 1995.

Kipling D, Wynford-Thomas D, Jones CJ, Akbar A, Aspinall R, Bacchetti S, Blasco MA, Broccoli D, DePinho RA, Edwards DR, Effros RB, Harley CB, Lansdorp PM, Linskens MH, Prowse

KR, Newbold RF, Olovnikov AM, Parkinson EK, Pawelec G, Ponten J, Shall S, Zijlmans M, Faragher RG. Telomere-dependent senescence. *Nat Biotechnol* 17:313–314, 1999.

Kirk KL. Dietary restriction and aging: comparative tests of evolutionary hypotheses. *J Gerontol A Biol Sci Med Sci* 56A:B123–129, 2001.

Kirkland JL. The biology of senescence: potential for prevention of disease. *Clin Geriatr Med* 18:383–405, 2002.

Kirkwood T. *Time of our Lives: The Science of Human Aging*. Oxford University Press, Oxford, 1999.

Kirkwood T. Evolution of aging: how genetic factors affect the end of life. *Generations* 24:12–18, 2000.

Kirkwood T. *The End of Age: Why Everything about Ageing is Changing*. Profile Books, London, 2001.

Kirkwood TB. Evolution of ageing. *Nature* 270:301–304, 1977.

Kirkwood TB. Towards a unified theory of cellular ageing. *Monogr Dev Biol* 17:9–20, 1984.

Kirkwood TB. Immortality of the germ-line versus disposability of the soma. *Basic Life Sci* 42:209–218, 1987.

Kirkwood TB. DNA, mutations and aging. *Mutat Res* Sept:7–13, 1988a.

Kirkwood TB. The nature and causes of ageing. *Ciba Found Symp* 134:193–207, 1988b.

Kirkwood TB. DNA, mutations and aging. *Mutat Res* 219:1–7, 1989.

Kirkwood TB. Comparative life spans of species: why do species have the life spans they do? *Am J Clin Nutr* 55(6 Suppl):1191S–1195S, 1992.

Kirkwood TB. Human senescence. *Bioessays* 18:1009–1016, 1996.

Kirkwood TB. The origins of human ageing. *Philos Trans R Soc Lond B Biol Sci* 352:1765–1772, 1997.

Kirkwood TB. Biological theories of aging: an overview. *Aging (Milano)* 10:144–146, 1998.

Kirkwood TB. Molecular gerontology. *J Inherit Metab Dis* 25:189–196, 2002.

Kirkwood TB, Austad SN. Why do we age? *Nature* 408:233–238, 2000.

Kirkwood TB, Cremer T. Cytogerontology since 1881: a reappraisal of August Weismann and a review of modern progress. *Hum Genet* 60:101–121, 1982.

Kirkwood TB, Franceschi C. Free radicals: only part of the story? *Aging (Milano)* 5:1–2, 1993.

Kirkwood TB, Kowald A. Network theory of aging. *Exp Gerontol* 32:395–399, 1997.

Kirkwood TB, Rose MR. Evolution of senescence: late survival sacrificed for reproduction. *Philos Trans R Soc Lond B Biol Sci* 332:15–24, 1991.

Kirkwood TBL, Holliday R. Commitment to senescence: a model for the finite and infinite growth of diploid and transformed human fibroblasts in culture. *J Theor Biol* 53:481–496, 1975.

Kirkwood TBL, Holliday R. Evolution of ageing and longevity. *Proc R Soc Lond B Biol Sci* 205:531–546, 1979.

Kirn D, Hermiston T, McCormick F. ONYX-015: clinical data are encouraging. *Nat Med* 4:1341–1342, 1998.

Kishi S, Lu KP. A critical role for Pin2/TRF1 in ATM-dependent regulation: inhibition of Pin2/TRF1 function complements telomere shortening, the radiosensitivity and G2/M checkpoint defect of ataxia-telangiectasia cells. *J Biol Chem* 277:7420–7429, 2002.

Kishi S, Wulf G, Nakamura M, Lu KP. Telomeric protein Pin2/TRF1 induces mitotic entry and apoptosis in cells with short telomeres and is down-regulated in human breast tumors. *Oncogene* 20:1497–1508, 2001.

Kishimoto K, Fujimoto J, Takeuchi M, Yamamoto H, Ueki T, Okamoto E. Telomerase activity in hepatocellular carcinoma and adjacent liver tissues. *J Surg Oncol* 69:119–124, 1998.

Kitagawa Y, Kyo S, Takakura M, Kanaya T, Koshida K, Namiki M, Inoue M. Demethylating reagent 5-azacytidine inhibits telomerase activity in human prostate cancer cells through transcriptional repression of hTERT. *Clin Cancer Res* 6:2868–2875, 2000.

Kitamoto M, Ide T. Telomerase activity in precancerous hepatic nodules. *Cancer* 85:245–248, 1999.

Kiyono T, Foster SA, Koop JI, McDougall JK, Galloway DA, Klingelhutz AJ. Both Rb/p16INK4a inactivation and telomerase activity are required to immortalize human epidermal cells. *Nature* 396:84–88, 1998.

Kiyozuka Y, Asai A, Yamamoto D, Senzaki H, Yoshioka S, Takahashi H, Hioki K, Tsubura A. Establishment of novel human esophageal cancer cell line in relation to telomere dynamics and telomerase activity. *Dig Dis Sci* 45:870–879, 2000a.

Kiyozuka Y, Yamamoto D, Yang J, Uemura Y, Senzaki H, Adachi S, Tsubura A. Correlation of chemosensitivity to anticancer drugs and telomere length, telomerase activity and telomerase RNA expression in human ovarian cancer cells. *Anticancer Res* 20:203–212, 2000b.

Klapper W, Parwaresch R, Krupp G. Telomere biology in human aging and aging syndromes. *Mech Aging Dev* 122:695–712, 2001.

Klein BE, Klein R, Lee KE, Jensen SC. Measures of obesity and age-related eye diseases. *Ophthalmic Epidemiol* 8:251–262, 2001.

Klein HL, Kreuzer KN. Replication, recombination, and repair: going for the gold. *Mol Cell* 9:471–480, 2002.

Kleinschmidt-DeMasters BK, Evans LC, Bitter MA, Shroyer AL, Shroyer KR. Part II. Telomerase expression in cerebrospinal fluid specimens as an adjunct to cytologic diagnosis. *J Neurol Sci* 161:124–134, 1998a.

Kleinschmidt-DeMasters BK, Hashizumi TL, Sze CI, Lillehei KO, Shroyer AL, Shroyer KR. Telomerase expression shows differences across multiple regions of oligodendroglioma versus high grade astrocytomas but shows correlation with Mib-1 labelling. *J Clin Pathol* 51:284–293, 1998b.

Kleinschmidt-DeMasters BK, Shroyer AL, Hashizumi TL, Evans LC, Markham N, Kindt G, Shroyer KR. Part I. Telomerase levels in human metastatic brain tumors show four-fold logarithmic variability but no correlation with tumor type or interval to patient demise. *J Neurol Sci* 161:116–123, 1998c.

Klingelhutz AJ. The roles of telomeres and telomerase in cellular immortalization and the development of cancer. *Anticancer Res* 19:4823–4830, 1999.

Klingelhutz AJ, Foster SA, McDougall JK. Telomerase activation by the E6 gene product of human papillomavirus type 16. *Nature* 380:79–82, 1996.

Klinman DM, Conover J, Bloom ET, Weiss W. Immunogenicity and efficacy of a DNA vaccine in aged mice. *J Gerontol A Biol Sci Med Sci* 53:B281–286, 1998.

Klobutcher LA, Gygax SE, Podoloff JD, Vermeesch JR, Price CM, Tebeau CM, Jahn CL. Conserved DNA sequences adjacent to chromosome fragmentation and telomere addition sites in *Euplotes crassus*. *Nucl Acids Res* 26:4230–4240, 1998.

Knopman D, Donohue JA, Gutterman EM. Patterns of care in the early stages of Alzheimer's disease: impediments to a timely diagnosis. *J Am Geriatr Soc* 48:300–304, 2000.

Kobayashi S, Gibo H, Sugita K, Komiya I, Yamada T. Werner's syndrome associated with meningioma. *Neurosurgery* 7:517–520, 1980.

Kobryn K, Chaconas G. The circle is broken: telomere resolution in linear replicons. *Curr Opin Microbiol* 4:558–564, 2001.

Kobryn K, Chaconas G. ResT, a telomere resolvase encoded by the Lyme disease spirochete. *Mol Cell* 9:195–201, 2002.

Koenig W. Inflammation and coronary heart disease: an overview. *Cardiol Rev* 9:31–35, 2001.

Koeppel F, Riou JF, Laoui A, Mailliet P, Arimondo PB, Labit D, Petitgenet O, Helene C, Mergny JL. Ethidium derivatives bind to G-quartets, inhibit telomerase and act as fluorescent probes for quadruplexes. *Nucleic Acids Res* 29:1087–1096, 2001.

Koering CE, Pollice A, Zibella MP, Bauwens S, Puisieux A, Brunori M, Brun C, Martins L, Sabatier L, Pulitzer JF, Gilson E. Human telomeric position effect is determined by chromosomal context and telomeric chromatin integrity. *EMBO Rep* 3:1055–1061, 2002.

Koetz K, Bryl E, Spickschen K, O'Fallon WM, Goronzy JJ, Weyand CM. T cell homeostasis in patients with rheumatoid arthritis. *Proc Natl Acad Sci USA* 97:9203–9208, 2000.

Koga S, Hirohata S, Kondo Y, Komata T, Takakura M, Inoue M, Kyo S, Kondo S. A novel telomerase-specific gene therapy: gene transfer of caspase-8 utilizing the human telomerase catalytic subunit gene promoter. *Hum Gene Ther* 11:1397–1406, 2000.

Koga S, Hirohata S, Kondo Y, Komata T, Takakura M, Inoue M, Kyo S, Kondo S. FADD gene therapy using the human telomerase catalytic subunit (hTERT) gene promoter to restrict induction of apoptosis to tumors in vitro and in vivo. *Anticancer Res* 21:1937–1943, 2001a.

Koga S, Kondo Y, Komata T, Kondo S. Treatment of bladder cancer cells in vitro and in vivo with 2–5A antisense telomerase RNA. *Gene Ther* 8:654–658, 2001b.

Kohara K, Jiang Y, Hiwada K. Carotid wall shear stress and aging [letter]. *J Am Geriatr Soc* 48:1349–1350, 2000.

Kohn RR. Aging and cell division [letter]. *Science* 188:203–204, 1975.

Kohn RR. Heart and cardiovascular system. In Finch CE, Hayflick L (eds). *Handbook of the Biology of Aging.* Van Nostrand Reinhold, New York, 1977, pp 281–317.

Kohrt WM. Osteoprotective benefits of exercise: more pain, less gain? *J Am Geriatr Soc* 49:1565–1567, 2001.

Koizumi H, Ohkawara A. Regulation of transmembrane signalling system during senescence of human epidermal keratinocytes. *Arch Dermatol Res* 288:611–614, 1996.

Kojima H, Miyazaki H, Shiwa M, Tanaka Y, Moriyama H. Molecular biological diagnosis of congenital and acquired cholesteatoma on the basis of differences in telomere length. *Laryngoscope* 111:867–873, 2001.

Kojima H, Yokosuka O, Imazeki F, Saisho H, Omata M. Telomerase activity and telomere length in hepatocellular carcinoma and chronic liver disease. *Gastroenterology* 112:493–500, 1997.

Kojima H, Yokosuka O, Kato N, Shiina S, Imazeki F, Saisho H, Shiratori Y, Omata M Quantitative evaluation of telomerase activity in small liver tumors: analysis of ultrasonography-guided liver biopsy specimens. *J Hepatol* 31:514–520, 1999.

Kolesnikova OA, Entelis NS, Mireau H, Fox TD, Martin RP, Tarassov IA. Suppression of mutations in mitochondrial DNA by tRNAs imported from the cytoplasm. *Science* 289:1931–1933, 2000.

Kolodner RD. Guarding against mutation. *Science* 407:687–689, 2000.

Kolquist KA, Ellisen LW, Counter CM, Meyerson M, Tan LK, Weinberg RA, Haber DA, Gerald WL. Expression of TERT in early premalignant lesions and a subset of cells in normal tissues. *Nat Genet* 19:182–186, 1998.

Komata T, Koga S, Hirohata S, Takakura M, Germano IM, Inoue M, Kyo S, Kondo S, Kondo Y. A novel treatment of human malignant gliomas in vitro and in vivo: FADD gene transfer under the control of the human telomerase reverse transcriptase gene promoter. *Int J Oncol* 19:1015–1020, 2001a.

Komata T, Kondo Y, Kanzawa T, Hirohata S, Koga S, Sumiyoshi H, Srinivasula SM, Barna BP, Germano IM, Takakura M, Inoue M, Alnemri ES, Shay JW, Kyo S, Kondo S. Treatment of malignant glioma cells with the transfer of constitutively active caspase-6 using the human telomerase catalytic subunit (human telomerase reverse transcriptase) gene promoter. *Cancer Res* 61:5796–5802, 2001b.

Komiya T, Kawase I, Nitta T, Yasumitsu T, Kikui M, Fukuoka M, Nakagawa K, Hirashima T. Prognostic significance of hTERT expression in non–small cell lung cancer. *Int J Oncol* 16:1173–1177, 2000.

Kondo T, Raff M. Oligodendrocyte precursor cells reprogrammed to become multipotential CNS stem cells. *Science* 289:1754–1757, 2000.

Kondo Y, Koga S, Komata T, Kondo S. Treatment of prostate cancer in vitro and in vivo with 2–5A-anti-telomerase RNA component. *Oncogene* 19:2205–2211, 2000.

Kondo Y, Komata T, Kondo S Combination therapy of 2–5A antisense against telomerase RNA and cisplatin for malignant gliomas. *Int J Oncol* 18:1287–1292, 2001.

Konety BR, Getzenberg RH. Urine based markers of urological malignancy. *J Urol* 165:600–611, 2001.

Kontogeorgos G, Kovacs K. Telomeres and telomerase in endocrine pathology. *Endocrine* 9:133–138, 1998.

Kordower JH, Emborg ME, Bloch J, Ma SY, Chu Y, Leventhal L, McBride J, Chen EY, Palfi S, Roitberg BZ, Brown WD, Holden JE, Pyzalski R, Taylor MD, Carvey P, Ling Z, Trono D, Hantraye P, Deglog N, Aebischer P. Neurodegeneration prevented by lentiviral vector delivery of GDNF in primate models of Parkinson's disease. *Science* 290:767–773, 2000.

Kornak DR, Rakic P. Cell proliferation without neurogenesis in adult primate neurocortex. *Science* 294:2127–2130, 2001.

Korniszewski L, Nowak R, Okninska-Hoffmann E, Skorka A, Gieruszczak-Bialek D, Sawadro-Rochowska M. Wiedemann-Rautenstrauch (neonatal progeroid) syndrome: new case with normal telomere length in skin fibroblasts. *Am J Med Genet* 103:144–148, 2001.

Korr H, Kurz C, Seidler TO, Sommer D, Schmitz C. Mitochondrial DNA synthesis studied autoradiographically in various cell types in vivo. *Braz J Med Biol Res* 31:289–28, 1998.

Koscielny S, Dahse R, Sonntag J, Riese U, Theuer C, Hofmann ME, von Eggeling F, Claussen U, Beleites E, Ernst G, Fiedler W. Clinical implications of telomerase activity and inactivation of the tumor suppressor gene *p16* (*CDKN2A*) in head and neck cancer. *Otolaryngol Pol* 54:291–295, 2000a.

Koscielny S, Fiedler W, Dahse R, Beleites E. Reactivation of telomerase in squamous epithelial carcinomas in the area of the head and neck [in German]. *Laryngorhinootologie* 79:551–556, 2000b.

Koudinova NV, Berezov TT, Koudinov AR. Beta-amyloid: Alzheimer's disease and brain beta-amyloidoses. *Biochemistry (Mosc)* 64:752–757, 1999.

Kounnas MZ, Moir RD, Rebeck GW, Bush AI, Argraves WS, Tanzi RE, Hyman BT, Strickland DK. LDL receptor–related protein, a multifunctional ApoE receptor, binds secreted beta-amyloid precursor protein and mediates its degradation. *Cell* 82:331–340, 1995.

Kousteni S, Chen JR, Bellido T, Han L, Ali AA, O'Brien CA, Plotkin L, Fu Q, Mancino AT, Wen Y, Vertino AM, Powers CC, Stewart SA, Ebert R, Parfitt AM, Weinstein RS, Jilka RL, Manolagas SC. Reversal of bone los in mice by nongenotropic signaling of sex steroids. *Science* 298:843–846, 2002.

Kovacs DM, Fausett HJ, Page KJ, Kim TW, Moir RD, Merriam DE, Hollister RD, Hallmark OG, Mancini R, Felsenstein KM, Hyman BT, Tanzi RE, Wasco W. Alzheimer-associated presenilins 1 and 2: neuronal expression in brain and localization to intracellular membranes in mammalian cells. *Nat Med* 2:224–229, 1996.

Kovalenko SA, Kopsidas G, Islam MM, Heffernan D, Fitzpatrick J, Caragounis A, Gingold E, Linnane AW. The age-associated decrease in the amount of amplifiable full-length mitochondrial DNA in human skeletal muscle. *Biochem Mol Biol Int* 46:1233–1241, 1998.

Kowald A. The mitochondrial theory of aging: do damaged mitochondria accumulate by delayed degradation? *Exp Gerontol* 34:605–162, 1999.

Kowald A, Kirkwood TB. Explaining fruit fly longevity. *Science* 260:1664–516; discussion 1665–1666, 1993a.

Kowald A, Kirkwood TB. Mitochondrial mutations, cellular instability and ageing: modeling the population dynamics of mitochondria. *Mutat Res* 295:93–103, 1993b.

Kowald A, Kirkwood TB. Towards a network theory of aging: a model combining the free radical theory and the protein error theory. *J Theor Biol* 168:75–94, 1994.

Kowald A, Kirkwood TB. A network theory of ageing: the interactions of defective mitochondria, aberrant proteins, free radicals and scavengers in the ageing process. *Mutat Res* 316:209–236, 1996.

Kowald A, Kirkwood TBL. Modeling the role of mitochondrial mutations in cellular aging. *J Anti-Aging Med* 2:243–253, 1999.

Kowald A, Kirkwood TB. Accumulation of defective mitochondria through delayed degradation of damaged organelles and its possible role in the ageing of post-mitotic and dividing cells. *J Theor Biol* 202:145–160, 2000.

Koyanagi K, Ozawa S, Ando N, Mukai M, Kitagawa Y, Ueda M, Kitajima M. Telomerase activity as an indicator of malignant potential in iodine-nonreactive lesions of the esophagus. *Cancer* 88:1524–1529, 2000.

Kraemer R. Regulation of cell migration in atherosclerosis. *Curr Atheroscler Rep* 2:445–452, 2000.

Krajnak K, Kashon ML, Rosewell KL, Wise PM. Aging alters the rhythmic expression of vasoactive intestinal polypeptide mRNA but not arginine vasopressin mRNA in the suprachiasmatic nuclei of female rats. *J Neurosci* 18:4767–4774, 1998.

Krall WJ, Sramek JJ, Cutler NR. Cholinesterase inhibitors: a therapeutic strategy for Alzheimer disease. *Ann Pharmacother* 33:441–450, 1999.

Krams M, Claviez A, Heidorn K, Krupp G, Parwaresch R, Harms D, Rudolph P. Regulation of telomerase activity by alternate splicing of human telomerase reverse transcriptase mRNA in a subset of neuroblastomas. *Am J Pathol* 159:1925–1932, 2001.

Krauskopf A, Blackburn EH. Control of telomere growth by interactions of RAP1 with the most distal telomeric repeats. *Nature* 383:354–357, 1996.

Krauskopf A, Blackburn EH. Rap1 protein regulates telomere turnover in yeast. *Proc Natl Acad Sci USA* 95:12486–12491, 1998.

Kremer JM. Rational use of new and existing disease-modifying agents in rheumatoid arthritis. *Ann Intern Med* 134:695–706, 2001.

Krieglstein CF, Granger DN. Adhesion molecules and their role in vascular disease. *Am J Hypertens* 14:44S-54S, 2001.

Kriz W, Elger M, Hosser H, Hahnel B, Provoost A, Kranzlin B, Gretz N. How does podocyte damage result in tubular damage? *Kidney Blood Press Res* 22:26–36, 1999.

Kriz W, Gretz N, Lemley KV. Progression of glomerular diseases: is the podocyte the culprit? *Kidney Int* 54:687–697, 1998.

Kriz W, Lemley KV. The role of the podocyte in glomerulosclerosis. *Curr Opin Nephrol Hypertens* 8:489–497, 1999.

Krogan NJ, Dover J, Khorrami S, Greenblatt JF, Schneider J, Johnston M, Shilatifard A. COM-PASS, a histone H3 (Lysine 4) methyltransferase required for telomeric silencing of gene expression. *J Biol Chem* 277:10753–10755, 2002.

Krohn PL. Transplantation and aging. In Krohn PL (ed). *Topics in the Biology of Aging*. Interscience, New York, 1962, pp 125–148.

Krtolica A, Parrinello S, Lockett S, Desprez PY, Campisi J. Senescent fibroblasts promote epithelial cell growth and tumorigenesis: a link between cancer and aging. *Proc Natl Acad Sci USA* 98:12072–12077, 2001.

Kruk PA, Rampino NJ, Bohr VA. DNA damage and repair in telomeres: relation to aging. *Proc Natl Acad Sci USA* 92:258–262, 1995.

Krupp G, Bonatz G, Parwaresch R. Telomerase, immortality and cancer. *Biotechnol Annu Rev* 6:103–140, 2000a.

Krupp G, Klapper W, Parwaresch R. Cell proliferation, carcinogenesis and diverse mechanisms of telomerase regulation. *Cell Mol Life Sci* 57:464–486, 2000b.

Kruse FE, Volcker HE. Stem cells, wound healing, growth factors, and angiogenesis in the cornea. *Curr Opin Ophthalmol* 8:46–54, 1997.

Kubota C, Yamakuchi H, Todoroki J, Mizoshita K, Tabara N, Barber M, Yang X. Six cloned calves produced from adult fibroblast cells after long-term culture. *Proc Natl Acad Sci USA* 97:990–995, 2000a.

Kubota T, Hisatake J, Hisatake Y, Said JW, Chen SS, Holden S, Taguchi H, Koeffler HP. PC-SPES: a unique inhibitor of proliferation of prostate cancer cells in vitro and in vivo. *Prostate* 42:163–171, 2000b.

Kucherlapati R, DePinho RA. Cancer. Telomerase meets its mismatch. *Nature* 411:647–648, 2001.

Kudielka BM, Schmidt-Reinwald AK, Hellhammer DH, Kirschbaum C. Psychological and endocrine responses to psychosocial stress and dexamethasone/corticotropin-releasing hormone in healthy postmenopausal women and young controls: the impact of age and a two-week estradiol treatment. *Neuroendocrinology* 70:422–430, 1999.

Kuether K, Arking R. *Drosophila* selected for extended longevity are more sensitive to heat shock. *J Am Aging Assoc* 22:175–180, 1999.

Kugler JP, Hustead T. Hyponatremia and hypernatremia in the elderly. *Am Fam Physician* 61:3623–3630, 2000.

Kugoh H, Shigenami K, Funaki K, Barrett JC, Oshimura M. Human chromosome 5 carries a putative telomerase repressor gene. *Genes Chromosomes Cancer* 36:37–47, 2003.

Kumaki F, Kawai T, Hiroi S, Shinomiya N, Ozeki Y, Ferrans VJ, Torikata C. Telomerase activity and expression of human telomerase RNA component and human telomerase reverse transcriptase in lung carcinomas. *Hum Pathol* 32:188–195, 2001.

Kumata M, Shimizu M, Oshimura M, Uchida M, Tsutsui T. Induction of cellular senescence in a telomerase negative human immortal fibroblast cell line, LCS-AF 1-3, by human chromosome 6. *Int J Oncol* 21:851–856, 2002.

Kumazaki T. Modulation of gene expression during aging of human vascular endothelial cells. *Hiroshima J Med Sci* 42:97, 1993.

Kunifuji Y, Gotoh S, Abe T, Miura M, Karasaki Y. Down-regulation of telomerase activity by anticancer drugs in human ovarian cancer cells. *Anticancer Drugs* 13:595–598, 2002.

Kuniyasu H, Yasui W, Yokozaki H, Tahara E. *Helicobacter pylori* infection and carcinogenesis of the stomach. *Langenbecks Arch Surg* 385:69–74, 2000.

Kunz J. Initial lesions of vascular aging disease (arteriosclerosis). *Gerontology* 46:295–299, 2000.

Kuranaga N, Shinomiya N, Mochizuki H. Long-term cultivation of colorectal carcinoma cells with anti-cancer drugs induces drug resistance and telomere elongation: an in vitro study. *BMC Cancer* 1:10, 2001.

Kurapati R, Passananti HB, Rose MR, Tower J. Increased hsp22 RNA levels in *Drosophila* lines genetically selected for increased longevity. *J Gerontol A Biol Sci Med Sci* 55:B552–559, 2000.

Kurenova EV, Champion L, Biessmann H, Mason JM. Directional gene silencing induced by a complex subtelomeric satellite from *Drosophila*. *Chromosoma* 107:311–20, 1998.

Kurenova EV, Mason JM. Telomere functions. A review. *Biochemistry (Mosc)* 62:1242–1253, 1997.

Kurzrock R. The role of cytokines in cancer-related fatigue. *Cancer* 92:1684–1688, 2001.

Kushner DM, Paranjape JM, Bandyopadhyay B, Cramer H, Leaman DW, Kennedy AW, Silverman RH, Cowell JK. 2–5A antisense directed against telomerase RNA produces apoptosis in ovarian cancer cells. *Gynecol Oncol* 76:183–192, 2000.

Kveiborg M, Flyvbjerg A, Rattan SIS, Kassem M. Changes in the insulin-like growth factor system may contribute to in vitro age-related impaired osteoblast functions. *Exp Gerontol* 35:1061–1074, 2000.

Kveiborg M, Gravholt CH, Kassem M. Evidence of a normal mean telomere fragment length in patients with Ullrich-Turner syndrome. *Eur J Hum Genet* 9:877–879, 2001a.

Kveiborg M, Kassem M, Langdahl B, Eriksen ER, Clark BF, Rattan SI. Telomere shortening during ageing of human osteoblasts in vitro and leukocytes in vivo: lack of excessive telomere loss in osteoporotic patients. *Mech Ageing Dev* 106:261–271, 1999.

Kveiborg, M, Rattan SI, Clark BF, Eriksen EF, Kassem M. Treatment with 1,25-dihydroxyvitamin D(3) reduces impairment of human osteoblast functions during cellular aging in culture. *J Cell Physiol* 186:298–306, 2001b.

Kvitko O. Participation theory of aging. *Biogerontology* 2:67–71, 2001.

Kwak B, Mulhaupt F, Myit S, Mach F. Statins as a newly recognized type of immunomodulator. *Nat Med* 6:1399–1402, 2000.

Kwon ED, Foster BA, Hurwitz AA, Madias C, Allison JP, Greenberg NM, Burg MB. Elimination of residual metastatic prostate cancer after surgery and adjunctive cytotoxic T lymphocyte–associated antigen 4 (CTLA-4) blockade immunotherapy. *Proc Natl Acad Sci USA* 96:15074–15079, 1999.

Kwong LK, Sohal RS. Age-related changes in activities of mitochondrial electron transport complexes in various tissues of the mouse. *Arch Biochem Biophys* 373:16–22, 2000.

Kyo S, Inoue M. Telomerase inhibitor [in Japanese]. *Gan To Kagaku Ryoho* 28:614–621, 2001.

Kyo S, Kanaya T, Ishikawa H, Ueno H, Inoue M. Telomerase activity in gynecological tumors. *Clin Cancer Res* 2:2023–2028, 1996.

Kyo S, Kanaya T, Takakura M, Tanaka M, Inoue M. Human telomerase reverse transcriptase as a critical determinant of telomerase activity in normal and malignant endometrial tissues. *Int J Cancer* 80:60–63, 1999a.

Kyo S, Kanaya T, Takakura M, Tanaka M, Yamashita A, Inoue H, Inoue M. Expression of human telomerase subunits in ovarian malignant, borderline and benign tumors. *Int J Cancer* 80:804–809, 1999b.

Kyo S, Kunimi K, Uchibayashi T, Namiki M, Inoue M. Telomerase activity in human urothelial tumors. *Am J Clin Pathol* 107:555–560, 1997a.

Kyo S, Takakura M, Inoue M. Telomerase activity in cancer as a diagnostic and therapeutic target. *Histol Histopathol* 15:813–824, 2000a.

Kyo S, Takakura M, Ishikawa H, Sasagawa T, Satake S, Tateno M, Inoue M. Application of telomerase assay for the screening of cervical lesions. *Cancer Res* 57:1863–1867, 1997b.

Kyo S, Takakura M, Kanaya T, Zhuo W, Fujimoto K, Nishio Y, Orimo A, Inoue M. Estrogen activates telomerase. *Cancer Res* 59:5917–5921, 1999c.

Kyo S, Takakura M, Kohama T, Inoue M. Telomerase activity in human endometrium. *Cancer Res* 57:610–614, 1997c.

Kyo S, Takakura M, Taira T, Kanaya T, Itoh H, Yutsudo M, Ariga H, Inoue M. Sp1 cooperates with c-Myc to activate transcription of the human telomerase reverse transcriptase gene (hTERT). *Nucleic Acids Res* 28:669–677, 2000b.

Kyo S, Takakura M, Tanaka M, Kanaya T, Inoue M. Telomerase activity in cervical cancer is quantitatively distinct from that in its precursor lesions. *Int J Cancer* 79:66–70, 1998a.

Kyo S, Takakura M, Tanaka M, Kanaya T, Sagawa T, Kohama T, Ishikawa H, Nakano T, Shimoya K, Inoue M. Expression of telomerase activity in human chorion. *Biochem Biophys Res Commun* 241:498–503, 1997d.

Kyo S, Takakura M, Tanaka M, Murakami K, Saitoh R, Hirano H, Inoue M. Quantitative differences in telomerase activity among malignant, premalignant, and benign ovarian lesions. *Clin Cancer Res* 4:399–405, 1998b.

Laan RF, van Riel PL, van de Putte LB. Leflunomide and methotrexate. *Curr Opin Rheumatol* 13:159–163, 2001.

LaFountain JR Jr, Cole RW, Rieder CL. Partner telomeres during anaphase in crane-fly spermatocytes are connected by an elastic tether that exerts a backward force and resists poleward motion. *J Cell Sci* 115:1541–1549, 2002.

Laguno M, Miro O, Perea M, Picon M, Urbano-Marquez A, Grau JM. Muscle diseases in elders: a 10-year retrospective study. *J Gerontol* 57A:M378–384, 2002.

Laible G, Wolf A, Dorn R, Reuter G, Nislow C, Lebersorger A, Popkin D, Pillus L, Jenuwein T. Mammalian homologues of the Polycomb-group gene *Enhancer* of zeste mediate gene silencing in *Drosophila* heterochromatin and at *S. cerevisiae* telomeres. *EMBO J* 16:3219–3232, 1997.

Laine K, Palovaara S, Tapanainen P, Manninen P. Plasma tacrine concentrations are significantly increased by concomitant hormone replacement therapy. Clin *Pharmacol Ther* 66:602–608, 1999.

Lakatta EG. Alterations in circulatory function. In *Principles of Geriatric Medicine and Gerontology, 3rd ed.* 1994, pp 493–508.

Lakatta EG, Boluyt MO. Age-associated changes in the cardiovascular system in the absence of cardiovascular disease. In Hosenpud JD, Greenberg BH (eds). *Congestive Heart Failure.* Lippincott Williams & Wilkins, Philadelphia, 2000, pp 137–156.

Lakowski B, Hekimi S. Determination of life-span in *Caenorhabditis elegans* by four clock genes. *Science* 272:1010–1013, 1996.

Lakowski B, Hekimi S. The genetics of caloric restriction in *Caenorhabditis elegans. Proc Natl Acad Sci USA* 95:13091–13096, 1998.

Lal SB, Ramsey JJ, Monemdjou S, Weindruch R, Harper M-E. Effects of caloric restriction on skeletal muscle mitochondrial proton leak in aging rats. *J Gerontol A Biol Sci Med Sci* 56A:B116–122, 2001.

Lam KY, Lo CY, Fan ST, Luk JM. Telomerase activity in pancreatic endocrine tumours: a potential marker for malignancy. *Mol Pathol* 53:133–136, 2000.

Lamb MJ. *Biology of Aging.* Halsted (Wiley), New York, 1977.

Lamers MH, Perrakis A, Enzlin JH, Winterwerp HHK, de Wind N, Sixma TK. The crystal structure of DNA mismatch repair protein MutS binding to a G-T mismatch. *Nature* 407:711–717, 2000.

Lamoureux EL, Sparrow WA, Murphy A, Newton RU. Differences in the neuromuscular capacity and lean muscle tissue in old and older community-dwelling adults. *J Gerontol A Biol Sci Med Sci* 56:M381–385, 2001.

Lancelin F, Anidjar M, Villette JM, Soliman A, Teillac P, Le Duc A, Fiet J, Cussenot O. Telomerase activity as a potential marker in preneoplastic bladder lesions. *BJU Int* 85:526–531, 2000.

Landis SH, Murray T, Bolden S, Wingo PA. Cancer statistics, 1999. *CA Cancer J Clin* 49:8–31, 1999.

Landmesser U, Hornig B, Drexler H. Endothelial dysfunction in hypercholesterolemia: mechanisms, pathophysiological importance, and therapeutic interventions. *Semin Thromb Hemost* 26:529–537, 2000.

Lane MA. Metabolic mechanisms of longevity: caloric restriction in mammals and longevity mutations in *Caenorhabditis elegans*: a common pathway? *J Am Aging Assoc* 23:1–7, 2000.

Lane MA, Baer DJ, Rumpler WV, Weindruch R, Ingram DK, Tilmont EM, Cutler RG, Roth GS. Calorie restriction lowers body temperature in rhesus monkeys, consistent with a postulated anti-aging mechanism in rodents. *Proc Natl Acad Sci USA* 93:4159–4164, 1996.

Lane MA, Ball SS, Ingram DK, Cutler RG, Engel J, Read V, Roth GS. Diet restriction in rhesus monkeys lowers fasting and glucose-stimulated glucoregulatory end points. *Am J Physiol* 268:E941–948, 1995.

Lane MA, Black A, Ingram DK, Roth GS. Calorie restriction in nonhuman primates: implications for age-related disease risk. *J Anti-Aging Med* 1:315–326, 1998a.

Lane MA, Ingram DK, Ball SS, Roth GS. Dehydroepiandrosterone sulfate: a biomarker of primate aging slowed by calorie restriction. *J Clin Endocrinol Metab* 82:2093–2096, 1997a.

Lane MA, Ingram DK, Cutler RG, Knapka JJ, Barnard DE, Roth GS. Dietary restriction in nonhuman primates: progress report on the NIA study. *Ann NY Acad Sci* 673:36–45, 1992.

Lane MA, Ingram DK, Roth GS. Beyond the rodent model: calorie restriction in rhesus monkeys. *Age Ageing* 20:45–56, 1997b.

Lane MA, Ingram DK, Roth GS. 2-deoxy-D-glucose feeding in rats mimics physiological effects of calorie restriction. *J Anti-Aging Med* 1:327–3337, 1998b.

Lane MA, Ingram DK, Roth GS. Calorie restriction in nonhuman primates: effects on diabetes and cardiovascular disease risk. *Toxicol Sci* 52:41–48, 1999.

Lane MA, Ingram DK, Roth GS. Easy to swallow: the serious search for an anti-aging pill. *Sci Am* 287:36–41, 2002.

Lane MA, Tilmont EM, De Angelis H, Handy A, Ingram DK, Kemnitz JW, Roth GS. Short-term calorie restriction improves disease-related markers in older male rhesus monkeys. *Mech Ageing Dev* 112:185–196, 2000.

Lang A, Brenner DA. Gene regulation in hepatic stellate cell. *Ital J Gastroenterol Hepatol* 31:173–179, 1999.

Langford LA, Piatyszek MA, Xu R, Schold SC Jr, Shay JW. Telomerase activity in human brain tumours. *Lancet* 346:1267–1268, 1995.

Langford LA, Piatyszek MA, Xu R, Schold SC Jr, Wright WE, Shay JW. Telomerase activity in ordinary meningiomas predicts poor outcome. *Hum Pathol* 28:416–420, 1997.

Lansdorp PM. Stem cell biology for the transfusionist. *Vox Sang* 74(Suppl 2):91–94, 1998.

Lansdorp PM. Repair of telomeric DNA prior to replicative senescence. *Mech Ageing Dev* 118:23–34, 2000.

Lansdorp PM, Poon S, Chavez E, Dragowska V, Zijlmans M, Bryan T, Reddel R, Egholm M, Bacchetti S, Martens U. Telomeres in the haemopoietic system. *Ciba Found Symp* 211:209–218; discussion 219–222, 1997.

Lanza RP, Caplan AL, Silver LM, Cibelli JB, West MD, Green RM. The ethical validity of using nuclear transfer in human transplantation. *JAMA* 284:3175–3179, 2000a.

Lanza RP, Cibelli JB, Blackwell C, Cristofalo VJ, Francis MK, Baerlocher GM, Mak J, Schertzer M, Chavez EA, Sawyer N, Lansdorp PM, West MD. Extension of cell life-span and telomere length in animals cloned from senescent somatic cells. *Science* 288:665–669, 2000b.

Lanza RP, Cibelli JB, Faber D, Sweeney RW, Henderson B, Nevala W, West MD, Wettstein PJ. Cloned cattle can be healthy and normal. *Science* 294:1893–1894, 2001.

Lanza RP, Cibelli JB, West MD. Human therapeutic cloning. *Nat Med* 5:975–977, 1999a.

Lanza RP, Cibelli JB, West MD. Prospects for the use of nuclear transfer in human transplantation. *Nat Biotechnol* 17:1171–1174, 1999b.

Lanzendorf SE, Boyd CA, Wright DL, Muasher S, Oehninger S, Hodgen GD. Use of human gametes obtained from anonymous donors for the production of human embryonic stem cell lines. *Fertil Steril* 76:132–137, 2001.

Laroche T, Martin SG, Tsai-Pflugfelder M, Gasser SM. The dynamics of yeast telomeres and silencing proteins through the cell cycle. *J Struct Biol* 129:159–174, 2000.

Larsen CJ. Telomerase and cancer: a therapeutic breakthrough or a cul-de-sac? [in French]. *Bull Cancer* 87:305–306, 2000.

Larsen PL. Aging and resistance to oxidative damage in *Caenorhabditis elegans*. *Proc Natl Acad Sci USA* 90:8905–8909, 1993.

Larsen PL, Albert PS, Riddle DL. Genes that regulate both development and longevity in *Caenorhabditis elegans. Genetics* 139:1567–1583, 1995.

Larsen PL, Clarke CF. Extension of life span in *Caenorhabditis elegans* by a diet lacking coenzyme Q. *Science* 295:120–123, 2002.

Lass A, Sohal BH, Weindruch R, Forster MJ, Sohal RS. Caloric restriction prevents age-associated accrual of oxidative damage to mouse skeletal muscle mitochondria. *Free Radic Biol Med* 25:1089–1097, 1998.

Lass JH, Greiner JV, Merchant TE, Glonek T. The effects of age on phosphatic metabolites of the human cornea. *Cornea* 14:89–94, 1995.

Latham RE. *Marco Polo. The Travels.* Penguin Classics, London, 1958.

Latil A, Vidaud D, Valeri A, Fournier G, Vidaud M, Lidereau R, Cussenot O, Biache I. hTERT expression correlates with MYC over-expression in human prostate cancer. *Int J Cancer* 89:172–176, 2000.

Lau D, Xue L, Hu R, Liaw T, Wu R, Reddy S. Expression and regulation of a molecular marker, SPR1, in multistep bronchial carcinogenesis. *Am J Respir Cell Mol Biol* 22:92–96, 2000.

Laux I, Khoshnan A, Tindell C, Bae D, Zhu X, June CH, Effros RB, Nel A. Response differences between human CD4(+) and CD8(+) T-cells during CD28 costimulation: implications for immune cell-based therapies and studies related to the expansion of double-positive T-cells during aging. *Clin Immunol* 96:187–197, 2000.

Lauzon W, Sanchez Dardon J, Cameron DW, Badley AD. Flow cytometric measurement of telomere length. *Cytometry* 42:159–164, 2000.

Lavelle F, Riou JF, Laoui A, Mailliet P. Telomerase: a therapeutic target for the third millennium? *Crit Rev Oncol Hematol* 34:111–126, 2000.

Lavranos TC, Mathis JM, Latham SE, Kalionis B, Shay JW, Rodgers RJ. Evidence for ovarian granulosa stem cells: telomerase activity and localization of the telomerase ribonucleic acid component in bovine ovarian follicles. *Biol Reprod* 61:358–366, 1999.

Lawton AJ, Mead GM. Staging and prognostic factors in testicular cancer. *Semin Surg Oncol* 17:223–229, 1999.

Layne JE, Nelson ME. The effects of progressive resistance training on bone density: a review. *Med Sci Sports Exerc* 31:25–30, 1999.

Lazaris ACh, Rigopoulou A, Tseleni-Balafouta S, Kavantzas N, Thimara I, Zorzos HS, Eutychiadis CA, Petraki K, Kandiloros D, Davaris P. Immunodetection and clinico-pathological correlates of two tumour growth regulators in laryngeal carcinoma. *Histol Histopathol* 17:131–138, 2002.

Lazarus HM. Hematopoietic progenitor cell transplantation in breast cancer: current status and future directions. *Cancer Invest* 16:102–126, 1998.

Le DL, Hoeffel CC, Nguyen QK, Nguyen HN. Gilford progeria. A case report [in French]. *Ann Med Interne (Paris)* 150:512–518, 1999a.

Le S, Moore JK, Haber JE, Greider CW. RAD50 and RAD51 define two pathways that collaborate to maintain telomeres in the absence of telomerase. *Genetics* 152:143–152, 1999b.

Le S, Sternglanz R, Greider CW. Identification of two RNA-binding proteins associated with human telomerase RNA. *Mol Biol Cell* 11:999–1010, 2000.

Le S, Zhu JJ, Anthony DC, Greider CW, Black PM. Telomerase activity in human gliomas. *Neurosurgery* 42:1120–1124, 1998.

Lea JS, Miller DS. Optimum screening interventions for gynecologic malignancies. *Tex Med* 97:49–55, 2001.

Leakey R. *Origins Reconsidered: In Search of What Makes Us Human.* Doubleday, New York, 1992.

Lear TL. Chromosomal distribution of the telomere sequence (TTAGGG)(n) in the *Equidae. Cytogenet Cell Genet* 93:127–130, 2001.

Learner N, Day HJ, Weiss L, DiGeorge A. Chromosomes in Werner's syndrome. *Lancet* 1:536–537, 1962.

Leber B, Bacchetti S. Telomeres and telomerase in normal and malignant haematologic cells. *Leuk Lymphoma* 24:1–9, 1996.

Lebkowski JS, Philip R, Okarma TB. Breast cancer: cell and gene therapy. *Cancer Invest* 15:568–576, 1997.

LeBlanc ES, Janowsky J, Chan BKS, Nelson HD. Hormone replacement therapy and cognition: systematic review and meta-analysis. *JAMA* 285:1489–1499, 2001.

Leblond CP. Classification of cell populations on the basis of their proliferative behaviour. *Natl Cancer Inst Monogr* 14:119–149, 1964.

Le Bourg E. Gerontologists and the media in a time of gerontology expansion. *Biogerontology* 1:89–92, 2000.

Le Bourg E. Applying hormesis in aging research and therapy: a sensible hope? *Belle Newsletter* 9:13–14, 2001.

Le Bras J, Longuet C, Charmot G. Human transmission and plasmodium resistance [in French]. *Rev Prat* 48:258–263, 1998.

Lee CC, Huang TS. A novel topoisomerase II poison GL331 preferentially induces DNA cleavage at (C/G)T sites and can cause telomere DNA damage. *Pharm Res* 18:846–851, 2001.

Lee CK, Klopp RG, Weindruch R, Prolla TA. Gene expression profile of aging and its retardation by caloric restriction. *Science* 285:1390–1393, 1999a.

Lee CM, Aspnes LE, Chung SS, Weindruch R, Aiken JM. Influences of caloric restriction on age-associated skeletal muscle fiber characteristics and mitochondrial changes in rats and mice. *Ann NY Acad Sci* 854:182–191, 1998a.

Lee CM, Eimon P, Weindruch R, Aiken JM. Direct repeat sequences are not required at the breakpoints of age-associated mitochondrial DNA deletions in rhesus monkeys. *Mech Ageing Dev* 75:69–79, 1994a.

Lee CM, Lopez ME, Weindruch R, Aiken JM. Association of age-related mitochondrial abnormalities with skeletal muscle fiber atrophy. *Free Radic Biol Med* 25:964–972, 1998b.

Lee CM, Weindruch R, Aiken JM. Age-associated alterations of the mitochondrial genome. *Free Radic Biol Med* 22:1259–1269, 1997.

Lee DM, Friend DS, Gurish MF, Benoist C, Mathis D, Brenner MB. Mast cells: a cellular link between autoantibodies and inflammatory arthritis. *Science* 297:1689–1692, 2002a.

Lee G, Park BS, Han SE, Oh JE, You YO, Baek JH, Kim GS, Min BM. Concurrence of replicative senescence and elevated expression of p16(INK4A) with subculture-induced but not calcium-induced differentiation in normal human oral keratinocytes. *Arch Oral Biol* 45:809–818, 2000a.

Lee HC, Pang CY, Hsu HS, Wei YH. Differential accumulations of 4977–bp deletion in mitochondrial DNA of various tissues in human ageing. *Biochim Biophys Acta* 1226:37–43, 1994b.

Lee HC, Wei YH. Mutation and oxidative damage of mitochondrial DNA and defective turnover of mitochondria in human aging. *J Formos Med Assoc* 96:770–777, 1997.

Lee HC, Wei YH. Mitochondrial alterations, cellular response to oxidative stress and defective degradation of proteins in aging. *Biogerontology* 2:231–244, 2001.

Lee HW, Blasco MA, Gottlieb GJ, Horner JW 2nd, Greider CW, DePinho RA. Essential role of mouse telomerase in highly proliferative organs. *Nature* 392:569–574, 1998c.

Lee IM, Blair SN, Allison DB, Folsom AR, Harris TB, Manson JE, Wing RR. Epidemiologic data on the relationships of caloric intake, energy balance, and weight gain over the life span with longevity and morbidity. *J Gerontol A Biol Sci Med Sci* 56A:B7–19, 2001a.

Lee IM, Rexrode KM, Cook NR, Manson JE, Buring JE. Physical activity and coronary heart disease in women: is "no pain, no gain" passe? *JAMA* 285:1447–1454, 2001b.

Lee J, Duan W, Long JM, Ingram DK, Mattson MP. Dietary restriction increases the number of newly generated neural cells, and induces BDNF expression, in the dentate gyrus of rats. *J Mol Neurosci* 15:99–108, 2000b.

Lee J, Herman JP, Mattson MP. Dietary restriction selectively decreases glucocorticoid receptor expression in the hippocampus and cerebral cortex of rats. *Exp Neurol* 166:435–441, 2000c.

Lee KH, Rudolph KL, Ju YJ, Greenberg RA, Cannizzaro L, Chin L, Weiler SR, DePinho RA. Telomere dysfunction alters the chemotherapeutic profile of transformed cells. *Proc Natl Acad Sci USA* 98:3381–3386, 2001c.

Lee SHJ, Suh I, Kim IS, Appel LJ. Smoking and atherosclerotic cardiovascular disease in men with low levels of serum cholesterol: the Korea Medical Insurance Corporation study. *JAMA* 282:2149–2155, 1999b.

Lee SJ, Benveniste EN. Adhesion molecule expression and regulation on cells of the central nervous system. *J Neuroimmunol* 98:77–88, 1999.

Lee VMY. Tauists and βaptists united—well almost! *Science* 293:1446–1447, 2001.

Lee WW, Nam KH, Terao K, Yoshikawa Y. Age-related telomere length dynamics in peripheral blood mononuclear cells of healthy cynomolgus monkeys measured by Flow FISH. *Immunology* 105:458–465, 2002b.

Lees JA, Weinberg RA. Tossing monkey wrenches into the clock: new ways of treating cancer. *Proc Natl Acad Sci USA* 96:4221–4223, 1999.

Leevy CB. Abnormalities of liver regeneration: a review. *Dig Dis* 16:88–98, 1998.

Lefkowitz RJ, Willerson JT. Prospects for cardiovascular research. *JAMA* 285:581–593, 2001.

Leissring MA, Akbari Y, Fanger CM, Cahalan MD, Mattson MP, LaFerla FM. Capacitative calcium entry deficits and elevated luminal calcium content in mutant presenilin-1 knockin mice. *J Cell Biol* 149:793–798, 2000.

Lemke MR, Glatzel M, Henneberg AE. Antimicroglia antibodies in sera of Alzheimer's disease patients. *Biol Psychiatry* 45:508–511, 1999.

Lenfant F, Mann RK, Thomsen B, Ling X, Grunstein M All four core histone N-termini contain sequences required for the repression of basal transcription in yeast. *EMBO J* 15:3974–3985, 1996.

Leopold JA, Loscalzo J. Clinical importance of understanding vascular biology. *Cardiol Rev* 8:115–123, 2000.

Leri A, Malhotra A, Liew CC, Kajstura J, Anversa P. Telomerase activity in rat cardiac myocytes is age and gender dependent. *J Mol Cell Cardiol* 32:385–390, 2000.

Leslie KK, Kumar NS. Endocrine cancer risks for women during the perimenopause and beyond. *Semin Reprod Endocrinol* 17:359–370, 1999.

Leung JK, Pereira-Smith OM. Identification of genes involved in cell senescence and immortalization: potential implications for tissue ageing. *Novartis Found Symp* 235:105–110, 2001.

Leveugle B, Ding W, Buee L, Fillit HM. Interleukin-1 and nerve growth factor induce hypersecretion and hypersulfation of neuroblastoma proteoglycans which bind beta-amyloid. *J Neuroimmunol* 60:151–160, 1995.

Leveugle B, Ding W, Durkin JT, Mistretta S, Eisle J, Matic M, Siman R, Greenberg BD, Fillit HM. Heparin promotes beta-secretase cleavage of the Alzheimer's amyloid precursor protein. *Neurochem Int* 30:543–548, 1997.

Leveugle B, Ding W, Laurence F, Dehouck MP, Scanameo A, Cecchelli R, Fillit H. Heparin oligosaccharides that pass the blood–brain barrier inhibit beta-amyloid precursor protein secretion and heparin binding to beta-amyloid peptide. *J Neurochem* 70:736–744, 1998.

Levis RW. Viable deletions of a telomere from a *Drosophila* chromosome. *Cell* 58:791–801, 1989.

Levrero M, De Laurenzi V, Costanzo A, Gong J, Wang JY, Melino G. The p53/p63/p73 family of transcription factors: overlapping and distinct functions. *J Cell Sci* 113:1661–1670, 2000.

Levy MZ, Allsopp RC, Futcher AB, Greider CW, Harley CB. Telomere end-replication problem and cell aging. *J Mol Biol* 225:951–960, 1992.

LeWinter MM, Decena B, Tischler MD. Abonromalities in myocardial relaxation and filling: diastolic dysfunction. In Hosenpud JD, Greenberg BH (eds). *Congestive Heart Failure.* Lippincott Williams & Wilkins, Philadelphia, 2000, pp 83–100.

Lewis J, Dickson DW, Lin WL, Chisholm L, Corral A, Jones G, Yen SH, Sahara N, Skipper L, Yager D, Eckman C, Hardy J, Hutton M, McGowan E. Enhanced neurofibrillary degeneration in transgenic mice expressing mutant tau and APP. *Science* 293:1487–1491, 2001.

Lewis JF. Clinical and echocardiographic features of hypertrophic cardiomyopathy in the elderly. *Am J Geriatr Cardiol* 10:11–17, 2001.

Lewis LK, Karthikeyan G, Westmoreland JW, Resnick MA. Differential suppression of DNA repair deficiencies of yeast rad50, mre11 and xrs2 mutants by EXO1 and TLC1 (the RNA component of telomerase). *Genetics* 160:49–62, 2002.

Lewis M. PRELP, collagen, and a theory of Hutchinson-Gilford progeria. *Ageing Res Rev* 2:95–105, 2003.

Lezhava T. Chromosome and aging: genetic conception of aging. *Biogerontology* 2:253–260, 2001a.

Lezhava TA. Human chromosome functional characteristics and aging [in Russian]. *Adv Gerontol* 8:34–43, 2001b.

Lezza AMS, Mecocci P, Cormio A, Flint Beal M, Cherubini A, Cantatore P, Semin U, Gadaleta MN. Area-specific differences of OH8dG and mtDNA4977 levels in AD patients and aged controls. *J Anti-Aging Med* 2:209–216, 1999.

Li B, Oestreich S, de Lange T. Identification of human Rap1: implications for telomere evolution. *Cell* 101:471–483, 2000a.

Li B, Yang J, Andrews C, Chen YX, Toofanfard P, Huang RW, Horvath E, Chopra H, Raza A, Preisler HD. Telomerase activity in preleukemia and acute myelogenous leukemia. *Leuk Lymphoma* 36:579–587, 2000b.

Li B, Yang J, Tao M, Nayini J, Horvath E, Chopra H, Meyer P, Venugopal P, Preisler HD. Poor prognosis acute myelogenous leukemia 2—biological and molecular biological characteristics and treatment outcome. *Leuk Res* 24:777–789, 2000c.

Li C, Liang Y, Wu M, Xu L, Cai W. Telomerase activity analysis of esophageal carcinoma using microdissection-TRAP assay. *Chin Med J (Engl)* 115:1405–1408, 2002.

Li D, Friedman SL. Liver fibrogenesis and the role of hepatic stellate cells: new insights and prospects for therapy. *J Gastroenterol Hepatol* 14:618–633, 1999.

Li F, Altieri DC. The cancer antiapoptosis mouse survivin gene: characterization of locus and transcriptional requirements of basal and cell cycle–dependent expression. *Cancer Res* 59:3143–3151, 1999.

Li GZ, Eller MS, Firoozabadi R, Gilchrest BA. Evidence that exposure of the telomere 3* overhang sequence induces senescence. *PNAS* 100:527–551, 2003.

Li H, Cao Y, Berndt MC, Funder JW, Liu JP. Molecular interactions between telomerase and the tumor suppressor protein p53 in vitro. *Oncogene* 18:6785–6794, 1999a.

Li H, Liu JP. Signaling on telomerase: a master switch in cell aging and immortalization. *Biogerontology* 3:107–116, 2002.

Li JJ, Dickson D, Hof PR, Vlassara H. Receptors for advanced glycosylation end products in human brain: role in brain homeostasis. *Mol Med* 4:46–60, 1998a.

Li JL, Harrison RJ, Reszka AP, Brosh RM Jr, Bohr VA, Neidle S, Hickson ID. Inhibition of the Bloom's and Werner's syndrome helicases by G-quadruplex interacting ligands. *Biochemistry* 40:15194–15202, 2001.

Li K, Tamai K, Tan EML, Uitto J. Cloning of type XVII collagen. Complementary and genomic DNA sequences of mouse 180-kilodalton bullous pemphigoid antigen (BPAG2) predict an interrupted collagenous domain, a transmembrane segment, and unusual features in the 5'-end of the gene and the 3'-untranslated region of the mRNA. *J Biol Chem* 268:8825–8834, 1993.

Li W, Yanoff M, Li Y, He Z. Artificial senescence of bovine retinal pigment epithelial cells induced by near-ultraviolet in vitro. *Mech Ageing Dev* 110:137–155, 1999b.

Li Y, Nichols MA, Shay JW, Xiong Y. Transcriptional repression of the D-type cyclin-dependent kinase inhibitor p16 by the retinoblastoma susceptibility gene product pRb. *Cancer Res* 54:6078–6082, 1994.

Li Y, Wolf NS. Effects of age and long-term caloric restriction on the aqueous collecting channel in the mouse eye. *J Glaucoma* 6:18–22, 1997.

Li Y, Yan Q, Pendergrass WR, Wolf NS. Response of lens epithelial cells to hydrogen peroxide stress and the protective effect of caloric restriction. *Exp Cell Res* 239:254–263, 1998b.

Li Y, Yan Q, Wolf NS. Long-term caloric restriction delays age-related decline in proliferation capacity of murine lens epithelial cells in vitro and in vivo. *Invest Ophthalmol Vis Sci* 95:13097–13102, 1997.

Libby P, Aikawa M, Kinlay S, Selwyn A, Ganz P. Lipid lowering improves endothelial functions. *Int J Cardiol* 74(Suppl 1):S3–S10, 2000.

Lieber CS. Prevention and treatment of liver fibrosis based on pathogenesis. *Alcohol Clin Exp Res* 23:944–949, 1999.

Lim CS, Mian IS, Dernburg AF, Campisi J. *C. elegans clk-2*, a gene that limits life span, encodes a telomere length regulator similar to yeast telomere binding protein Tel2p. *Curr Biol* 11:1706–1710, 2001.

Lin JJ, Zakian VA. Isolation and characterization of two *Saccharomyces cerevisiae* genes that encode proteins that bind to (TG1-3)n single strand telomeric DNA in vitro. *Nucleic Acids Res* 22:4906–4913, 1994.

Lin JJ, Zakian VA. An in vitro assay for *Saccharomyces* telomerase requires EST1. *Cell* 81:1127–1135, 1995.

Lin JJ, Zakian VA. The *Saccharomyces* CDC13 protein is a single-strand TG1–3 telomeric DNA-binding protein in vitro that affects telomere behavior in vivo. *Proc Natl Acad Sci USA* 93:13760–13765, 1996.

Lin K, Dorman JB, Rodan A, Kenyon C. daf-16: An HNF-3/forkhead family member that can function to double the life span of *Caenorhabditis elegans*. *Science* 278:1319–1322, 1997.

Lin SJ, Defossez PA, Guarente L. Requirement of NAD and SIR2 for life span extension by calorie restriction in *Saccharomyces cerevisiae*. *Science* 289:2126–2128, 2000a.

Lin X, Koelsch G, Wu S, Downs D, Dashti A, Tang J. Human aspartic protease memapsin 2 cleaves the beta-secretase site of beta-amyloid precursor protein. *Proc Natl Acad Sci USA* 97:1456–1460, 2000b.

Lin YC, Shih JW, Hsu CL, Lin JJ. Binding and partial denaturing of G-quartet DNA by Cdc13p of *Saccharomyces cerevisiae*. *J Biol Chem* 276:47671–47674, 2001.

Lindahl T, Barnes DE, Klungland A, Mackenney VJ, Schar P. Repair and processing events at DNA ends. *Ciba Found Symp* 211:198–205; discussion 205–208, 1997.

Lindahl T, Wood RD. Quality control by DNA repair. *Science* 286:1897–1905, 1999.

Lindeman RD, Tobin J, Shock NW. Longitudinal studies on the rate of decline in renal function with age. *J Am Geriatr Soc* 33:278–285, 1985.

Lindop GB, Boyle JJ, McEwan P, Kenyon CJ. Vascular structure, smooth muscle cell phenotype and growth in hypertension. *J Hum Hypertens* 9:475–478, 1995.

Lindsay R, Cosman F, Herrington BS, Himmelstein S. Bone mass and body composition in normal women. *J Bone Miner Res* 7:55–63, 1992.

Lindsay R, Gallagher JC, Kleerekoper M, Pickar JH. Effect of lower doses of conjugated equine estrogens with and without medroxyprogesterone acetate on bone in early postmenopausal women. *JAMA* 287:2668–2676, 2002.

Lindsey J, McGill NI, Lindsey LA, Green DK, Cooke HJ. In vivo loss of telomeric repeats with age in humans. *Mutat Res* 256:45–48, 1991.

Lindstrom UM, Chandrasekaran RA, Orbai L, Helquist SA, Miller GP, Oroudjev E, Hansma HG, Kool ET. Artificial human telomeres from DNA nanocircle templates. *Proc Natl Acad Sci USA* 99:15953–15958, 2002.

Lingner J, Cech TR. Telomerase and chromosome end maintenance. *Curr Opin Genet Dev* 8:226–232, 1998.

Lingner J, Cooper JP, Cech TR. Telomerase and DNA end replication: no longer a lagging strand problem? *Science* 269:1533–1534, 1995.

Lingner J, Hughes TR, Shevchenko AJ, Mann M, Lundblad V, Cech TR. Reverse transcriptase motifs in the catalytic subunit of telomerase. *Science* 276:561–567, 1997.

Linnane AW, Baumer A, Maxwell RJ, Preston H, Zhang CF, Marzuki S. Mitochondrial gene mutation: the ageing process and degenerative diseases. *Biochem Int* 22:1067–1076, 1990.

Linnane AW, Zhang C, Baumer A, Nagley P. Mitochondrial DNA mutation and the ageing process: bioenergy and pharmacological intervention. *Mutat Res* 275:195–208, 1992.

Lino M, Goto K, Kakegawa W, Okado H, Sudo M, Ishiuchi S, Miwa A, Takayasu Y, Saito I, Tsuzuki K, Ozawa S. Glia–synapse interaction through Ca^{2+}-permeable AMPA receptors in Bergmann glia. *Science* 292:926–929, 2001.

Linskens MH, Feng J, Andrews WH, Enlow BE, Saati SM, Tonkin LA, Funk WD, Villeponteau B. Cataloging altered gene expression in young and senescent cells using enhanced differential display. *Nucleic Acids Res* 23:3244–3251, 1995a.

Linskens MH, Harley CB, West MD, Campisi J, Hayflick L. Replicative senescence and cell death. *Science* 267:17, 1995b.

Linton PJ, Haynes L, Tsui L, Zhang X, Swain S. From naive to effector: alterations with aging. *Immunol Rev* 160:9–18, 1997.

Lio D, D'Anna C, Gervasi F, Scola L, Potestio M, Di Lorenzo G, Listi F, Colombo A, Candore G, Caruso C. Interleukin 12-release by mitogen-stimulated mononuclear cells in the elderly. *Mech Ageing Dev* 102:211–219, 1998.

Lipman JM, Applegate-Stevens A, Soyka LA, Hart RW. Cell-cycle defect of DNA repair in progeria skin fibroblasts. *Mutat Res* 219:273–281, 1989.

Lipsitz R. Biology — cell death. One-hit wonder. *Sci Am* 283:26–27, 2000.

Lipsky PE. The clinical potential of cyclooxygenase-2-specific inhibitors. *Am J Med* 106:51S–57S, 1999.

Lithgow GJ. Hormesis — a new hope for aging studies or a poor second to genetics? *Belle Newsletter* 9:15–16, 2001.

Lithgow GJ, Kirkwood TB. Mechanisms and evolution of aging. *Science* 273:80, 1996.

Liu BC, Loughlin KR. Telomerase in human bladder cancer. *Urol Clin North Am* 27:115–123, 2000.

Liu H, Dong XP, Zhou W. The immortalized cell lines induced by human papillomavirus type 16. *Zhonghua Shi Yan He Lin Chuang Bing Du Xue Za Zhi* 14:205–208, 2000a.

Liu J, Head E, Gharib AM, Yuan W, Ingersoll RT, Hagen TM, Cotman CW, Ames BN. Memory loss in old rats is associated with brain mitochondrial decay and RNA/DNA oxidation: partial reversal by feeding acetyl-L-carnitine and/or *R*-lipoic acid. *Proc Natl Acad Sci USA* 99: 2356–2361, 2002a.

Liu J, Killilea DW, Ames BN. Age-associated mitochondrial oxidative decay: improvement of carnitine acetyltransferase substrate-binding affinity and activity in brain by feeding old rats acetyl-L-carnitine and/or *R*-lipoic acid. *Proc Natl Acad Sci USA* 99: 1876–1881, 2002b.

Liu JJ, Shay JW, Wilson SE. Characterization of a soluble KGF receptor cDNA from human corneal and breast epithelial cells. *Invest Ophthalmol Vis Sci* 39:2584–2593, 1998.

Liu JP. Studies of the molecular mechanisms in the regulation of telomerase activity. *FASEB J* 13:2091–1204, 1999.

Liu K, Hodes RJ, Weng NP. Cutting edge: telomerase activation in human T lymphocytes does not require increase in telomerase reverse transcriptase (hTERT) protein but is associated with hTERT phosphorylation and nuclear translocation. *J Immunol* 166:4826–4830, 2001a.

Liu K, Schoonmaker MM, Levine BL, June CH, Hodes RJ, Weng NP. Constitutive and regulated expression of telomerase reverse transcriptase (hTERT) in human lymphocytes. *Proc Natl Acad Sci USA* 96:5147–5152, 1999.

Liu L, Blasco M, Trimarchi J, Keefe D. An essential role for functional telomeres in mouse germ cells during fertilization and early development. *Dev Biol* 249:74–84, 2002c.

Liu L, Blasco MA, Keefe DL. Requirement of functional telomeres for metaphase chromosome alignments and integrity of meiotic spindles. *EMBO Rep* 3:230–234, 2002d.

Liu L, Sun B, Liang Y. Analysis of telomerase activity and telomere length in acute myelogenous leukemia [in Chinese]. *Zhonghua Xue Ye Xue Za Zhi* 22:592–594. Chinese, 2001b.

Liu SC, Meagher K, Hanawalt PC. Role of solar conditioning in DNA repair response and survival of human epidermal keratinocytes following UV irradiation. *J Invest Dermatol* 85:93–97, 1985.

Liu SC, Parsons CS, Hanawalt PC. DNA repair response in human epidermal keratinocytes from donors of different age. *J Invest Dermatol* 79:330–335, 1982.

Liu Y, Kha H, Ungrin M, Robinson MO, Harrington L. Preferential maintenance of critically short telomeres in mammalian cells heterozygous for mTert. *Proc Natl Acad Sci USA* 99:3597–3602, 2002e.

Liu Y, Snow BE, Hande MP, Baerlocher G, Kickhoefer VA, Yeung D, Wakeham A, Itie A, Siderovski DP, Lansdorp PM, Robinson MO, Harrington L. Telomerase-associated protein TEP1 is not essential for telomerase activity or telomere length maintenance in vivo. *Mol Cell Biol* 20:8178–8184, 2000b.

Liu Y, Snow BE, Hande MP, Yeung D, Erdmann NJ, Wakeham A, Itie A, Siderovski DP, Lansdorp PM, Robinson MO, Harrington L. The telomerase reverse transcriptase is limiting and necessary for telomerase function in vivo. *Curr Biol* 10:1459–1462, 2000c.

Livingston DM, Shivdasani R. Toward mechanism-based cancer care. *JAMA* 285:588–593, 2001.

Livingston G. The scale of the problem. In Burns A, Levy R (eds). *Dementia, 1st ed.* Chapman and Hall, London, 1994, pp 21–35.

Lloyd JM, Hoffman GE, Wise PM. Decline in immediate early gene expression in gonadotropin-releasing hormone neurons during proestrus in regularly cycling, middle-aged rats. *Endocrinology* 134:1800–1805, 1994.

Lo AW, Sabatier L, Fouladi B, Pottier G, Ricoul M, Murnane JP. DNA amplification by breakage/fusion/bridge cycles initiated by spontaneous telomere loss in a human cancer cell line. *Neoplasia* 4:531–538, 2002.

Lo YM, Chan WY, Ng EK, Chan LY, Lai PB, Tam JS, Chung SC. Circulating Epstein-Barr virus DNA in the serum of patients with gastric carcinoma. *Clin Cancer Res* 7:1856–1859, 2001.

Lockshin RA, Osborne B, Zakeri Z. Cell death in the third millenium. *Cell Death Differ* 7:2–7, 2000.

Lockshin RA, Zakeri ZF. Programmed cell death: new thoughts and relevance to aging. *J Gerontol* 45:B135–140, 1990.

Loeb C. Binswanger's disease is not a single entity. *Neurol Sci* 21:343–348, 2000.

Loeuillet C, Douay L, Herve P, Chalmers DE. Preservation of the myofibroblastic phenotype of human papilloma virus 16 E6/E7 immortalized human bone marrow cells using the lineage limited alpha-smooth muscle actin promoter. *Cell Growth Differ* 12:233–242, 2001.

Lokeshwar VB, Block NL. HA-HAase urine test. A sensitive and specific method for detecting bladder cancer and evaluating its grade. *Urol Clin North Am* 27:53–61, 2000.

Lokeshwar VB, Soloway MS. Current bladder tumor tests: does their projected utility fulfill clinical necessity? *J Urol* 165:1067–1077, 2001.

Lombard DB, Guarente L. Nijmegen breakage syndrome disease protein and MRE11 at PML nuclear bodies and meiotic telomeres. *Cancer Res* 60:2331–2334, 2000.

Lombardi VR, Garcia M, Cacabelos R. Microglial activation induced by factor(s) contained in sera from Alzheimer-related ApoE genotypes. *J Neurosci Res* 54:539–553, 1998.

Londono-Vallejo JA, DerSarkissian H, Cazes L, Thomas G. Differences in telomere length between homologous chromosomes in humans. *Nucleic Acids Res* 29:3164–3171, 2001.

Lord JM, Akbar AN, Kipling D. Telomere-based therapy for immunosenescence. *Trends Immunol* 23:175–176, 2002.

Lord RV, Salonga D, Danenberg KD, Peters JH, DeMeester TR, Park JM, Johansson J, Skinner KA, Chandrasoma P, DeMeester SR, Bremner CG, Tsai PI, Danenberg PV. Telomerase reverse transcriptase expression is increased early in the Barrett's metaplasia, dysplasia, adenocarcinoma sequence. *J Gastrointest Surg* 4:135–142, 2000.

Lorenz M, Saretzki G, Sitte N, Metzkow S, von Zglinicki T. BJ fibroblasts display high antioxidant capacity and slow telomere shortening independent of hTERT transfection. *Free Radic Biol Med* 31:824–831, 2001.

Loschen G, Azzi A, Richter C, Flohe L. Superoxide radicals as precursors of mitochondrial hydrogen peroxide. *FEBS Lett* 42:68–72, 1974.

Losi L, Dal Cin P. Telomeres: a review of the literature [in Italian]. *Pathologica* 91:121–123, 1999.

Loughran O, Clark LJ, Bond J, Baker A, Berry IJ, Edington KG, Ly IS, Simmons R, Haw R, Black DM, Newbold RF, Parkinson EK. Evidence for the inactivation of multiple replicative life span genes in immortal human squamous cell carcinoma keratinocytes. *Oncogene* 14:1955–1964, 1997.

Loughran O, Malliri A, Owens D, Gallimore PH, Stanley MA, Ozanne B, Frame MC, Parkinson EK. Association of CDKN2A/p16INK4A with human head and neck keratinocyte replicative senescence: relationship of dysfunction to immortality and neoplasia. *Oncogene* 13:561–568, 1996.

Loveday RL, Greenman J, Drew PJ, Monson JR, Kerin MJ. Genetic changes associated with telomerase activity in breast cancer. *Int J Cancer* 84:516–520, 1999.

Lovell MA, Ehmann WD, Butler SM, Markesbury WR. Elevated thiobarbituric acid–reactive substances and antioxidant enzyme activity in the brain in Alzheimer's disease. *Neurology* 45:1594–1601, 1995.

Lowell JE, Pillus L. Telomere tales: chromatin, telomerase and telomere function in *Saccharomyces cerevisiae*. *Cell Mol Life Sci* 54:32–49, 1998.

Lubbe J, Nakazawa H, Burg G. Telomerase [in German]. *Hautarzt* 48:615–621, 1997.

Luckinbill LS, Arking R, Clare MJ, Cirocco WC, Buck SA. Selection for delayed senescence in *Drosophila melanogaster*. *Evolution* 38:996–1003, 1984.

Luckinbill LS, Foley P. The role of metabolism in aging. *J Am Aging Assoc* 23:85–93, 2000.

Ludwig A, Saretzki G, Holm PS, Tiemann F, Lorenz M, Emrich T, Harley CB, von Zglinicki T. Ribozyme cleavage of telomerase mRNA sensitizes breast epithelial cells to inhibitors of topoisomerase. *Cancer Res* 61:3053–3061, 2001.

Lue LF, Brachova L, Civin WH, Rogers J. Inflammation, A beta deposition, and neurofibrillary tangle formation as correlates of Alzheimer's disease neurodegeneration. *J Neuropathol Exp Neurol* 55:1083–1088, 1996.

Lue LF, Rydel R, Brigham EF, Yang LB, Hampel H, Murphy GM Jr, Brachova L, Yan SD, Walker DG, Shen Y, Rogers J. Inflammatory repertoire of Alzheimer's disease and nondemented elderly microglia in vitro. *Glia* 35:72–79, 2001.

Luhtala TA, Roecker EB, Pugh T, Feuers RJ, Weindruch R. Dietary restriction attenuates age-related increases in rat skeletal muscle antioxidant enzyme activities. *J Gerontol* 49:B231–238, 1994.

Lukowiak AA, Narayanan A, Li ZH, Terns RM, Terns MP. The snoRNA domain of vertebrate telomerase RNA functions to localize the RNA within the nucleus. *RNA* 7:1833–1844, 2001.

Lumelsky N, Blondel O, Laeng P, Velasco I, Ravin R, McKay R. Differentiation of embryonic stem cells to insulin-secreting structures similar to pancreatic islets. *Science* 292:1389–1394, 2001.

Lumpkin CK, Knepper JE, Butel JS, Smith JR, Pereira-Smith OM. Mitogenic effects of the proto-oncogene and oncogene forms of c-H-ras DNA in human diploid fibroblasts. *Mol Cell Biol* 6:2990–2993, 1986a.

Lumpkin CK, McClung JK, Pereira-Smith OM, Smith JR. Existence of high abundance anti-proliferative mRNA's in senescent human diploid fibroblasts. *Science* 232:393–395, 1986b.

Lundberg AS, Weinberg RA. Control of the cell cycle and apoptosis. *Eur J Cancer* 35:531–539, 1999.

Lundblad V. Telomeres keep on rappin'. *Science* 288:2141–2142, 2000.

Lundblad V. Genome instability: McClintock revisited. *Curr Biol* 11:R957–960, 2001.

Lundblad V. Telomere maintenance without telomerase. *Oncogene* 21:522–531, 2002.

Lundblad V, Szostak JW. A mutant with a defect in telomere elongation leads to senescence in yeast. *Cell* 57:633–643, 1989.

Lundblad V, Wright WE. Telomeres and telomerase: a simple picture becomes complex. *Cell* 87:369–375, 1996.

Luo L, Chen H, Zirkin BR. Are Leydig cell steroidogenic enzymes differentially regulated with aging? *J Androl* 17:509–515, 1996.

Luo L, Chen H, Zirkin BR. Leydig cell aging: steroidogenic acute regulatory protein (StAR) and cholesterol side-chain cleavage enzyme. *J Androl* 22:149–156, 2001.

Luoto R, Manolio T, Meilahn E, Bhadelia R, Furberg C, Cooper L, Kraut M. Estrogen re-placement therapy and MRI-demonstrated cerebral infarcts, white matter changes, and brain atrophy in older women: the cardiovascular health study. *J Am Geriatr Soc* 48:467–472, 2000.

Lupien SJ, Nair NP, Briere S, Maheu F, Tu MT, Lemay M, McEwen BS, Meaney MJ. Increased cortisol levels and impaired cognition in human aging: implication for depression and dementia in later life. *Rev Neurosci* 10:117–139, 1999.

Lustig AJ. Mechanisms of silencing in Saccharomyces cerevisiae. *Curr Opin Genet Dev* 8:233–239, 1998.

Lustig AJ. Crisis intervention: the role of telomerase. *Proc Natl Acad Sci USA* 96:3339–3341, 1999.

Lustig AJ, Kurtz S, Shore D. Involvement of the silencer and UAS binding protein RAP1 in regulation of telomere length. *Science* 250:549–553, 1990.

Luterman JD, Haroutunian V, Yemul S, Ho L, Purohit D, Aisen PS, Mohs R, Pasinetti GM. Cytokine gene expression as a function of the clinical progression of Alzheimer disease dementia. *Arch Neurol* 57:1153–1160, 2000.

Ly DH, Lockhart DJ, Lerner RA, Schultz PG. Mitotic misregulation and human aging. *Science* 287:2486–2492, 2000.

Lynch CD, Cooney PT, Bennett SA, Thornton PL, Khan AS, Ingram RL, Sonntag WE. Effects of moderate caloric restriction on cortical microvascular density and local cerebral blood flow in aged rats. *Neurobiol Aging* 20:191–200, 1999.

Lynch HT, De La Chapelle A. Genetic susceptibility to non-polyposis colorectal cancer. *J Med Genet* 36:801–811, 1999.

Lyras L, Cairns NJ, Jenner A, Jenner P, Halliwell B. An assessment of oxidative damage to proteins, lipids, and DNA in brain from patients with Alzheimer's disease. *J Neurochem* 68:2061–2069, 1997.

Ma LP, Pan XY, Yan ZY, Zhang Y, Jiang B, Wang SW. A quantitative assay for telomerase activity in peripheral blood mononuclear cells from patients with acute leukemia [in Chinese]. *Zhongguo Shi Yan Xue Ye Xue Za Zhi* 10:191–194, 2002a.

Ma W, Wlaschek M, Brenneisen P, Schneider LA, Hommel C, Hellweg C, Sauer H, Wartenberg M, Herrmann G, Meewes C, Boukamp P, Scharffetter-Kochanek K. Human dermal fibroblasts escape from the long-term phenocopy of senescence induced by psoralen photoactivation. *Exp Cell Res* 274:299–309, 2002b.

Ma XY, Su YB, Zhang FR, Li JF. Effects of vitamin E on the blastogenic response of splenocytes and lipofuscin contents in the hearts and brains of aged mice. *J Environ Pathol Toxicol Oncol* 15:51–53, 1996.

Ma YY, Wei SJ, Lin YC, Lung JC, Chang TC, Whang-Peng J, Liu JM, Yang DM, Yang WK, Shen CY. *PIK3CA* as an oncogene in cervical cancer. *Oncogene* 19:2739–2744, 2000.

Macera-Bloch L, Houghton J, Lenahan M, Jha KK, Ozer HL. Termination of life span of SV40-transformed human fibroblasts in crisis is due to apoptosis. *J Cell Physiol* 190:332–344, 2002.

MacGibbon MF, Walls RS, Everitt AV. An age-related decline in melatonin secretion is not altered by food restriction. *J Gerontol A Biol Sci Med Sci* 56:21–26, 2001.

Machiavelli N. *The Prince*. Bantam Classic Edition Bantam Books, New York, 1981. Original publication, 1513.

Macieira-Coelho A. Changes in membrane properties associated with cellular aging. *Int Rev Cytol* 83:183–220, 1983.

Macieira-Coelho A. Ups and downs of aging studies in vitro: the crooked path of science. *Gerontology* 46:55–63, 2000.

Maciel AT. Evidence for autosomal recessive inheritance of progeria (Hutchinson Gilford). *Am J Med Genet* 31:483–487, 1988.

MacKenzie KL, Franco S, May C, Sadelain M, Moore MA. Mass cultured human fibroblasts overexpressing hTERT encounter a growth crisis following an extended period of proliferation. *Exp Cell Res* 259:336–350, 2000.

MacKenzie KL, Franco S, Naiyer AJ, May C, Sadelain M, Rafii S, Moore MA. Multiple stages of malignant transformation of human endothelial cells modeled by co-expression of telomerase reverse transcriptase, SV40 T antigen and oncogenic N-ras. *Oncogene* 21:4200–4211, 2002.

MacManus A, Ramsden M, Murray M, Henderson Z, Pearson HA, Campbell VA. Enhancement of (45)Ca($^{2+}$) influx and voltage-dependent Ca($^{2+}$) channel activity by β-amyloid-(1-40) in rat cortical synaptosomes and cultured cortical neurons. Modulation by the proinflammatory cytokine interleukin-1β. *J Biol Chem* 275:4713–4718, 2000.

MacNamara BG, Farn KT, Mitra AK, Lloyd JK, Fosbrooke AS. Progeria, case report with long-term studies of serum lipids. *Arch Dis Child* 45:553–560, 1970.

Maddar H, Ratzkovsky N, Krauskopf A. Role for telomere cap structure in meiosis. *Mol Biol Cell* 12:3191–3203, 2001.

Maddox GL (ed). *The Encyclopedia of Aging, Second Edition*. Springer Publishing Company, New York, 1995.

Maftah A, Ratinaud MH, Dumas M, Bonte F, Meybeck A, Julien R. Human epidermal cells progressively lose their cardiolipins during ageing without change in mitochondrial transmembrane potential. *Mech Ageing Dev* 77:83–96, 1994.

Magri F, Terenzi F, Ricciardi T, Fioravanti M, Solerte SB, Stabile M, Balza G, Gandini C, Villa M, Ferrari E. Association between changes in adrenal secretion and cerebral morphometric correlates in normal aging and senile dementia. *Dement Geriatr Cogn Disord* 11:90–99, 2000.

Mah AL, Perry G, Smith MA, Monteiro MJ. Identification of ubiquilin, a novel presenilin interactor that increases presenilin protein accumulation. *J Cell Biol* 151:847–862, 2000.

Mahadevia PJ, Fleisher LA, Frick KD, Eng J, Goodman SN, Powe NR. Lung cancer screening with helical computed tomography in older adult smokers: a decision and cost-effectiveness analysis. *JAMA* 289:313–322, 2003.

Mahmud N, Weiss P, Li F, Hoffman R. Primate skeletal muscle contains cells capable of sustaining in vitro hematopoiesis. *Exp Hematol* 30:925–936, 2002.

Maigne J, Deschatrette J, Sarrazin S, Hecquet B, Guerroui S, Wolfrom C. The time-pattern of rises and falls in proliferation fades with senescence of mortal lines and is perpetuated in immortal rat hepatoma Fao cell line. *In Vitro Cell Dev Biol Anim* 34:163–169, 1998.

Mailand N, Falck J, Lukas C, Syljuasen RG, Welcker M, Bartek J, Lukas J. Rapid destruction of human Cdc25A in response to DNA damage. *Science* 288:1425–1429, 2000.

Maitra A, Rathi A, Gazdar AF, Sagalowsky A, Ashfaq R. Expression of the RNA component of human telomerase (hTR) in ThinPrep preparations from bladder washings. *Cancer* 293:73–79, 2001.

Maitra A, Yashima K, Rathi A, Timmons CF, Rogers BB, Shay JW, Gazdar AF. The RNA component of telomerase as a marker of biologic potential and clinical outcome in childhood neuroblastic tumors. *Cancer* 85:741–749, 1999.

Majumdar AS, Hughes DE, Lichtsteiner SP, Wang Z, Lebkowski JS, Vasserot AP. The telomerase reverse transcriptase promoter drives efficacious tumor suicide gene therapy while preventing hepatotoxicity encountered with constitutive promoters. *Gene Ther* 8:568–578, 2001.

Makinodan T, Kay MM. Age influence on the immune system. *Adv Immunol* 29:287–330, 1980.

Makous N, Friedman S, Yakovac W, Maris EP. Cardiovascular manifestations in progeria. Report of clinical and pathologic findings in a patient with severe arteriosclerotic heart disease and aortic stenosis. *Am Heart J* 64:334–346, 1962.

Malek AM, Alper SL, Izumo S. Hemodynamic shear stress and its role in atherosclerosis. *JAMA* 282:2035–2042, 1999.

Malik NS, Meek KM. Vitamins and analgesics in the prevention of collagen ageing. *Age Ageing* 25:279–284, 1996.

Malik NS, Moss SJ, Ahmed N, Furth AJ, Wall RS, Meek KM. Ageing of the human corneal stroma: structural and biochemical changes. *Biochim Biophys Act* 1138:222–228, 1992.

Mangahas JL, Alexander MK, Sandell LL, Zakian VA. Repair of chromosome ends after telomere loss in *Saccharomyces*. *Mol Biol Cell* 12:4078–4089, 2001.

Mann MJ, Dzau VJ. Genetic manipulation of vein grafts. *Curr Opin Cardiol* 12:522–527, 1997.

Mann MJ, Gibbons GH, Kernoff RS, Diet FP, Tsao PS, Cooke JP, Kaneda Y, Dzau VJ. Genetic engineering of vein grafts resistant to atherosclerosis. *Proc Natl Acad Sci USA* 92:4502–4506, 1995.

Mann MJ, Gibbons GH, Tsao PS, von der Leyen HE, Cooke JP, Buitrago R, Kernoff R, Dzau VJ. Cell cycle inhibition preserves endothelial function in genetically engineered rabbit vein grafts. *J Clin Invest* 99:1295–1301, 1997a.

Mann MJ, Morishita R, Gibbons GH, von der Leyen HE, Dzau VJ. DNA transfer into vascular smooth muscle using fusigenic Sendai virus (HVJ)-liposomes. *Mol Cell Biochem* 172:3–12, 1997b.

Mann MJ, Whittemore AD, Donaldson MC, Belkin M, Conte MS, Polak JF, Orav EJ, Ehsan A, Dell'Acqua G, Dzau VJ. Ex-vivo gene therapy of human vascular bypass grafts with E2F decoy: the PREVENT single-centre, randomised, controlled trial. *Lancet* 354:1493–1498, 1999.

Manning EL, Crossland J, Dewey MJ, Van Zant G. Influences of inbreeding and genetics on telomere length in mice. *Mamm Genome* 13:234–238, 2002.

Mano Y, Shimizu T, Tanuma S, Takeda K. Synergistic down-regulation of telomerase activity and hTERT mRNA expression by combination of retinoic acid and GM-CSF in human myeloblastic leukemia ML-1 cells. *Anticancer Res* 20:1649–1652, 2000.

Manolagas SC. Birth and death of bone cells: basic regulatory mechanisms and implications for the pathogenesis and treatment of osteoporosis. *Endocr Rev* 21:115–137, 2000.

Mantell LL, Greider CW. Telomerase activity in germline and embryonic cells of *Xenopus*. *EMBO J* 13:3211–3217, 1994.

Maquart FX, Bellon G, Gillery P, Borel JP, Labeille B, Risbourg B, Denoeux JP. Increased secretion of fibronectin and collagen by progeria (Hutchinson-Gilford) fibroblasts. *Eur J Pediatr* 147:442, 1988.

Marcand S, Gasser SM, Gilson E. Chromatin: a sticky silence. *Curr Biol* 6:1222–1225, 1996.

Marcand S, Gilson E, Shore D. A protein-counting mechanism for telomere length regulation in yeast. *Science* 275:986–990, 1997a.

Marcand S, Wotton D, Gilson E, Shore D. Rap1p and telomere length regulation in yeast. *Ciba Found Symp* 211:76–93; discussion 93–103, 1997b.

Marciniak RA, Johnson FB, Guarente L. Dyskeratosis congenita, telomeres and human ageing. *Trends Genet* 16:193–195, 2000.

Marciniak RA, Lombard DB, Johnson FB, Guarente L. Nucleolar localization of the Werner syndrome protein in human cells. *Proc Natl Acad Sci USA* 95:6887–6892, 1998.

Marcotte R, Wang E. Replicative senescence revisited. *J Gerontol A Biol Sci Med Sci* 57A:B257–269, 2002.

Marcus R. Relationship of age-related decreases in muscle mass and strength to skeletal status. *J Gerontol A Biol Sci Med Sci* 50(Spec No):86–87, 1995.

Marder K, Tang MX, Mejia H, Alfaro B, Cote L, Louis E, Groves J, Mayeux R. Risk of Parkinson's disease among first-degree relatives: A community-based study. *Neurology* 47:155–160, 1996.

Margolin EG, Balko MG. The course of Binswanger's disease as chronicled over a period of seven years. *Ann Long Term Care* 9:22–29, 2001.

Margolis D, Bilker W, Hennessy S, Vittorio C, Santanna J, Strom BL. The risk of malignancy associated with psoriasis. *Arch Dermatol* 137:778–783, 2001.

Margolis DJ, Bilker W, Knauss J, Baumgarten M, Strom BL. The incidence and prevalence of pressure ulcers among elderly patients in general medical practice. *Ann Epidemiol* 12:321–325, 2002.

Margulis L. *Origin of Eukaryotic Cells*. Yale University Press, New Haven, 1970.

Mariotti S, Barbesino G, Chiovato L, Marino M, Pinchera A, Zuliani G, Mezzetti A, Fellin R. Circulating thyroid autoantibodies in a sample of Italian octo-nonagenarians: relationship to age, sex, disability, and lipid profile. *Aging (Milano)* 11:362–366, 1999.

Mark RJ, Blanc EM, Mattson MP. Amyloid beta-peptide and oxidative cellular injury in Alzheimer's disease. *Mol Neurobiol* 12:211–224, 1996.

Mark RJ, Pang Z, Geddes JW, Uchida K, Mattson MP. Amyloid beta-peptide impairs glucose transport in hippocampal and cortical neurons: involvement of membrane lipid peroxidation. *J Neurosci* 17:1046–5104, 1997.

Markell EK, Voge M. *Medical Parasitology*. W.B. Saunders Company, Philadelphia, 1976.

Marklund S, Nordensson I, Back O. Normal CuZn superoxide dismutase, Mn superoxide dismutase, catalase, and glutathione peroxidase in Werner's syndrome. *J Gerontol* 36:405–409, 1981.

Markman M. The genetics, screening, and treatment of epithelial ovarian cancer: an update. *Cleve Clin J Med* 67:294–298, 2000.

Markowska AL, Mooney M, Sonntag WE. Insulin-like growth factor-1 ameliorates age-related behavioral deficits. *Neuroscience* 87:559–569, 1998.

Marriott LK, Hauss-Wegrzyniak B, Benton RS, Vraniak PD, Wenk GL. Long-term estrogen therapy worsens the behavioral and neuropathological consequences of chronic brain inflammation. *Behav Neurosci* 116:902–911, 2002.

Marshall J. The susceptible visual apparatus. In Marshall J (ed). *Vision and Visual Dysfunction*, Vol. 16. Macmillan Press, London, 1991.

Martens UM, Brass V, Engelhardt M, Glaser S, Waller CF, Lange W, Schmoor C, Poon SS, Landsdorp PM. Measurement of telomere length in haematopoietic cells using in situ hybridization techniques. *Biochem Soc Trans* 28:245–250, 2000a.

Martens UM, Chavez EA, Poon SS, Schmoor C, Lansdorp PM. Accumulation of short telomeres in human fibroblasts prior to replicative senescence. *Exp Cell Res* 256:291–299, 2000b.

Martens UM, Brass V, Sedlacek L, Pantic M, Exner C, Guo Y, Engelhardt M, Lansdorp PM, Waller CF, Lange W. Telomere maintenance in human B lymphocytes. *Br J Haematol* 119(3):810–818, 2002.

Martin CL, Waggoner DJ, Wong A, Uhrig S, Roseberry JA, Hedrick JF, Pack SD, Russell K, Zackai E, Dobyns WB, Ledbetter DH. "Molecular rulers" for calibrating phenotypic effects of telomere imbalance. *J Med Genet* 39:734–740, 2002a.

Martin CL, Wong A, Gross A, Chung J, Fantes JA, Ledbetter DH. The evolutionary origin of human subtelomeric homologies—or where the ends begin. *Am J Hum Genet* 70:972–984, 2002.

Martin ER, Scott WK, Nance MA, Watts RL, Hubble JP, Koller WC, Lyons K, Pahwa R, Stern MB, Colcer A, Hiner BC, Jankovic J, Ondo WG, Allen FH, Goetz CG, Small GW, Masterman D, Mastaglia F, Laing NG, Stajich JM, Ribble RC, Booze MW, Rogala A, Hauser MA, Zhang F, Gibson RA, Middleton LT, Roses AD, Haines JL, Scott BL, Pericak-Vance MA, Vance JM. Association of single-nucleotide polymorphisms of the tau gene with late-onset Parkinson disease. *JAMA* 286:2245–2250, 2001.

Martin GM. Cellular aging—clonal senescence: a review (Part I). *Am J Pathol* 89:484–511, 1977a.

Martin GM. Cellular aging—postreplicative cells: a review (Part II). *Am J Pathol* 89:513–530, 1977b.

Martin GM. Genetic syndromes in man with potential relevance to the pathobiology of aging. *Birth Defects* 14:5–39, 1977c.

Martin GM. Genetics and the pathobiology of ageing. *Philos Trans R Soc Lond B Biol Sci* 352:1773–1780, 1997a.

Martin GM. The Werner mutation: does it lead to a "public" or "private" mechanism of aging? *Mol Med* 3:356–358, 1997b.

Martin GM. Genetic influences on late-life diseases. *Generations* 24:8–11, 2000.

Martin GM, Oshima J. Lessons from human progeroid syndromes. *Nature* 408:263–269, 2000.

Martin GM, Oshima J, Gray MD, Poot M. What geriatricians should know about the Werner syndrome. *J Am Geriatr Soc* 47:1136–1144, 1999.

Martin GM, Sprague CA, Epstein CJ. Replicative life-span of cultivate human cells: effects of donor's age, tissue, and genotype. *J Lab Invest* 23:86–92, 1970.

Martin JA, Buckwalter JA. Roles of articular cartilage aging and chondrocyte senescence in the pathogenesis of osteoarthritis. *Iowa Orthop J* 21:1–7, 2001a.

Martin JA, Buckwalter JA. Telomere erosion and senescence in human articular cartilage chondrocytes. *J Gerontol A Biol Sci Med Sci* 56:B172–B179, 2001b.

Martin JA, Mitchell CJ, Klingelhutz AJ, Buckwalter JA. Effects of telomerase and viral oncogene expression on the in vitro growth of human chondrocytes. *J Gerontol A Biol Sci Med Sci* 57:B48–53, 2002b.

Martin K. Estrogen therapy for menopause. *J Anti-Aging Med* 1:339–348, 1998.

Martin K, Kirkwood TB, Potten CS. Age changes in stem cells of murine small intestinal crypts. *Exp Cell Res* 241:316–323, 1998a.

Martin K, Potten CS, Roberts SA, Kirkwood TB. Altered stem cell regeneration in irradiated intestinal crypts of senescent mice. *J Cell Sci* 111(Pt 16):2297–3303, 1998b.

Martin M, Nabout ER, Lafuma C, Crechet F, Remy J. Fibronectin and collagen gene expression during in vitro ageing of pig skin fibroblasts. *Exp Cell Res* 191:8–13, 1990.

Martin-Du Pan RC. Are the hormones of youth carcinogenic? [in French]. *Ann Endocrinol (Paris)* 60:392–397, 1999.

Martinez JL, Edstrom JE, Morcillo G, Diez JL. Telomeres in *Chironomus thummi* are characterized by different subfamilies of complex DNA repeats. *Chromosoma* 110:221–227, 2001a.

Martinez JL, Sanchez-Elsner T, Morcillo G, Diez JL. Heat shock regulatory elements are present in telomeric repeats of *Chironomus thummi*. *Nucleic Acids Res* 29:4760–4766, 2001b.

Martinez-Hernandez A, Amenta PS. The extracellular matrix in hepatic regeneration. *FASEB J* 9:1401–1410, 1995.

Martin-Rivera L, Herrera E, Albar JP, Blasco MA. Expression of mouse telomerase catalytic subunit in embryos and adult tissues. *Proc Natl Acad Sci USA* 95:10471–10476, 1998.

Martins D, Adetola A, Norris KC. Emergency management of salt and water disturbances in the elderly. *Clin Geriatr* 9:39–46, 2001a.

Martins S, Soares RM, do Rosario L, Quininha J, Antunes AM. Early and medium term results of tailored therapy for heart failure [in Portuguese]. *Rev Port Cardiol* 20:261–282, 2001b.

Marusic L, Anton M, Tidy A, Wang P, Villeponteau B, Bacchetti S. Reprogramming of telomerase by expression of mutant telomerase RNA template in human cells leads to altered telomeres that correlate with reduced cell viability. *Mol Cell Biol* 17:6394–6401, 1997.

Maruyama H, Toji H, Harrington CR, Sasaki K, Izumi Y, Ohnuma T, Arai H, Yasuda M, Tanaka C, Emson PC, Nakamura S, Kawakami H. Lack of an association of estrogen receptor alpha gene polymorphisms and transcriptional activity with Alzheimer disease. *Arch Neurol* 57:236–240, 2000.

Marx F, Blasko I, Grubeck-Loebenstein B. Mechanisms of immune regulation in Alzheimer's disease: a viewpoint. *Arch Immunol Ther Exp (Warsz)* 47:205–209, 1999.

Marx J. Chipping away at the causes of aging. *Science* 287:2390, 2000.

Marx J. Chromosome end game draws a crowd. *Science* 295:2348–2351, 2002.

Marzabadi MR, Llvaas E. Spermine prevent iron accumulation and depress lipofuscin accumulation in cultured myocardial cells. *Free Radic Biol Med* 21:375–381, 1996.

Maser RS, DePinho RA. Connecting chromosomes, crisis, and cancer. *Science* 297:565–569, 2002.

Mason DX, Autexier C, Greider CW. Tetrahymena proteins p80 and p95 are not core telomerase components. *Proc Natl Acad Sci USA* 98:12368–12373, 2001.

Masoro EJ. Food restriction and the aging process. *J Am Geriatr Soc* 32:296–300, 1984.

Masoro EJ. Dietary restriction: an experimental approach to the study of the biology of aging. In Masoro EJ, Austad SN (eds). *Handbook of the Biology of Aging, 5th ed.* Academic Press, New York, 2001, pp. 346–395.

Masoro EJ, Austad SN. *Handbook of the Biology of Aging, 5th ed.* Academic Press, New York, 2001.

Masoro EJ, McCarter RJ, Katz MS, McMahan CA. Dietary restriction alters characteristics of glucose fuel use. *J Gerontol* 47:B202–208, 1992.

Masutomi K, Kaneko S, Hayashi N, Yamashita T, Shirota Y, Kobayashi K, Murakami S. Telomerase activity reconstituted in vitro with purified human telomerase reverse transcriptase and human telomerase RNA component. *J Biol Chem* 275:22568–22573, 2000.

Mather LH. *The Peripheral Nervous System.* Butterworths, Boston, 1985.

Mathioudakis G, Storb R, McSweeney PA, Torok-Storb B, Lansdorp PM, Brummendorf TH, Gass MJ, Bryant EM, Storek J, Flowers ME, Gooley T, Nash RA. Polyclonal hematopoiesis with variable telomere shortening in human long-term allogeneic marrow graft recipients. *Blood* 96:3991–3994, 2001.

Mathon NF, Lloyd AC. Cell senescence and cancer. *Nat Rev Cancer* 1:203–213, 2001.

Mathon NF, Malcolm DS, Harrisingh MC, Cheng L, Lloyd AC. Lack of replicative senescence in normal rodent glia. *Science* 291:872–876, 2001.

Matsui M, Miyasaka J, Hamada K, Ogawa Y, Hiramoto M, Fujimori R, Aioi A. Influence of aging and cell senescence on telomerase activity in keratinocytes. *J Dermatol Sci* 22:80–87, 2000.

Matsumura T, Pfendt EA, Hayflick L. DNA synthesis in the human diploid cell strain WI-38 during in vitro aging: an autoradiography study. *J Gerontol* 34:323–327, 1979a.

Matsumura T, Zerrudo Z, Hayflick L. Senescent human diploid cells in culture: survival, DNA synthesis and morphology. *J Gerontol* 34:328–334, 1979b.

Matsunaga H, Handa JT, Aotaki-Keen A, Sherwood SW, West MD, Hjelmeland LM. Beta-galactosidase histochemistry and telomere loss in senescent retinal pigment epithelial cells. *Invest Ophthalmol Vis Sci* 40:197–202, 1999a.

Matsunaga H, Handa JT, Gelfman CM, Hjelmeland LM. The mRNA phenotype of a human RPE cell line at replicative senescence. *Mol Vis* 5:39, 1999b.

Matsuo A, Walker DG, Terai K, McGeer PL. Expression of CD43 in human microglia and its downregulation in Alzheimer's disease. *J Neuroimmunol* 71:81–86, 1996.

Matsuo S, Takeuchi Y, Hayashi S, Kinugasa A, Sawada T. Patient with unusual Hutchinson-Gilford syndrome (progeria). *Pediatr Neurol* 10:237–240, 1994.

Matsushita H, Chang E, Glassford AJ, Cooke JP, Chiu CP, Tsao PS. eNOS activity is reduced in senescent human endothelial cells: preservation by hTERT immortalization. *Circ Res* 89:793–798, 2001.

Matsutani N, Yokozaki H, Tahara E, Tahara H, Kuniyasu H, Haruma K, Chayama K, Yasui W, Tahara E. Expression of telomeric repeat binding factor 1 and 2 and TRF1-interacting nuclear protein 2 in human gastric carcinomas. *Int J Oncol* 19:507–512, 2001a.

Matsutani N, Yokozaki H, Tahara E, Tahara H, Kuniyasu H, Kitadai Y, Haruma K, Chayama K, Tahara E, Yasui W. Expression of MRE11 complex (MRE11, RAD50, NBS1) and hRap1 and its relation with telomere regulation, telomerase activity in human gastric carcinomas. *Pathobiology* 69:219–224, 2001b.

Matsuzaki Y, Sato M, Saito Y, Karube M, Doy M, Shoda J, Abei M, Tanaka N, Hadama T, Kinoshita M. The role of previous infection of hepatitis B virus in Hbs antigen negative and anti-HCV negative Japanese patients with hepatocellular carcinoma: etiological and molecular biological study. *J Exp Clin Cancer Res* 18:379–389, 1999.

Matthews P, Jones CJ. Clinical implications of telomerase detection. *Histopathology* 38:485–498, 2001.

Matthews P, Jones CJ, Skinner J, Haughton M, de Micco C, Wynford-Thomas D. Telomerase activity and telomere length in thyroid neoplasia: biological and clinical implications. *J Pathol* 194:183–193, 2001.

Mattila KJ, Valtonen VV, Nieminen MS, Asikainen S. Role of infection as a risk factor for atherosclerosis, myocardial infarction, and stroke. *Clin Infect Dis* 26:719–734, 1998.

Mattson MP. Cellular actions of beta-amyloid precursor protein and its soluble and fibrillogenic derivatives. *Physiol Rev* 77:1081–1132, 1997.

Mattson MP. Emerging neuroprotective strategies for Alzheimer's disease: dietary restriction, telomerase activation, and stem cell therapy. *Exp Gerontol* 35:489–502, 2000a.

Mattson MP. Existing data suggest that Alzheimer's disease is preventable. *Ann NY Acad Sci* 924:153–159, 2000b.

Mattson MP. Neuroprotective signaling and the aging brain: take away my food and let me run. *Brain Res* 886:47–53, 2000c.

Mattson MP, Barger SW, Furukawa K, Bruce AJ, Wyss-Coray T, Mark RJ, Mucke L. Cellular signaling roles of TGF beta, TNF alpha and beta APP in brain injury responses and Alzheimer's disease. *Brain Res Brain Res Rev* 23:47–61, 1997a.

Mattson MP, Culmsee C, Yu Z, Camandola S. Roles of nuclear factor κB in neuronal survival and plasticity. *J Neurochem* 74:443–456, 2000a.

Mattson MP, Duan W, Chan SL, Camandola S. Par-4: an emerging pivotal player in neuronal apoptosis and neurodegenerative disorders. *J Mol Neurosci* 13:17–30, 1999a.

Mattson MP, Guo Q. Cell and molecular neurobiology of presenilins: a role for the endoplasmic reticulum in the pathogenesis of Alzheimer's disease? *J Neurosci Res* 50:505–513, 1997.

Mattson MP, Guo Q, Furukawa K, Pedersen WA. Presenilins, the endoplasmic reticulum, and neuronal apoptosis in Alzheimer's disease. *J Neurochem* 70:1–14, 1998a.

Mattson MP, Guo ZH, Geiger JD. Secreted form of amyloid precursor protein enhances basal glucose and glutamate transport and protects against oxidative impairment of glucose and glutamate transport in synaptosomes by a cyclic GMP-mediated mechanism. *J Neurochem* 73:532–537, 1999b.

Mattson MP, Partin J, Begley JG. Amyloid beta-peptide induces apoptosis-related events in synapses and dendrites. *Brain Res* 807:167–176, 1998b.

Mattson MP, Pedersen WA. Effects of amyloid precursor protein derivatives and oxidative stress on basal forebrain cholinergic systems in Alzheimer's disease. *Int J Dev Neurosci* 16:737–753, 1998.

Mattson MP, Pedersen WA, Duan W, Culmsee C, Camandola S. Cellular and molecular mechanisms underlying perturbed energy metabolism and neuronal degeneration in Alzheimer's and Parkinson's diseases. *Ann NY Acad Sci* 893:154–175, 1999c.

Mattson MP, Robinson N, Guo Q. Estrogens stabilize mitochondrial function and protect neural cells against the pro-apoptotic action of mutant presenilin-1. *Neuroreport* 8:3817–3821, 1997b.

Mattson MP, Zhu H, Yu J, Kindy MS. Presenilin-1 mutation increases neuronal vulnerability to focal ischemia in vivo and to hypoxia and glucose deprivation in cell culture: involvement of perturbed calcium homeostasis. *J Neurosci* 20:1358–1364, 2000b.

Maugeri D, Speciale S, Santangelo A, Motta M, Panebianco P. Altered laboratory thyroid parameters in elderly people. *J Endocrinol Invest* 22(10 Suppl):37, 1999.

Mayeux R, Saunders AM, Shea S, Mirra S, Evans D, Roses AD, Hyman BT, Crain B, Tang MX, Phelps CH. Utility of the apolipoprotein E genotype in the diagnosis of Alzheimer's disease. Alzheimer's Disease Centers Consortium on Apolipoprotein E and Alzheimer's Disease. *N Engl J Med* 338:506–511, 1998.

Mayeux R, Schofield PW. Alzheimer's disease. In Hazzard WR, Bierman EL, Blass JP, Ettinger WH Jr, Halter JB (eds). *Principles of Geriatric Medicine and Gerontology, 3rd ed.* McGraw-Hill, New York, 1994, pp 1035–1050.

Mayeux R, Tang MX, Jacobs DM, Manly J, Bell K, Merchant C, Small SA, Stern Y, Wisniewski HM, Mehta PD. Plasma amyloid beta-peptide 1-42 and incipient Alzheimer's disease. *Ann Neurol* 46:412–416, 1999.

Mayne LV, Priestley A, James MR, Burke JF. Efficent immortalization and morphological transformation of human fibroblasts by transfection with SV40 DNA linked to a dominant marker. *Exp Cell Res* 162:530–538, 1986.

Maytin M, Leopold J, Loscalzo J. Oxidant stress in the vasculature. *Curr Atheroscler Rep* 1:156–164, 1999.

Mazza E, Maccario M, Ramunni J, Gauna C, Bertagna A, Barberis AM, Patroncini S, Messina M, Ghigo E. Dehydroepiandrosterone sulfate levels in women. Relationships with age, body mass index and insulin levels. *J Endocrinol Invest* 22:681–687, 1999.

McArthur JC, Sacktor N, Selnes O. Human immunodeficiency virus–associated dementia. *Semin Neurol* 19:129–150, 1999.

McCarroll RM, Fangman WL. Time of replication of yeast centromeres and telomeres. *Cell* 54:505–513, 1988.

McCarter RJ. Role of caloric restriction in the prolongation of life. *Clin Geriatr Med* 11:553–565, 1995.

McCarter RJ, Palmer J. Energy metabolism and aging: a lifelong study of Fischer 344 rats. *Am J Physiol* 263(3 Pt 1):E448–452, 1992.

McCarter RJ, Shimokawa I, Ikeno Y, Higami Y, Hubbard GB, Yu BP, McMahan CA. Physical activity as a factor in the action of dietary restriction on aging: effects in Fischer 344 rats. *Aging (Milano)* 9:73–79, 1997.

McCaul JA, Gordon KE, Clark LJ, Parkinson EK. Telomerase inhibition and the future management of head-and-neck cancer. *Lancet Oncol* 3:280–288, 2002.

McCay CM, Crowell MF, Maynard LM. The effect of retarded growth upon the length of life span and upon the ultimate body size. *J Nutr* 10:63, 1935.

McCleary R, Dick MB, Buckwalter G, Henderson V, Shankle WR. Full-information models for multiple psychometric tests: annualized rates of change in normal aging and dementia. *Alzheimer Dis Assoc Disord* 10:216–223, 1996.

McClintock B. The stability of broken ends of chromosomes in *Zea mays*. *Genetics* 26:24–282, 1941.

McCormick A, Campisi J. Cellular aging and senescence. *Curr Opin Cell Biol* 3:230–234, 1991.

McCormick F. Cancer therapy based on p53. *Cancer J Sci Am* 5:139–144, 1999a.

McCormick F. Signalling networks that cause cancer. *Trends Cell Biol* 9:M53–56, 1999b.

McCormick F. Cancer therapy based on p53. Presented at Cancer and Molecular Genetics in the Twenty-first Century, Van Andel Research Institute, Grand Rapids, MI, September 5–9, 2000.

McCully KK, Posner JD. The application of blood flow measurements to the study of aging muscle. *J Gerontol A Biol Sci Med Sci* 50:130–136, 1995.

McCune SL, Gockerman JP, Rizzieri DA. Monoclonal antibody therapy in the treatment of non-Hodgkin lymphoma. *JAMA* 286:1149–1152, 2001.

McDermott MM, Greenland P, Liu K, Guralnik JM, Criqui MH, Dolan NC, Chan C, Celic L, Pearce WH, Schneider JR, Sharma L, Clark E, Gibson D, Martin GJ. Leg symptoms in peripheral arterial disease: associated clinical characteristics and functional impairment. *JAMA* 286:1599–1606, 2001.

McDougall JK. Telomerase activity and cellular immortalization. *Dev Biol (Basel)* 106:267–272, 2001.

McDougall JK, Klingelhutz A. Telomerase activity, expression of the RNA component and the catalytic subunit gene in human keratinocytes and in cervical cancer. Abstract presented at Telomeres and Telomerase: Implications for Cell Immortality, Cancer, and Age-related Disease. San Francisco, CA, June 1–3, 1998.

McEachern MJ, Blackburn EH. A conserved sequence motif within the exceptionally diverse telomeric sequences of budding yeasts. *Proc Nat Acad Sci USA* 91:3453–3457, 1994.

McEachern MJ, Blackburn EH. Runaway telomere elongation caused by telomerase RNA mutations. *Nature* 376:403–409, 1995.

McEachern MJ, Blackburn EH. Cap-prevented recombination between terminal telomeric repeat arrays (telomere CPR) maintains telomeres in *Kluyveromyces lactis* lacking telomerase. *Genes Dev* 10:1822–1834, 1996.

McEachern MJ, Underwood DH, Blackburn EH. Dynamics of telomeric DNA turnover in yeast. *Genetics* 160:63–73, 2002.

McGeer EG, McGeer PL. The future use of complement inhibitors for the treatment of neurological diseases. *Drugs* 55:739–746, 1998a.

McGeer EG, McGeer PL. The importance of inflammatory mechanisms in Alzheimer disease. *Exp Gerontol* 33:371–378, 1998b.

McGeer EG, McGeer PL. Brain inflammation in Alzheimer disease and the therapeutic implications. *Curr Pharm Des* 5:821–836, 1999a.

McGeer PL, Kawamata T, McGeer EG. Localization and possible functions of presenilins in brain. *Rev Neurosci* 9:1–15, 1998.

McGeer PL, McGeer EG. The inflammatory response system of brain: implications for therapy of Alzheimer and other neurodegenerative diseases. *Brain Res Brain Res Rev* 21:195–218, 1995.

McGeer PL, McGeer EG. Glial cell reactions in neurodegenerative diseases: pathophysiology and therapeutic interventions. *Alzheimer Dis Assoc Disord* 12(Suppl 2):S1–6, 1998c.

McGeer PL, McGeer EG. Mechanisms of cell death in Alzheimer disease—immunopathology. *J Neural Transm Suppl* 54:159–166, 1998d.

McGeer PL, McGeer EG. Inflammation of the brain in Alzheimer's disease: implications for therapy. *J Leukoc Biol* 65:409–415, 1999b.

McGill HC Jr, McMahan CA. Determinants of atherosclerosis in the young. Pathobiological Determinants of Atherosclerosis in Youth (PDAY) Research Group. *Am J Cardiol* 82:30T–36T, 1998.

McGuigan MRM, Bronks R, Newton RU, Sharman MJ, Graham JC, Cody DV, Kraemer WJ. Resistance training in patients with peripheral arterial disease: effects on myosin isoforms, fiber type distribution, and capillary supply to skeletal muscle. *J Gerontol A Biol Sci Med Sci* 56:B302–310, 2001.

McGuire WP. High-dose chemotherapy and autologous bone marrow or stem cell reconstitution for solid tumors. *Curr Probl Cancer* 22:135–177, 1998.

McIlrath J, Bouffler SD, Samper E, Cuthbert A, Wojcik A, Szumiel I, Bryant PE, Riches AC, Thompson A, Blasco MA, Newbold RF, Slijepcevic P. Telomere length abnormalities in mammalian radiosensitive cells. *Cancer Res* 61:912–915, 2001.

McKenzie KE, Umbricht CB, Sukumar S. Applications of telomerase research in the fight against cancer. *Mol Med Today* 5:114–122, 1999.

McKevitt TP, Nasir L, Devlin P, Argyle DJ. Telomere lengths in dogs decrease with increasing donor age. *J Nutr* 132:1604S–1606S, 2002.

McKnight TD, Fitzgerald MS, Shippen DE. Plant telomeres and telomerases. A review. *Biochemistry (Mosc)* 62:1224–1231, 1997.

McKnight TD, Riha K, Shippen DE. Telomeres, telomerase, and stability of the plant genome. *Plant Mol Biol* 48:331–337, 2002.

McNeal MG, Zareparsi S, Camicioli R, Dame A, Howieson D, Quinn J, Ball M, Kaye J, Payami H. Predictors of healthy brain aging. *J Gerontol A Biol Sci Med Sci* 56:B294–301, 2001.

McShane TM, Wise PM. Life-long moderate caloric restriction prolongs reproductive life span in rats without interrupting estrous cyclicity: effects on the gonadotropin-releasing hormone/luteinizing hormone axis. *Biol Reprod* 54:70–75, 1996.

McSharry BP, Jones CJ, Skinner JW, Kipling D, Wilkinson GW. Human telomerase reverse transcriptase–immortalized MRC-5 and HCA2 human fibroblasts are fully permissive for human cytomegalovirus. *J Gen Virol* 82(Pt 4):855–863, 2001.

Meagher EA, Barry OP, Lawson JA, Rokach J, FitzGerald GA. Effects of vitamin E on lipid peroxidation in healthy persons. *JAMA* 285:1178–1182, 2001.

Mecocci P, MacGarvey U, Flint Beal M. Oxidative damage to mitochondrial DNA is increased in Alzheimer's disease. *Ann Neurol* 36:747–751, 1994.

Medcalf AS, Klein-Szanto AJ, Cristofalo VJ. Expression of p21 is not required for senescence of human fibroblasts. *Cancer Res* 56:4582–4585, 1996.

Medical Letter. Drugs for rheumatoid arthritis. *Med Lett Drugs Ther* 42:57–64, 2000a.

Medical Letter. Drugs for prevention and treatment of postmenopausal osteoporosis. *Med Lett Drugs Ther* 42:97–100, 2000b.

Medical Letter. Rivastigmine (Exelon) for Alzheimer's disease. *Med Lett Drugs Ther* 42:93–94, 2000c.

Medical Letter. Cardiovascular safety of COX-2 inhibitors. *Med Lett Drugs Ther* 43:99–100, 2001a.

Medical Letter. Galantamine (Reminyl) for Alzheimer's disease. *Med Lett Drugs Ther* 43:53–54, 2001b.

Medical Letter. Screening for lung cancer. *Med Lett Drugs Ther* 43:61–62, 2001c.

Medical Letter. Update on glucosamine for osteoarthritis. *Med Lett Drugs Ther* 43:111–112, 2001d.

Medical Letter. Botulinum toxin (Botox cosmetic) for frown lines. *Med Lett Drugs Ther* 44:47–48, 2002.

Medical Letter. Teriparatide (Forteo) for osteoporosis. *Med Lett Drugs Ther* 45:9–10, 2003a.

Medical Letter. Adalimumab (*Humira*) for rheumatoid arthritis. *Med Lett Drugs Ther* 45:9–25–27, 2003b.

Meeker AK, Coffey DS. Telomerase: a promising marker of biological immortality of germ, stem, and cancer cells. A review. *Biochemistry (Mosc)* 62:1323–1331, 1997.

Meeker AK, Gage WR, Hicks JL, Simon I, Coffman JR, Platz EA, March GE, De Marzo AM. Telomere length assessment in human archival tissues: combined telomere fluorescence in situ hybridization and immunostaining. *Am J Pathol* 160:1259–1268, 2002a.

Meeker AK, Hicks JL, Platz EA, March GE, Bennett CJ, Delannoy MJ, De Marzo AM. Telomere shortening is an early somatic DNA alteration in human prostate tumorigenesis. *Cancer Res* 62:6405–6409, 2002b.

Mefford HC, Trask BJ. The complex structure and dynamic evolution of human subtelomeres. *Nat Rev Genet* 3:91–102, 2002.

Mehle C, Lindblom A, Ljungberg B, Stenling R, Roos G. Loss of heterozygosity at chromosome 3p correlates with telomerase activity in renal cell carcinoma. *Int J Oncol* 13:289–295, 1998.

Mehle C, Piatyszek MA, Ljungberg B, Shay JW, Roos G. Telomerase activity in human renal cell carcinoma. *Oncogene* 13:161–166, 1996.

Mehta JL, Saldeen TG, Rand K J. Mehta JL, Saldeen TG, Rand K. Interactive role of infection, inflammation and traditional risk factors in atherosclerosis and coronary artery disease. *Am Coll Cardiol* 31:1217–1225, 1998.

Mehta S, Yusuf S: Acute myocardial infarction. *Clinical Evidence* 3:1–11, 2000.

Meid FH, Gygi CM, Leisinger HJ, Bosman FT, Benhattar J. The use of telomerase activity for the detection of prostatic cancer cells after prostatic massage. *J Urol* 165:1802–1805, 2001.

Meier CR, Schlienger RG, Kraenzlin ME, Schlegel B, Jick H. HMG-CoA reductase inhibitors and the risk of fractures. *JAMA* 283:3205–3210, 2000.

Melk A, Ramassar V, Helms LM, Moore R, Rayner D, Solez K, Halloran PF. Telomere shortening in kidneys with age. *J Am Soc Nephrol* 11:444–453, 2000.

Melov S. Mitochondrial oxidative stress. Physiologic consequences and potential for a role in aging. *Ann NY Acad Sci* 908:219–225, 2000.

Melov S, Ravenscroft J, Malik S, Gill MS, Walker DW, Clayton PE, Wallace DC, Malfroy B, Doctrow SR, Lithgow GJ. Extension of life span with superoxide dismutase/catalase mimetics. *Science* 289:1567–1569, 2000.

Melton LJ III. Perspectives: how many women have osteoporosis now? *J Bone Miner Res* 10:175–177, 1995.

Melton LJ III, Atkinson EJ, O'Connor MK, O'Fallon WM, Riggs BL. Bone density and fracture risk in men. *J Bone Miner Res* 13:1915–1923, 1998.

Melton LJ III, Khosla S, Crowson CS, O'Connor MK, O'Fallon WM, Riggs BL. Epidemiology of sarcopenia. *J Am Geriatr Soc* 48:625–630, 2000.

Melville H. *Moby Dick*. 1851.

Meme JS, Kimemiah SG, Oduori ML. Hutchinson-Gilford progeria syndrome: report of a case presenting with hypertensive cerebrovascular disease. *East Afr Med J* 55:442–443, 1978.

Mendoza C, Sato H, Hiyama K, Ishioka S, Isobe T, Maeda H, Hiyama E, Inai K, Yamakido M. Allelotype and loss of heterozygosity around the L-myc gene locus in primary lung cancers. *Lung Cancer* 28:117–125, 2000.

Mendoza-Nunez VM, Retana-Ugalde R, Sanchez-Rodriguez MA, Altamirano-Lozano MA. DNA damage in lymphocytes of elderly patients in relation with total antioxidant levels. *Mech Ageing Dev* 108:9–23, 1999.

Menon U, Jacobs IJ. Recent developments in ovarian cancer screening. *Curr Opin Obstet Gynecol* 12:39–42, 2000.

Menzies RA, Gold PH. The turnover of mitochondria in a variety of tissues of young adult and aged rats. *J Biol Chem* 246:2425–2429, 1971.

Mera SL. The role of telomeres in ageing and cancer. *Br J Biomed* Sci 55:221–225, 1998.

Mercadier JJ. Progression from cardiac hypertrophy to heart failure. In Hosenpud JD, Greenberg BH (eds). *Congestive Heart Failure*. Lippincott Williams & Wilkins, 2000, pp 4–66.

Merchant C, Tang MX, Albert S, Manly J, Stern Y, Mayeux R. The influence of smoking on the risk of Alzheimer's disease. *Neurology* 52:1408–1412, 1999.

Mergny JL, Lacroix L, Teulade-Fichou MP, Hounsou C, Guittat L, Hoarau M, Arimondo PB, Vigneron JP, Lehn JM, Riou JF, Garestier T, Helene C. Telomerase inhibitors based on quadruplex ligands selected by a fluorescence assay. *Proc Natl Acad Sci USA* 98:3062–3067, 2001.

Merly F, Magras-Resch C, Rouaud T, Fontaine-Perus J, Gardahaut MF Comparative analysis of satellite cell properties in heavy- and light-weight strains of turkey. *J Muscle Res Cell Motil* 19:257–270, 1998.

Metter EJ, Talbot LA, Schrager M, Conwit R. Skeletal muscle strength as a predictor of all-cause mortality in healthy men. *J Gerontol A Biol Sci Med Sci* 57:359–365, 2002.

Meyerson M. Role of telomerase in normal and cancer cells. *J Clin Oncol* 18:2626–2634, 2000.

Meyerson M, Counter CM, Eaton EN, Ellisen LW, Steiner P, Caddle SD, Ziaugra L, Beijersbergen RL, Davidoff MJ, Liu Q, Bacchetti S, Haber DA, Weinberg RA. hEST2, the putative human telomerase catalytic subunit gene, is up-regulated in tumor cells and during immortalization. *Cell* 90:785–795, 1997.

Mezey E, Chandross KJ, Harta G, Maki RA, McKercher SR. Turning blood into brain: cells bearing neuronal antigens generated in vivo from bone marrow. *Science* 290:1779–1782, 2000.

Mezzetti A, Zuliani G, Romano F, Costantini F, Pierdomenico SD, Cuccurullo F, Fellin R, and the Associazione Medica Sabin. Vitamin E and lipid peroxide plasma levels predict the risk of cardiovascular events in a group of healthy very old people. *J Am Geriatr Soc* 49:533–537, 2001.

Michaels DD. The eye. In Hazzard WR, Bierman EL, Blass JP, Ettinger WH Jr, Halter JB (eds). *Principles of Geriatric Medicine and Gerontology, 3rd ed.* McGraw-Hill, New York, 1994, pp 441–456.

Michaud DS, Giovannucci E, Willett WC, Colditz GA, Stampfer MJ, Fuchs CS. Physical activity, obesity, height, and the risk of pancreatic cancer. *JAMA* 286:921–929, 2001.

Michel M, L'Heureux N, Auger FA, Germain L. From newborn to adult: phenotypic and functional properties of skin equivalent and human skin as a function of donor age. *J Cell Physiol* 171:179–189, 1997.

Michel M, Torok N, Godbout MJ, Lussier M, Gaudreau P, Royal A, Germain L. Keratin 19 as a biochemical marker of skin stem cells in vivo and in vitro: keratin 19 expressing cells are differentially localized in function of anatomic sites, and their number varies with donor age and culture stage. *J Cell Sci* 109:1017–1028, 1996.

Michikawa Y, Mazzucchelli F, Bresolin N, Scarlato G, Attardi G. Aging-dependent large accumulation of point mutations in the human mtDNA control region for replication. *Science* 286:774–779, 1999.

Michishita E, Nakabayashi K, Suzuki T, Kaul SC, Ogino H, Fujii M, Mitsui Y, Ayusawa D. 5-bromodeoxyuridine induces senescence-like phenomena in mammalian cells regardless of cell type or species. *J Biochem (Tokyo)* 126:1052–1059, 1999.

Middleton RG, Thompson IM, Austenfeld MS, Cooner WH, Correa RJ, Gibbons RP, Miller HC, Oesterling JE, Resnick MI, Smalley SR, et al. Prostate cancer clinical guidelines panel summary report on the management of clinically localized prostate cancer. *J Urol* 154:2144–2148, 1995.

Middleton SB, Pack K, Phillips RK. Telomere length in familial adenomatous polyposis-associated desmoids. *Dis Colon Rectum* 43:1535–1539, 2000.

Migliaccio E, Giorgio M, Mele S, Pelicci G, Reboldi P, Pandolfi PP, Lanfrancone L, Pelicci PG. The p66^{shc} adaptor protein controls oxidative stress response and life span in mammals. *Nature* 402:309–313, 1999.

Migliaccio M, Amacker M, Just T, Reichenbach P, Valmori D, Cerottini JC, Romero P, Nabholz M. Ectopic human telomerase catalytic subunit expression maintains telomere length but is not sufficient for CD8+ T lymphocyte immortalization. *J Immunol* 165:4978–4984, 2000.

Mignon-Ravix C, Depetris D, Delobel B, Croquette MF, Mattei MG. A human interstitial telomere associates in vivo with specific TRF2 and TIN2 proteins. *Eur J Hum Genet* 10:107–112, 2002.

Mikhelson VM. Replicative mosaicism might explain the seeming contradictions in the telomere theory of aging. *Mech Ageing Dev* 122:1361–1365, 2001.

Mikuls TR, Saag KG. Comorbidity in rheumatoid arthritis. *Rheum Dis Clin North Am* 27:283–303, 2001.

Milas M, Yu D, Sun D, Pollock RE. Telomerase activity of sarcoma cell lines and fibroblasts is independent of p53 status. *Clin Cancer Res* 4:1573–1579, 1998.

Miller CJ, Stein GH. Human diploid fibroblasts that undergo a senescent-like differentiation have elevated ceramide and diacylglycerol. *J Gerontol A Biol Sci Med Sci* 56:8–19, 2001.

Miller MC, Collins K. Telomerase recognizes its template by using an adjacent RNA motif. *Proc Natl Acad Sci USA* 99:6585–6590, 2002.

Miller RA. The aging immune system: primer and prospectus. *Science* 273:70–74, 1996.

Miller RA. Kleemeier award lecture: are there genes for aging? *J Gerontol A Biol Sci Med Sci* 54:B297–307, 1999.

Miller RA. Telomere diminution as a cause of immune failure in old age: an unfashionable demurral. *Biochem Soc Trans* 28:241–245, 2000.

Miller RA. Genetics of longevity and aging in mice. In Masoro EJ, Austad SN (eds). *Handbook of the Biology of Aging, 5th ed.* Academic Press, New York, 2001, pp. 369–395.

Miller RJ, Meucci O. AIDS and the brain: is there a chemokine connection? *Trends Neurosci* 22:471–479, 1999.

Millis AT, Hoyle M, McCue HM, Martini H. Differential expression of metalloproteinase and tissue inhibitor of metalloproteinase in aged human fibroblasts. *Exp Cell Res* 201:373–379, 1992.

Millis AT, Sottile J, Hoyle M, Mann DM, Diemer V. Collagenase production by early and late passage cultures of human fibroblasts. *Exp Gerontol* 24:559–575, 1989.

Mills KD, Sinclair DA, Guarente L. MEC1–dependent redistribution of the Sir3 silencing protein from telomeres to DNA double-strand breaks. *Cell* 97:609–620, 1999a.

Mills W, Critcher R, Lee C, Farr CJ. Generation of an approximately 2.4 Mb human X centromere-based minichromosome by targeted telomere-associated chromosome fragmentation in DT40. *Hum Mol Genet* 8:751–761, 1999b.

Milton J. *On His Blindness.* 1652; cited on p 341a, Beck, 1968.

Milyavsky M, Mimran A, Senderovich S, Zurer I, Erez N, Shats I, Goldfinger N, Cohen I, Rotter V. Activation of p53 protein by telomeric (TTAGGG)n repeats. *Nucleic Acids Res* 29:5207–5215, 2001.

Minaker KL, Rowe JW, Tonino R, Pallotta JA. Influence of age on clearance of insulin in man. *Diabetes* 31:851–855, 1982a.

Minaker KL, Rowe JW, Young JB, Sparrow D, Pallotta JA, Landsberg L. Effect of age on insulin stimulation of sympathetic nervous system activity in man. *Metabolism* 31:1181–1184, 1982b.

Minami K, Yamaguchi Y, Yoshida K, Quan CP, Toge T. Dysregulation of telomerase activity and expression in lymphokine-activated killer cells from advanced cancer patients: possible involvement in cancer-associated immunosuppression mechanism. *Oncol Rep* 8:649–653, 2001.

Minamino T, Komuro I. Role of telomere in endothelial dysfunction in atherosclerosis. *Curr Opin Lipidol* 13:537–543, 2002.

Minamino T, Miyauchi H, Yoshida T, Ishida Y, Yoshida H, Komuro I. Endothelial cell senescence in human atherosclerosis: role of telomere in endothelial dysfunction. *Circulation* 105:1541–1544, 2002.

Minev B, Hipp J, Firat H, Schmidt JD, Langlade-Demoyen P, Zanetti M. Cytotoxic T cell immunity against telomerase reverse transcriptase in humans. *Proc Natl Acad Sci USA* 97:4796–4801, 2000.

Minghetti L, Nicolini A, Polazzi E, Greco A, Perretti M, Parente L, Levi G. Down-regulation of microglial cyclo-oxygenase-2 and inducible nitric oxide synthase expression by lipocortin 1. *Br J Pharmacol* 126:1307–1314, 1999.

Miracco C, Margherita De Santi M, Schurfeld K, Santopietro R, Lalinga AV, Fimiani M, Biagioli M, Brogi M, De Felice C, Luzi P, Andreassi L. Quantitative in situ evaluation of telomeres in fluorescence in situ hybridization–processed sections of cutaneous melanocytic lesions and correlation with telomerase activity. *Br J Dermatol* 146:399–408, 2002.

Mirowsky J. Age, subjective life expectancy, and the sense of control: the horizon hypothesis. *J Gerontol* 52B:S125–134, 1997.

Misawa M, Tauchi T, Sashida G, Nakajima A, Abe K, Ohyashiki JH, Ohyashiki K. Inhibition of human telomerase enhances the effect of chemotherapeutic agents in lung cancer cells. *Int J Oncol* 21:1087–1092, 2002.

Mishima K, Handa JT, Aotaki-Keen A, Lutty GA, Morse LS, Hjelmeland LM. Senescence-associated β-galactosidase histochemistry for the primate eye. *Invest Ophthalmol Vis Sci* 40:1590–1593, 1999.

Mishima S. Clinical investigations on the corneal endothelium. *Am J Ophthalmol* 93:1–29, 1982.

Mishra OP, Delivoria-Papadopoulos M. Cellular mechanisms of hypoxic injury in the developing brain. *Brain Res Bull* 48:233–238, 1999.

Misiti S, Nanni S, Fontemaggi G, Cong YS, Wen J, Hirte HW, Piaggio G, Sacchi A, Pontecorvi A, Bacchetti S, Farsetti A. Induction of hTERT expression and telomerase activity by estrogens in human ovary epithelium cells. *Mol Cell Biol* 20:3764–3771, 2000.

Mitchell AR, Jeppesen P, Nicol L, Morrison H, Kipling D. Epigenetic control of mammalian centromere protein binding: does DNA methylation have a role? *J Cell Sci* 109(Pt 9):2199–2206, 1996.

Mitchell EC, Goltman DW. Progeria: report of a classic case with a review of the literature since 1929. *Am J Dis Child* 59:379–385, 1940.

Mitchell JR, Wood E, Collins K. A telomerase component is defective in the human disease dyskeratosis congenita. *Nature* 402:551–555, 1999.

Mitka M. New advice for women patients about hormone therapy and the heart. *JAMA* 286:907, 2001.

Mitton-Fry RM, Anderson EM, Hughes TR, Lundblad V, Wuttke DS. Conserved structure for single-strand telomeric DNA recognition. *Science* 296:145–147, 2002.

Miura M, Karasaki Y, Abe T, Higashi K, Ikemura K, Gotoh S. Prompt activation of telomerase by chemical carcinogens in rats detected with a modified TRAP assay. *Biochem Biophys Res Commun* 246:13–19, 1998.

Miura N, Horikawa I, Nishimoto A, Ohmura H, Ito H, Hirohashi S, Shay JW, Oshimura M. Progressive telomere shortening and telomerase reactivation during hepatocellular carcinogenesis. *Cancer Genet Cytogenet* 93:56–62, 1997.

Miyashita N, Shiga K, Yonai M, Kaneyama K, Kobayashi S, Kojima T, Goto Y, Kishi M, Aso H, Suzuki T, Sakaguchi M, Nagai T. Remarkable differences in telomere lengths among cloned cattle derived from different cell types. *Biol Reprod* 66:1649–1655, 2002.

Mizumoto I, Ogawa Y, Niiyama H, Nagai E, Sato I, Urashima T, Matsumoto T, Iida M, Tanaka I. Possible role of telomerase activation in the multistep tumor progression of periampullary lesions in patients with familial adenomatous polyposis. *Am J Gastroenterol* 96:1261–1265, 2001.

Mizushina Y, Iida A, Ohta K, Sugawara F, Sakaguchi K. Novel triterpenoids inhibit both DNA polymerase and DNA topoisomerase. *Biochem J* 350:757–763, 2000.

Mobbs CV, Bray GA, Atkinson RL, Bartke A, Finch CE, Maratos-Flier E, Crawley JN, Nelson JF. Neuroendocrine and pharmacological manipulations to assess how caloric restriction increases life span. *J Gerontol A Biol Sci Med Sci* 56A:B34–44, 2001.

Mockett RJ, Orr WC, Rahmandar JJ, Benes JJ, Radyuk SN, Klichko VI, Sohal RS. Overexpression of Mn-containing superoxide dismutase in transgenic *Drosophila melanogaster*. *Arch Biochem Biophys* 371:260–269, 1999.

Modino S, Slijepcevic P. Telomere shortening in mouse strains with constitutional chromosomal aberrations. *Int J Radiat Biol* 78:757–764, 2002.

Moehlig RC. Progeria with nanism and congenital cataracts in a five-year-old child. *JAMA* 132:640–642, 1946.

Moen C. Orthopedic aspects of progeria. *J Bone Joint Surg* 64:542–546, 1982.

Mohaghegh P, Hickson ID. Premature aging in RecQ helicase–deficient human syndromes. *Int J Biochem Cell Biol* 34:1496–1501, 2002.

Moine H, Mandel JL. Do G quartets orchestrate fragile X pathology? *Science* 294:2487–2488, 2002.

Mokbel K. The role of telomerase in breast cancer. *Eur J Surg Oncol* 26:509–514, 2000.

Mokbel KM, Parris CN, Ghilchik M, Amerasinghe CN, Newbold RF. Telomerase activity and lymphovascular invasion in breast cancer. *Eur J Surg Oncol* 26:30–633, 2000.

Molineaux L. Malaria and mortality: some epidemiological considerations. *Ann Trop Med Parasitol* 91:811–825, 1997.

Moll R, Moll I, Franke WW. Identification of Merkel cells in human skin by specific cytokeratin antibodies: changes of cell density and distribution in fetal and adult plantar epidermis. *Differentiation* 28:136–154, 1984.

Mollee P, Woodward N, Durrant S, Lockwood L, Gillett EA, Morton J, Rowell J. Single institution outcomes of treatment of severe aplastic anemia. *Int Med J* 31:337–342, 2001.

Mollenbeck M, Klobutcher LA. De novo telomere addition to spacer sequences prior to their developmental degradation in Euplotes crassus. *Nucleic Acids Res* 30:523–531, 2002.

Moller-Pederson T. A comparative study of human corneal keratocyte and endothelial cell density during aging. *Cornea* 16:333–338, 1997.

Molyneux DH. Patterns of change in vector-borne diseases. *Ann Trop Med Parasitol* 91:827–839, 1997.

Molyneux DH. Vector-borne parasitic diseases—an overview of recent changes. *Int J Parasitol* 28:927–934, 1998.

Monajemi H, Arkenbout EK, Pannekoek H. Gene expression in atherogenesis. *Thromb Haemost* 86:404–412, 2001.

Monserrat AJ, Benavides SH, Berra A, Farina S, Vicario SC, Porta EA. Lectin histochemistry of lipofuscin and certain ceroid pigments. *Histochem Cell Biol* 103:435–445, 1995.

Monson EK, de Bruin D, Zakian VA. The yeast Cac1 protein is required for the stable inheritance of transcriptionally repressed chromatin at telomeres. *Proc Natl Acad Sci USA* 94:13081–13086, 1997.

Monteiro J, Batliwalla F, Ostrer H, Gregersen PK. Shortened telomeres in clonally expanded CD28(–)CD8(+) T cells imply a replicative history that is distinct from their CD28(+)CD8(+) counterparts. *J Immunol* 156:3587–3590, 1996.

Montuenga LM, Mulshine JL. New molecular strategies for early lung cancer detection. *Cancer Invest* 18:555–563, 2000.

Monu JU, Benka-Coker LB, Fatunde Y. Hutchinson-Gilford progeria syndrome in siblings. Report of three new cases. *Skeletal Radiol* 19:585–590, 1990.

Moon MS, Lee CJ, Um SJ, Park JS, Yang JM, Hwang ES. Effect of BPV1 E2-mediated inhibition of E6/E7 expression in HPV16-positive cervical carcinoma cells. *Gynecol Oncol* 80:168–175, 2001.

Moore JK, Haber JE. Capture of retrotransposon DNA at the sites of chromosomal double-stranded breaks. *Nature* 383:644–645 1996.

Moore MA. Stem cell proliferation: ex vivo and in vivo observations. *Stem Cells* 15:239–248, 1997.

Moore RA. The total number of glomeruli in the normal human kidney. *Anat Rec* 48:153–168, 1958.

Moore RA, Topping A. Young men's knowledge of testicular cancer and testicular self-examination: a lost opportunity? *Eur J Cancer Care (Engl)* 8:137–142, 1999.

Moore WA, Davey VA, Weindruch R, Walford R, Ivy GO. The effect of caloric restriction on lipofuscin accumulation in mouse brain with age. *Gerontology* 41(Suppl 2):173–185, 1995.

Mor G, Nilsen J, Horvath T, Bechmann I, Brown S, Garcia-Segura LM, Naftolin F. Estrogen and microglia: a regulatory system that affects the brain. *J Neurobiol* 40:484–496, 1999.

Morales A, Heaton JP, Carson CC 3rd. Andropause: a misnomer for a true clinical entity. *J Urol* 163:705–712, 2000.

Morales CP, Burdick JS, Saboorian MH, Wright WE, Shay JW. In situ hybridization for telomerase RNA in routine cytologic brushings for the diagnosis of pancreaticobiliary malignancies. *Gastrointest Endosc* 48:402–405, 1998a.

Morales CP, Holt SE, Ouellette M, Kaur KJ, Yan Y, Wilson KS, White MA, Wright WE, Shay JW. Absence of cancer-associated changes in human fibroblasts immortalized with telomerase. *Nat Genet* 21:115–118, 1999.

Morales CP, Lee EL, Shay JW. In situ hybridization for the detection of telomerase RNA in the progression from Barrett's esophagus to esophageal adenocarcinoma. *Cancer* 83:652–659, 1998b.

Moreau S, Morgan EA, Symington LS. Overlapping functions of the *Saccharomyces cerevisiae* Mre11, Exo1 and Rad27 nucleases in DNA metabolism. *Genetics* 159:1423–1433, 2001.

Morel DW, DiCorleto PE, Chisolm GM. Endothelial and smooth muscle cells alter low density lipoprotein in vitro by free radical oxidation. *Arteriosclerosis* 4:357–364, 1984.

Moreto M. Diagnosis of esophagogastric tumors. *Endoscopy* 33:1–7, 2001.

Moretti P, Shore D. Multiple interactions in Sir protein recruitment by Rap1p at silencers and telomeres in yeast. *Mol Cell Biol* 21:8082–8094, 2001.

Mori H, Sugie S, Yoshimi N, Hara A, Tanaka T. Control of cell proliferation in cancer prevention. *Mutat Res* 428:291–298, 1999.

Mori N, Oka M, Hazama S, Iizuka N, Yamamoto K, Yoshino S, Tangoku A, Noma T, Hirose K. Detection of telomerase activity in peritoneal lavage fluid from patients with gastric cancer using immunomagnetic beads. *Br J Cancer* 83:1026–1032, 2000.

Morin GB. The human telomere terminal transferase enzyme is a ribonucleoprotein that synthesizes TTAGGG repeats. *Cell* 59:521–529, 1989.

Morin GB. Is telomerase a universal cancer target? *J Natl Cancer Inst* 87:859–861, 1995.

Morin GB. Telomere integrity and cancer. *J Natl Cancer Inst* 88:1095–1096, 1996a.

Morin GB. The structure and properties of mammalian telomerase and their potential impact on human disease. *Cell Dev Biol* 7:5–13, 1996b.

Morin GB. Telomere control of replicative life span. *Exp Gerontol* 32:375–382, 1997a.

Morin GB. The implications of telomerase biochemistry for human disease. *Eur J Cancer* 33:750–760, 1997b.

Morin GB. Endothelial cell rescue using telomerase. "Experimental Gerontology in the Next Millennium: New Models, Mechanisms and Manipulations." 28th Annual Meeting of the American Aging Association. June 4–8, 1999; Seattle, Washington, 1999.

Morin GB, Cech TR. Mitochondrial telomeres: surprising diversity of repeated telomeric DNA sequences among six species of tetrahymena. *Cell* 52:367–374, 1988.

Morisaki H, Ando A, Nagata Y, Pereira-Smith O, Smith JR, Ikeda K, Nakanishi M. Complex mechanisms underlying impaired activation of Cdk4 and Cdk2 in replicative senescence: roles of p16, p21, and cyclin D1. *Exp Cell Res* 253:503–510, 1999.

Morishita R, Gibbons GH, Dzau VJ. Potential for transcatheter application of antisense oligo-nucleotides for the treatment of vascular diseases. *J Intervent Cardiol* 8:377–381, 1995a.

Morishita R, Gibbons GH, Ellison KE, Nakajima M, von der Leyen H, Zhang L, Kaneda Y, Ogihara T, Dzau VJ. Intimal hyperplasia after vascular injury is inhibited by antisense cdk 2 kinase oligonucleotides. *J Clin Invest* 93:1458–1464, 1994.

Morishita R, Gibbons GH, Horiuchi M, Ellison KE, Nakama M, Zhang L, Kaneda Y, Ogihara T, Dzau VJ. A gene therapy strategy using a transcription factor decoy of the E2F binding site inhibits smooth muscle proliferation in vivo. *Proc Natl Acad Sci USA* 92:5855–5859, 1995b.

Morishita R, Gibbons GH, Horiuchi M, Nakajima M, Ellison KE, Lee W, Kaneda Y, Ogihara T, Dzau VJ. Molecular delivery system for antisense oligonucleotides: enhanced effectiveness of antisense oligonucleotides by HVJ-liposome mediated transfer. *J Cardiovasc Pharmacol Ther* 2:213–222, 1997.

Morishita R, Gibbons GH, Tomita N, Zhang L, Kaneda Y, Ogihara T, Dzau VJ. Antisense oligodeoxynucleotide inhibition of vascular angiotensin-converting enzyme expression attenuates neointimal formation: evidence for tissue angiotensin-converting enzyme function. *Arterioscler Thromb Vasc Biol* 20:915–922, 2000.

Moritz T, Mackay W, Glassner BJ, Williams DA, Samson L. Retrovirus-mediated expression of a DNA repair protein in bone marrow protects hematopoietic cells from nitrosourea-induced toxicity in vitro and in vivo. *Cancer Res* 55:2608–2614, 1995.

Moriwaki S, Ray S, Tarone RE, Kraemer KH, Grossman L. The effect of donor age on the processing of UV-damaged DNA by cultured human cells: reduced DNA repair capacity and increased DNA mutability. *Mutat Res* 364:117–123, 1996.

Morley JE. Growth hormone: fountain of youth or death hormone? *J Am Geriatr Soc* 47:1475–1476, 1999.

Morley JE. Diabetes mellitus: a major disease of older persons. *J Gerontol A Biol Sci Med Sci* 55:M255–256, 2000a.

Morley JE. Tithonusism: is it reversible? In Morley JE, van den Berg L (eds). *Endocrinology of Aging.* Humana Press, Totowa, NJ, 2000b, pp 11–22.

Morley JE. Andropause: is it time for the geriatrician to treat it? *J Gerontol A Biol Sci Med Sci* 56:263–265, 2001a.

Morley JE. Decreased food intake with aging. *J Gerontol A Biol Sci Med Sci* 56:81–88, 2001b.

Morley JE, Kaiser FE. Hypogonadism in the elderly man. *Adv Endocrinol Metab* 4:241, 1993.

Morley JE, Kaiser FE, Perry HM 3rd, Patrick P, Morley PM, Stauber PM, Vellas B, Baumgartner RN, Garry PJ. Longitudinal changes in testosterone, luteinizing hormone, and follicle-stimulating hormone in healthy older men. *Metabolism* 46:410–413, 1997.

Morris ED, Chefer SI, Lane MA, Muzic RF Jr, Wong DF, Dannals RF, Matochik JA, Bonab AA, Villemagne VL, Grant SJ, Ingram DK, Roth GS, London ED. Loss of D2 receptor binding with age in rhesus monkeys: importance of correction for differences in striatal size. *J Cereb Blood Flow Metab* 19:218–229, 1999.

Morris M, Hepburn P, Wynford-Thomas D. Sequential extension of proliferative life span in human fibroblasts induced by over-expression of CDK4 or 6 and loss of p53 function. *Oncogene* 21:4277–4288, 2002a.

Morris MC, Evans DA, Bienias JL, Tangney CC, Bennett DA, Aggarwal N, Wilson RS, Scherr PA. Dietary intake of antioxidant nutrients and the risk of incident Alzheimer disease in a biracial community study. *JAMA* 287:3230–3237, 2002b.

Morris MC, Evans DA, Bienias JL, Tangney CC, Wilson RS. Vitamin E and cognitive decline in older persons. *Arch Neurol* 59:1125–1132, 2002c.

Morrison LK, Harrison A, Krishnaswamy P, Kazanegra R, Clopton P, Maisel A. Utility of a rapid B-natriuretic peptide assay in differentiating congestive heart failure from lung disease in patients presenting with dyspnea. *J Am Coll Cardiol* 39:202–209, 2002.

Morrison SJ, Prowse KR, Ho P, Weissman IL. Telomerase activity in hematopoietic cells is associated with self-renewal potential. *Immunity* 5:207–216, 1996.

Morse MA, Lyerly HK, Clinical applications of dendritic cell vaccines. *Curr Opin Mol Ther* 2:20–28, 2000.

Morse RH. RAP, RAP, open up! New wrinkles for RAP1 in yeast. *Trends Genet* 16:51–53, 2000.

Mosekilde L, Thomsen JS, Orhii PB, McCarter RJ, Mejia W, Kalu DN. Additive effect of voluntary exercise and growth hormone treatment on bone strength assessed at four different skeletal sites in an aged rat model. *Bone* 24:71–80, 1999.

Moser MJ, Kamath-Loeb AS, Jacob JE, Bennett SE, Oshima J, Monnat RJ Jr. WRN helicase expression in Werner syndrome cell lines. *Nucleic Acids Res* 28:648–654, 2000.

Moser MJ, Oshima J, Monnat RJ Jr. WRN mutations in Werner syndrome. *Hum Mutat* 13:271–279, 1999.

Mosquera A, Fernandez JL, Campos A, Goyanes VJ, Ramiro-Diaz J, Gosalvez J. Simultaneous decrease of telomere length and telomerase activity with ageing of human amniotic fluid cells. *J Med Genet* 36:494–496, 1999.

Moss NS, Benditt EP. Human atherosclerotic plaque cells and leiomyoma cells: comparison of in vitro growth characteristics. *Am J Pathol* 78:175–190, 1975.

Mossi R, Hubscher U. Clamping down on clamps and clamp loaders—the eukaryotic replication factor C. *Eur J Biochem* 254:209–216, 1998.

Mostafa AH, Gabr M. Hereditary progeria: with a follow-up of two affected sisters. *Arch Pediatr* 71:163–172, 1954.

Motulsky AG, Schultz A, Priest J. Werner's syndrome: chromosomes, genes, and the ageing process. *Lancet* 1:160, 1962.

Moulias R, Meaume S, Raynaud-Simon A. Sarcopenia, hypermetabolism, and aging. *Z Gerontol Geriatr* 32:425–432, 1999.

Mountcastle VB. *Medical Physiology, 13th ed.* CV Mosby Company, St. Louis, 1974.

Movahed MR. Infection with *Chlamydia pneumoniae* and atherosclerosis: a review. *J S C Med Assoc* 95:303–308, 1999.

Moyzis RK. The human telomere. *Sci Am* 274:48–55, 1991.

Moyzis RK, Buckingham JM, Cram LS, Dani M, Deaven LL, Jones MD, Meyne J, Ratliff RL, Wu JR. A highly conserved repetitive DNA sequence, (TTAGGG)n, present at the telomeres of human chromosomes. *Proc Natl Acad Sci USA* 85:6622–6626, 1988.

Mrak RE, Griffin ST, Graham DI. Aging-associated changes in human brain. *J Neuropathol Exp Neurol* 56:1269–1275, 1997.

Mu J, Wei LX. Telomere and telomerase in oncology. *Cell Res* 12:1–7, 2002.

Mueller LD, Nusbaum TJ, Rose MR. The Gompertz equation as a predictive tool in demography. *Exp Gerontol* 30:553–569, 1995.

Mueller LD, Rose MR. Evolutionary theory predicts late-life mortality plateaus. *Proc Natl Acad Sci USA* 93:15249–15253, 1996.

Muhlestein JB. Bacterial infections and atherosclerosis. *J Invest Med* 46:396–402, 1998.

Mukherjee AB, Costello C. Aneuploidy analysis in fibroblasts of human premature aging syndromes by FISH during in vitro cellular aging. *Mech Ageing Dev* 103:209–222, 1998.

Mukherjee D, Nissen SE, Topol EJ. Risk of cardiovascular events associated with selective COX-2 inhibitors. *JAMA* 286:954–959, 2001.

Mukhopadhyay T, Multani AS, Roth JA, Pathak S. Reduced telomeric signals and increased telomeric associations in human lung cancer cell lines undergoing p53–mediated apoptosis. *Oncogene* 17:901–906, 1998.

Muller F. The nature and mechanism of superoxide production by the electron transport chain: its relevance to aging. *J Am Aging Assoc* 23:227–253, 2001.

Muller F, Wicky C, Spicher A, Tobler H. New telomere formation after developmentally regulated chromosomal breakage during the process of chromatin diminution in *Ascaris lumbricoides*. *Cell* 67:815–822, 1991.

Muller HJ. The remaking of chromosomes. *Collecting Net* 8:182–195, 1938.

Muller M, Krause H, Heicappell R, Tischendorf J, Shay JW, Miller K. Comparison of human telomerase RNA and telomerase activity in urine for diagnosis of bladder cancer. *Clin Cancer Res* 4:1949–1954, 1998.

Muller MM, Griesmacher A. Markers of endothelial dysfunction. *Clin Chem Lab Med* 38:77–85, 2000.

Mulligan T, Iranmanesh A, Kerzner R, Demers LW, Veldhuis JD. Two-week pulsatile gonadotropin releasing hormone infusion unmasks dual (hypothalamic and Leydig cell) defects in the healthy aging male gonadotropic axis. *Eur J Endocrinol* 141:257–266, 1999a.

Mulligan T, Jaen-Vinuales A, Godschalk M, Iranmanesh A, Veldhuis JD. Synthetic somatostatin analog (octreotide) suppresses daytime growth hormone secretion equivalently in young and older men: preserved pituitary responsiveness to somatostatin's inhibition in aging. *J Am Geriatr Soc* 47:1422–1424, 1999b.

Mulnard RA, Cotman CW, Kawas C, van Dyck CH, Sano M, Doody R, Koss E, Pfeiffer E, Jin S, Gamst A, Grundman M, Thomas R, Thal LJ. Estrogen replacement therapy for treatment of mild to moderate Alzheimer disease: a randomized controlled trial. *JAMA* 283:1007–1015, 2000.

Multani AS, Li C, Ozen M, Imam AS, Wallace S, Pathak S. Cell-killing by paclitaxel in a metastatic murine melanoma cell line is mediated by extensive telomere erosion with no decrease in telomerase activity. *Oncol Rep* 6:39–44, 1999a.

Multani AS, Narayan S, Jaiswal AS, Zhao YJ, Barkley RA, Furlong CL, Pathak S. Telomere dynamics, aging, and cancer: study of human syndromes characteristic of premature aging. *J Anti-Aging Med* 5:271–281, 2002.

Multani AS, Ozen M, Narayan S, Kumar V, Chandra J, McConkey DJ, Newman RA, Pathak S. Caspase-dependent apoptosis induced by telomere cleavage and TRF2 loss. *Neoplasia* 2:339–345, 2000.

Multani AS, Ozen M, Sen S, Mandal AK, Price JE, Fan D, Radinsky R, Ali-Osman F, Von Eschenbach AC, Fidler IJ, Pathak S. Amplification of telomeric DNA directly correlates with metastatic potential of human and murine cancers of various histological origin. *Int J Oncol* 15:423–429, 1999b.

Multani AS, Worth LL, Jeha S, Chan KW, Pathak S. Human bone marrow transplant rejection is associated with telomere cleavage. *Int J Mol Med* 8:607–610, 2001.

Mundel P, Shankland SJ. Glomerular podocytes and adhesive interaction with glomerular basement membrane. *Exp Nephrol* 7:160–166, 1999.

Muniyappa K, Kironmai KM. Telomere structure, replication and length maintenance. *Crit Rev Biochem Mol Biol* 33:297–336, 1998.

Munro J, Steeghs K, Morrison V, Ireland H, Parkinson EK. Human fibroblast replicative senescence can occur in the absence of extensive cell division and short telomeres. *Oncogene* 20:3541–3552, 2001.

Murakami S, Johnson TE. Life extension and stress resistance in *Caenorhabditis elegans* modulated by the tkr-1 gene. *Curr Biol* 8:1091–1094, 1998.

Murnane JP, Sabatier L, Marder BA, Morgan WF. Telomere dynamics in an immortal human cell line. *EMBO J* 13:4953–4962, 1994.

Murphy C, Alvarado J, Juster R, Maglio M. Prenatal and postnatal cellularity of the human corneal endothelium. *Invest Ophthalmol Vis Sci* 25:312–322, 1984.

Murry CE, Gipaya CT, Bartosek T, Benditt EP, Schwartz SM. Monoclonality of smooth muscle cells in human atherosclerosis. *Am J Pathol* 151:697–705, 1997.

Muscari C, Giaccari A, Giordano E, Clo C, Guarnieri C, Caldarera CM. Role of reactive oxygen species in cardiovascular aging. *Mol Cell Biochem* 160–161:159–166, 1996.

Muskhelishvili L, Hart RW, Turturro A, James SJ. Age-related changes in the intrinsic rate of apoptosis in livers of diet-restricted and ad libitum-fed B6C3F1 mice. *Am J Pathol* 147:20–24, 1995.

Myung SJ, Kim MH, Kim YS, Kim HJ, Park ET, Yoo KS, Lim BC, Wan Seo D, Lee SK, Min YI, Kim JY. Telomerase activity in pure pancreatic juice for the diagnosis of pancreatic cancer may be complementary to K-*ras* mutation. *Gastrointest Endosc* 51:708–713, 2000.

Naasani I, Seimiya H, Tsuruo T. Telomerase inhibition, telomere shortening, and senescence of cancer cells by tea catechins. *Biochem Biophys Res Commun* 249:391–396, 1998.

Naasani I, Yamori T, Tsuruo T. Screening with COMPARE analysis for telomerase inhibitors. In Double JA, Thompson MJ (eds). *Telomeres and Telomerase: Methods and Protocols.* Humana Press, Totowa, NJ, 2002, pp. 197–208.

Nagai N, Oshita T, Murakami J, Ohama K. Semiquantitative analysis of telomerase activity in cervical cancer and precancerous lesions. *Oncol Rep* 6:325–328, 1999.

Nagane M, Lin H, Cavenee WK, Huang HJ. Aberrant receptor signaling in human malignant gliomas: mechanisms and therapeutic implications. *Cancer Lett* 162(Suppl):S17–S21, 2001.

Naganuma Y, Konishi T, Hongou K, Murakami M, Yamatani M, Okada T. A case of progeria syndrome with cerebral infarction [in Japanese]. *No To Hattatsu* 22:71–76, 1990.

Nagao K, Tomimatsu M, Endo H, Hisatomi H, Hikiji K. Telomerase reverse transcriptase mRNA expression and telomerase activity in hepatocellular carcinoma. *J Gastroenterol* 34:83–87, 1999.

Nagata T, Ito M, Liang Y, Gao F. Study of the effects of aging on macromolecular synthesis in mouse steroid secreting cells using microscopic radioautography. *Methods Find Exp Clin Pharmacol* 22:5–18, 2000.

Nagy Z. Mechanisms of neuronal death in Down's syndrome. *J Neural Transm Suppl* 57:233–245, 1999.

Nair KS. Muscle protein turnover: methodological issues and the effect of aging. *J Gerontol A Biol Sci Med Sci* 50(Spec No):107–112, 1995.

Nair KS. Age-related changes in muscle. *Mayo Clin Proc* 75(Suppl):S14–18, 2000.

Nair P, Jayaprakash PG, Nair MK, Pillai MR. Telomerase, p53 and human papillomavirus infection in the uterine cervix. *Acta Oncol* 39:65–70, 2000a.

Nair SK, Heiser A, Boczkowski D, Majumdar A, Naoe M, Lebkowski JS, Vieweg J, Gilboa E. Induction of cytotoxic T cell responses and tumor immunity against unrelated tumors using telomerase reverse transcriptase RNA transfected dendritic cells. *Nat Med* 6:1011–1917, 2000b.

Najemnik C, Sinzinger H, Kritz H. Endothelial dysfunction, atherosclerosis and diabetes. *Acta Med Austriaca* 26:148–153, 1999.

Nakamura E, Lane MA, Roth GS, Ingram DK. A strategy for identifying biomarkers of aging: further evaluation of hematology and blood chemistry data from a calorie restriction study in rhesus monkeys. *Exp Gerontol* 33:421–443, 1998.

Nakamura K, Furugori E, Esaki Y, Arai T, Sawabe M, Okayasu I, Fujiwara M, Kammori M, Mafune K, Kato M, Oshimura M, Sasajima K, Takubo K. Correlation of telomere lengths in normal and cancers tissue in the large bowel. *Cancer Lett* 158:179–184, 2000.

Nakamura K, Izumiyama-Shimomura N, Sawabe M, Arai T, Aoyagi Y, Fujiwara M, Tsuchiya E, Kobayashi Y, Kato M, Oshimura M, Sasajima K, Nakachi K, Takubo K. Comparative analysis of telomere lengths and erosion with age in human epidermis and lingual epithelium. *J Invest Dermatol* 119:1014–1019, 2002a.

Nakamura KD, Turturro A, Hart RW. Elevated c-myc expression in progeria fibroblasts. *Biochem Biophys Res Commun* 155:996–1000, 1988.

Nakamura M, Saito H, Ebinuma H, Wakabayashi K, Saito Y, Takagi T, Nakamoto N, Ishii H. Reduction of telomerase activity in human liver cancer cells by a histone deacetylase inhibitor. *J Cell Physiol* 187:392–401, 2001a.

Nakamura M, Zhen Zhou X, Kishi S, Ping Lu K. Involvement of the telomeric protein Pin2/TRF1 in the regulation of the mitotic spindle. *FEBS Lett* 514:193–198, 2002b.

Nakamura M, Zhou XZ, Kishi S, Kosugi I, Tsutsui Y, Lu KP. A specific interaction between the telomeric protein Pin2/TRF1 and the mitotic spindle. *Curr Biol* 11:1512–1516, 2001b.

Nakamura TM, Morin GB, Chapman KB, Weinrich SL, Andrews WH, Lingner J, Harley CB, Cech TR. Telomerase catalytic subunit homologs from fission yeast and human. *Science* 277:955–959, 1997.

Nakanishi M, Adami GR, Robetorye RS, Noda A, Venable SF, Dimitrov D, Pereira-Smith OM, Smith JR. Exit from G0 and entry into the cell cycle of cells expressing p21Sdi1 antisense RNA. *Proc Natl Acad Sci USA* 92:4352–4356, 1995a.

Nakanishi M, Robetorye RS, Adami GR, Pereira-Smith OM, Smith JR. Identification of the active region of the DNA synthesis inhibitory gene *p21Sdi1/CIP1/WAF1*. *EMBO J* 14:555–563, 1995b.

Nakanishi M, Robetorye RS, Pereira-Smith OM, Smith JR. The C-terminal region of p21SDI1/WAF1/CIP1 is involved in proliferating cell nuclear antigen binding but does not appear to be required for growth inhibition. *J Biol Chem* 270:17060–17063, 1995c.

Nakano K, Watney E, McDougall JK. Telomerase activity and expression of telomerase RNA component and telomerase catalytic subunit gene in cervical cancer. *Am J Pathol* 153:857–864, 1998.

Nakao Y, Hattori T, Takatsuki K, Kuroda Y, Nakaji T, Fujiwara Y, Kishihara M, Baba Y, Fujita T. Immunological studies on Werner's syndrome. *Clin Exp Immunol* 42:10–19, 1980.

Nakao Y, Kishihara M, Yoshimi H, Inoue Y, Tanaka K, Sakamoto N, Matsukura S, Imura H, Ichihashi M, Fujiwara Y. Werner's syndrome: in vivo and in vitro characteristics as a model of aging. *Am J Med* 65:919–932, 1978.

Nakashio R, Kitamoto M, Nakanishi T, Takaishi H, Takahashi S, Kajiyama G. Telomere length and telomerase activity in hepatocellular carcinoma [in Japanese]. *Nippon Rinsho* 56:1239–1243, 1998.

Nakashio R, Kitamoto M, Tahara H, Nakanishi T, Ide T, Kajiyama G. Significance of telomerase activity in the diagnosis of small differentiated hepatocellular carcinoma. *Int J Cancer* 74:141–147, 1997.

Nakayama J, Ishikawa F. Stretch PCR assay. In Double JA, Thompson MJ (eds). *Telomeres and Telomerase: Methods and Protocols.* Humana Press, Totowa, NJ, 2002, pp 125–136.

Nakayama J, Tahara H, Tahara E, Saito M, Ito K, Nakamura H, Nakanishi T, Ide T, Ishikawa F. Telomerase activation by hTRT in human normal fibroblasts and hepatocellular carcinomas. *Nat Genet* 18:65–68, 1998.

Nakayama Y, Sakamoto H, Satoh K, Yamamoto T. Tamoxifen and gonadal steroids inhibit colon cancer growth in association with inhibition of thymidylate synthase, survivin and telomerase expression through estrogen receptor beta mediated system. *Cancer Lett* 161:63–71, 2000.

Narada MT. *A Manual of Abhidhamma.* Buddhist Publication Society, Kandy, 1968.

Narayan S, Jaiswal AS, Multani AS, Pathak S. DNA damage-induced cell cycle checkpoints involve both p53-dependent and -independent pathways: role of telomere repeat binding factor 2. *Br J Cancer* 85:898–901, 2001.

Nardi M, Di Bari M, Grasso L, Chiovato L, Martino E, Pinchera A, Briganti MP, Masotti G, Marchionni N. The "low-T3 syndrome" in unselected elderly home-dwellers: an epidemiological study in Dicomano, Italy. *J Endocrinol Invest* 22(10 Suppl):40–41, 1999.

Nasir L, Devlin P, Mckevitt T, Rutteman G, Argyle DJ. Telomere lengths and telomerase activity in dog tissues: a potential model system to study human telomere and telomerase biology. *Neoplasia* 3:351–359, 2001.

Naslund J, Haroutunian V, Mohs R, Davis KL, Davies P, Greengard P, Buxbaum JD. Correlation between elevated levels of amyloid -peptide in the brain and cognitive decline. *JAMA* 283:1571–1577, 2000.

Natarajan S, McEachern MJ. Recombinational telomere elongation promoted by DNA circles. *Mol Cell Biol* 22:4512–4521, 2002.

Natarajan V, Lempicki RA, Sereti I, Badralmaa Y, Adelsberger JW, Metcalf JA, Prieto DA, Stevens R, Baseler MW, Kovacs JA, Lane HC. Increased peripheral expansion of naive CD4+ T cells in vivo after IL-2 treatment of patients with HIV infection. *Proc Natl Acad Sci USA* 99:10712–10717, 2002.

Nautiyal S, DeRisi JL, Blackburn EH. The genome-wide expression response to telomerase deletion in *Saccharomyces cerevisiae. Proc Natl Acad Sci USA* 99:9316–9321, 2002.

Nee LE, Lippa CF. Alzheimer's disease in 22 twin pairs — 13-year follow-up: hormonal, infectious and traumatic factors. *Dement Geriatr Cogn Disord* 10:148–151, 1999.

Neidle S, Harrison RJ, Reszka AP, Read MA. Structure–activity relationships among guanine-quadruplex telomerase inhibitors. *Pharmacol Ther* 85:133–139, 2000.

Neidle S, Kelland LR. Telomerase as an anti-cancer target: current status and future prospects. *Anticancer Drug Des* 14:341–347, 1999.

Neidle S, Parkinson G. Telomere maintenance as a target for anticancer drug discovery. *Nat Rev Drug Discov* 1:383–393, 2002.

Neidle S, Read MA. G-quadruplexes as therapeutic targets. *Biopolymers* 56:195–208, 2000–2001.

Neill CA, Dingwall MM. A syndrome resembling progeria: a review of two cases. *Arch Dis Child* 25:213–221, 1950.

Nelson HD. Assessing benefits and harms of hormone replacement therapy — clinical applications. *JAMA* 288:882–884, 2002.

Nelson HD, Humphrey LL, Nygren P, Teutsch SM, Allan JD. Postmenopausal hormone replacement therapy — scientific review. *JAMA* 288:872–880, 2002.

Nemoto K, Kondo Y, Himeno S, Suzuki Y, Hara S, Akimoto M, Imura N. Modulation of telomerase activity by zinc in human prostatic and renal cancer cells. *Biochem Pharmacol* 59:401–495, 2000.

Ness J, Aronow WS, Ahn C. Risk factors for symptomatic peripheral arterial disease in older persons in an academic hospital–based geriatrics practice. *J Am Geriatr Soc* 48:312–314, 2000a.

Ness RB, Grisso JA, Klapper J, Schlesselman JJ, Silberzweig S, Vergona R, Morgan M, Wheeler JE. Risk of ovarian cancer in relation to estrogen and progestin dose and use characteristics of oral contraceptives. *Am J Epidemiol* 152:233–241, 2000b.

Netzer C, Rieger L, Brero A, Zhang CD, Hinzke M, Kohlhase J, Bohlander SK. *SALL1*, the gene mutated in Townes-Brocks syndrome, encodes a transcriptional repressor which interacts with TRF1/PIN2 and localizes to pericentromeric heterochromatin. *Hum Mol Genet* 10:3017–3024, 2001.

Neumeister P, Albanese C, Balent B, Greally J, Pestell RG. Senescence and epigenetic dysregulation in cancer. *Int J Biochem Cell Biol* 34:1475–1490, 2002.

Newbold RF. Genetic control of telomerase and replicative senescence in human and rodent cells. *Ciba Found Symp* 211:177–189, 1997.

Newbold RF. Telomerase as an anti-cancer drug target: will it fulfil its early promise? *Anticancer Drug Des* 14:349–354, 1999.

Newbold RF. The significance of telomerase activation and cellular immortalization in human cancer. Mutagenesis 17:539–550, 2002.

Newby AC, Zaltsman AB. Molecular mechanisms in intimal hyperplasia. *J Pathol* 190:300–309, 2000.

Newman AB. Peripheral arterial disease: insights from population studies of older adults. *J Am Geriatr Soc* 48:1157–1162, 2000.

Newman AB, Yanez D, Harris T, Duxbury A, Enright PL, Fried LP, for the Cardiovascular Study Research Group. Weight change in old age and its association with mortality. *J Am Geriatr Soc* 49:1309–1318, 2001.

Niblock MM, Brunso-Bechtold JK, Lynch CD, Ingram RL, McShane T, Sonntag WE. Distribution and levels of insulin-like growth factor I mRNA across the life span in the Brown Norway X Fischer 344 rat brain. *Brain Res* 804:79–86, 1998.

Nichols NR. Glial responses to steroids as markers of brain aging. *J Neurobiol* 40:585–601, 1999.

Nickoloff BJ. Creation of psoriatic plaques: the ultimate tumor suppressor pathway. A new model for an ancient T-cell–mediated skin disease. Viewpoint. *J Cutan Pathol* 28:57–64, 2001.

Niiyama H, Mizumoto K, Sato N, Nagai E, Mibu R, Fukui T, Kinoshita M, Tanaka M. Quantitative analysis of hTERT mRNA expression in colorectal cancer. *Am J Gastroenterol* 96:1895–1900, 2001.

Nikaido R, Haruyama T, Watanabe Y, Iwata H, Iida M, Sugimura H, Yamada N, Ishikawa F. Presence of telomeric G-strand tails in the telomerase catalytic subunit TERT knockout mice. *Genes Cells* 4:563–572, 1999.

Nilsberth C, Westlind-Danielsson A, Eckman CB, Condron MM, Axelman K, Forsell C, Stenh C, Luthman J, Teplow DB, Younkin SG, Naslund J, Lannfelt L. The 'Arctic' *APP* mutation (E693G) causes Alzheimer's disease by enhanced Abeta protofibril formation. *Nat Neurosci* 4:887–893, 2001.

Nilsen J, Mor G, Naftolin F. Estrogen-regulated developmental neuronal apoptosis is determined by estrogen receptor subtype and the Fas/Fas ligand system. *J Neurobiol* 43:64–78, 2000.

Nilsson L, Rogers J, Potter H. The essential role of inflammation and induced gene expression in the pathogenic pathway of Alzheimer's disease. *Front Biosci* 3:d436–446, 1998.

Nilsson M, Perfilieva E, Johansson U, Orwar O, Eriksson PS. Enriched environment increases neurogenesis in the adult rat dentate gyrus and improves spatial memory. *J Neurobiol* 39:569–578, 1999.

Ning Y, Pereira-Smith OM. Molecular genetic approaches to the study of cellular senescence. *Mutat Res* 256:303–310, 1991.

Ning Y, Shay JW, Lovell M, Taylor L, Ledbetter DH, Pereira-Smith OM. Tumor suppression by chromosome 11 is not due to cellular senescence. *Exp Cell Res* 192:220–226, 1991a.

Ning Y, Weber JL, Killary AM, Ledbetter DH, Smith JR, Pereira-Smith OM. Genetic analysis of indefinite division in human cells: evidence for a cell senescence-related gene(s) on human chromosome 4. *Proc Natl Acad Sci USA* 88:5635–5639, 1991b.

Nippoldt TB, Nair KS. Is there a case for DHEA replacement? *Baillieres Clin Endocrinol Metab* 12:507–520, 1998.

Nishi R. Neurotrophic factors: two are better than one. *Science* 265:1052–1053, 1994.

Nishikawa T, Okamura H, Nagadoi A, Konig P, Rhodes D, Nishimura Y. Solution structure of a telomeric DNA complex of human TRF1. *Structure (Camb)* 9:1237–1251, 2001.

Nishimoto A, Miura N, Horikawa I, Kugoh H, Murakami Y, Hirohashi S, Kawasaki H, Gazdar AF, Shay JW, Barrett JC, Oshimura M. Functional evidence for a telomerase repressor gene on human chromosome 10p15.1. *Oncogene* 20:828–835, 2001.

Nishimoto A, Miura N, Oshimura M. Clinical significance of telomerase activity in precancerous lesion of the liver [in Japanese]. *Nippon Rinsho* 56:1244–1247, 1998.

Niyaz H, Zhao C, Li Y. Detection and significance of HPV16, 18 infection, P53 overexpression and telomerase activity in patients with lung cancer [in Chinese]. *Zhonghua Jie He He Hu Xi Za Zhi* 23:679–682, 2000.

Nnodim JO. Satellite cell numbers in senile rat levator ani muscle. *Mech Ageing Dev* 112:99–111, 2000.

Nochlin D, Shaw CM, Campbell LA, Kuo CC. Failure to detect *Chlamydia pneumoniae* in brain tissues of Alzheimer's disease. *Neurology* 53:1888, 1999.

Noda A, Ning Y, Venable SF, Pereira-Smith OM, Smith JR. Cloning of senescent cell-derived inhibitors of DNA synthesis using an expression screen. *Exp Cell Res* 211:90–98, 1994.

Nohria A, Lewis E, Stevenson LW. Medical management of advanced heart failure. *JAMA* 287:628–640, 2002.

Noller KL. Estrogen replacement therapy and risk of ovarian cancer. *JAMA* 288:368–369, 2002.

Nonet GH, Stampfer MR, Chin K, Gray JW, Collins CC, Yaswen P. The *ZNF217* gene amplified in breast cancers promotes immortalization of human mammary epithelial cells. *Cancer Res* 61:1250–1254, 2001.

Nordberg A, Svensson AL. Cholinesterase inhibitors in the treatment of Alzheimer's disease: a comparison of tolerability and pharmacology [published erratum in *Drug Saf* 20:146, 1999]. *Drug Saf* 19:465–480, 1998.

Nordstrom CK, Dwyer KM, Merz CN, Shircore A, Dwyer JH. Work-related stress and early atherosclerosis. *Epidemiology* 12:180–185, 2001.

Nordstrom L, Arulkumaran S. Intrapartum fetal hypoxia and biochemical markers: a review. *Obstet Gynecol Surv* 53:645–657, 1998.

Norrback KF, Hultdin M, Dahlenborg K, Osterman P, Carlsson R, Roos G. Telomerase regulation and telomere dynamics in germinal centers. *Eur J Haematol* 67:309–317, 2001.

Norsgaard H, Clark BF, Rattan SI. Distinction between differentiation and senescence and the absence of increased apoptosis in human keratinocytes undergoing cellular aging in vitro. *Exp Gerontol* 31:563–570, 1996.

Norton JC, Holt SE, Wright WE, Shay JW. Enhanced detection of human telomerase activity. *DNA Cell Biol* 17:217–219, 1998.

Norton JC, Piatyszek MA, Wright WE, Shay JW, Corey DR. Inhibition of human telomerase activity by peptide nucleic acids. *Nat Biotechnol* 14:615–619, 1996.

Norwood TH, Pendergrass WR, Sprague CA, Martin GM. Dominance of the senescent phenotype in heterokaryons between replicative and post-replicative human fibroblast-like cells. *Proc Natl Acad Sci USA* 71:2231–2235, 1974.

Norwood TH, Smith JR, Stein GH. Aging at the cellular level: the human fibroblast like cell model. In Schneider EL, Rowe JW, Birren E (eds). *The Handbook of the Biology of Aging, 3rd ed*. New York, Academic Press, 1990a, pp 131–154.

Norwood TH, Stein G, Smith JR. The cultured fibroblast-like cell as a model for the study of aging. In Schneider EL, Rowe JW, Birren E (eds). *The Handbook of the Biology of Aging. 3rd ed*. New York, Academic Press, 1990b, pp 291–321.

Nosek J, Tomaska L, Fukuhara H, Suyama Y, Kovac L. Linear mitochondrial genomes: 30 years down the line. *Trends Genet* 14:184–188, 1998.

Nosek J, Tomaska L, Rycovska A, Fukuhara H. Mitochondrial telomeres as molecular markers for identification of the opportunistic yeast pathogen *Candida parapsilosis*. *J Clin Microbiol* 40:1283–1289, 2002.

Nouso K, Urabe Y, Higashi T, Nakatsukasa H, Hino N, Ashida K, Kinugasa N, Yoshida K, Uematsu S, Tsuji T. Telomerase as a tool for the differential diagnosis of human hepatocellular carcinoma. *Cancer* 78:232–236, 1996.

Nowak JA. Telomerase, cervical cancer, and human papillomavirus. *Clin Lab Med* 20:369–382, 2000.

Nowak R, Siwicki JK, Chechlinska M, Markowicz S. Telomere shortening and atherosclerosis. *Lancet* 359:976; discussion 976–977, 2002.

Nozawa K, Kurumiya Y, Yamamoto A, Isobe Y, Suzuki M, Yoshida S. Up-regulation of telomerase in primary cultured rat hepatocytes. *J Biochem (Tokyo)* 126:361–367, 1999.

Nozawa K, Maehara K, Isobe K. Mechanism for the reduction of telomerase expression during muscle cell differentiation. *J Biol Chem* 276:22016–22023, 2001.

Nozawa K, Suzuki M, Takemura M, Yoshida S. In vitro expansion of mammalian telomere repeats by DNA polymerase alpha-primase. *Nucleic Acids Res* 28:3117–3124, 2000.

Nugent CI, Lundblad V. The telomerase reverse transcriptase: components and regulation. *Genes Dev* 12:1073–1085, 1998.

Nunomura A, Perry G, Pappolla MA, Friedland RP, Hirai K, Chiba S, Smith MA. Neuronal oxidative stress precedes amyloid-beta deposition in Down syndrome. *J Neuropathol Exp Neurol* 59:1011–1017, 2000.

Nunomura A, Perry G, Zhang J, Montine TJ, Takeda A, Chiba S, Smith MA. RNA oxidation in Alzheimer and Parkinson diseases. *J Anti-Aging Med* 2:227–230, 1999.

Nusbaum TJ, Graves JL, Mueller LD, Rose MR. Fruit fly aging and mortality. *Science* 260:1567; discussion 1567–1569, 1993.

Nusbaum TJ, Mueller LD, Rose MR. Evolutionary patterns among measures of aging. *Exp Gerontol* 31:507–516, 1996.

Nusbaum TJ, Rose MR. Aging in *Drosophila*. *Comp Biochem Physiol* 109:33–38, 1994.

Nusbaum TJ, Rose MR. The effects of nutritional manipulation and laboratory selection on life span in *Drosophila melanogaster*. *J Gerontol A Biol Sci Med Sci* 54:B192–198, 1999.

Nybo H, Gaist D, Jeune B, McGue M, Vaupel JW, Christensen K. Functional status and self-rated health in 2, 262 nonagenarians: the Danish 1905 cohort study. *J Am Geriatr Soc* 49:601–609, 2001.

Obeid LM, Venable ME. Signal transduction in cellular senescence. *J Am Geriatr Soc* 45:361–366, 1997.

O'Brien ME, Jensen S, Weiss AS. Hutchinson-Gilford progeria: faithful DNA maintenance, inheritance and allelic transcription of beta(1–4) galactosyltransferase. *Mech Ageing Dev* 101:43–56, 1998.

O'Brien ME, Weiss AS. Hutchinson-Gilford progeria fibroblasts exhibit metabolically normal uridine uptake and RNA synthetic rates. *Biochem Biophys Res Commun* 210:225–230, 1995.

O'Connor KG, Harman SM, Stevens TE, Jayme JJ, Bellantoni MF, Busby-Whitehead MJ, Christmas C, Munzer T, Tobin JD, Roy TA, Cottrell E, St Clair C, Pabst KM, Blackman MR. Interrelationships of spontaneous growth hormone axis activity, body fat, and serum lipids in healthy elderly women and men. *Metabolism* 48:1424–1431, 1999.

Oeppen J, Vaupel JW. Broken limits to life expectancy. *Science* 296:1029–1031, 2002.

Oexle K, Kohlschutter A. Cause of progression in Duchenne muscular dystrophy: impaired differentiation more probable than replicative aging. *Neuropediatrics* 32:123–129, 2001.

Ogami M, Ikura Y, Nishiguchi S, Kuroki T, Ueda M, Sakurai M. Quantitative analysis and in situ localization of human telomerase RNA in chronic liver disease and hepatocellular carcinoma. *Lab Invest* 79:15–26, 1999.

Ogburn CE, Carlberg K, Ottinger MA, Holmes DJ, Martin GM, Sustad SN. Exceptional cellular resistance to oxidative damage in long-lived birds requires active gene expression. *J Gerontol A Biol Sci Med Sci* 56:468–474, 2001.

Ogg S, Paradis S, Gottlieb S, Patterson GI, Lee L, Tissenbaum HA, Ruvkun G. The Forkhead transcription factor DAF-16 transduces insulin-like metabolic and longevity signals in *C. elegans*. *Nature* 389:994–999, 1997.

Ogihara T, Hata T, Tanaka K, Fukuchi K, Tabuchi Y, Kumahara Y. Hutchinson-Gilford progeria syndrome in a 45-year-old man. *Am J Med* 81:135–138, 1986.

Ogino M, Hisatomi H, Hanazono M. Effectiveness of indomethacin as an antitumor agent in colon 26–bearing conventional and nude mice, and telomerase activity in the tumors. *Exp Anim* 48:15–21, 1999a.

Ogino M, Hisatomi H, Murata M, Hanazono M. Indomethacin suppresses the growth of colon 26, Meth-A and FM3A tumors in mice by reducing the prostaglandin E2 content and telomerase activity in tumor tissues. *Jpn J Cancer Res* 90:758–764, 1999b.

Ogino M, Nakabayashi K, Suzuki M, Takahashi E, Fujii M, Suzuki T, Ayusawa D. Release of telomeric DNA from chromosomes in immortal human cells lacking telomerase activity. *Biochem Biophys Res Commun* 248:223–227, 1998.

Ognibene A, Petruzzi E, Troiano L, Pini G, Franceschi C, Monti D, Masotti G, Messeri G, Cilotti A, Forti G. Age-related changes of thyroid function in both sexes. *J Endocrinol Invest* 22(10 Suppl):38–39, 1999.

Ogoshi M, Le T, Shay JW, Taylor RS. In situ hybridization analysis of the expression of human telomerase RNA in normal and pathologic conditions of the skin. *J Invest Dermatol* 110:818–823, 1998.

Oh H, Taffet GE, Youker KA, Entman ML, Overbeek PA, Michael LH, Schneider MD. Telomerase reverse transcriptase promotes cardiac muscle cell proliferation, hypertrophy, and survival. *Proc Natl Acad Sci USA* 98:10308–10313, 2001a.

Oh S, Kyo S, Laimins LA. Telomerase activation by human papillomavirus type 16 E6 protein: induction of human telomerase reverse transcriptase expression through Myc and GC-rich Sp1 binding sites. *J Virol* 75:5559–5566, 2001b.

Oh S, Song YH, Kim UJ, Yim J, Kim TK. In vivo and in vitro analyses of Myc for differential promoter activities of the human telomerase (hTERT) gene in normal and tumor cells. *Biochem Biophys Res Commun* 263:361–365, 1999a.

Oh S, Song Y, Yim J, Kim TK. The Wilms' tumor 1 tumor suppressor gene represses transcription of the human telomerase reverse transcriptase gene. *J Biol Chem* 274:37473–37378, 1999b.

Oh S, Song Y, Yim J, Kim TK. Identification of Mad as a repressor of the human telomerase (hTERT) gene. *Oncogene* 19:1485–1490, 2000.

O'Hagan RC, Chang S, Maser RS, Mohan R, Artandi SE, Chin L, DePinho RA. Telomere dysfunction provokes regional amplification and deletion in cancer genomes. *Cancer Cell* 2:149–155, 2002.

O'Hare MJ, Bond J, Clarke C, Takeuchi Y, Atherton AJ, Berry C, Moody J, Silver AR, Davies DC, Alsop AE, Neville AM, Jat PS. Conditional immortalization of freshly isolated human mammary fibroblasts and endothelial cells. *Proc Natl Acad Sci USA* 98:646–651, 2001.

Ohki R, Tsurimoto T, Ishikawa F. In vitro reconstitution of the end replication problem. *Mol Cell Biol* 21:5753–5766, 2001.

Ohmido N, Kijima K, Ashikawa I, de Jong JH, Fukui K. Visualization of the terminal structure of rice chromosomes 6 and 12 with multicolor FISH to chromosomes and extended DNA fibers. *Plant Mol Biol* 47:413–421, 2001.

Ohmura H, Tahara H, Suzuki M, Ide T, Shimizu M, Yoshida MA, Tahara E, Shay JW, Barrett JC, Oshimura M. Restoration of the cellular senescence program and repression of telomerase by human chromosome 3. *Jpn J Cancer Res* 86:899–904, 1995.

Ohmura Y, Aoe M, Andou A, Shimizu N. Telomerase activity and Bcl-2 expression in non-small cell lung cancer. *Clin Cancer Res* 6:2980–2987, 2000.

Ohno M, Cooke JP, Dzau VJ, Gibbons GH. Fluid shear stress induces endothelial transforming growth factor beta-1 transcription and production. Modulation by potassium channel blockade. *J Clin Invest* 95:1363–1369, 1995.

Ohshima K, Sugihara M, Haraoka S, Suzumiya J, Kanda M, Kawasaki C, Shimazaki K, Kikuchi M. Possible immortalization of Hodgkin and Reed-Sternberg cells: telomerase expression, lengthening of telomere, and inhibition of apoptosis by nf-κb expression. *Leuk Lymphoma* 41:367–376, 2001.

Ohta K, Kanamaru T, Morita Y, Hayashi Y, Ito H, Yamamoto M. Telomerase activity in hepatocellular carcinoma as a predictor of postoperative recurrence. *J Gastroenterol* 32:791–796, 1997.

Ohta K, Kanamaru T, Yamamoto M, Saitoh Y. Clinical significance of telomerase activity in hepatocellular carcinoma. *Kobe J Med Sci* 42:207–217, 1996.

Ohtsuka T, Yamakage A, Yamazaki S. The polymorphism of telomerase RNA component gene in patients with systemic sclerosis. *Br J Dermatol* 147:250–254, 2002.

Ohya T, Kawasaki Y, Hiraga SI, Kanbara S, Nakajo K, Nakashima N, Suzuki A, Sugino A. The DNA polymerase domain of Pol epsilon is required for rapid, efficient and highly accurate chromosomal DNA replication, telomere length maintenance, and normal cell senescence in *Saccharomyces cerevisiae. J Biol Chem* 277:28099–28108, 2002.

Ohyashiki JH, Iwama H, Yahata N, Ando K, Hayashi S, Shay JW, Ohyashiki K. Telomere stability is frequently impaired in high-risk groups of patients with myelodysplastic syndromes. *Clin Cancer Res* 5:1155–1160, 1999.

Ohyashiki JH, Ohyashiki K, Iwama H, Hayashi S, Toyama K, Shay JW. Clinical implications of telomerase activity levels in acute leukemia. *Clin Cancer Res* 3:619–625, 1997a.

Ohyashiki JH, Ohyashiki K, Toyama K, Shay JW. A nonradioactive, fluorescence-based telomeric repeat amplification protocol to detect and quantitate telomerase activity. *Trends Genet* 12:395–396, 1996.

Ohyashiki JH, Sashida G, Tauchi T, Ohyashiki K. Telomeres and telomerase in hematologic neoplasia. *Oncogene* 21:680–687, 2002.

Ohyashiki K, Iwama H, Yahata N, Tauchi T, Kawakubo K, Shimamoto T, Ohyashiki JH. Telomere dynamics in myelodysplastic syndromes and acute leukemic transformation. *Leuk Lymphoma* 42:291–299, 2001.

Ohyashiki K, Ohyashiki JH. In situ TRAP assay detection of telomerase activity in cytological preparations. In Double JA, Thompson MJ (eds). *Telomeres and Telomerase: Methods and Protocols.* Humana Press, Totowa, NJ, 2002, pp 159–164.

Ohyashiki K, Ohyashiki JH, Iwama H, Hayashi S, Shay JW, Toyama K. Telomerase activity and cytogenetic changes in chronic myeloid leukemia with disease progression. *Leukemia* 11:190–194, 1997b.

Ohyashiki K, Ohyashiki JH, Nishimaki J, Toyama K, Ebihara Y, Kato H, Wright WE, Shay JW. Cytological detection of telomerase activity using an in situ telomeric repeat amplification protocol assay. *Cancer Res* 57:2100–2103, 1997c.

Okarma TB. Human primordial stem cells. *Hastings Cent Rep* 29:30, 1999.

Okatani Y, Morioka N, Wakatsuki A. Changes in nocturnal melatonin secretion in perimenopausal women: correlation with endogenous estrogen concentrations. *J Pineal Res* 28:111–118, 2000.

Okimoto T, Imazu M, Hayashi Y, Fujiwara H, Ueda H, Kohno N. Atherosclerotic plaque characterization by quantitative analysis using intravascular ultrasound correlation with histological and immunohistochemical findings. *Circ J* 66:173–177, 2002.

Okubo M, Tsurukubo Y, Higaki T, Kawabe T, Goto M, Murase T, Ide T, Furuichi Y, Sugimoto M. Clonal chromosomal aberrations accompanied by strong telomerase activity in immortalization of human B-lymphoblastoid cell lines transformed by Epstein-Barr virus. *Cancer Genet Cytogenet* 129:30–34, 2001.

Okuda K, Bardeguez A, Gardner JP, Rodriguez P, Ganesh V, Kimura M, Skurnick J, Awad G, Aviv A. Telomere length in the newborn. *Pediatr Res* 52:377–381, 2002.

Okusa Y, Ichikura T, Mochizuki H, Shinomiya N. Clinical significance of telomerase activity in biopsy specimens of gastric cancer. *J Clin Gastroenterol* 30:61–63, 2000.

Okusa Y, Shinomiya N, Ichikura T, Mochizuki H. Correlation between telomerase activity and DNA ploidy in gastric cancer. *Oncology* 55:258–264, 1998.

Oliet SHR, Piet R, Poulain DA. Control of glutamate clearance and synaptic efficacy by glial coverage of neurons. *Science* 292:923–926, 2001.

Olovnikov AM,. Principle of marginotomy in template synthesis of polynucleotides [in Russian]. *Doklady Akademii Nauk SSSR* 201:1496–1499, 1971.

Olovnikov AM. The telomere shortening signal may be explained by a fountain mechanism modulating the expression of eukaryotic genes. *J Anti-Aging Med* 2:59–74, 1999.

Olshansky SJ, Hayflick L, Carnes BA. No truth to the fountain of youth. *Sci Am* 286:92–95, 2002a.

Olshansky SJ, Hayflick L, Carnes BA. Position statement on human aging. *J Gerontol A Biol Sci Med Sci* 57A:B292–297, 2002b.

Olson DJ, Gibo DM. Antisense wnt-5a mimics wnt-1-mediated c57mg mammary epithelial cell transformation. *Exp Cell Res* 241:134–141, 1998.

Olson DJ, Oshimura M, Otte AP, Kumar R. Ectopic expression of wnt-5a in human renal cell carcinoma cells suppresses in vitro growth and telomerase activity. *Tumour Biol* 19:244–252, 1998.

Olson L. Combating Parkinson's disease—step three. *Science* 290:721–724, 2000.

Omar A. A case of the Hutchinson-Gilford progeria syndrome. *Med J Malaysia* 37:362–364, 1982.

Omata M, Tada M. General rules for the study of pancreatic cancer by molecular biological aspect [in Japanese]. *Nippon Geka Gakkai Zasshi* 101:233–236, 2000.

O'Neill MJ, Ingram RS, Vrana PB, Tilghman SM. Allelic expression of IGF2 in marsupials and birds. *Dev Genes Evol* 210:18–20, 2000.

Opitz OG, Suliman Y, Hahn WC, Harada H, Blum HE, Rustgi AK. Cyclin D1 overexpression and p53 inactivation immortalize primary oral keratinocytes by a telomerase-independent mechanism. *J Clin Invest* 108:725–732, 2001.

Oppenheimer BS, Kugel VH. Werner's syndrome: a heredofamilial disorder with scleroderma, bilateral juvenile cataract, precocious graying of the hair and endocrine stigmatization. *Trans Assoc Am Physicians* 49:358–370, 1934.

Opresko PL, Laine JP, Brosh RM Jr, Seidman MM, Bohr VA. Coordinate action of the helicase and 3' to 5' exonuclease of Werner syndrome protein. *J Biol Chem* 276:44677–44687, 2001.

Opresko PL, von Kobbe C, Laine JP, Harrigan J, Hickson ID, Bohr VA. Telomere-binding protein TRF2 binds to and stimulates the Werner and Bloom syndrome helicases. *J Biol Chem* 277:41110–41119, 2002.

O'Riordan VB, Burnell, AM. Intermediary metabolism in the dauer larva of the nematode Caenorhabditis elegans. I. Glycolysis, gluconeogenesis, oxidative phosphorylation and the tricarboxylic acid cycle. *Comp Biochem Physiol* 92:233–238, 1989.

Ornish D, Scherwitz LW, Billings JH, Brown SE, Gould KL, Merritt TA, Sparler S, Armstrong WT, Ports TA, Kirkeeide RL, Hogeboom C, Brand RJ. Intensive lifestyle changes for reversal of coronary heart disease. *JAMA* 280:2001–2007, 1998.

Orren DK, Theodore S, Machwe A. The Werner syndrome helicase/exonuclease (WRN) disrupts and degrades D-loops in vitro. *Biochemistry* 41:13483–3488, 2002.

Oshima H, Rochat A, Kedzia C, Kobayashi K, Barrandon Y. Morphogenesis and renewal of hair follicles from adult multipotent stem cells. *Cell* 104:233–245, 2001.

Oshima J, Brown WT, Martin GM. No detectable mutations at Werner helicase locus in progeria. *Lancet* 348:1106, 1996a.

Oshima J, Campisi J, Tannock TC, Martin GM. Regulation of c-fos expression in senescing Werner syndrome fibroblasts differs from that observed in senescing fibroblasts from normal donors. *J Cell Physiol* 162:277–283, 1995.

Oshima J, Yu CE, Piussan C, Klein G, Jabkowski J, Balci S, Miki T, Nakura J, Ogihara T, Ells J, Smith M, Melaragno MI, Fraccaro M, Scappaticci S, Matthews J, Ouais S, Jarzebowicz A, Schellenberg GD, Martin GM. Homozygous and compound heterozygous mutations at the Werner syndrome locus. *Hum Mol Genet* 5:1909–1913, 1996b.

Oshita T, Nagai N, Ohama K. Expression of telomerase reverse transcriptase mRNA and its quantitative analysis in human endometrial cancer. *Int J Oncol* 17:1225–1230, 2000.

Osiewacz HD, Hamann A. DNA reorganization and biological aging. A review. Biochemistry (Moscow) 62:1275–1284, 1997.

Ostler EL, Wallis CV, Sheerin AN, Faragher RG. A model for the phenotypic presentation of Werner's syndrome. *Exp Gerontol* 37:285–292, 2002.

O'Sullivan JN, Bronner MP, Brentnall TA, Finley JC, Shen WT, Emerson S, Emond MJ, Gollahon KA, Moskovitz AH, Crispin DA, Potter JD, Rabinovitch PS. Chromosomal instability in ulcerative colitis is related to telomere shortening. *Nat Genet* 32:280–284, 2002.

Otsuka T, Uchida N, Arima F, Shigematsu H, Fukuyama T, Maeda M, Sugio Y, Itoh Y, Niho Y. Down-regulation of human telomeric protein TRF1 gene expression during myeloid differentiation in human hematopoietic cells. *Int J Hematol* 71:334–339, 2000.

Ouellette MM, Aisner DL, Savre-Train I, Wright WE, Shay JW. Telomerase activity does not always imply telomere maintenance. *Biochem Biophys Res Commun* 254:795–803, 1999.

Ouellette MM, Liao M, Herbert BS, Johnson M, Holt SE, Liss HS, Shay JW, Wright WE. Subsenescent telomere lengths in fibroblasts immortalized by limiting amounts of telomerase. *J Biol Chem* 275:10072–10076, 2000a.

Ouellette MM, McDaniel LD, Wright WE, Shay JW, Schultz RA. The establishment of telomerase-immortalized cell lines representing human chromosome instability syndromes. *Hum Mol Genet* 9:403–411, 2000b.

Oulton R, Harrington L. Telomeres, telomerase, and cancer: life on the edge of genomic stability. *Curr Opin Oncol* 12:74–81, 2000.

Ourednik V, Ourednik J, Flax JD, Zawada WM, Hutt C, Yang C, Park KI, Kim SU, Sidman RL, Freed CR, Snyder EY. Segregation of human neural stem cells in the developing primate forebrain. *Science* 293:1820–1824, 2001.

Ourednik V, Ourednik J, Park KI, Snyder EY. Neural stem cells—a versatile tool for cell replacement and gene therapy in the central nervous system. *Clin Genet* 56:267–278, 1999.

Ouriel K. Detection of peripheral arterial disease in primary care. *JAMA* 286:1380–1381, 2001.

Ozaki S, Harada K, Sanzen T, Watanabe K, Tsui W, Nakanuma Y. In situ nucleic acid detection of human telomerase in intrahepatic cholangiocarcinoma and its preneoplastic lesion. *Hepatology* 30:914–919, 1999.

Ozen H, Hall MC. Bladder cancer. *Curr Opin Oncol* 12:255–259, 2000.

Ozen M, Imam SA, Datar RH, Multani AS, Narayanan R, Chung LW, von Eschenbach AC, Pathak S. Telomeric DNA: marker for human prostate cancer development? *Prostate* 36:264–271, 1998.

Ozen M, Pathak S. Genetic alterations in human prostate cancer: a review of current literature. *Anticancer Res* 20:1905–1912, 2000.

Ozonoff MB, Clemett AR. Progressive osteolysis in progeria. *AJR Am J Roentgenol* 100:75–79, 1967.

Paganini-Hill A, Henderson VW. Estrogen replacement therapy and risk of Alzheimer disease. *Arch Intern Med* 156:2213–2217, 1996.

Page K, Hollister R, Tanzi RE, Hyman BT. In situ hybridization analysis of presenilin 1 mRNA in Alzheimer disease and in lesioned rat brain. *Proc Natl Acad Sci USA* 93:14020–14024, 1996.

Palacios S, Cifuentes I, Menendez C, von Helde S. The central nervous system and HRT. *Int J Fertil Womens Med* 45:13–21, 2000.

Palli D. Epidemiology of gastric cancer: an evaluation of available evidence. *J Gastroenterol* 35(Suppl 12):84–89, 2000.

Pallotta R, Morgese G. Mandibuloacral dysplasia: a rare progeroid syndrome. *Clin Genet* 26:133–138, 1984.

Palmer LD, Weng N, Levine BL, June CH, Lane HC, Hodes RJ. Telomere length, telomerase activity, and replicative potential in HIV infection: analysis of CD4+ and CD8+ T cells from HIV-discordant monozygotic twins. *J Exp Med* 185:1381–1386, 1997.

Pandit B, Bhattacharyya NP. In vitro and in vivo inhibition of telomerase activity from Chinese hamster V79 cells. *Indian J Biochem Biophys* 38:42–47, 2001.

Pandita TK. The role of ATM in telomere structure and function. *Radiat Res* 156:642–647, 2001.

Pandita TK. ATM function and telomere stability. *Oncogene* 21:611–618, 2002.

Pandita TK, Benvenuto JA, Shay JW, Pandita RK, Rakovitch E, Geard CR, Antman KH, Newman RA. Effect of penclomedine (NSC-338720) on telomere fusions, chromatin blebbing, and cell viability with and without telomerase activity and abrogated p53 function. *Biochem Pharmacol* 53:409–415, 1997.

Pandita TK, Dhar S. Influence of ATM function on interactions between telomeres and nuclear matrix. *Radiat Res* 154:133–139, 2000.

Pandita TK, Hall EJ, Hei TK, Piatyszek MA, Wright WE, Piao CQ, Pandita RK, Willey JC, Geard CR, Kastan MB, Shay JW. Chromosome end-to-end associations and telomerase activity during cancer progression in human cells after treatment with alpha-particles simulating radon progeny. *Oncogene* 13:1423–1430, 1996.

Pandita TK, Pathak S, Geard CR. Chromosome end associations, telomeres and telomerase activity in ataxia telangiectasia cells. *Cytogenet Cell Genet* 71:86–93, 1995.

Pang JH, Good LF, Chen KY. The age-dependent binding of CBP/tk, a CCAAT binding protein, is deregulated in transformed and immortalized mammalian cells but absent in premature aging cells. *Exp Gerontol* 31:97–109, 1996.

Panossian LA, Porter VR, Valenzuela HF, Zhu X, Reback E, Masterman D, Cummings L, Effros RB. Telomere shortening in T cells correlates with Alzheimer's disease status. *Neurobiol Aging* 24:77–84, 2003.

Pao CC, Tseng CJ, Lin CY, Yang FP, Hor JJ, Yao DS, Hsueh S. Differential expression of telomerase activity in human cervical cancer and cervical intraepithelial neoplasia lesions. *J Clin Oncol* 15:1932–1937, 1997.

Pappolla M, Bozner P, Soto C, Shao H, Robakis NK, Zagorski M, Frangione B, Ghiso J. Inhibition of Alzheimer beta-fibrillogenesis by melatonin. *J Biol Chem* 273:7185–7188, 1998a.

Pappolla MA, Chyan YJ, Omar RA, Hsiao K, Perry G, Smith MA, Bozner P. Evidence of oxidative stress and in vivo neurotoxicity of beta-amyloid in a transgenic mouse model of Alzheimer's disease: a chronic oxidative paradigm for testing antioxidant therapies in vivo. *Am J Pathol* 152:871–877, 1998b.

Paradis S, Ailion M, Toker A, Thomas JH, Ruvkun G. A PDK1 homolog is necessary and sufficient to transduce AGE-1 PI3 kinase signals that regulate diapause in *Caenorhabditis elegans. Genes Dev* 13:1438–52, 1999.

Paradis S, Ruvkun G. *Caenorhabditis elegans* Akt/PKB transduces insulin receptor–like signals from AGE-1 PI3 kinase to the DAF-16 transcription factor. *Genes Dev* 12:2488–2498, 1998.

Pardue ML, Danilevskaya ON, Lowenhaupt K, Slot F, Traverse KL. Drosophila telomeres: new views on chromosome evolution. *Trends Genet* 12:48–52, 1996.

Pardue ML, DeBaryshe PG. Telomeres and telomerase: more than the end of the line. *Chromosoma* 108:73–82, 1999.

Parikh SA, Edelman ER. Endothelial cell delivery for cardiovascular therapy. *Adv Drug Deliv Rev* 42:139–161, 2000.

Paris F, Fuks Z, Kang A, Capodieci P, Juan G, Ehleiter D, Haimovitz-Friedman A, Cordon-Cardo C, Kolesnick R. Endothelial apoptosis as the primary lesion initiating intestinal radiation damage in mice. *Science* 293:293–297, 2001.

Park JK, Kim BH, Han YS, Park IK. The effect of telomerase expression on the escape from M2 crisis in virus-transformed human retinal pigment epithelial cells. *Exp Mol Med* 34:107–113, 2002a.

Park MJ, Jang YK, Choi ES, Kim HS, Park SD. Fission yeast Rap1 homolog is a telomere-specific silencing factor and interacts with Taz1p. *Mol Cells* 13:327–333, 2002b.

Park PU, Defossez PA, Guarente L. Effects of mutations in DNA repair genes on formation of ribosomal DNA circles and life span in *Saccharomyces cerevisiae. Mol Cell Biol* 19:3848–3856, 1999.

Park YM, Choi JY, Byun BH, Cho CH, Kim HS, Kim BS. Telomerase is strongly activated in hepatocellular carcinoma but not in chronic hepatitis and cirrhosis. *Exp Mol Med* 30:35–40, 1998.

Parkash H, Sidhu SS, Raghavan R, Deshmukh RN. Hutchinson-Gilford progeria: familial occurrence. *Am J Med Genet* 36:431–433, 1990.

Parker CR Jr. Dehydroepiandrosterone and dehydroepiandrosterone sulfate production in the human adrenal during development and aging. *Steroids* 64:640–647, 1999.

Parker CR Jr, Slayden SM, Azziz R, Crabbe SL, Hines GA, Boots LR, Bae S. Effects of aging on adrenal function in the human: responsiveness and sensitivity of adrenal androgens and cortisol to adrenocorticotropin in premenopausal and postmenopausal women. *J Clin Endocrinol Metab* 85:48–54, 2000.

Parkinson EK, Munro J, Steeghs K, Morrison V, Ireland H, Forsyth N, Fitzsimmons S, Bryce S. Replicative senescence as a barrier to human cancer. *Biochem Soc Trans* 28:226–233, 2000.

Parkinson EK, Newbold RF, Keith WN. The genetic basis of human keratinocyte immortalisation in squamous cell carcinoma development: the role of telomerase reactivation. *Eur J Cancer* 33:727–734, 1997.

Parkinson GN, Lee MP, Neidle S. Crystal structure of parallel quadruplexes from human telomeric DNA. *Nature* 417:876–880, 2002.

Parris CN, Jezzard S, Silver A, MacKie R, McGregor JM, Newbold RF. Telomerase activity in melanoma and non-melanoma skin cancer. *Br J Cancer* 79:47–53, 1999.

Parsch D, Brummendorf TH, Richter W, Fellenberg J. Replicative aging of human articular chondrocytes during ex vivo expansion. *Arthritis Rheum* 46:2911–2916, 2002.

Parseghian MH, Newcomb RL, Hamkalo BA. Distribution of somatic H1 subtypes is non-random on active vs. inactive chromatin II: distribution in human adult fibroblasts. *J Cell Biochem* 83:643–659, 2001.

Pashko LL, Fairman DK, Schwartz AG. Inhibition of proteinuria development in aging Sprague-Dawley rats and C57BL/6 mice by long-term treatment with dehydroepitandrosterone. *J Gerontol* 41:433–438, 1986.

Patel MM, Parekh LJ, Jha FP, Sainger RN, Patel JB, Patel DD, Shah PM, Patel PS. Clinical usefulness of telomerase activation and telomere length in head and neck cancer. *Head Neck* 24:1060–1067, 2002.

Patel VB, Robbins MA, Topol EJ. C-reactive protein: a 'golden marker' for inflammation and coronary artery disease. *Cleve Clin J Med* 68:521–524, 527–534, 2001.

Pathak S, Multani AS, Furlong CL, Sohn SH. Telomere dynamics, aneuploidy, stem cells, and cancer [review]. *Int J Oncol* 20:637–641, 2002.

Pathak S, Multani AS, McConkey DJ, Imam AS, Amoss MS Jr. Spontaneous regression of cutaneous melanoma in sinclair swine is associated with defective telomerase activity and extensive telomere erosion. *Int J Oncol* 17:1219–1224, 2000.

Pathak S, Multani AS, Ozen M, Richardson MA, Newman RA. Dolastatin-10 induces polyploidy, telomeric associations and apoptosis in a murine melanoma cell line. *Oncol Rep* 5:373–376, 1998.

Pavenstadt H. The charge for going by foot: modifying the surface of podocytes. *Exp Nephrol* 6:98–103, 1998.

Pavenstadt H. Roles of the podocyte in glomerular function. *Am J Physiol* (*Renal Physiol*) 278:F173–F179, 2000.

Pawelec G. Immunosenescence: impact in the young as well as the old? *Mech Ageing Dev* 108:1–7, 1999a.

Pawelec G. Importance of T-cell replicative senescence for the adoptive immunotherapy of cancer in humans? *J Anti-Aging Med* 2:115–120, 1999b.

Pawelec G. Tumour escape from the immune response: the last hurdle for successful immunotherapy of cancer? *Cancer Immunol Immunother* 48:343–345, 1999c.

Pawelec G, Adibzadeh M, Pohla H, Schaudt K. Immunosenescence: ageing of the immune system. *Immunol Today* 16:420–422, 1995.

Pawelec G, Adibzadeh M, Rehbein A, Hahnel K, Wagner W, Engel A. In vitro senescence models for human T lymphocytes. *Vaccine* 18:1666–1674, 2000a.

Pawelec G, Adibzadeh M, Solana R, Beckman I. The T cell in the ageing individual. *Mech Ageing Dev* 93:35–45, 1997a.

Pawelec G, Barnett Y, Forsey R, Frasca D, Globerson A, McLeod J, Caruso C, Franceschi C, Fulop T, Gupta S, Mariani E, Mocchegiani E, Solana R. T cells and aging, January 2002 update. *Front Biosci* 7:d1056–1183, 2002a.

Pawelec G, Barnett Y, Mariani E, Solana R. Human CD4+ T cell clone longevity in tissue culture: lack of influence of donor age or cell origin. *Exp Gerontol* 37:265–269, 2002b.

Pawelec G, Effros RB, Caruso C, Remarque E, Barnett Y, Solana R. T cells and aging (update February 1999). *Front Biosci* 4:D216–269, 1999a.

Pawelec G, Effros RB, Globerson A. A multidisciplinary approach to immunity and ageing: ImAginEering. *Mech Ageing Dev* 121:1–4, 2000b.

Pawelec G, Engel A, Adibzadeh M. Prerequisites for the immunotherapy of cancer. *Cancer Immunol Immunother* 48:214–217, 1999b.

Pawelec G, Muller R, Rehbein A, Hahnel K, Ziegler BL. Extrathymic T cell differentiation in vitro from human CD34+ stem cells. *J Leukoc Biol* 64:733–739, 1998a.

Pawelec G, Muller R, Rehbein A, Hahnel K, Ziegler BL. Finite life spans of T cell clones derived from CD34+ human haematopoietic stem cells in vitro. *Exp Gerontol* 34:69–77, 1999c.

Pawelec G, Rees RC, Kiessling R, Madrigal A, Dodi A, Baxevanis C, Gambacorti-Passerini C, Masucci G, Zeuthen J. Cells and cytokines in immunotherapy and gene therapy of cancer. *Crit Rev Oncog* 10:83–127, 1999d.

Pawelec G, Rehbein A, Haehnel K, Merl A, Adibzadeh M. Human T cell clones as a model for immunosenescence. *Immunol Rev* 160:31–43, 1997b.

Pawelec G, Remarque E, Barnett Y, Solana R. T cells and aging. *Front Biosci* 3:d59–99, 1998b.

Pawelec G, Sansom D, Rehbein A, Adibzadeh M, Beckman I. Decreased proliferative capacity and increased susceptibility to activation-induced cell death in late-passage human CD4+ TCR2+ cultured T cell clones. *Exp Gerontol* 31:655–668, 1996.

Pawelec G, Solana R. Immunosenescence. *Immunol Today* 18:514–516, 1997.

Pawelec G, Solana R, Remarque E, Mariani E. Impact of aging on innate immunity. *J Leukoc Biol* 64:703–712, 1998c.

Pawelec G, Wagner W, Adibzadeh M, Engel A. T cell immunosenescence in vitro and in vivo. *Exp Gerontol* 34:419–429, 1999e.

Peacocke M, Campisi J. Cellular senescence: a reflection of normal growth control, differentiation, or aging? *J Cell Biochem* 45:147–155, 1991.

Peacocke M, Yaar M, Gilchrest BA. Interferon and the epidermis: implications for cellular senescence. *Exp Gerontol* 24:415–421, 1989.

Pearce L, Brown WH. Hereditary premature senescence of the rabbit: I. Chronic form; general features. *J Exp Med* 111:485–503 (plates ff), 1960a.

Pearce L, Brown WH. Hereditary premature senescence of the rabbit: II. Acute form; general features. *J Exp Med* 111:505–515 (plates ff), 1960b.

Pearson AS, Chiao P, Zhang L, Zhang W, Larry L, Katz RL, Evans DB, Abbruzzese JL. The detection of telomerase activity in patients with adenocarcinoma of the pancreas by fine needle aspiration. *Int J Oncol* 17:381–385, 2000.

Pearson AS, Gollahon LS, O'Neal NC, Saboorian H, Shay JW, Fahey TJ 3rd. Detection of telomerase activity in breast masses by fine-needle aspiration. *Ann Surg Oncol* 5:186–193, 1998.

Pearson JD. Normal endothelial cell function. *Lupus* 9:183–188, 2000.

Pedersen NL. Genetics of human aging: Swedish twin studies. *Generations* 24:31–35, 2000.

Pedersen WA, Chan SL, Mattson MP. A mechanism for the neuroprotective effect of apolipoprotein E: isoform-specific modification by the lipid peroxidation product 4-hydroxynonenal. *J Neurochem* 74:1426–1433, 2000.

Pedersen WA, Culmsee C, Ziegler D, Herman JP, Mattson MP. Aberrant stress response associated with severe hypoglycemia in a transgenic mouse model of Alzheimer's disease. *J Mol Neurosci* 13:159–165, 1999.

Pegram MD, Konecny G, Slamon DJ. The molecular and cellular biology of HER2/neu gene amplification/overexpression and the clinical development of herceptin (Trastuzumab) therapy for breast cancer. *Cancer Treat Res* 103:57–75, 2000.

Peitl P, Mello SS, Camparoto ML, Passos GA, Hande MP, Cardoso RS, Sakamoto-Hojo ET. Chromosomal rearrangements involving telomeric DNA sequences in Balb/3T3 cells transfected with the Ha-*ras* oncogene. *Mutagenesis* 17:67–72, 2002.

Pendergrass WR, Gray M, Wold MS, Luo P, Norwood TH. Analysis of the capacity of extracts from normal human young and senescent fibroblasts to support DNA synthesis in vitro. *J Cell Biochem* 73:176–187, 1999a.

Pendergrass WR, Lane MA, Bodkin NL, Hansen BC, Ingram DK, Roth GS, Yi L, Bin H,Wolf NS. Cellular proliferation potential during aging and caloric restriction in rhesus monkeys (*Macaca mulatta*). *J Cell Physiol* 180:123–130, 1999b.

Pendergrass WR, Li Y, Jiang D, Fei RG, Wolf NS. Caloric restriction: conservation of cellular replicative capacity in vitro accompanies life-span extension in mice. *Exp Cell Res* 217:309–316, 1995.

Pendergrass WR, Li Y, Jiang D, Wolf NS. Decrease in cellular replicative potential in "giant" mice transfected with the bovine growth hormone gene correlates to shortened life span. *J Cell Physiol* 156:96–103, 1993.

Pendergrass WR, Penn PE, Li J, Wolf NS. Age-related telomere shortening occurs in lens epithelium from old rats and is slowed by caloric restriction. *Exp Eye Res* 73:221–228, 2001.

Pera M. Epidemiology of esophageal cancer, especially adenocarcinoma of the esophagus and esophagogastric junction. *Recent Results Cancer Res* 155:1–14, 2000.

Pereira-Smith OM. Molecular genetic approaches to the study of cellular aging. *Exp Gerontol* 27:441–445, 1992.

Pereira-Smith OM. Genetic theories on aging. *Aging (Milano)* 9:429–430, 1997.

Pereira-Smith OM, Fisher SF, Smith JR. Senescent and quiescent cell inhibitors of DNA synthesis. Membrane-associated proteins. *Exp Cell Res* 160:297–306, 1985.

Pereira-Smith OM, Ning Y. Molecular genetic studies of cellular senescence. *Exp Gerontol* 27:519–522, 1992.

Pereira-Smith OM, Robetorye S, Ning Y, Orson FM. Hybrids from fusion of normal human T lymphocytes with immortal human cells exhibit limited life span. *J Cell Physiol* 144:546–549, 1990a.

Pereira-Smith OM, Smith JR. Expression of SV40 T antigen in finite life-span hybrids of normal and SV40–transformed fibroblasts. *Somatic Cell Genet* 7:411–421, 1981.

Pereira-Smith OM, Smith JR. Phenotype of low proliferative potential is dominant in hybrids of normal human fibroblasts. *Somatic Cell Genet* 8:731–742, 1982.

Pereira-Smith OM, Smith JR. Evidence for the recessive nature of cellular immortality. *Science* 221:964–966, 1983.

Pereira-Smith OM, Smith JR. Functional simian virus 40 T antigen is expressed in hybrid cells having finite proliferative potential. *Mol Cell Biol* 7:1541–1544, 1987.

Pereira-Smith OM, Smith JR. Genetic analysis of indefinite division in human cells: identification of four complementation groups. *Proc Natl Acad Sci USA* 85:6042–6046, 1988.

Pereira-Smith OM, Stein GH, Robetorye S, Meyer-Demarest S. Immortal phenotype of the HeLa variant D98 is recessive in hybrids formed with normal human fibroblasts. *J Cell Physiol* 143:222–225, 1990b.

Perfect JR, Wong B, Chang YC, Kwon-Chung KJ, Williamson PR. *Cryptococcus neoformans*: virulence and host defences. *Med Mycol* 36(Suppl 1):79–86, 1998.

Perillo NL, Naeim F, Walford RL, Effros RB. In vitro cellular aging in T-lymphocyte cultures: analysis of DNA content and cell size. *Exp Cell Res* 207:131–135, 1993a.

Perillo NL, Naeim F, Walford RL, Effros RB. The in vitro senescence of human T lymphocytes: failure to divide is not associated with a loss of cytolytic activity or memory T cell phenotype. *Mech Ageing Dev* 67:173–185, 1993b.

Perls T, Kunkel LM, Puca AA. The genetics of exceptional human longevity. *J Am Geriatr Soc* 50:359–368, 2002.

Perls T, Shea-Drinkwater M, Bowen-Flynn J, Ridge SB, Kang S, Joyce E, Daly M, Brewster SJ, Kunkel L, Puca AA. Exceptional familial clustering for extreme longevity in humans. *J Am Geriatr Soc* 48:1483–1485, 2000.

Perrem K, Bryan TM, Englezou A, Hackl T, Moy EL, Reddel RR. Repression of an alternative mechanism for lengthening of telomeres in somatic cell hybrids. *Oncogene* 18:3383–3390, 1999.

Perrem K, Colgin LM, Neumann AA, Yeager TR, Reddel RR. Coexistence of alternative lengthening of telomeres and telomerase in hTERT-transfected GM847 cells. *Mol Cell Biol* 21:3862–3875, 2001.

Perrem K, Reddel RR. Telomeres and cell division potential. *Prog Mol Subcell Biol* 24:173–189, 2000.

Perricone N. *The Wrinkle Cure*. Rodale Books, Emmaus, PA, 2000.

Perrod S, Cockell MM, Laroche T, Renauld H, Ducrest AL, Bonnard C, Gasser SM. A cytosolic NAD-dependent deacetylase, Hst2p, can modulate nucleolar and telomeric silencing in yeast. *EMBO J* 20:197–209, 2001.

Perry D. Patients' voices: the powerful sound in the stem cell debate. *Science* 287:1423, 2000.

Perry G, Nunomura A, Hirai K, Takeda A, Aliev G, Smith MA. Oxidative damage in Alzheimer's disease: the metabolic dimension. *Int J Dev Neurosci* 18:417–421, 2000.

Perry HM 3rd. The endocrinology of aging. *Clin Chem* 45(8 Pt 2):1369–1376, 1999.

Perry PJ, Arnold JR, Jenkins TC. Telomerase inhibitors for the treatment of cancer: the current perspective. *Expert Opin Invest Drugs* 10:2141–2156, 2001.

Pershouse MA, Ligon AH, Pereira-Smith OM, Killary AM, Yung WK, Steck PA. Suppression of transformed phenotype and tumorigenicity after transfer of chromosome 4 into U251 human glioma cells. *Genes Chromosomes Cancer* 20:260–267, 1997.

Peterson SE, Stellwagen AE, Diede SJ, Singer MS, Haimberger ZW, Johnson CO, Tzoneva M, Gottschling DE. The function of a stem-loop in telomerase RNA is linked to the DNA repair protein Ku. *Nat Genet* 27:64–67, 2001.

Petitti DB. Hormone replacement therapy for prevention. *JAMA* 288:99–101, 2002.

Petricoin EF, Ardekani AM, Hitt BA, Levine PJ, Fusaro VA, Steinberg SM, Mills GB, Simone C, Fishman DA, Kohn EC, Liotta LA. Use of proteomic patterns in serum to identify ovarian cancer. *Lancet* 359:572–577, 2002.

Petronis A. Alzheimer's disease and down syndrome: from meiosis to dementia. *Exp Neurol* 158:403–413, 1999.

Petty TL. Screening strategies for early detection of lung cancer. *JAMA* 284:1987–1980, 2000.

Pfeifer C, Thomsen PD, Scherthan H. Centromere and telomere redistribution precedes homologue pairing and terminal synapsis initiation during prophase I of cattle spermatogenesis. *Cytogenet Cell Genet* 93:304–314, 2001.

Phan AT, Mergny JL. Human telomeric DNA: G-quadruplex, I-motif and Watson-Crick double helix. *Nucleic Acids Res* 30:4618–4625, 2002.

Phillips A, Janssen U, Floege J. Progression of diabetic nephropathy. Insights from cell culture studies and animal models. *Kidney Blood Press Res* 22:81–97, 1999.

Phillips PA, Rolls BJ, Ledingham JG, Forsling ML, Morton JJ, Crowe MJ, Wollner L. Reduced thirst after water deprivation in healthy elderly men. *N Engl J Med* 311:753–759, 1984.

Phillips PD, Doggett DL, Cristofalo VJ. Growth factors and cell aging. *Annu Rev Gerontol Geriatr* 10:43–52, 1990.

Piera-Velazquez S, Jimenez SA, Stokes D. Increased life span of human osteoarthritic chondrocytes by exogenous expression of telomerase. *Arthritis Rheum* 46:683–693, 2002.

Pierpaoli W, Bulian. The pineal gland and death program: 1. Grafting of old pineals in young mice accelerates their aging. *J Anti-Aging Med* 4:31–38, 2001.

Pierpaoli W, Bulian D, Arrighi S. Transferrin treatment corrects aging-related immunologic and hormonal decay in old mice. *Exp Gerontol* 35:401–408, 2000.

Pierpaoli W, Regelson W. *The Melatonin Miracle*. Simon and Schuster, New York, 1995.

Pietras RJ, Pegram MD, Finn RS, Maneval DA, Slamon DJ. Remission of human breast cancer xenografts on therapy with humanized monoclonal antibody to HER-2 receptor and DNA-reactive drugs. *Oncogene* 17:2235–2249, 1998.

Pignolo RJ, Cristofalo VJ, Rotenberg MO Senescent WI-38 cells fail to express EPC-1, a gene induced in young cells upon entry into the G0 state. *J Biol Chem* 268:8949–8957, 1993.

Pignolo RJ, Martin BG, Horton JH, Kalbach AN, Cristofalo VJ. The pathway of cell senescence: WI-38 cells arrest in late G1 and are unable to traverse the cell cycle from a true G0 state. *Exp Gerontol* 33:67–80, 1998a.

Pignolo RJ, Masoro EJ, Nichols WW, Bradt CI, Cristofalo VJ. Skin fibroblasts from aged Fischer 344 rats undergo similar changes in replicative life span but not immortalization with caloric restriction of donors. *Exp Cell Res* 201:16–22, 1992.

Pignolo RJ, Rotenberg MO, Cristofalo VJ. Alterations in contact and density-dependent arrest state in senescent WI-38 cells. *In Vitro Cell Dev Biol Anim* 30A:471–476, 1994.

Pignolo RJ, Rotenberg MO, Horton JH, Cristofalo VJ. Senescent WI-38 fibroblasts overexpress LPC-1, a putative transmembrane shock protein. *Exp Cell Res* 240:305–311, 1998b.

Pillai MR, Nair MK. Development of a condemned mucosa syndrome and pathogenesis of human papillomavirus-associated upper aerodigestive tract and uterine cervical tumors. *Exp Mol Pathol* 69:233–241, 2000.

Pincus G, Dorfman RI, Romanoff LP, Rubin BL, Bloch E, Carlo J, Freeman H. Steroid metabolism in aging men and women. *Recent Prog Hormone Res* 11:307–341, 1955.

Pinzani M, Gentilini P. Biology of hepatic stellate cells and their possible relevance in the pathogenesis of portal hypertension in cirrhosis. *Semin Liver Dis* 19:397–410, 1999.

Pinzani M, Marra F, Carloni V. Signal transduction in hepatic stellate cells. *Liver* 18:2–13, 1998.

Pisetsky DS, St. Clair EW. Progress in the treatment of rheumatoid arthritis. *JAMA* 286:2787–2790, 2001.

Pitchumoni SS, Doraiswamy PM. Current status of antioxidant therapy for Alzheimer's disease. *J Am Geriatr Soc* 46:1566–1572, 1998.

Pletcher SD, Khazaeli AA, Curtsinger JW. Why do life spans differ? Partitioning mean longevity differences in terms of age-specific mortality parameters. *J Gerontol A Biol Sci Med Sci* 55:B381–389, 2000.

Plunkett ER, Sawtelle WE, Hamblen EC. Report of a patient with typical progeria, including data from urinary hormone studies. *J Clin Endocrinol Metab* 14:735–741, 1954.

Pluta AF, Zakian VA. Recombination occurs during telomere formation in yeast. *Nature* 337:429–433, 1989.

Plutzky J. Peroxisome proliferator-activated receptors in endothelial cell biology. *Curr Opin Lipidol* 12:511–518, 2001.

Podesta M. Transplantation hematopoiesis. *Curr Opin Hematol* 8:331–336, 2001.

Poehlman ET, Turturro A, Bodkin N, Cefalu W, Heymsfield S, Holloszy J, Kemnitz J. Caloric restriction mimetics: physical activity and body composition changes. *J Gerontol A Biol Sci Med Sci* 56A:B45–54, 2001.

Poetsch M, Woenckhaus C, Dittberner T, Pambor M, Lorenz G, Herrmann FH. Significance of the small subtelomeric area of chromosome 1 (1p36.3) in the progression of malignant melanoma: FISH deletion screening with YAC DNA probes. *Virchows Arch* 435:105–111, 1999.

Pollack M, Leeuwenburgh C. Apoptosis and aging: role of mitochondria. *J Gerontol A Biol Sci Med Sci* 56:B475–482, 2001.

Polse KA, Brand R, MandellR, Vastine D, Demartini D, Flom R. Age differences in corneal hydration control. *Invest Ophthalmol Vis Sci* 30:392–399, 1989.

Pomerantz RJ. Initiating antiretroviral therapy during HIV infection: confusion and clarity. *JAMA* 286:2597–2599, 2001.

Pommier JP, Sabatier L. Telomere length distribution: digital image processing and statistical analysis. In Double JA, Thompson MJ (eds). *Telomeres and Telomerase: Methods and Perotocols.* Humana Press, Totowa, NJ, 2002, pp 33–64.

Poole JC, Andrews LG, Tollefsbol TO. Activity, function, and gene regulation of the catalytic subunit of telomerase (hTERT). *Gene* 269:1–12, 2001.

Poole-Wilson PA. Treatment of acute heart failure: out with the old,in with the new. *JAMA* 287:1578–1580, 2002.

Poon SS, Lansdorp PM. Measurements of telomere length on individual chromosomes by image cytometry. Methods Cell Biol 64:69–96, 2001.

Porter MB, Pereira-Smith OM, Smith JR. Novel monoclonal antibodies identify antigenic determinants unique to cellular senescence. *J Cell Physiol* 142:425–433, 1990.

Porter MB, Pereira-Smith OM, Smith JR. Common senescent cell-specific antibody epitopes on fibronectin in species and cells of varied origin. *J Cell Physiol* 150:545–551, 1992.

Porter R. *The Greatest Benefit: A Medical History of Humanity.* W.W. Norton & Company, New York, 1997.

Porter RK, Joyce OJ, Farmer MK, Heneghan R, Tipton KF, Andrews JF, McBennett SM, Lund MD, Jensen CH, Melia HP. Indirect measurement of mitochondrial proton leak and its application. *Int J Obes Relat Metab Disord* 23(Suppl 6):S12–18, 1999.

Porter VR, Greendale GA, Schocken M, Zhu X, Effros RB. Immune effects of hormone replacement therapy in post-menopausal women. *Exp Gerontol* 36:311–326, 2001.

Post SG. Future scenarios for the prevention and delay of Alzheimer disease onset in high-risk groups. An ethical perspective. *Am J Prev Med* 16:105–110, 1999.

Post WS, Goldschmidt-Clermont PJ, Wilhide CC, Heldman AW, Sussman MS, Ouyang P, Milliken EE, Issa JP. Methylation of the estrogen receptor gene is associated with aging and atherosclerosis in the cardiovascular system. *Cardiovasc Res* 43:985–991, 1999.

Poston RS, Tran KP, Mann MJ, Hoyt EG, Dzau VJ, Robbins RC. Prevention of ischemically induced neointimal hyperplasia using ex vivo antisense oligodeoxynucleotides. *J Heart Lung Transplant* 17:349–355, 1998.

Potestio M, Pawelec G, Di Lorenzo G, Candore G, D'Anna C, Gervasi F, Lio D, Tranchida G, Caruso C, Romano GC. Age-related changes in the expression of CD95 (APO1/FAS) on blood lymphocytes. *Exp Gerontol* 34:659–673, 1999.

Potten CS. Regeneration in epithelial proliferative units as exemplified by small intestinal crypts. *Ciba Found Symp* 160:54–71; discussion 71–76, 1991.

Potten CS. Stem cells in gastrointestinal epithelium: numbers, characteristics and death. *Philos Trans R Soc Lond B Biol Sci* 353:821–830, 1998.

Potten CS, Booth C. The role of radiation-induced and spontaneous apoptosis in the homeostasis of the gastrointestinal epithelium: a brief review. *Comp Biochem Physiol B Biochem Mol Biol* 118:473–478, 1997.

Potten CS, Booth C, Pritchard DM. The intestinal epithelial stem cell: the mucosal governor. *Int J Exp Pathol* 78:219–243, 1997a.

Potten CS, Loeffler M. Stem cells: attributes, cycles, spirals, pitfalls and uncertainties. Lessons for and from the crypt. *Development* 110:1001–1020, 1990.

Potten CS, Wilson JW, Booth C. Regulation and significance of apoptosis in the stem cells of the gastrointestinal epithelium. *Stem Cells* 15:82–93, 1997b.

Pradhan AD, Manson JE, Rossouw JE, Siscovick DS, Mouton CP, Rifai N, Wallace RB, Jackson RD, Pettinger MB, Ridker PM. Inflammatory biomarkers, hormone replacement therapy, and incident coronary heart disease. *JAMA* 288:980–987, 2003.

Prather RS. Pigs is pigs. *Science* 289:1886–1887, 2000.

Pratt RE, Dzau VJ. Genomics and hypertension: concepts, potentials, and opportunities. *Hypertension* 33:238–247, 1999.

Pratt S. Dietary prevention of age-related macular degeneration. *J Am Optom Assoc* 70:39–47, 1999.

Preisler HD, Li B, Yang BL, Huang RW, Devemy E, Venugopal P, Tao M, Chopra H, Gregory SA, Adler S, Sivaraman S, Toofanfard P, Jajeh A, Galvez A, Robin E. Suppression of telomerase activity and cytokine messenger RNA levels in acute myelogenous leukemia cells in vivo in patients by amifostine and interleukin 4. *Clin Cancer Res* 6:807–812, 2000.

Prescott JC, Blackburn EH. Telomerase: Dr. Jekyll or Mr. Hyde? *Curr Opin Genet Dev* 9:368–373, 1999.

Prescott JC, Blackburn EH. Telomerase RNA template mutations reveal sequence-specific requirements for the activation and repression of telomerase action at telomeres. *Mol Cell Biol* 20:2941–2948, 2000.

Pretzlaff R, Arking R. Patterns of amino acid incorporation in long-lived genetic strains of *Drosophila melanogaster*. *Exp Gerontol* 24:67–81, 1989.

Price CM. Telomeres and telomerase: broad effects on cell growth. *Curr Opin Genet Dev* 9:218–224, 1999.

Price CM, Skopp R, Krueger J, Williams D. DNA recognition and binding by the Euplotes telomere protein. *Biochemistry* 31:10835–10843, 1992.

Price DL, Tanzi RE, Borchelt DR, Sisodia SS. Alzheimer's disease: genetic studies and transgenic models. *Annu Rev Genet* 32:461–43, 1998.

Price JL, Ko AI, Wade MJ, Tsou SK, McKeel DW, Morris JC. Neuron number in the entorhinal cortex and CA1 in preclinical Alzheimer disease. *Arch Neurol* 58:1395–1402, 2001.

Prince LS, Launspach JL, Geller DS, Lifton RP, Pratt JH, Zabner J, Welsh MJ. Absence of amiloride-sensitive sodium absorption in the airway of an infant with pseudohypoaldosteronism. *J Pediatr* 135:786–789, 1999.

Pritchard DE, Ceryak S, Ha L, Fornsaglio JL, Hartman SK, O'Brien TJ, Patierno SR. Mechanism of apoptosis and determination of cellular fate in chromium(VI)-exposed populations of telomerase-immortalized human fibroblasts. *Cell Growth Differ* 12:487–496, 2001.

Proctor CJ, Kirkwood TB. Modelling telomere shortening and the role of oxidative stress. *Mech Ageing Dev* 123:351–363, 2002.

Proctor DN, Balagopal P, Nair KS. Age-related sarcopenia in humans is associated with reduced synthetic rates of specific muscle proteins. *J Nutr* 128:351S–355S, 1998.

Prokofeva VV, Pleskach NM, Bozhkov VM, Demin VG, Liashko VN Cellular DNA repair, proliferative activity and biochemical characteristics in the human premature aging syndrome [in Russian]. *Tsitologiia* 24:592–603, 1982.

Prothero J, Gallant JA. A model of clonal attenuation. *Proc Natl Acad Sci USA* 78:333–337, 1981.

Prowse KR. Detection of telomerase activity in neural cells. *Methods Mol Biol* 198:137–147, 2002.

Prowse KR, Avilion AA, Greider CW. Identification of a nonprocessive telomerase activity from mouse cells. *Proc Natl Acad Sci USA* 90:1493–1497, 1993.

Prowse KR, Greider CW. Developmental and tissue-specific regulation of mouse telomerase and telomere length. *Proc Natl Acad Sci USA* 92:4818–4822, 1995.

Pryde FE, Gorham HC, Louis EJ. Chromosome ends: all the same under their caps. *Curr Opin Genet Dev* 7:822–828, 1997.

Pryde FE, Louis EJ. *Saccharomyces cerevisiae* telomeres. A review. *Biochemistry (Mosc)* 62:1232–1241, 1997.

Psaty BM, Smith NL, Lemaitre RN, Vos HL, Heckbert SR, LaCroix AZ, Rosendaal FR. Hormone replacement therapy, prothrombotic mutations, and the risk of incident nonfatal myocardial infarction in postmenopausal women. *JAMA* 285:906–913, 2001.

Puddu P, Puddu GM, Muscari A. HMG-CoA reductase inhibitors: is the endothelium the main target? *Cardiology* 95:9–13, 2001.

Puddu P, Puddu GM, Zaca F, Muscari A. Endothelial dysfunction in hypertension. *Acta Cardiol* 55:221–232, 2000.

Pugh TD, Klopp RG, Weindruch R. Controlling caloric consumption: protocols for rodents and rhesus monkeys. *Neurobiol Aging* 20:157–165, 1999a.

Pugh TD, Oberley TD, Weindruch R. Dietary intervention at middle age: caloric restriction but not dehydroepiandrosterone sulfate increases lifespan and lifetime cancer incidence in mice. *Cancer Res* 59:1642–1648, 1999b.

Putnam CT, Sultan KR, Wassmer T, Bamford JA, Skorjanc D, Pette D. Fiber-type transitions and satellite cell activation in low-frequency-stimulated muscles of young and aging rats. *J Gerontol A Biol Sci Med Sci* 56:B510–519, 2001.

Qiu WQ, Walsh DM, Ye Z, Vekrellis K, Zhang J, Podlisny MB, Rosner MR, Safavi A, Hersh LB, Selkoe DJ. Insulin-degrading enzyme regulates extracellular levels of amyloid beta-protein by degradation. *J Biol Chem* 273:32730–32738, 1998.

Qu Y, Liu SQ, Peng WZ, Liu BL. Inhibition of telomerase activity by ribozyme targeted to human telomerase transcriptase [in Chinese]. *Sheng Wu Hua Xue Yu Sheng Wu Wu Li Xue Bao (Shanghai)* 34:323–328, 2002.

Quaini F, Urbanek K, Beltrami AP, Finato N, Beltrami CA, Nadal-Ginard B, Kajstura J, Leri A, Anversa P. Chimerism of the transplanted heart. *N Engl J Med* 346:5–15, 2002.

Rabchevsky AG, Streit WJ. Grafting of cultured microglial cells into the lesioned spinal cord of adult rats enhances neurite outgrowth. *J Neurosci Res* 47:34–48, 1997.

Radak Z, Taylor AW, Sasvari M, Ohno H, Horkay B, Furesz J, Gaal D, Kanel T. Telomerase activity is not altered by regular strenuous exercise in skeletal muscle or by sarcoma in liver of rats. *Redox Rep* 6:99–103, 2001.

Rader DJ, Dugi KA. The endothelium and lipoproteins: insights from recent cell biology and animal studies. *Semin Thromb Hemost* 26:521–528, 2000.

Radig K, Schneider-Stock R, Mittler U, Neumann HW, Roessner A. Genetic instability in osteoblastic tumors of the skeletal system. *Pathol Res Pract* 194:669–677, 1998.

Rafalowska J. Genetically determined vascular diseases. *Folia Neuropathol* 37:210–216, 1999.

Raff H, Raff JL, Duthie EH, Wilson CR, Sasse EA, Rudman I, Mattson D. Elevated salivary cortisol in the evening in healthy elderly men and women: correlation with bone mineral density. *J Gerontol A Biol Sci Med Sci* 54:M479–483, 1999.

Raina AK, Pardo P, Rottkamp CA, Zhu X, Pereira-Smith OM, Smith MA. Neurons in Alzheimer disease emerge from senescence. *Mech Ageing Dev* 123:3–9, 2001.

Raina AK, Zhu X, Monteiro M, Takeda A, Smith MA. Abortive oncogeny and cell cycle–mediated events in Alzheimer disease. *Prog Cell Cycle Res* 4:235–242, 2000a.

Raina AK, Zhu X, Rottkamp CA, Monteiro M, Takeda A, Smith MA. Cyclin' toward dementia: cell cycle abnormalities and abortive oncogenesis in Alzheimer disease. *J Neurosci Res* 61:1281–1233, 2000b.

Rainfray M, Richard-Harston S, Salles-Montaudon N, Emeriau JP. Effects of aging on kidney function and implications for medical practice [in French]. *Presse Med* 29:1373–1378, 2000.

Raitakari OT, Celermajer DS. Testing for endothelial dysfunction. *Ann Med* 32:293–304, 2000.

Raman SV, Cooke GE, Binkley PF. Evidence that human cardiac myocytes divide after myocardial infarction. *N Engl J Med* 345:1130–1131, 2001.

Rambhatla L, Chiu CP, Glickman RD, Rowe-Rendleman C. In vitro differentiation capacity of telomerase immortalized human RPE cells. *Invest Ophthalmol Vis Sci* 43:1622–1630, 2002.

Ramirez RD, D'Atri S, Pagani E, Faraggiana T, Lacal PM, Taylor RS, Shay JW. Progressive increase in telomerase activity from benign melanocytic conditions to malignant melanoma. *Neoplasia* 1:42–49, 1999.

Ramirez RD, Morales CP, Herbert BS, Rohde JM, Passons C, Shay JW, Wright WE. Putative telomere-independent mechanisms of replicative aging reflect inadequate growth conditions. *Genes Dev* 15:398–403, 2001.

Ramirez RD, Wright WE, Shay JW, Taylor RS. Telomerase activity concentrates in the mitotically active segments of human hair follicles. *J Invest Dermatol* 108:113–117, 1997.

Ramos-Estebanez C, Rebollo Alvarez-Amandi MR. Binswanger disease: a common type of vascular dementia [in Spanish]. *Rev Neurol* 31:53–58, 2000.

Ramsey JJ, Colman RJ, Swick AG, Kemnitz JW. Energy expenditure, body composition, and glucose metabolism in lean and obese rhesus monkeys treated with ephedrine and caffeine. *Am J Clin Nutr* 68:42–51, 1998.

Ramsey JJ, Roecker EB, Weindruch R, Kemnitz JW. Energy expenditure of adult male rhesus monkeys during the first 30 mo of dietary restriction. *Am J Physiol* 272:E901–907, 1997.

Ramsey MJ, Moore DH 2nd, Briner JF, Lee DA, Olsen La, Senft JR, Tucker JD. The effects of age and lifestyle factors on the accumulation of cytogenetic damage as measured by chromosome painting. *Mutat Res* 338:95–106, 1995.

Ran Q, Pereira-Smith OM. Genetic approaches to the study of replicative senescence. *Exp Gerontol* 35:7–13, 2000.

Ran Q, Wadhwa R, Bischof O, Venable S, Smith JR, Pereira-Smith OM. Characterization of a novel zinc finger gene with increased expression in nondividing normal human cells. *Exp Cell Res* 263:156–162, 2001.

Ranganathan V, Heine WF, Ciccone DN, Rudolph KL, Wu X, Chang S, Hai H, Ahearn IM, Livingston DM, Resnick I, Rosen F, Seemanova E, Jarolim P, DePinho RA, Weaver DT. Rescue of a telomere length defect of Nijmegen breakage syndrome cells requires NBS and telomerase catalytic subunit. *Curr Biol* 11:962–966, 2001.

Ranganathan VK, Siemionow V, Sahgal V, Yue GH. Effects of aging on hand function. *J Am Geriatr Soc* 49:1478–1484, 2001.

Rao RN. Targets for cancer therapy in the cell cycle pathway. *Curr Opin Oncol* 8:516–524, 1996.

Rapoport SI. In vivo PET imaging and postmortem studies suggest potentially reversible and irreversible stages of brain metabolic failure in Alzheimer's disease. *Eur Arch Psychiatry Clin Neurosci* 249:46–55, 1999.

Rapp L, Chen JJ. The papillomavirus E6 proteins. *Biochim Biophys Acta* 1378:F1–19, 1998.

Rattan SIS. Repeated mild heat shock delays ageing in cultured human skin fibroblasts. *Biochem Mol Biol Int* 45:753–759, 1998a.

Rattan SIS. The nature of gerontogenes and vitagenes: antiaging effects of repeated heat shock on human fibroblasts. *Ann NY Acad Sci* 854:54–60, 1998b.

Rattan SIS. Ageing, gerontogenes, and hormesis. *Indian J Exp Biol* 38:1–5, 2000a.

Rattan SIS. Biogerontology: the next step. *Mol Cell Gerontol* 908:282–290, 2000b.

Rattan SIS. Applying hormesis in aging research and therapy. *Belle Newsletter* 9:2–5, 2001.

Rattan SIS, Clark BFC. Protein synthesis, post-translational modifications and aging. *Mol Biol Aging* 44:316–327, 1999.

Ravaglia G, Forti P, Maioli F, Nesi B, Pratelli L, Cucinotta D, Bastagli L, Cavalli G. Body composition, sex steroids, IGF-1, and bone mineral status in aging men. *J Gerontol A Biol Sci Med Sci* 55:M516–521, 2000.

Ravin NV, Strakhova TS, Kuprianov VV. The protelomerase of the phage-plasmid N15 is responsible for its maintenance in linear form. *J Mol Biol* 312:899–906, 2001.

Rawes V, Kipling D, Kill IR, Faragher RGA. The kinetics of senescence in retinal pigmented epithelial cells: a test for the telomere hypothesis of aging? *Biochemistry* (*Mosc*) 62:1291–1295, 1997.

Ray S, Karamysheva Z, Wang L, Shippen DE, Price CM. Interactions between telomerase and primase physically link the telomere and chromosome replication machinery. *Mol Cell Biol* 22:5859–5868, 2002.

Raymond E, Soria JC, Izbicka E, Boussin F, Hurley L, Von Hoff DD. DNA G-quadruplexes, telomerase-specific proteins and telomere-associated enzymes as potential targets for new anticancer drugs. *Invest New Drugs* 18:123–137, 2000.

Raymond E, Sun D, Izbicka E, Mangold G, Silvas E, Windle B, Sharma S, Soda H, Laurence R, Davidson K, Von Hoff DD. A human breast cancer model for the study of telomerase inhibitors based on a new biotinylated-primer extension assay. *Br J Cancer* 80:1332–1341, 1999.

Raza A. Consilience across evolving dysplasias affecting myeloid, cervical, esophageal, gastric and liver cells: common themes and emerging patterns. *Leuk Res* 24:63–72, 2000.

Re MC, Monari P, Gibellini D, Ciancianaini P, Dall'Aglio PP, Vignoli M, Furlini G, Ramazzotti E, Bertazzoni U, Casoli C. Human T cell leukemia virus type II increases telomerase activity in uninfected CD34+ hematopoietic progenitor cells. *J Hematother Stem Cell Res* 9:481–487, 2000.

Rea MA, Rice RH. Telomerase deregulation in immortalized human epidermal cells: modulation by cellular microenvironment. *Int J Cancer* 94:669–673, 2001.

Read M, Harrison RJ, Romagnoli B, Tanious FA, Gowan SH, Reszka AP, Wilson WD, Kelland LR, Neidle S. Structure-based design of selective and potent G quadruplex-mediated telomerase inhibitors. *Proc Natl Acad Sci USA* 98:4844–4849, 2001.

Read MA, Neidle S. Structural characterization of a guanine-quadruplex ligand complex. *Biochemistry* 39:13422–13432, 2000.

Reddel RR. A reassessment of the telomere hypothesis of senescence. *Bioessays* 20:977–984, 1998a.

Reddel RR. Genes involved in the control of cellular proliferative potential. *Ann NY Acad Sci* 854:8–19, 1998b.

Reddel RR. The role of senescence and immortalization in carcinogenesis. *Carcinogenesis* 21:477–484, 2000.

Reddel RR. An alternative lifestyle for immortalized oral keratinocytes. *J Clin Invest* 108:665–667, 2001.

Reddel RR, Bryan TM, Colgin LM, Perrem KT, Yeager TR. Alternative lengthening of telomeres in human cells. *Radiat Res* 155:194–200, 2001.

Reddel RR, Bryan TM, Murnane JP. Immortalized cells with no detectable telomerase activity. A review. *Biochemistry (Mosc)* 62:1254–1262, 1997.

Reddy VG, Khanna N, Jain SK, Das BC, Singh N. Telomerase-A molecular marker for cervical cancer screening. *Int J Gynecol Cancer* 11:100–106, 2001.

Reed MJ, Penn PE, Li Y, Birnbaum R, Vernon RB, Johnson TS, Pendergrass WR, Sage EH, Abrass IB, Wolf NS. Enhanced cell proliferation and biosynthesis mediate improved wound repair in refed, caloric-restricted mice. *Mech Ageing Dev* 89:21–43, 1996.

Reesink-Peters N, Helder MN, Wisman GB, Knol AJ, Koopmans S, Boezen HM, Schuuring E, Hollema H, De Vries EG, De Jong S, Van Der Zee AG. Detection of telomerase, its components, and human papillomavirus in cervical scrapings as a tool for triage in women with cervical dysplasia. *J Clin Pathol* 56:31–35, 2003.

Regan JD, Setlow RB. DNA repair in progeroid cells. *Biochem Biophys Res Commun* 59:858–864, 1974.

Reichel W, Garcia-Bunuel R, Dilallo J. Progeria and Werner's syndrome as models for the study of normal human aging. *J Am Geriatr Soc* 19:369–375, 1971.

Reid IR, Brown JP, Burckhardt P, Horowitz Z, Richardson P, Trechsel U, Widmer A, Devogelaer JP, Kaufman JM, Jaeger P, Body JJ, Brandi ML, Broell J, Di Micco R, Genazzani AR, Felsenberg D, Happ J, Hooper MJ, Ittner J, Leb G, Mallmin H, Murray T, Ortolani S, Rubinacci A, Saaf M, Samsioe G, Verbruggen L, Meunier PJ. Intravenous zoledronic acid in postmenopausal women with low bone mineral density. *N Engl J Med* 346:653–661, 2002.

Reiter RJ, Tan D, Kim SJ, Cabrera J, D'Arpa D. A perspective on the proposed association of melatonin and aging. *J Anti-Aging Med* 1:229–237, 1998.

Reiter RJ, Tan D, Kim SJ, Manchester LC, Qi W, Garcia JJ, Cabrera JC, El-Sokkary G, Rouvier-Garay V. Augmentation of indices of oxidative damage in life-long melatonin-deficient rats. *Mech Ageing Dev* 110:157–173, 1999.

Rejeski WJ, Mihalko SL. Physical activity and quality of life in older adults. *J Gerontol A Biol Sci Med Sci* 56:B23–35, 2001.

Remarque EJ. Influenza vaccination in elderly people. *Exp Gerontol* 34:445–452, 1999.

Remes K, Norrback KF, Rosenquist R, Mehle C, Lindh J, Roos G. Telomere length and telomerase activity in malignant lymphomas at diagnosis and relapse. *Br J Cancer* 82:601–607, 2000.

Ren J, Qu X, Trent JO, Chaires JB. Tiny telomere DNA. *Nucleic Acids Res* 30:2307–2315, 2002.

Ren JG, Xia HL, Tian YM, Just T, Cai GP, Dai YR. Expression of telomerase inhibits hydroxyl radical-induced apoptosis in normal telomerase negative human lung fibroblasts. *FEBS Lett* 488:133–138, 2001.

Renauld H, Aparicio OM, Zierath PD, Billington BL, Chhablani SK, Gottschling DE. Silent domains are assembled continuously from the telomere and are defined by promoter distance and strength, and by SIR3 dosage. *Genes Dev* 7:1133–1145, 1993.

Renault V, Thornell LE, Butler-Browne G, Mouly V. Human skeletal muscle satellite cells: aging, oxidative stress and the mitotic clock. *Exp Gerontol* 37:1229–1236, 2002.

Rensing L, Meyer-Grahle U, Ruoff P. Biological timing and the clock metaphor: oscillatory and hourglass mechanisms. *Chronobiol Int* 18:329–369, 2001.

Renvoize EB, Awad IO, Hambling MH. A sero-epidemiological study of conventional infectious agents in Alzheimer's disease. *Age Ageing* 16:311–314, 1987.

Resnick SM, Henderson VW. Hormone therapy and risk of Alzheimer disease. *JAMA* 288:2170–2172, 2002.

Resnick SM, Maki PM, Golski S, Kraut MA, Zonderman AB. Effects of estrogen replacement therapy on PET cerebral blood flow and neuropsychological performance. *Horm Behav* 34:171–182, 1998.

Resnick SM, Metter EJ, Zonderman AB Estrogen replacement therapy and longitudinal decline in visual memory. A possible protective effect? *Neurology* 49:1491–1497, 1997.

Revskoy S, Redei E. Decreased in vitro sensitivity to dexamethasone in corticotropes from middle-age rats. *Exp Gerontol* 35:237–242, 2000.

Rexrode KM, Manson JE. Postmenopausal hormone therapy and the quality of life: no cause for celebration. *JAMA* 287:641–642, 2002.

Rezaie P, Male D. Colonisation of the developing human brain and spinal cord by microglia: a review. *Microsc Res Tech* 45:359–382, 1999.

Rezler EM, Bearss DJ, Hurley LH. Telomeres and telomerases as drug targets. *Curr Opin Pharmacol* 2:415–423, 2002.

Rha SY, Izbicka E, Lawrence R, Davidson K, Sun D, Moyer MP, Roodman GD, Hurley L, Von Hoff D. Effect of telomere and telomerase interactive agents on human tumor and normal cell lines. *Clin Cancer Res* 6:987–993, 2000.

Rheinwald JG, Hahn WC, Ramsey MR, Wu JY, Guo Z, Tsao H, De Luca M, Catricala C, O'Toole KM. A two-stage, p16(INK4A)- and p53-dependent keratinocyte senescence mechanism that limits replicative potential independent of telomere status. *Mol Cell Biol* 22:5157–5172, 2002.

Rhodes D, Fairall L, Simonsson T, Court R, Chapman L. Telomere architecture. *EMBO Rep* 3:1139–1145, 2002.

Rich JN, Guo C, McLendon RE, Bigner DD, Wang XF, Counter CM. A genetically tractable model of human glioma formation. *Cancer Res* 61:3556–3560, 2001.

Richards EJ, Ausubel FM. Isolation of a higher eukaryotic telomere from *Arabidopsis thaliana*. *Cell* 53:127–136, 1988.

Richardson MW, Sverstiuk A, Hendel H, Cheung TW, Zagury JF, Rappaport J. Analysis of telomere length and thymic output in fast and slow/non-progressors with HIV infection. *Biomed Pharmacother* 54:21–31, 2000.

Richter C. Do mitochondrial DNA fragments promote cancer and ageing? *FEBS Lett* 241:1–5, 1988.

Richter C. Reactive oxygen and DNA damage in mitochondria. *Mutat Res* 275:249–255, 1992.

Richter C. Mitochondrial DNA oxidation. *J Anti-Aging Med* 2:217–225, 1999.

Rico H, Revilla M, Villa LF, Alvarez de Buergo M. Age-related differences in total and regional bone mass: a cross-sectional study with DXA in 429 normal women. *Osteoporos Int* 3:154–159, 1993.

Rideout WM 3rd, Eggan K, Jaenisch R. Nuclear cloning and epigenetic reprogramming of the genome. *Science* 293:1093–1098, 2001.

Rideout WM 3rd, Wakayama T, Wutz A, Eggan K, Jackson-Grusby L, Dausman J, Yanagimachi R, Jaenisch R. Generation of mice from wild-type and targeted ES cells by nuclear cloning. *Nat Genet* 24:109–110, 2000.

Ridker PM, Stampfer MJ, Rifai N. Novel risk factors for systemic atherosclerosis: a comparison of C-reactive protein, fibrinogen, homocysteine, lipoprotein(a), and standard cholesterol screening as predictors of peripheral arterial disease. *JAMA* 285:2481–2485, 2001.

Riedel H. Morphologic contribution to a progeria syndrome (Hutchinson-Gilford) [in German]. *Zentralbl Allg Pathol* 124:410–415, 1980.

Riemenschneider M, Lautenschlager N, Wagenpfeil S, Diehl J, Drzezga A, Kurz A. Cerebrospinal fluid tau and β-amyloid 42 proteins identify Alzheimer disease in subjects with mild cognitive impairment. *Arch Neurol* 59:1729–1734, 2002.

Riha K, McKnight TD, Griffing LR, Shippen DE. Living with genome instability: plant responses to telomere dysfunction. *Science* 291:1979–1800, 2001.

Riha K, Watson JM, Parkey J, Shippen DE. Telomere length deregulation and enhanced sensitivity to genotoxic stress in Arabidopsis mutants deficient in Ku70. *EMBO J* 21:2819–2826, 2002.

Rio M, Molinari F, Heuertz S, Ozilou C, Gosset P, Raoul O, Cormier-Daire V, Amiel J, Lyonnet S, Le Merrer M, Turleau C, de Blois MC, Prieur M, Romana S, Vekemans M, Munnich A, Colleaux L. Automated fluorescent genotyping detects 10% of cryptic subtelomeric rearrangements in idiopathic syndromic mental retardation. *J Med Genet* 39:266–270, 2002.

Riou JF, Guittat L, Mailliet P, Laoui A, Renou E, Petitgenet O, Megnin-Chanet F, Helene C, Mergny JL. Cell senescence and telomere shortening induced by a new series of specific G-quadruplex DNA ligands. *Proc Natl Acad Sci USA* 99:2672–2677, 2002.

Ripple MO, Henry WF, Schwarze SR, Wilding G, Weindruch R. Effect of antioxidants on androgen-induced AP-1 and NF-kappaB DNA-binding activity in prostate carcinoma cells. *J Natl Cancer Inst* 91:1227–1232, 1999.

Rippmann JF, Damm K, Schnapp A. Functional characterization of the poly(ADP-ribose) polymerase activity of tankyrase 1, a potential regulator of telomere length. *J Mol Biol* 323:217–224, 2002.

Rizki A, Lundblad V. Defects in mismatch repair promote telomerase-independent proliferation. *Nature* 411:713–716, 2001.

Robbins SL. *Pathologic Basis of Disease*. W.B. Saunders, Philadelphia, 1974.

Robert AM, Schaeverbeke M, Schaeverbeke J, Robert L. Aging and brain circulation. Role of the extracellular matrix of brain microvessels [in French]. *C R Seances Soc Biol Fil* 191:253–260, 1997.

Robert L, Robert AM, Jacotot B. Elastin-elastase-atherosclerosis revisited. *Atherosclerosis* 140:281–295, 1998.

Roberts SB, Pi-Sunyer X, Kuller L, Lane MA, Ellison P, Prior JC, Shapses S. Physiologic effects of lowering caloric intake in nonhuman primates and nonobese humans. *J Gerontol A Biol Sci Med Sci* 56A:B66–75, 2001.

Robertson JD, Gale RE, Wynn RF, Dougal M, Linch DC, Testa NG, Chopra R. Dynamics of telomere shortening in neutrophils and T lymphocytes during ageing and the relationship to skewed X chromosome inactivation patterns. *Br J Haematol* 109:272–279, 2000.

Robertson JD, Testa NG, Russell NH, Jackson G, Parker AN, Milligan DW, Stainer C, Chakrabarti S, Dougal M, Chopra R. Accelerated telomere shortening following allogeneic transplantation is independent of the cell source and occurs within the first year post transplant. *Bone Marrow Transplant* 27:1283–1286, 2001.

Robinson MO. Telomerase and cancer. *Genet Eng (NY)* 22:209–222, 2000.

Robinzon B, Cutolo M. Should dehydroepiandrosterone replacement therapy be provided with glucocorticoids? *Rheumatology (Oxford)* 38:488–495, 1999.

Rockwood K, Mintzer J, Truyen L, Wessel T, Wilkinson D. Effects of a flexible galantamine dose in Alzheimer's disease: a randomized, controlled trial. *J Neurol Neurosurg Psychiatry* 71:589–595, 2001.

Rodan GA, Martin TJ. Therapeutic approaches to bone disease. *Science* 289:1508–1514, 2000.

Rodriguez C, Patel AV, Calle EE, Jacob EJ, Thun MJ. Estrogen replacement therapy and ovarian cancer mortality in a large prospective study of US women. *JAMA* 285:1460–1465, 2001.

Rodriguez JI, Perez-Alonso P, Funes R, Perez-Rodriguez J. Lethal neonatal Hutchinson-Gilford progeria syndrome. *Am J Med Genet* 82:242–248, 1999.

Roecker EB, Kemnitz JW, Ershler WB, Weindruch R. Reduced immune responses in rhesus monkeys subjected to dietary restriction. *J Gerontol A Biol Sci Med Sci* 51:B276–279, 1996.

Roelofs H, De Pauw ES, Zwinderman AH, Opdam SM, Willemze R, Tanke HJ, Fibbe WE. Homeostasis of telomere length rather than telomere shortening after allogeneic peripheral blood stem cell transplantation. *Blood* 101:358–362, 2003.

Roffe C. Ageing of the heart. *Br J Biomed Sci* 55:136–148, 1998.

Rogan EM, Bryan TM, Hukku B, Maclean K, Chang AC, Moy EL, Englezou A, Warneford SG, Dalla-Pozza L, Reddel RR. Alterations in p53 and p16INK4 expression and telomere length during spontaneous immortalization of Li-Fraumeni syndrome fibroblasts. *Mol Cell Biol* 15:4745–4753, 1995.

Rogers GS, Gilchrest BA. The senile epidermis: environmental influences on skin ageing and cutaneous carcinogenesis. *Br J Dermatol* 122(Suppl 35):55–60, 1990.

Rogers J, Webster S, Lue LF, Brachova L, Civin WH, Emmerling M, Shivers B, Walker D, McGeer P. Inflammation and Alzheimer's disease pathogenesis. *Neurobiol Aging* 17:681–686, 1996.

Rogers JT, Leiter LM, McPhee J, Cahill CM, Zhan SS, Potter H, Nilsson LN. Translation of the alzheimer amyloid precursor protein mRNA is up-regulated by interleukin-1 through 5'-untranslated region sequences. *J Biol Chem* 274:6421–6431, 1999.

Rogers MA, Evans WJ. Changes in skeletal muscle with aging: effects of exercise training. *Exerc Sport Sci Rev* 21:65–102, 1993.

Rogina B, Helfand SL, Frankel S. Longevity regulation by Drosophila Rpd3 deacetylase and caloric restriction. *Science* 298:1745, 2002.

Rogina B, Reenan RA, Nilsen SP, Helfand SL. Extended life-span conferred by cotransporter gene mutations in *Drosophila*. *Science* 290:2137–2140, 2000.

Rohde V, Sattler HP, Bund T, Bonkhoff H, Fixemer T, Bachmann C, Lensch R, Unteregger G, Stoeckle M, Wullich B. Expression of the human telomerase reverse transcriptase is not related to telomerase activity in normal and malignant renal tissue. *Clin Cancer Res* 6:4803–4809, 2000.

Rohrbach JM, Riedinger C, Wild M, Partsch M. Telomerase activity in uveal melanomas [in German]. *Ophthalmologe* 97:359–363, 2000.

Roman GC. Vascular dementia today. *Rev Neurol (Paris)* 155(Suppl 4):S64–72, 1999.

Romaniukha AA, Iashin AI. Mathematical model of the age-related changes in peripheral T cells population [in Russian]. *Adv Gerontol* 8:58–69, 2001.

Romanoff LP, Morris CW, Welch P, Rodrigues RM, Pincus G. The metabolism of crtisol-4-C14 in young and elderly men. I. Secretion rate of cortisol and daily secretion of tetrahydrocortisol (allotetrahydrocortisol), tetrahydrocortisone, and cortolone (20α and 20β). *J Clin Endocrinol Metab* 21:1413, 1961.

Romanov SR, Kozakiewicz BK, Holst CR, Stampfer MR, Haupt LM, Tlsty TD. Normal human mammary epithelial cells spontaneously escape senescence and acquire genomic changes. *Nature* 409:633–637, 2001.

Romas SN, Mayeux R, Tang MX, Lantigua R, Medrano M, Tycko B, Knowles J. No association between a presenilin 1 polymorphism and Alzheimer disease. *Arch Neurol* 57:699–702, 2000.

Romero MT, Silverman AJ, Wise PM, Witkin JW. Ultrastructural changes in gonadotropin-releasing hormone neurons as a function of age and ovariectomy in rats. *Neuroscience* 58:217–225, 1994.

Romney CA, Paulauskis JD, Nagasawa H, Little JB. Multiple manifestations of X-ray-induced genomic instability in Chinese hamster ovary (CHO) cells. *Mol Carcinog* 32:118–127, 2001.

Roque RS, Agarwal N, Wordinger RJ, Brun AM, Xue Y, Huang LC, Nguyen LP, Shay JW. Human papillomavirus-16 E6/E7 transfected retinal cell line expresses the Muller cell phenotype. *Exp Eye Res* 64:519–527, 1997.

Roques CN, Boyer JC, Farber RA. Microsatellite mutation rates are equivalent in normal and telomerase-immortalized human fibroblasts. *Cancer Res* 61:8405–8407, 2001.

Rose M. Laboratory evolution of postponed senescence in *Drosophila melanogaster*. *Evolution* 38:1004–1010, 1984.

Rose M, Charlesworth B. A test of evolutionary theories of senescence. *Nature* 287:141–42, 1980.

Rose MR. Genetics of increased life span in *Drosophila*. *Bioessays* 11:132–135, 1989.

Rose MR. *Evolutionary Biology of Aging*. Oxford University Press, New York, 1991.

Rose MR. Can human aging be postponed? *Sci Am* 281:106–111, 1999a.

Rose MR. Genetics of aging in *Drosophila*. *Exp Gerontol* 34:577–585, 1999b.

Rose MR, Archer MA. Genetic analysis of mechanisms of aging. *Curr Opin Genet Dev* 6:366–370, 1996.

Rose MR, Charlesworth B. Genetics of life history in *Drosophila melanogaster*. II. Exploratory selection experiments. *Genetics* 97:187–196, 1981.

Rose MR, Finch CE. The Janiform genetics of aging. *Genetica* 91:3–10, 1993.

Rose MR, Graves JL Jr. What evolutionary biology can do for gerontology. *J Gerontol* 44:B27–29, 1989.

Rose MR, Nusbaum TJ. Prospects for postponing human aging. *FASEB J* 8:925–928, 1994.

Rose MR, Nusbaum TJ, Fleming JE. *Drosophila* with postponed aging as a model for aging research. *Lab Anim Sci* 42:114–118, 1992a.

Rose MR, Vu LN, Park SU, Graves JL Jr. Selection on stress resistance increases longevity in *Drosophila melanogaster*. *Exp Gerontol* 27:241–250, 1992b.

Rosenberg IH. Summary comments. *Am J Clin Nutr* 50:1231–1233, 1989.

Rosenberg IH. Sarcopenia: origins and clinical relevance. *J Nutr* 127:990S–991S, 1997.

Rosenberg MJ, Killoran C, Dziadzio L, Chang S, Stone DL, Meck J, Aughton D, Bird LM, Bodurtha J, Cassidy SB, Graham JM Jr, Grix A, Guttmacher AE, Hudgins L, Kozma C, Michaelis RC, Pauli R, Peters KF, Rosenbaum KN, Tifft CJ, Wargowski D, Williams MS, Biesecker LG. Scanning for telomeric deletions and duplications and uniparental disomy using genetic markers in 120 children with malformations. *Hum Genet* 109:311–318, 2001.

Rosenberg R. The molecular and genetic basis of AD: the end of the beginning. *Neurology* 54:2045–2054, 2000.

Rosenberg R. Evolutionary time and human memory. *JAMA* 288:3045–3047, 2002.

Rosenbloom AL, Kappy MS, DeBusk FL, Francis GL, Philpot TJ, Maclaren NK. Progeria: insulin resistance and hyperglycemia. *J Pediatr* 102:400–402, 1983.

Rosenthal AN, Jacobs IJ. The role of CA 125 in screening for ovarian cancer. *Int J Biol Markers* 13:216–220, 1998.

Rosenthal IM, Bronstein IP, Dallenbach FD, Pruzansky S, Rosewald AK. Progeria: report of a case with cephalometric roentgenograms in abnormally high concentrations of lipoproteins in the serum. *Pediatrics* 18:565–577, 1956.

Ross GRT. Translation of Aristotle's *De Lontiudine et Brevitate Vitae*. Clarendon Press, Oxford, 1908.

Ross KS, Carter HB, Pearson JD, Guess HA. Comparative efficiency of prostate-specific antigen screening strategies for prostate cancer detection. *JAMA* 284:1399–1405, 2000.

Ross JS, Cohen MB. Ancillary methods for the detection of recurrent urothelial neoplasia. *Cancer* 90:75–86, 2000.

Ross JS, Cohen MB. Biomarkers for the detection of bladder cancer. *Adv Anat Pathol* 8:37–45, 2001.

Ross OA, Hyland P, Curran MD, McIlhatton BP, Wikby A, Johansson B, Tompa A, Pawelec G, Barnett CR, Middleton D, Barnett YA. Mitochondrial DNA damage in lymphocytes: a role in immunosenescence? *Exp Gerontol* 37:329–340, 2002.

Roth GS. Changes in tissue responsiveness to hormones and neurotransmitters during aging. *Exp Gerontol* 30:361–368, 1995.

Roth GS. Age changes in signal transduction and gene expression. *Mech Ageing Dev* 98:231–238, 1997.

Roth GS, Ingram DK, Lane MA. Slowing ageing by caloric restriction. *Nat Med* 1:414–415, 1995a.

Roth GS, Ingram DK, Lane MA. Calorie restriction in primates: will it work and how will we know? *J Am Geriatr Soc* 47:896–903, 1999.

Roth GS, Joseph JA, Mason RP. Membrane alterations as causes of impaired signal transduction in Alzheimer's disease and aging. *Trends Neurosci* 18:203–206, 1995b.

Roth GS, Kowatch MA, Hengemihle J, Ingram DK, Spangler EL, Johnson LK, Lane MA. Effect of age and caloric restriction on cutaneous wound closure in rats and monkeys. *J Gerontol A Biol Sci Med Sci* 52:B98–102, 1997.

Roth GS, Lane MA, Ingram DK, Mattison JA, Elahi D, Tobin JD, Muller D, Metter EJ. Biomarkers of caloric restriction may predict longevity in humans. *Science* 297:811, 2003.

Roth SM, Ivey FM, Martel GF, Lemmer JT, Hurlbut DE, Siegel EL, Metter EJ, Fleg JL, Fozard JL, Kostek MC, Wernick DM, Hurley BF. Muscle size responses to strength training in young and older men and women. *J Am Geriatr Soc* 49:1428–1433, 2001a.

Roth SM, Martel GF, Ivey FM, Lemmer JT, Tracy BL, Metter EJ, Hurley BF, Rogers MA. Skeletal muscle satellite cell characteristics in young and older men and women after heavy resistance strength training. *J Gerontol A Biol Sci Med Sci* 56:B240–247, 2001b.

Rothman JH. Aging: from radiant youth to an abrupt end. *Curr Biol* 12:R239–241, 2002.

Rothstein M. Lipids. In Maddox GL (ed). *The Encyclopedia of Aging, Second Edition.* Springer Publishing Company, New York, 1995, pp 565–566.

Rothstein M, Evans JG. Proteins. In Maddox GL (ed). *The Encyclopedia of Aging, Second Edition.* Springer Publishing Company, New York, 1995, pp 769–771.

Rottkamp CA, Nunomura A, Raina AK, Sayre LM, Perry G, Smith MA. Oxidative stress, antioxidants, and Alzheimer disease. *Alzheimer Dis Assoc Disord* 14(Suppl 1):S62–66, 2000.

Roubenoff R, Castaneda C. Sarcopenia—understanding the dynamics of aging muscle. *JAMA* 286:1230–1231, 2001.

Roubenoff R, Hughes V. Sarcopenia: current concepts. *J Gerontol A Biol Sci Med Sci* 55:716–724, 2000.

Roubenoff R, Rall LC, Veldhuis JD, Kehayias JJ, Rosen C, Nicolson M, Lundgren N, Reichlin S. The relationship between growth hormone kinetics and sarcopenia in postmenopausal women: the role of fat mass and leptin. *J Clin Endocrinol Metab* 83:1502–1506, 1998.

Roukos DH. Current status and future perspectives in gastric cancer management. *Cancer Treat Rev* 26:243–255, 2000.

Roupe G. Skin of the aging human being [in Swedish]. *Lakartidningen* 98:1091–1095, 2001.

Rouse J, Jackson SP. Interfaces between the detection, signaling, and repair of DNA damage. *Science* 297:547–551, 2002.

Rousseau R, Soria JC. Telomerase, a universal target in immunotherapy strategies against tumor [in French]. *Bull Cancer* 87:895–901, 2000.

Rowe JW, Andres R, Tobin JD, Norris AH, Shock NW. The effect of age on creatinine clearance in men: a cross-sectional and longitudinal study. *J Gerontol* 31:155–163, 1976.

Rowe JW, Kahn RL. Successful aging. *Gerontologist* 37:433–440, 1997.

Rowe JW, Kahn RL. Successful aging and disease prevention. *Adv Ren Replace Ther* 7:70–77, 2000.

Roy J, Fulton TB, Blackburn EH. Specific telomerase RNA residues distant from the template are essential for telomerase function. *Genes Dev* 12:3286–3300, 1998.

Roy N, Runge KW. Two paralogs involved in transcriptional silencing that antagonistically control yeast life span. *Curr Biol* 10:111–114, 2000.

Rubelj I, Pereira-Smith OM. SV40–transformed human cells in crisis exhibit changes that occur in normal cellular senescence. *Exp Cell Res* 211:82–89, 1994.

Rubelj I, Venable SF, Lednicky J, Butel JS, Bilyeu T, Darlington G, Surmacz E, Campisi J, Pereira-Smith OM. Loss of T-antigen sequences allows SV40-transformed human cells in crisis to acquire a senescent-like phenotype. *J Gerontol A Biol Sci Med Sci* 52:B229–234, 1997.

Rubin E, Lieber CS. Alcohol-induced hepatic injury in nonalcoholic volunteers. *N Engl J Med* 282:869, 1968.

Rubin H. Telomerase and cellular life span: ending the debate? *Nat Biotechnol* 16:396–397, 1998.

Rubin H. The disparity between human cell senescence in vitro and lifelong replication in vivo. *Nat Biotechnol* 20:675–681, 2002a.

Rubin MA. Understanding disease cell by cell. *Science* 296:1329–1330, 2002b.

Rubin MA, Zhou M, Dhanasekaran SM, Varambally S, Barrette TR, Sanda MG, Pienta KJ, Ghosh D, Chinnaiyan AM. α-methylacyl coenzyme A racemase as a tissue biomarker for prostate cancer. *JAMA* 287:1662–1670, 2002.

Rubin SA. The molecular and cellular biology of cardiac failure. In Hosenpud JD, Greenberg BH (eds). *congestive Heart Failure*. Lippincott Williams & Wilkins, Philadelphia, 2000, pp 9–40.

Rubio MA, Kim SH, Campisi J. Reversible manipulation of telomerase expression and telomere length. Implications for the ionizing radiation response and replicative senescence of human cells. *J Biol Chem* 277:28609–28617, 2002.

Rudman D, Kutner M, Rogers C, Lubin M, Fleming G, Bain R. Impaired growth hormone secretion in the adult population: relation to age and adiposity. *J Clin Invest* 67:1361–1369, 1981.

Rudolph KL, Chang S, Lee HW, Blasco M, Gottlieb GJ, Greider C, DePinho RA. Longevity, stress response, and cancer in aging telomerase-deficient mice. *Cell* 96:701–712, 1999.

Rudolph KL, Chang S, Millard M, Schreiber-Agus N, DePinho RA. Inhibition of experimental liver cirrhosis in mice by telomerase gene delivery. *Science* 287:1253–1258, 2000.

Rudolph KL, Millard M, Bosenberg MW, DePinho RA. Telomere dysfunction and evolution of intestinal carcinoma in mice and humans. *Nat Genet* 28:155–159, 2001.

Rufer N, Breummendorf TH, Kolvraa S, Bischoff C, Christensen K, Wadsworth L, Schulzer M, Lansdorp P. Telomere fluorescence measurements in granulocytes and T lymphocyte subsets point to a high turnover of hematopoetic stem cells and memory T cells in early childhood. *J Exp Med* 190:157–167, 1999.

Rufer N, Migliaccio M, Antonchuk J, Humphries RK, Roosnek E, Lansdorp PM. Transfer of the human telomerase reverse transcriptase (TERT) gene into T lymphocytes results in extension of replicative potential. *Blood* 98:597–603, 2001.

Ruggero D, Grisendi S, Piazza F, Rego E, Mari F, Rao PH, Cordon-Carod C, Pandolfi PP. Dyskeratosis congenita and cancer in mice deficient in ribosomal RNA modification. *Science* 299:259–262, 2003.

Runge KW, Wellinger RJ, Zakian VA. Effects of excess centromeres and excess telomeres on chromosome loss rates. *Mol Cell Biol* 11:2919–2928, 1991.

Runge KW, Zakian VA. Properties of the transcriptional enhancer in *Saccharomyces cerevisiae* telomeres. *Nucleic Acids Res* 18:1783–1787, 1990.

Runge KW, Zakian VA. *Saccharomyces cerevisiae* linear chromosome stability (lcs) mutants increase the loss rate of artificial and natural linear chromosomes. *Chromosoma* 102:207–217, 1993.

Runge KW, Zakian VA. *TEL2*, an essential gene required for telomere length regulation and telomere position effect in *Saccharomyces cerevisiae*. *Mol Cell Biol* 16:3094–3105, 1996.

Runge P, Asnis MS, Brumley GW, Grossman H. Hutchinson-Gilford progeria syndrome. *South Med J* 71:877–879, 1978.

Rushing EJ, Yashima K, Brown DF, White CL 3rd, Shay JW, Risser RC, Gazdar AF. Expression of telomerase RNA component correlates with the MIB-1 proliferation index in ependymomas. *J Neuropathol Exp Neurol* 56:1142–1146, 1997.

Russell B, Dix DJ, Haller DL, Jacobs-El J. Repair of injured skeletal muscle: a molecular approach. *Med Sci Sports Exerc* 24:189–196, 1992.

Russell-Aulet M, Jaffe CA, Demott-Friberg R, Barkan AL. In vivo semiquantification of hypothalamic growth hormone-releasing hormone (GHRH) output in humans: evidence for relative GHRH deficiency in aging. *J Clin Endocrinol Metab* 84:3490–3497, 1999.

Russo I, Silver AR, Cuthbert AP, Griffin DK, Trott DA, Newbold RF. A telomere-independent senescence mechanism is the sole barrier to Syrian hamster cell immortalization. *Oncogene* 17:3417–3426, 1998.

Russo J, Russo IH. The pathway of neoplastic transformation of human breast epithelial cells. *Radiat Res* 155:151–154, 2001.

Rusting RL. Hair: why it grows, why it stops. *Sci Am* 284:70–79, 2001

Ruvalcaba RHA, Churesigaew S, Myhre SA, Kelley VC, Martin GM. Children who are rapidly progeroid syndromes: case report of a new variant. *Clin Pediatr* 16:248–252, 1977.

Sabbah HN, Sharov VG, Goldstein S. Programmed cell death in the progression of heart failure. *Ann Med* 30(Suppl 1):33–38, 1998.

Sachais BS. Platelet-endothelial interactions in atherosclerosis. *Curr Atheroscler Rep* 3:412–416, 2001.

Sachsinger J, Gonzalez-Suarez E, Samper E, Heicappell R, Muller M, Blasco MA. Telomerase inhibition in RenCa, a murine tumor cell line with short telomeres, by overexpression of a dominant negative mTERT mutant, reveals fundamental differences in telomerase regulation between human and murine cells. *Cancer Res* 61:5580–5586, 2001.

Saeki T, Takashima S, Tachibana M, Koga M, Hiyama E, Salomon DS, Holland JF, Ohnuma T. Inhibitory effect of telomere-mimic phosphorothioate oligodeoxy nucleotides (S-ODNS) on human tumor cell lines. *Oncology* 57(Suppl 2):27–36, 1999.

Sagawa Y, Nishi H, Isaka K, Fujito A, Takayama M. The correlation of TERT expression with c-myc expression in cervical cancer. *Cancer Lett* 168:45–50, 2001.

Saito H, Moses RE. Immortalization of Werner syndrome and progeria fibroblasts. *Exp Cell Res* 192:373–379, 1991.

Saito K, Yagihashi A, Nasu S, Izawa Y, Nakamura M, Kobayashi D, Tsuji N, Watanabe N. Gene expression for suppressors of telomerase activity (telomeric-repeat binding factors) in breast cancer. *Jpn J Cancer Res* 93:253–258, 2002.

Sakamoto M, Toyoizumi T, Kikuchi Y, Okamoto A, Nakayama H, Aoki D, Yamamoto K, Hata H, Sugishita T, Tenjin Y. Telomerase activity in gynecological tumors. *Oncol Rep* 7:1003–1009, 2000.

Sakoff JA, De Waal E, Garg MB, Denham J, Scorgie FE, Enno A, Lincz LF, Ackland SP. Telomere length in haemopoietic stem cells can be determined from that of mononuclear blood cells or whole blood. *Leuk Lymphoma* 43:2017–2020, 2002.

Sakr WA, Partin AW. Histological markers of risk and the role of high-grade prostatic intra-epithelial neoplasia. *Urology* 57:115–120, 2001.

Salla S, Redbrake C, Franz A, Reim M. Changes of human donor corneas preserved for longer than 4 weeks. *Vision Res* 36s:81, 1996.

Salonga DS, Danenberg KD, Grem J, Park JM, Danenberg PV. Relative gene expression in normal and tumor tissue by quantitative RT-PCR. In Double JA, Thompson MJ (eds). *Telomeres and Telomerase: Methods and Protocols*. Humana Press, Totowa, NJ, 2002, pp 83–98.

Samani NJ, Boultby R, Butler R, Thompson JR, Goodall AH. Telomere shortening in athero-sclerosis. *Lancet* 358:472–473, 2001.

Samantray SK, Samantray S, Johnson SC, Bhaktaviziam A. Werner syndrome. *Aust NZ J Med* 7:309–311, 1977.

Samper E, Fernandez P, Eguia R, Martin-Rivera L, Bernad A, Blasco MA, Aracil M. Long-term repopulating ability of telomerase-deficient murine hematopoietic stem cells. *Blood* 99:2767–2775, 2002.

Samper E, Flores JM, Blasco MA. Restoration of telomerase activity rescues chromosomal instability and premature aging in Terc–/– mice with short telomeres. *EMBO Rep* 2:800–807, 2001.

Samper E, Goytisolo FA, Slijepcevic P, van Buul PP, Blasco MA. Mammalian Ku86 protein prevents telomeric fusions independently of the length of TTAGGG repeats and the G-strand overhang. *EMBO Rep* 1:244–252, 2000.

Sanchez-Ramos J, Song S, Cardozo-Pelaez F, Hazzi C, Stedeford T, Willing A, Freeman TB, Saporta S, Janssen W, Patel N, Cooper DR, Sanberg PR. Adult bone marrow stromal cells differentiate into neural cells in vitro. *Exp Neurol* 164:247–256, 2000.

Sandars NK. *The Epic of Gilgamesh. An English Version with an Introduction*. Penguin Books, London, 1960.

Sandell LL, Gottschling DE, Zakian VA. Transcription of a yeast telomere alleviates telomere position effect without affecting chromosome stability. *Proc Natl Acad Sci USA* 91:12061–12065, 1994.

Sandell LL, Zakian VA. Loss of a yeast telomere: arrest, recovery, and chromosome loss. *Cell* 75:729–739, 1993.

Sanderson JP, Binkley N, Roecker EB, Champ JE, Pugh TD, Aspnes L, Weindruch R. Influence of fat intake and caloric restriction on bone in aging male rats. *J Gerontol A Biol Sci Med Sci* 52:B20–25, 1997.

Sandstrom O, El-Salhy M. Ageing and endocrine cells of human duodenum. *Mech Ageing Dev* 108:39–48, 1999a.

Sandstrom O, el-Salhy M. Human rectal endocrine cells and aging. *Mech Ageing Dev* 108:219–226, 1999b.

Sansoni P, Cossarizza A, Brianti V, Fagnoni F, Snelli G, Monti D, Marcato A, Passeri G, Ortolani C, Forti E, et al. Lymphocyte subsets and natural killer cell activity in healthy old people and centenarians. *Blood* 82:2767–2773, 1993.

Santos Ruiz A, Cascales Angosto M. Physiopathologic implications of telomerase [in Spanish]. *An R Acad Nac Med (Madr)* 117:427–444, 2000.

Sapolsky R. *Stress, the Aging Brain, and the Mechanisms of Neuron Death.* MIT Press, Cambridge, MA, 1992.

Sapolsky RM. Glucocorticoids, stress, and their adverse neurological effects: relevance to aging. *Exp Gerontol* 34:721–732, 1999.

Saretzki G, Feng J, von Zglinicki T, Villeponteau B. Similar gene expression pattern in senescent and hyperoxic-treated fibroblasts. *J Gerontol Ser A Biol Sci Med* 53:B438–B442, 1998.

Saretzki G, Ludwig A, von Zglinicki T, Runnebaum IB. Ribozyme-mediated telomerase inhibition induces immediate cell loss but not telomere shortening in ovarian cancer cells. *Cancer Gene Ther* 8:827–834, 2001.

Saretzki G, Sitte N, Merkel U, Wurm RE, von Zglinicki T. Telomere shortening triggers a p53–dependent cell cycle arrest via accumulation of G-rich single stranded DNA fragments. *Oncogene* 18:5148–5158, 1999.

Saretzki G, Von Zglinicki T. Replicative aging, telomeres, and oxidative stress. *Ann NY Acad Sci* 959:24–29, 2002.

Sasaki S, Ehara T, Sakata I, Fujino Y, Harada N, Kimura J, Nakamura H, Maeda M. Development of novel telomerase inhibitors based on a bisindole unit. *Bioorg Med Chem Lett* 11:583–585, 2001.

Sasgary S, Wieser M, Cerni C. Targeted inhibition of telomerase in human cancer: will it be a double-edged sword? *Onkologie* 24:22–26, 2001.

Sashiyama H, Shino Y, Kawamata Y, Tomita Y, Ogawa N, Shimada H, Kobayashi S, Asano T, Ochiai T, Shirasawa H. Immortalization of human esophageal keratinocytes by E6 and E7 of human papillomavirus type 16. *Int J Oncol* 19:97–103, 2001.

Satish S, Freeman DH, Ray L, Goodwin JS. The relationship between blood pressure and mortality in the oldest old. *J Am Geriatr Soc* 49:367–374, 2001.

Sato N, Maehara N, Mizumoto K, Nagai E, Yasoshima T, Hirata K, Tanaka M. Telomerase activity of cultured human pancreatic carcinoma cell lines correlates with their potential for migration and invasion. *Cancer* 91:496–504, 2001.

Sato N, Mizumoto K, Beppu K, Maehara N, Kusumoto M, Nabae T, Morisaki T, Katano M, Tanaka M. Establishment of a new human pancreatic cancer cell line, NOR-P1, with high angiogenic activity and metastatic potential. *Cancer Lett* 155:153–161, 2000a.

Sato N, Mizumoto K, Kusumoto M, Nishio S, Maehara N, Urashima T, Ogawa T, Tanaka M. Up-regulation of telomerase activity in human pancreatic cancer cells after exposure to etoposide. *Br J Cancer* 82:1819–1826, 2000b.

Saunders NA, Smith RJ, Jetten AM. Regulation of proliferation-specific and differentiation-specific genes during senescence of human epidermal keratinocyte and mammary epithelial cells. *Biochem Biophys Res Commun* 197:46–54, 1993.

Savine R, Sonksen PH. Is the somatopause an indication for growth hormone replacement? *J Endocrinol Invest* 22(5 Suppl):142–149, 1999.

Savitsky M, Kravchuk O, Melnikova L, Georgiev P. Heterochromatin protein 1 is involved in control of telomere elongation in *Drosophila melanogaster*. *Mol Cell Biol* 22:3204–3218, 2002.

Savre-Train I, Gollahon LS, Holt SE. Clonal heterogeneity in telomerase activity and telomere length in tumor-derived cell lines. *Proc Soc Exp Biol Med* 223:379–388, 2000.

Sawa A. Neuronal cell death in Down's syndrome. *J Neural Transm Suppl* 57:87–97, 1999.

Sawyer JR, Husain M, Pravdenkova S, Krisht A, Al-Mefty O. A role for telomeric and centromeric instability in the progression of chromosome aberrations in meningioma patients. *Cancer* 88:440–453, 2000.

Sayama K, Shirakata Y, Midorikawa K, Hanakawa Y, Hashimoto K. Possible involvement of p21 but not of p16 or p53 in keratinocyte senescence. *J Cell Physiol* 179:40–44, 1999.

Sayeed-Shah U, Mann MJ, Martin J, Grachev S, Reimold S, Laurence R, Dzau V, Cohn LH. Complete reversal of ischemic wall motion abnormalities by combined use of gene therapy with transmyocardial laser revascularization. *J Thorac Cardiovasc Surg* 116:763–769, 1998.

Schachter F, Cohen D, Kirkwood T. Prospects for the genetics of human longevity. *Hum Genet* 91:519–526, 1993.

Schaniel C, Gottar M, Roosnek E, Melchers F, Rolink AG. Extensive in vivo self-renewal, long-term reconstitution capacity, and hematopoietic multipotency of *Pax5*-deficient precursor B-cell clones. *Blood* 99:2760–2766, 2002.

Scheel C, Poremba C. Telomere lengthening in telomerase-negative cells: the ends are coming together. *Virchows Arch* 440:573–582, 2002.

Scheffer GL, Schroeijers AB, Izquierdo MA, Wiemer EA, Scheper RJ. Lung resistance-related protein/major vault protein and vaults in multidrug-resistant cancer. *Curr Opin Oncol* 12:550–556, 2000.

Scher AM. Absence of atherosclerosis in human intramyocardial coronary arteries: a neglected phenomenon. *Atherosclerosis* 149:1–3, 2000.

Scherf A, Figueiredo LM, Freitas-Junior LH. Plasmodium telomeres: a pathogen's perspective. *Curr Opin Microbiol* 4:409–414, 2001.

Scherthan H. A bouquet makes ends meet. *Nat Rev Mol Cell Biol* 2:621–627, 2001.

Scherthan H. Detection of chromosome ends by telomere FISH. In Double JA, Thompson MJ (eds). *Telomeres and Telomerase: Methods and Protocols*. Humana Press, Totowa, NJ, 2002, pp 13–32.

Scherthan H, Jerratsch M, Dhar S, Wang YA, Goff SP, Pandita TK. Meiotic telomere distribution and Sertoli cell nuclear architecture are altered in Atm- and Atm-p53-deficient mice. *Mol Cell Biol* 20:7773–7783, 2000.

Schiemann B, Gommerman JL, Vora K, Cachero TG, Shulga-Morskaya S, Dobles M, Frew E, Scott ML. An essential role for BAFF in the normal development of B cells through a BCMA-independent pathway. *Science* 293:2111–2114, 2001.

Schindler A, Fiedler U, Meye A, Schmidt U, Fussel S, Pilarsky C, Herrmann J, Wirth MP. Human telomerase reverse transcriptase antisense treatment downregulates the viability of prostate cancer cells in vitro. *Int J Oncol* 19:25–30, 2001.

Schipper HM, Liang JJ, Wang E. Quiescent and cycling cell compartments in the senescent and Alzheimer-diseased human brain. *Neurology* 43:87–94, 1993.

Schlecht NF, Kulaga S, Robitaille J, Ferreira S, Santos M, Miyamura RA, Duarte-Franco E, Rohan TE, Ferenczy A, Villa LI, Franco EI. Persistent human papillomavirus infection as a predictor of cervical intraepithelial neoplasia. *JAMA* 286:3106–3114, 2001.

Schmidt JV, Matteson PG, Jones BK, Guan XJ, Tilghman SM. The *dlk1* and *gtl2* genes are linked and reciprocally imprinted. *Genes Dev* 14:1997–2002, 2000.

Schmidt PM, Lehmann C, Matthes E, Bier FF. Detection of activity of telomerase in tumor cells using fiber optical biosensors. *Biosens Bioelectron* 17:1081–1087, 2002.

Schnabl B, Choi YH, Olsen JC, Hagedorn CH, Brenner DA. Immortal activated human hepatic stellate cells generated by ectopic telomerase expression. *Lab Invest* 82:323–333, 2002.

Schneider EL, Mitsui Y. The relationship between in vitro cellular aging and in vivo human age. *Proc Natl Acad Sci USA* 73:3584–3588, 1976.

Schneider LS, Farlow MR, Henderson VW, Pogoda JM. Effects of estrogen replacement therapy on response to tacrine in patients with Alzheimer's disease. *Neurology* 46:1580–1584, 1996.

Schneider-Stock R, Epplen C, Radig K, Oda Y, Dralle H, Hoang-Vu C, Epplen JT, Roessner A. On telomere shortening in soft-tissue tumors. *J Cancer Res Clin Oncol* 124:165–171, 1998a.

Schneider-Stock R, Epplen JT, Walter H, Radig K, Rys J, Epplen C, Hoang-Vu C, Niezabitowski A, Roessner A. Telomeric lengths and telomerase activity in liposarcomas. *Mol Carcinog* 24:144–151, 1999.

Schneider-Stock R, Eppler C, Walter H, Radig K, Haeckel C, Hoang-Vu C, Epplen JT, Roessner A. Telomere lengths and telomerase activity in liposarcomas [in German]. *Verh Dtsch Ges Pathol* 82:226–231, 1998b.

Schofield PW, Tang M, Marder K, Bell K, Dooneief G, Chun M, Sano M, Stern Y, Mayeux R. Alzheimer's disease after remote head injury: an incidence study. *J Neurol Neurosurg Psychiatry* 62:119–124, 1997.

Schopenhauer A. *On the Basis of Morality.* The Bobbs-Merrill Company, Indianapolis, 1965.

Schraermeyer U, Heimann K. Current understanding on the role of retinal pigment epithelium and its pigmentation. *Pigment Cell Res* 12:219–236, 1999.

Schroder CP, Wisman GB, de Jong S, van der Graaf WT, Ruiters MH, Mulder NH, de Leij LF, van der Zee AG, de Vries EG. Telomere length in breast cancer patients before and after chemotherapy with or without stem cell transplantation. *Br J Cancer* 84:1348–1353, 2001.

Schubert HD. Ocular manifestations of systemic hypertension. *Curr Opin Ophthalmol* 9:69–72, 1998.

Schubert P, Morino T, Miyazaki H, Ogata T, Nakamura Y, Marchini C, Ferroni S. Cascading glia reactions: a common pathomechanism and its differentiated control by cyclic nucleotide signaling. *Ann NY Acad Sci* 903:24–33, 2000.

Schubert P, Ogata T, Miyazaki H, Marchini C, Ferroni S, Rudolphi K. Pathological immunoreactions of glial cells in Alzheimer's disease and possible sites of interference. *J Neural Transm Suppl* 54:167–174, 1998a.

Schubert P, Rudolphi K. Interfering with the pathologic activation of microglial cells and astrocytes in dementia. *Alzheimer Dis Assoc Disord* 12(Suppl 2):S21–28, 1998b.

Schultz E, Lipton BH. Skeletal muscle satellite cells: changes in proliferation as a function of age. *Mech Ageing Dev* 20:377–383, 1982.

Schultz E, McCormick KM. Skeletal muscle satellite cells. *Rev Physiol Biochem Pharmacol* 123:213–257, 1994.

Schultz G, Cipolla L, Whitehouse A, Eiferman R, Woost P, Jumblatt M. Growth factors and corneal endothelial cell. III: Stimulation of adult human corneal endothelial cell mitosis in vitro by defined mitogenic agents. *Cornea* 11:20–27, 1992.

Schultze JL, Maecker B, von Bergwelt-Baildon MS, Anderson KS, Vonderheide RH. Tumour immunotherapy: new tools, new treatment modalities and new T-cell antigens. *Vox Sang* 80:81–89, 2001.

Schulz VP, Zakian VA. The saccharomyces PIF1 DNA helicase inhibits telomere elongation and de novo telomere formation. *Cell* 76:145–155, 1994.

Schulz VP, Zakian VA, Ogburn CE, McKay J, Jarzebowicz AA, Edland SD, Martin GM. Accelerated loss of telomeric repeats may not explain accelerated replicative decline of Werner syndrome cells. *Hum Genet* 97:750–754, 1996.

Schwartz AG. Inhibition of spontaneous breast cancer formation in female C3H(Avy/A) mice by long-term treatment with dehydroepiandrosterone. *Cancer Res* 39:1129–1132, 1979.

Schwartz HS, Eskew JD, Butler MG. Clonality studies in giant cell tumor of bone. *J Orthop Res* 20:387–390, 2002.

Schwartz JL, Jordan R, Evans HH. Characteristics of chromosome instability in the human lymphoblast cell line WTK1. *Cancer Genet Cytogenet* 129:124–130, 2001.

Schwartz MM. The role of podocyte injury in the pathogenesis of focal segmental glomerulosclerosis. *Ren Fail* 22:663–684, 2000.

Schwarze SR, Lee CM, Chung SS, Roecker EB, Weindruch R, Aiken JM. High levels of mitochondrial DNA deletions in skeletal muscle of old rhesus monkeys. *Mech Ageing Dev* 83:91–101, 1995.

Schwarze SR, Weindruch R, Aiken JM. Decreased mitochondrial RNA levels without accumulation of mitochondrial DNA deletions in aging *Drosophila melanogaster. Mutat Res* 382:99–107, 1998a.

Schwarze SR, Weindruch R, Aiken JM. Oxidative stress and aging reduce COX I RNA and cytochrome oxidase activity in *Drosophila. Free Radic Biol Med* 25:740–747, 1998b.

Schwenke DC. Aging, menopause, and free radicals. *Semin Reprod Endocrinol* 16:281–308, 1998.

Scopacasa F, Wishart JM, Need AG, Horowitz M, Morris HA, Nordin BEC. Bone density and bone-related biochemical variables in normal men: a longitudinal study. *J Gerontol Med Sci* 57A:M385–391, 2002.

Scott WK, Nance MA, Watts RL, Hubble JP, Koller WC, Lyons K, Pahwa R, Stern MB, Colcer A, Hiner BC, Jankovic J, Ondo WG, Allen FH, Goetz CG, Small GW, Masterman D, Mastaglia F, Laing NG, Stajich JM, Slotterbeck B, Booze MW, Ribble RC, Rampersaud E, West SG, Gibson RA, Middleton LT, Roses AD, Haines JL, Scott BL, Vance JM, Pericak-Vance MA. Complete genomic screen in Parkinson disease: evidence for multiple genes. *JAMA* 286:2239–2244, 2001.

Scully C, Field JK, Tanzawa H. Genetic aberrations in oral or head and neck squamous cell carcinoma (SCCHN): 1. Carcinogen metabolism, DNA repair and cell cycle control. *Oral Oncol* 36:256–263, 2000.

Seachrist L. Telomeres draw a crowd at Toronto cancer meeting. *Science* 268:29–30, 1995.

Seddon JM, Rosner B, Sperduto RD, Yannuzzi L, Haller JA, Blair NP, Willett W. Dietary fat and risk for advanced age-related macular degeneration. *Arch Ophthalmol* 119:1191–1199, 2001.

Sedivy JM. Can ends justify the means?: telomeres and the mechanisms of replicative senescence and immortalization in mammalian cells. *Proc Natl Acad Sci USA* 95:9078–9081, 1998.

Seeger M, Nordstedt C, Petanceska S, Kovacs DM, Gouras GK, Hahne S, Fraser P, Levesque L, Czernik AJ, George-Hyslop PS, Sisodia SS, Thinakaran G, Tanzi RE, Greengard P, Gandy S. Evidence for phosphorylation and oligomeric assembly of presenilin 1. *Proc Natl Acad Sci USA* 94:5090–5094, 1997.

Seger YR, Garcia-Cao M, Piccinin S, Cunsolo CL, Doglioni C, Blasco MA, Hannon GJ, Maestro R. Transformation of normal human cells in the absence of telomerase activation. *Cancer Cell* 2:401–413, 2002.

Seidman MD, Khan MJ, Bai U, Shirwany N, Quirk WS. Biologic activity of mitochondrial metabolites on aging and age-related hearing loss. *Am J Otol* 21:161–167, 2000.

Seidman SN, Walsh BT. Testosterone and depression in aging men. *Am J Geriatr Psychiatry* 7:18–33, 1999.

Seigneurin-Venin S, Bernard V, Moisset PA, Ouellette MM, Mouly V, Di Donna S, Wright WE, Tremblay JP. Transplantation of normal and DMD myoblasts expressing the telomerase gene in SCID mice. *Biochem Biophys Res Commun* 272:362–369, 2000.

Seimiya H, Oh-hara T, Suzuki T, Naasani I, Shimazaki T, Tsuchiya K, Tsuruo T. Telomere shortening and growth inhibition of human cancer cells by novel synthetic telomerase inhibitors MST-312, MST-295, and MST-1991. *Mol Cancer Ther* 1:657–665, 2002.

Seimiya H, Sawada H, Muramatsu Y, Shimizu M, Ohko K, Yamane K, Tsuruo T. Involvement of 14–3–3 proteins in nuclear localization of telomerase. *EMBO J* 19:2652–2661, 2000.

Seimiya H, Smith S. The telomeric poly(ADP-ribose) polymerase, tankyrase 1, contains multiple binding sites for telomeric repeat binding factor 1 (TRF1) and a novel acceptor, 182-kDa tankyrase-binding protein (TAB182). *J Biol Chem* 277:14116–14126, 2002.

Seimiya H, Tanji M, Oh-hara T, Tomida A, Naasani I, Tsuruo T. Hypoxia up-regulates telomerase activity via mitogen-activated protein kinase signaling in human solid tumor cells. *Biochem Biophys Res Commun* 260:365–370, 1999.

Sekine M, Tanaka K. Familial ovarian cancer [in Japanese]. *Nippon Rinsho* 58:1409–1412, 2000.

Sela B. On telomeres and telomerases: the key to cell senescence or immortality [in Hebrew]. *Harefuah* 138:24–27, 2000.

Selkoe DJ. Alzheimer's disease: genotypes, phenotype, and treatments. *Science* 275:630–631, 1997.

Sell C, Ptasznik A, Chang CD, Swantek J, Cristofalo VJ, Baserga R. IGF-1 receptor levels and the proliferation of young and senescent human fibroblasts. *Biochem Biophys Res Commun* 194:259–265, 1993.

Selmanowitz VJ. Cutaneous changes associated with aging. *J Dermatol Surg Oncol* 3:628–634, 1977.

Selye H, Strebel R, Mikulaj L. A progeria-like syndrome produced by dihydrotachysterol and its prevention by methyltesterone and ferric dextran. *J Am Geriatr Soc* 11:1–16, 1963.

Selzman CH, Miller SA, Harken AH. Therapeutic implications of inflammation in atherosclerotic cardiovascular disease. *Ann Thorac Surg* 71:2066–2074, 2001.

Sen D, Gilbert W. Novel DNA superstructures formed by telomere-like oligomers. *Biochemistry* 31:65–70, 1992.

Sen S, Reddy VG, Khanna N, Guleria R, Kapila K, Singh N. A comparative study of telomerase activity in sputum, bronchial washing and biopsy specimens of lung cancer. *Lung Cancer* 33:41–49, 2001.

Sen S, Talukder G, Sharma A. Age-related alterations in human chromosome composition and DNA content in vitro during senescence. *Biol Rev* 62:25–44, 1987.

Senior K. Telomerase: are we expecting too much? *Lancet* 355:2226, 2000.

Sephel GC, Sturrock A, Giro MG, Davidson JM. Increased elastin production by progeria skin fibroblasts is controlled by the steady-state levels of elastin mRNA. *J Invest Dermatol* 90:643–647, 1988.

Serakinci N, Krejci K, Koch J Telomeric repeat organization—a comparative in situ study between man and rodent. *Cytogenet Cell Genet* 86:204–211, 1999.

Serakinci N, Ostergaard M, Larsen H, Madsen B, Pedersen B, Koch J. Multiple telomeric aberrations in a telomerase-positive leukemia patient. *Cancer Genet Cytogenet* 138:11–16, 2002.

Serebrovs'ka TV, Safronova OS, Hordii SK. Free-radical processes under different conditions of body oxygen allowance [in Ukrainian]. *Fiziol Zh* 45:92–103, 1999.

Serra V, von Zglinicki T. Human fibroblasts in vitro senesce with a donor-specific telomere length. *FEBS Lett* 516:71–74, 2002.

Serra V, von Zglinicki T, Lorenz M, Saretzki G. Extracellular superoxide dismutase is a major antioxidant in human fibroblasts and slows down telomere shortening. *J Biol Chem* 278:6824–6830, 2003.

Serrano M, Blasco MA. Putting the stress on senescence. *Curr Opin Cell Biol* 13:748–753, 2001.

Serrano M, Lin AW, McCurrach ME, Beach D, Lowe S. Oncogenic *ras* provokes premature cell senescence associated with accumulation of p53 and p16INC4a. *Cell* 88:593–602, 1997.

Serruys, PW, de Feyter P, Macaya C, Kokott N, Puel J, Vrolix M, Branzi A, Bertolami MC, Jackson G, Strauss B, Meier B; Lescol Intervention Prevention Study (LIPS) Investigators. Fluvastatin for prevention of cardiac events following successful first percutaneous coronary intervention: a randomized controlled trial. *JAMA* 287:3215–3222, 2002.

Service RF. Tissue engineers build new bone. *Science* 289:1498–1500, 2000.

Seshadri T, Uzman JA, Oshima J, Campisi J. Identification of a transcript that is down-regulated in senescent human fibroblasts. Cloning, sequence analysis, and regulation of the human L7 ribosomal protein gene. *J Biol Chem* 268:18474–18480, 1993.

Severino J, Allen RG, Balin S, Balin A, Cristofalo VJ. Is beta-galactosidase staining a marker of senescence in vitro and in vivo? *Exp Cell Res* 257:162–171, 2000.

Shafer RH, Smirnov I. Biological aspects of DNA/RNA quadruplexes. *Biopolymers* 56:209–227, 2001.

Shah GN, Mooradian AD. Age-related changes in the blood–brain barrier. *Exp Gerontol* 32:501–519, 1997.

Shah PK. Plaque disruption and thrombosis: potential role of inflammation and infection. *Cardiol Rev* 8:31–39, 2000.

Shah S, Ravindranath Y. Neuroblastoma. *Indian J Pediatr* 65:691–705, 1998.

Shall S. The limited reproductive life span of normal human cells in culture. *Ciba Found Symp* 211:112–124; discussion 124–128, 1997.

Shall S, Stein WD. A mortalization theory for the control of the cell proliferation and for the origin of immortal cell lines. *J Theor Biol* 76:219–231, 1979.

Shammas MA, Shmookler Reis RJ. Recombination and its roles in DNA repair: cellular immortalization and cancer. *AGE* 22:71–88, 1999.

Shammas MA, Simmons C, Corey DR, Shmookler Reis RJ. Telomerase inhibition by peptide nucleic acids reverses "immortality" of transformed human cells. *Oncogene* 18:6191–6200, 1999.

Shamsi FA, Nagaraj RH. Immunochemical detection of dicarbonyl-derived imidazolium protein crosslinks in human lenses. *Curr Eye Res* 19:276–284, 1999.

Shapira AHV. Oxidative stress and mitochondrial dysfunction in neurodegeneration. *Curr Opin Neurol* 9:260–264, 1996.

Sharpe DN. Cardiac remodeling in congestive heart failure. In Hosenpud JD, Greenberg BH (eds). *Congestive Heart Failure*. Lippincott Williams & Wilkins, Philadelphia, 2000, pp 101–110.

Sharpless NE, DePinho RA. p53: good cop/bad cop. *Cell* 110:9–12, 2002.

Shay JW. Aging and cancer: are telomeres and telomerase the connection? *Mol Med Today* 1:378–384, 1995.

Shay JW. Molecular pathogenesis of aging and cancer: are telomeres and telomerase the connection? *J Clin Pathol* 50:799–800, 1997a.

Shay JW. Telomerase in human development and cancer. *J Cell Physiol* 173:266–270, 1997b.

Shay JW. Aging and cancer: are telomeres and telomerase the connection? Presented at Telomeres and Telomerase: Implications for Cell Immortality, Cancer, and Age-related Disease. San Francisco, CA, June 1–3, 1998a.

Shay JW. Telomerase in cancer: diagnostic, prognostic, and therapeutic implications. *Cancer J Sci Am* 4(Suppl 1):S26–34, 1998b.

Shay JW. At the end of the millennium, a view of the end. *Nat Genet* 23:382–383, 1999a.

Shay JW. Toward identifying a cellular determinant of telomerase repression. *J. Natl Cancer Inst* 91:4–6, 1999b.

Shay JW, Bacchetti S. A survey of telomerase activity in human cancer. *Eur J Cancer* 33:787–791, 1997.

Shay JW, Gazdar AF. Telomerase in the early detection of cancer. *J Clin Pathol* 50:106–109, 1997.

Shay JW, Pereira-Smith OM, Wright WE. A role for both RB and p53 in the regulation of human cellular senescence. *Exp Cell Res* 196:33–39, 1991a.

Shay JW, Tomlinson G, Piatyszek MA, Gollahon LS. Spontaneous in vitro immortalization of breast epithelial cells from a patient with Li-Fraumeni syndrome. *Mol Cell Biol* 15:425–432, 1995a.

Shay JW, Van Der Haegen BA, Ying Y, Wright WE. The frequency of immortalization of human fibroblasts and mammary epithelial cells transfected with SV40 large T-antigen. *Exp Cell Res* 209:45–52, 1993.

Shay JW, Werbin H. New evidence for the insertion of mitochondrial DNA into the human genome: significance for cancer and aging. *Mutat Res* 275:227–235, 1992.

Shay JW, Werbin H, Funk WD, Wright WE. Cellular and molecular advances in elucidating p53 function. *Mutat Res* 277:163–171, 1992a.

Shay JW, Werbin H, Wright WE. Telomere shortening may contribute to aging and cancer. *Mol Cell Differ* 2:1–21, 1994.

Shay JW, Werbin H, Wright WE. You haven't heard the end of it: telomere loss may link human aging with cancer. *Can J Aging* 14:511–524, 1995b.

Shay JW, Werbin H, Wright WE. Telomeres and telomerase in human leukemias. *Leukemia* 10:1255–1261, 1996.

Shay JW, Werbin H, Wright WE. Telomerase assays in the diagnosis and prognosis of cancer. *Ciba Found Symp* 211:148–155, 1997.

Shay JW, West MD, Wright WE. Re-expression of senescent markers in deinduced reversibly immortalized cells. *Exp Gerontol* 27:477–492, 1992b.

Shay JW, Wright. Quantitation of the frequency of immortalization of normal diploid fibroblasts by SV40 large T-antigen. *Exp Cell Res* 1874:109–118, 1989.

Shay JW, Wright. The reactivation of telomerase activity in cancer progression. *Trends Genet* 12:129–131, 1996a.

Shay JW, Wright WE. Telomerase activity in human cancer. *Curr Opin Oncol* 8:66–71, 1996b.

Shay JW, Wright W. Mutant dyskerin ends relationship with telomerase. *Science* 286:2284–2286, 1999.

Shay JW, Wright WE. Hayflick, his limit, and cellular ageing. *Nat Rev* 1:72–76, 2000a.

Shay JW, Wright WE. Implications of mapping the human telomerase gene (hTERT) as the most distal gene on chromosome 5p. *Neoplasia* 2:195–196, 2000b.

Shay JW, Wright WE. The use of telomerized cells for tissue engineering. *Nat Biotechnol* 18:22–23, 2000c.

Shay JW, Wright WE. Ageing and cancer: the telomere and telomerase connection. *Novartis Found Symp* 235:116–125, 2001a.

Shay JW, Wright WE. Telomeres and telomerase: implications for cancer and aging. *Radiat Res* 155:188–193, 2001b.

Shay JW, Wright WE. When do telomeres matter? *Science* 291:839–840, 2001c.

Shay JW, Wright WE, Werbin H. Defining the molecular mechanisms of human cell immortalization. *Biochim Biophys Acta* 1072:1–7, 1991b.

Shay JW, Zou Y, Hiyama E, Wright WE. Telomerase and cancer. *Hum Mol Genet* 10:677–685, 2001.

Sheen F, Levis RW. Transposition of the LINE-like retrotransposon TART to *Drosophila* chromosome termini. *Proc Natl Acad Sci USA* 91:12510–12514, 1994.

Shelton DN, Chang E, Whittier PS, Choi D, Funk WD. Microarray analysis of replicative senescence. *Curr Biol* 9:939–945, 1999.

Shen ZY, Xu LY, Chen XH, Cai WJ, Shen J, Chen JY, Huang TH, Zeng Y. The genetic events of HPV-immortalized esophageal epithelium cells. *Int J Mol Med* 8:537–542, 2001.

Shen ZY, Xu LY, Li EM, Cai WJ, Chen MH, Shen J, Zeng Y. Telomere and telomerase in the initial stage of immortalization of esophageal epithelial cell. *World J Gastroenterol* 8:357–362, 2002.

Sherr CJ. Cancer cell cycles. *Science* 274:1672–1677, 1996.

Sherr CJ. G1 progression: accelerators and brakes. Presented at Cancer and Molecular Genetics in the Twenty-first Century, Van Andel Research Institute, Grand Rapids, MI, September 5–9, 2000a.

Sherr CJ. The Pezcoller lecture: cancer cell cycles revisited. *Cancer Res* 60:3689–3695, 2000b.

Sherr CJ, DePinho RA. Cellular senescence: mitotic clock or culture shock? *Cell* 102:407–410, 2000.

Sheshadri T, Campisi J. Repression of c-fos and an altered genetic programme in senescent human fibroblasts. *Science* 247:205–209, 1990.

Sheu JC. Molecular mechanism of hepatocarcinogenesis. *J Gastroenterol Hepatol* 12:S309–313, 1997.

Shi J, Perry G, Smith MA, Friedland RP. Vascular abnormalities: the insidious pathogenesis of Alzheimer's disease. *Neurobiol Aging* 21:357–361, 2000.

Shi S, Gronthos S, Chen S, Reddi A, Counter CM, Robey PG, Wang CY. Bone formation by human postnatal bone marrow stromal stem cells is enhanced by telomerase expression. *Nat Biotechnol* 20:587–591, 2002.

Shibanuma M, Mochizuki E, Maniwa R, Mashimo J, Nishiya N, Imai S, Takano T, Oshimura M, Nose K. Induction of senescence-like phenotypes by forced expression of hic-5, which encodes a novel LIM motif protein, in immortalized human fibroblasts. *Mol Cell Biol* 17:1224–1235, 1997.

Shiels PG, Kind AJ, Campbell KH, Waddington D, Wilmut I, Colman A, Schnieke AE. Analysis of telomere lengths in cloned sheep. *Nature* 399:316–317, 1999.

Shifren JL, Schiff I. The aging ovary. *J Womens Health Gend Based Med* 9(Suppl 1):S3–7, 2000.

Shihabuddin LS, Palmer TD, Gage FH. The search for neural progenitor cells: prospects for the therapy of neurodegenerative disease. *Mol Med Today* 5:474–480, 1999.

Shimamoto H. Telomerase activity in oral squamous cell carcinoma and leukoplakia [in Japanese]. *Kokubyo Gakkai Zasshi* 68:125–133, 2001.

Shimazui T, Ami Y, Miyanaga N, Ideyama Y, Nakahara T, Akaza H. Telomerase is upregulated in irreversible preneoplastic lesions during bladder carcinogenesis in rats. *Jpn J Cancer Res* 93:495–500, 2002.

Shimura H, Schlossmacher MG, Hattori N, Frosch MP, Trockenbacher A, Schneider R, Mizuno Y, Kosik KS, Selkoe DJ. Ubiquitination of a new form of α-synuclein by Parkin from human brain: implications for Parkinson's disease. *Science* 293:263–269, 2001.

Shirotani Y, Hiyama K, Ishioka S, Inyaku K, Awaya Y, Yonehara S, Yoshida Y, Inai K, Hiyama E, Hasegawa K, et al. Alteration in length of telomeric repeats in lung cancer. *Lung Cancer* 11:29–41, 1994.

Shmookler Reis RJ, Goldstein S, Harley CB. Is cellular aging a stochastic process? *Mech Ageing Dev* 13:393–395, 1980.

Shoeman RL, Wadle S, Sherbarth A, Traub P. The binding in vitro of the intermediate filament protein vimentin to synthetic oligonucleotides containing telomere sequences. *J Biol Chem* 263:18744–18749, 1988.

Shoji Y, Yoshinaga K, Inoue A, Iwasaki A, Sugihara K. Quantification of telomerase activity in sporadic colorectal carcinoma: association with tumor growth and venous invasion. *Cancer* 88:1304–1309, 2000.

Shor A, Phillips JI. *Chlamydia pneumoniae* and atherosclerosis. *JAMA* 282:2071–2073, 1999.

Shore D. Telomere position effects and transcriptional silencing in the yeast *Saccharomyces cerevisiae*. In Blackburn EH, Greider CW (eds). *Telomeres*. Cold Spring Harbor Laboratory Press, Cold Spring Harbor, NY, 1995, pp 139–191.

Shore D. Different means to common ends. *Nature* 385:676–677, 1997a.

Shore D. Telomerase and telomere-binding proteins: controlling the endgame. *Trends Biochem Sci* 22:233–235, 1997b.

Shore D. Cellular senescence: lessons from yeast for human aging? *Curr Biol* 8:R192–195, 1998a.

Shore D. Telomeres—unsticky ends. *Science* 281:1818–1819, 1998b.

Short KR, Nair KS. Mechanisms of sarcopenia of aging. *J Endocrinol Invest* 22(5 Suppl):95–105, 1999.

Short KR, Nair KS. The effect of age on protein metabolism. *Curr Opin Clin Nutr Metab Care* 3:39–44, 2000.

Shroyer KR. Analysis of telomerase expression as an adjunct in cervical cytopathology. Presented at Telomeres and Telomerase: Implications for Cell Immortality, Cancer, and Age-related Disease. San Francisco, CA, June 1–3, 1998.

Shroyer KR, Thompson LC, Enomoto T, Eskens JL, Shroyer AL, McGregor JA. Telomerase expression in normal epithelium, reactive atypia, squamous dysplasia, and squamous cell carcinoma of the uterine cervix. *Am J Clin Pathol* 109:153–162, 1998

Shroyer NF, Lewis RA, Allikmets R, Singh N, Dean M, Leppert M, Lupski JR. The rod photoreceptor ATP-binding cassette transporter gene, ABCR, and retinal disease: from monogenic to multifactorial. *Vision Res* 39:2537–2544, 1999.

Siddiqui MT, Greene KL, Clark DP, Xydas S, Udelsman R, Smallridge RC, Zeiger MA, Saji M. Human telomerase reverse transcriptase expression in Diff-Quik-stained FNA samples from thyroid nodules. *Diagn Mol Pathol* 10:123–129, 2001.

Sidorov IA, Hirsch KS, Harley CB, Dimitrov DS. Cancer cell dynamics in presence of telomerase inhibitors: analysis of in vitro data. *J Theor Biol* 219:225–233, 2002.

Sikora E, Kaminska B, Radziszewska E, Kazmarek L. Loss of transcription factor AP1 DNA binding activity during lymphocyte aging in vivo. *FEBS Lett* 312:179–182, 1992.

Silverman DHS, Small GW, Chang CY, Lu CS, Kung de Aburto MA, Chen W, Czernin J, Rapoport SI, Pietrini P, Alexander GE, Schapiro MB, Jagust WJ, Hoffman JM, Welsh-Bohmer KA, Alavi A, Clark CM, Salmon E, de Leon MJ, Mielke R, Cummoings JL, Kowell AP, Gambhir SS, Hoh CK, Phelps ME. Positron emission tomography in evaluation of dementia. *JAMA* 286:2120–2127, 2001.

Silverstein FE, Faich G, Goldstein JL, Simon LS, Pincus T, Whelton A, Makuch R, Eisen G, Agrawal NM, Stenson WF, Bur AM, Zhao WW, Kent JD, Lefkowith JB, Verburg KM, Geis GS. Gastrointestinal toxicity with celecoxib vs nonsterioidal anti-inflammatory drugs for osteoarthritis and rheumatoid arthritis. *JAMA* 284:1247–1255, 2000.

Silvestri G. Age-related macular degeneration: genetics and implications for detection and treatment. *Mol Med Today* 3:84–91, 1997.

Simbulan-Rosenthal CM, Ly DH, Rosenthal DS, Konopka G, Luo R, Wang ZQ, Schultz PG, Smulson ME. Misregulation of gene expression in primary fibroblasts lacking poly(ADP-ribose) polymerase. *Proc Natl Acad Sci USA* 97:11274–11279, 2000.

Simickova M, Nekulova M, Pecen L, Cernoch M, Vagundova M, Pacovsky Z. Quantitative determination of telomerase activity in breast cancer and benign breast diseases. *Neoplasma* 48:267–273, 2001.

Simon JA, Hsia J, Cauley JA, Richards C, Harris F, Fong J, Barrett-Connor E, Hulley SB. Postmenopausal hormone therapy and risk of stroke: The Heart and Estrogen-progestin Replacement Study (HERS). *Circulation* 103:638–642, 2001.

Simonsen JL, Rosada C, Serakinci N, Justesen J, Stenderup K, Rattan SI, Jensen TG, Kassem M. Telomerase expression extends the proliferative life span and maintains the osteogenic potential of human bone marrow stromal cells. *Nat Biotechnol* 20:592–596, 2002.

Simonsson T. The human TINF2 gene organisation and chromosomal localization. *Biochimie* 83:433–435, 2001.

Simonsson T, Henriksson M. c-myc suppression in Burkitt's lymphoma cells. *Biochem Biophys Res Commun* 290:11–15, 2002.

Sinclair DA, Mills K, Guarente L. Accelerated aging and nucleolar fragmentation in yeast *sgs1* mutants. *Science* 277:1313–1316, 1997.

Sinclair DA, Mills K, Guarente L. Aging in *Saccharomyces cerevisiae*. *Annu Rev Microbiol* 52:533–560, 1998a.

Sinclair DA, Mills K, Guarente L. Molecular mechanisms of yeast aging. *Trends Biochem Sci* 23:131–134, 1998b.

Singal DP, Goldstein S. Absence of detectable HL-A antigens on cultured fibroblasts in progeria. *J Clin Invest* 52:2259–2263, 1973.

Singer M, Berg P. *Genes and Genomes.* University *Science* Books, Mill Valley, CA, 1991.

Singer MS, Gottschling DE. TLC1: template RNA component of *Saccharomyces cerevisiae* telomerase. *Science* 266:404–409, 1994.

Singer MS, Kahana A, Wolf AJ, Meisinger LL, Peterson SE, Goggin C, Mahowald M, Gottschling DE. Identification of high-copy disruptors of telomeric silencing in *Saccharomyces cerevisiae*. *Genetics* 150:613–632, 1998.

Singh NP, Danner DB, Tice RR, Brant L, Schneider EL. DNA damage and repair with age in individual human lymphocytes. *Mutat Res* 237:123–130, 1990.

Singh NP, Danner DB, Tice RR, Pearson JD, Brant LJ, Morrell CH, Schneider EL. Basal DNA damage in individual human lymphocytes with age. *Mutat Res* 256:1–6, 1991.

Siriaco GM, Cenci G, Haoudi A, Champion LE, Zhou C, Gatti M, Mason JM. Telomere elongation (Tel), a new mutation in *Drosophila melanogaster* that produces long telomeres. *Genetics* 160:235–245, 2002.

Siris ES, Miller PD, Barrett-Connor E, Faulkner KG, Wehren LE, Abbott TA, Berger ML, Santora AC, Sherwood LM. Identification and fracture outcomes of undiagnosed low bone mineral density in postmenopausal women: results from the National Osteoporosis Risk Assessment. *JAMA* 286:2815–2822, 2001.

Sismani C, Armour JA, Flint J, Girgalli C, Regan R, Patsalis PC. Screening for subtelomeric chromosome abnormalities in children with idiopathic mental retardation using multiprobe telomeric FISH and the new MAPH telomeric assay. *Eur J Hum Genet* 9:527–532, 2001.

Sivaraman, Thappa DM, D'Souza M, Ratnakar C. Progeria (Hutchinson-Gilford): a case report. *J Dermatol* 26:324–328, 1999.

Siwicki JK, Hedberg Y, Nowak R, Loden M, Zhao J, Landberg G, Roos G. Long-term cultured IL-2-dependent T cell lines demonstrate p16(INK4a) overexpression, normal pRb/p53, and upregulation of cyclins E or D2. *Exp Gerontol* 35:375–388, 2000.

Skammelsrud N, Martin ER, Murphy P, Khuu C, Frengen E, Kolsto AB. The gene for human transcription factor TCF11 is located telomeric to D17S1827, BTR and HP1Hsβ on chromosome 17q22. *Genet Anal* 15:217–222, 1999.

Skorjanc D, Dunstl G, Pette D. Mitochondrial enzyme defects in normal and low-frequency-stimulated muscles of young and aging rats. *J Gerontol A Biol Sci Med Sci* 56:B503–509, 2001.

Skulachev VP. Aging is a specific biological function rather than the result of a disorder in complex living systems: biochemical evidence in support of Weismann's hypothesis. *Biochemistry (Mosc)* 62:1191–1195, 1997.

Slack JMW. Stem cells in epithelial tissues. *Science* 287:1431–1433, 2000.

Slagboom PE, Droog S, Boomsma DI. Genetic determination of telomere size in humans: a twin study of three age groups. *Am J Hum Genet* 55:876–882, 1994.

Slamon DJ. Use of anti HER2/neu antibody Herceptin in the treatment of human breast cancer; biologic rationale and clinical results. Presented at Cancer and Molecular Genetics in the Twenty-first Century, Van Andel Research Institute, Grand Rapids, MI, September 5–9, 2000.

Slavkin HC, Baum BJ. Relationship of dental and oral pathology to systemic illness. *JAMA* 284:1215–1217, 2000.

Slijepcevic P. Telomeres and mechanisms of Robertsonian fusion. *Chromosoma* 107:136–140, 1998a.

Slijepcevic P. Telomere length regulation—a view from the individual chromosome perspective. *Exp Cell Res* 244:268–274, 1998b.

Slijepcevic P. Telomere length measurement by Q-FISH. *Methods Cell Sci* 23:17–22, 2001.

Slijepcevic P, Bryant PE. Chromosome healing, telomere capture and mechanisms of radiation-induced chromosome breakage. *Int J Radiat Biol* 73:1–13, 1998.

Slijepcevic P, Hande MP. Chinese hamster telomeres are comparable in size to mouse telomeres. *Cytogenet Cell Genet* 85:196–199, 1999.

Slijepcevic P, Hande MP, Bouffler SD, Lansdorp P, Bryant PE. Telomere length, chromatin structure and chromosome fusigenic potential. *Chromosoma* 106:413–421, 1997.

Slominski A, Wortsman J, Carlson AJ, Matsuoka LY, Balch CM, Mihm MC. Malignant melanomas: an update. *Arch Pathol Lab Med* 125:1295–1306, 2001.

Slooter AJ, Tang MX, van Duijn CM, Stern Y, Ott A, Bell K, Breteler MM, Van Broeckhoven C, Tatemichi TK, Tycko B, Hofman A, Mayeux R. Apolipoprotein E epsilon4 and the risk of dementia with stroke. A population-based investigation. *JAMA* 277:818–821, 1997.

Smith CD, Blackburn EH. Uncapping and deregulation of telomeres lead to detrimental cellular consequences in yeast. *J Cell Biol* 145:203–214, 1999.

Smith D, Gupta S, Kaski JC. Chronic infections and coronary heart disease. *Int J Clin Pract* 53:460–466, 1999.

Smith DWE. *Human Longevity*. Oxford University Press, New York, 1993.

Smith JR, Nakanishi M, Robetorye RS, Venable SF, Pereira-Smith OM. Studies demonstrating the complexity of regulation and action of the growth inhibitory gene *SDI1*. *Exp Gerontol* 31:327–335, 1996a.

Smith JR, Ning Y, Pereira-Smith OM. Why are transformed cells immortal? Is the process reversible? *Am J Clin Nutr* 55:1215S–1221S, 1992.

Smith JR, Pereira-Smith OM. Altered gene expression during cellular aging. *Genome* 31:386–389, 1989a.

Smith JR, Pereira-Smith OM. Further studies on the genetic and biochemical basis of cellular senescence. *Exp Gerontol* 24:377–381, 1989b.

Smith JR, Pereira-Smith OM. Genetic and molecular studies of cellular immortalization. *Adv Cancer Res* 54:63–77, 1990.

Smith JR, Pereira-Smith OM. Replicative senescence: implications for in vivo aging and tumor suppression. *Science* 273:63–67, 1996.

Smith JR, Pereira-Smith OM, Braunschweiger KI, Roberts TW, Whitney RG. A general method for determining the replicative age of normal animal cell cultures. *Mech Ageing Dev* 12:355–365, 1980.

Smith JR, Pereira-Smith OM, Schneider EL. Colony size distributions as a measure of in vivo and in vitro aging. *Proc Natl Acad Sci USA* 75:1353–1356, 1978.

Smith JR, Venable S, Roberts TW, Metter EJ, Monticone R, Schneider EL. Relationship between in vivo age and in vitro aging: assessment of 669 cell cultures derived from members of The Baltimore Longitudinal Study of Aging. *J Gerontol A Biol Sci Med Sci* 57A:B239–246, 2002.

Smith JR, Whitney RG. Intraclonal variation in proliferative potential of human diploid fibroblasts: stochastic mechanism for cellular aging. *Science* 207:82–84, 1980.

Smith KJ, Germain M, Skelton H. Perspectives in dermatopathology: telomeres and telomerase in ageing and cancer; with emphasis on cutaneous disease. *J Cutan Pathol* 27:2–18, 2000a.

Smith MA, Joseph JA, Perry G. Arson. Tracking the culprit in Alzheimer's disease. *Ann NY Acad Sci* 924:35–38, 2000b.

Smith MA, Nunomura A, Zhu X, Takeda A, Perry G. Metabolic, metallic, and mitotic sources of oxidative stress in Alzheimer disease. *Antioxid Redox Signal* 2:413–420, 2000c.

Smith MA, Perry G, Richey PL, Sayre LM, Anderson VE, Beal MF, Kowall N. Oxidative damage in Alzheimer's. *Nature* 382:120–121, 1996b.

Smith MA, Rottkamp CA, Nunomura A, Raina AK, Perry G. Oxidative stress in Alzheimer's disease. *Biochim Biophys Acta* 1502:139–144, 2000d.

Smith RG. The aging process: where are the drug opportunities? *Curr Opin Chem Biol* 4:371–376, 2000.

Smith S, de Lange T. Cell cycle dependent localization of the telomeric PARP, tankyrase, to nuclear pore complexes and centrosomes. *J Cell Sci* 112:3649–3656, 1999.

Smith S, Giriat I, Schmitt A, de Lange T. Tankyrase, a poly(ADP-ribose) polymerase at human telomeres. *Science* 282:1484–1487, 1998.

Smith SD, Wheeler MA, Plescia J, Colberg JW, Weiss RM, Altieri DC. Urine detection of survivin and diagnosis of bladder cancer. *JAMA* 285:324–328, 2001.

Smith SE. The role of antioxidants in AMD: ongoing research. *J Ophthalmic Nurs Technol* 18:68–70, 1999.

Smith ZE, Higgs DR. The pattern of replication at a human telomeric region (16p13.3): its relationship to chromosome structure and gene expression. *Hum Mol Genet* 8:1373–1386, 1999.

Smogorzewska A, de Lange T. Different telomere damage signaling pathways in human and mouse cells. *EMBO J* 21:4338–4348, 2002.

Smogorzewska A, van Steensel B, Bianchi A, Oelmann S, Schaefer MR, Schnapp G, de Lange T. Control of human telomere length by TRF1 and TRF2. *Mol Cell Biol* 20:1659–1668, 2000.

Smoyer WE, Mundel P. Regulation of podocyte structure during the development of nephrotic syndrome. *J Mol Med* 76:172–183, 1998.

Snijders PJ, van Duin M, Walboomers JM, Steenbergen RD, Risse EK, Helmerhorst TJ, Verheijen RH, Meijer CJ. Telomerase activity exclusively in cervical carcinomas and a subset of cervical intraepithelial neoplasia grade III lesions: strong association with elevated messenger RNA levels of its catalytic subunit and high-risk human papillomavirus DNA. *Cancer Res* 58:3812–3818, 1998.

Snow KK, Seddon JM. Do age-related macular degeneration and cardiovascular disease share common antecedents? *Ophthalmic Epidemiol* 6:125–143, 1999.

Snow RW, Craig MH, Deichmann U, le Sueur D. A preliminary continental risk map for malaria mortality among African children. *Parasitol Today* 15:99–104, 1999.

Snowden JA, Brooks PM. Hematopoietic stem cell transplantation in rheumatic diseases. *Curr Opin Rheumatol* 11:167–172, 1999.

Soares MV, Borthwick NJ, Maini MK, Janossy G, Salmon M, Akbar AN. IL-7-dependent extrathymic expansion of CD45RA+ T cells enables preservation of a naive repertoire. *J Immunol* 161:5909–5917, 1998.

Soares MV, Maini MK, Beverley PC, Salmon M, Akbar AN. Regulation of apoptosis and replicative senescence in CD8+ T cells from patients with viral infections. *Biochem Soc Trans* 28:255–258, 2000.

Soda H, Raymond E, Sharma S, Lawrence R, Davidson K, Oka M, Kohno S, Izbicka E, Von Hoff DD. Effects of androgens on telomerase activity in normal and malignant prostate cells in vitro. *Prostate* 43:161–168, 2000.

Soder AI, Hoare SF, Muir S, Going JJ, Parkinson EK, Keith WN. Amplification, increased dosage and in situ expression of the telomerase RNA gene in human cancer. *Oncogene* 14:1013–1021, 1997.

Sohal RS, Weindruch R. Oxidative stress, caloric restriction, and aging. *Science* 273:59–63, 1996.

Sohn SH, Multani AS, Gugnani PK, Pathak S. Telomere erosion-induced mitotic catastrophe in continuously grown chinese hamster don cells. *Exp Cell Res* 279:271–276, 2002.

Solana R, Pawelec G. Molecular and cellular basis of immunosenescence. *Mech Ageing Dev* 102:115–129, 1998.

Solerte SB, Gornati R, Cravello L, Albertelli N, Oberti S, Perotta D, Rossi G, Cuzzoni G, Ferrari E, Fioravanti M. Dehydroepiandrosterone-sulfate (DHEA-S) restores the release of IGF-I from natural killer (NK) immune in old patients with dementia of Alzheimer's type (DAT). *J Endocrinol Invest* 22(10 Suppl):32–34, 1999.

Soliman A, Hawkins D. The link between Down's syndrome and Alzheimer's disease: 1. *Br J Nurs* 7:779–784, 1998a.

Soliman A, Hawkins D. The link between Down's syndrome and Alzheimer's disease: 2. *Br J Nurs* 7:847–850, 1998b.

Solomon PR, Adams F, Silver A, Zimmer J, DeVeaux R. Ginkgo for memory enhancement: a randomized controlled trial. *JAMA* 288:835–840, 2002.

Sommerfeld HJ, Meeker AK, Piatyszek MA, Bova GS, Shay JW, Coffey DS. Telomerase activity: a prevalent marker of malignant human prostate tissue. *Cancer Res* 56:218–222, 1996.

Son NH, Murray S, Yanovski J, Hodes RJ, Weng N. Lineage-specific telomere shortening and unaltered capacity for telomerase expression in human T and B lymphocytes with age. *J Immunol* 165:1191–1196, 2000.

Sondergaard SR, Essen MV, Schjerling P, Ullum H, Pedersen BK. Proliferation and telomere length in acutely mobilized blood mononuclear cells in HIV infected patients. *Clin Exp Immunol* 127:499–506, 2002.

Song S, Morgan M, Ellis T, Poirier A, Chesnut K, Wang J, Brantly M, Muzyczka N, Byrne BJ, Atkinson M, Flotte TR. Sustained secretion of human alpha-1–antitrypsin from murine muscle transduced with adeno-associated virus vectors. *Proc Natl Acad Sci USA* 95:14384–14388, 1998.

Sonntag WE, Lynch CD, Bennett SA, Khan AS, Thornton PL, Cooney PT, Ingram RL, McShane T, Brunso-Bechtold JK. Alterations in insulin-like growth factor-1 gene and protein expression and type 1 insulin-like growth factor receptors in the brains of ageing rats. *Neuroscience* 88:269–279, 1999a.

Sonntag WE, Lynch CD, Cefalu WT, Ingram RL, Bennett SA, Thornton PL, Khan AS. Pleiotropic effects of growth hormone and insulin-like growth factor (IGF)-1 on biological aging: inferences from moderate caloric-restricted animals. *J Gerontol A Biol Sci Med Sci* 54:B521–538, 1999b.

Sonntag WE, Lynch CD, Cooney PT, Hutchins PM. Decreases in cerebral microvasculature with age are associated with the decline in growth hormone and insulin-like growth factor 1. *Endocrinology* 138:3515–3520, 1997.

Sonntag WE, Xu X, Ingram RL, D'Costa A. Moderate caloric restriction alters the subcellular distribution of somatostatin mRNA and increases growth hormone pulse amplitude in aged animals. *Neuroendocrinology* 61:601–608, 1995.

Sonoda Y, Zhu J, Pieper RO. Exogenous hTERT prevents immortalization-induced aberrant cpg island methylation in normal human fibroblasts. *Proceedings of the 91st Annual Meeting of the American Association for Cancer Research*, Vol. 41, Abstract #1437, March 2000.

Sopher BL, Fukuchi K, Kavanagh TJ, Furlong CE, Martin GM. Neurodegenerative mechanisms in Alzheimer disease. A role for oxidative damage in amyloid beta protein precursor–mediated cell death. *Mol Chem Neuropathol* 29:153–68, 1996.

Sopher BL, Fukuchi K, Smith AC, Leppig KA, Furlong CE, Martin GM. Cytotoxicity mediated by conditional expression of a carboxyl-terminal derivative of the beta-amyloid precursor protein. *Brain Res Mol Brain Res* 26:207–217, 1994.

Sopko G. Preventing cardiac events and restenosis after percutaneous coronary intervention. *JAMA* 287:3259–3261, 2002.

Soria JC, Morat L, Commo F, Dabit D, Perie S, Sabatier L, Fouret P. Telomerase activation cooperates with inactivation of p16 in early head and neck tumorigenesis. *Br J Cancer* 84:504–511, 2001.

Soria JC, Vielh P, el-Naggar AK. Telomerase activity in cancer: a magic bullet or a mirage? *Adv Anat Pathol* 5:86–94, 1998.

Sorrentino JA, Millis AJT. Structural comparisons of fibronectin isolated from early and late passage cells. *Mech Ageing Dev* 28:83–97, 1984.

Sosunov AA, Krugliakov PP, SHvalev VN, Guski G, Postnov IuV. Age-related changes in the autonomic ganglia [in Russian]. *Arkh Patol* 59:32–37, 1997.

Southern SA, Herrington CS. Molecular events in uterine cervical cancer. *Sex Transm Infect* 74:101–109, 1998.

Southern SA, Herrington CS. Disruption of cell cycle control by human papillomaviruses with special reference to cervical carcinoma. *Int J Gynecol Cancer* 10:263–274, 2000.

Sowers MF, Pope S, Welch G, Sternfeld B, Albrecht G. The association of menopause and physical functioning in women at midlife. *J Am Geriatr Soc* 49:1485–1492, 2001.

Sozou PD, Kirkwood TB. A stochastic model of cell replicative senescence based on telomere shortening, oxidative stress, and somatic mutations in nuclear and mitochondrial DNA. *J Theor Biol* 213:573–586, 2001.

Span JP, Pieters GF, Sweep CG, Swinkels LM, Smals AG. Plasma IGF-I is a useful marker of growth hormone deficiency in adults. *J Endocrinol Invest* 22:446–450, 1999.

Spaulding C, Guo W, Effros RB. Resistance to apoptosis in human CD8+ T cells that reach replicative senescence after multiple rounds of antigen-specific proliferation. *Exp Gerontol* 34:633–644 , 1999.

Spaulding CC, Walford RL, Effros RB. Calorie restriction inhibits the age-related dysregulation of the cytokines TNF-alpha and IL-6 in C3B10RF1 mice. *Mech Ageing Dev* 93:87–94, 1997a.

Spaulding CC, Walford RL, Effros RB. The accumulation of non-replicative, non-functional, senescent T cells with age is avoided in calorically restricted mice by an enhancement of T cell apoptosis. *Mech Ageing Dev* 93:25–33, 1997b.

Speiser DE, Migliaccio M, Pittet MJ, Valmori D, Lienard D, Lejeune F, Reichenbach P, Guillaume P, Luscher I, Cerottini JC, Romero P. Human CD8(+) T cells expressing HLA-DR and CD28 show telomerase activity and are distinct from cytolytic effector T cells. *Eur J Immunol* 31:459–466, 2001.

Spiering AL, Pereira-Smith OM, Smith JR. Correlation between complementation group for immortality and DNA synthesis inhibitors. *Exp Cell Res* 195:541–545, 1991.

Spiering AL, Smith JR, Pereira-Smith OM. A potent DNA synthesis inhibitor expressed by the immortal cell line SUSM-1. *Exp Cell Res* 179:159–167, 1988.

Spillantini MG, Goedert M. Tau and Parkinson disease. *JAMA* 286:2324–2326, 2001.

Spitkovsky DM. Telomere DNA sequences and the concept of ontogenetic reserve cells. *Biochemistry (Mosc)* 62:1285–1290, 1997.

Spruill MD, Nelson DO, Ramsey MJ, Nath J, Tucker JD. Lifetime persistence and clonality of chromosome aberrations in the peripheral blood of mice acutely exposed to ionizing radiation. *Radiat Res* 153:110–121, 2000.

Sprung CN, Bryan TM, Reddel RR, Murnane JP. Normal telomere maintenance in immortal ataxia telangiectasia cell lines. *Mutat Res* 379:177–184, 1997.

Sramek JJ, Alexander BD, Cutler NR. Acetylcholinesterase inhibitors for the treatment of Alzheimer's disease. *Ann Long Term Care* 9:15–22, 2001.

Stadtman ER. Protein oxidation and aging. *Science* 257:1220–1224, 1992.

Stamey TA, Johnstone IM, McNeal JE, Lu AY, Yemoto CM. Preoperative serum prostate specific antigen levels between 2 and 22 ng/ml correlate poorly with post-radical prostatectomy canccer morphology: prostate specific antigen cure rates appear constant between 2 and 9 ng/ml. *J Urol* 167:103–111, 2002.

Stamler J. A radical vascular connection. *Nature* 380:108–110, 1996.

Stamler J, Daviglus ML, Garside DB, Dyer AR, Greenland P, Neaton JD. Relationship of baseline serum cholesterol levels in 3 large cohorts of younger men to long-term coronary, cardiovascular, and all-cause mortality and to longevity. *JAMA* 284:311–318, 2000.

Staniforth M. *Marcus Aurelius: Meditations.* Penguin Classics, Penguin Books, New York, 1964.

Stansel RM, de Lange T, Griffith JD. T-loop assembly in vitro involves binding of TRF2 near the 3' telomeric overhang. *EMBO J* 20:5532–5540, 2001.

Stansel RM, Subramanian D, Griffith JD. p53 binds telomeric single strand overhangs and t-loop junctions in vitro. *J Biol Chem* 277:11625–11628, 2002.

Stanta G, Bonin S, Niccolini B, Raccanelli A, Baralle F. Catalytic subunit of telomerase expression is related to RNA component expression. *FEBS Lett* 460:285–288, 1999.

Stanulis-Praeger BM, Gilchrest BA. Growth factor responsiveness declines during adulthood for human skin-derived cells. *Mech Ageing Dev* 35:185–198, 1986.

Stavenhagen JB, Zakian VA. Internal tracts of telomeric DNA act as silencers in *Saccharomyces cerevisiae*. *Genes Dev* 8:1411–1422, 1994.

Stavenhagen JB, Zakian VA. Yeast telomeres exert a position effect on recombination between internal tracts of yeast telomeric DNA. *Genes Dev* 12:3044–3058, 1998.

Stavropoulos DJ, Bradshaw PS, Li X, Pasic I, Truong K, Ikura M, Ungrin M, Meyn MS. The Bloom syndrome helicase BLM interacts with TRF2 in ALT cells and promotes telomeric DNA synthesis. *Hum Mol Genet* 11:3135–144, 2002.

St. Croix B, Rago C, Velculescu V, Traverso G, Romans KD, Montgomery E, Lal A, Riggins GJ, Lengauer C, Vogelstein B, Kinzler KW. Genes expressed in human tumor endothelium. *Science* 289:1197–1202, 2000.

Steenbergen RD, Kramer D, Meijer CJ, Walboomers JM, Trott DA, Cuthbert AP, Newbold RF, Overkamp WJ, Zdzienicka MZ, Snijders PJ. Telomerase suppression by chromosome 6 in a human papillomavirus type 16-immortalized keratinocyte cell line and in a cervical cancer cell line. *J Natl Cancer Inst* 93:865–872, 2001.

Steenbergen RD, Walboomers JM, Meijer CJ, van der Raaij-Helmer EM, Parker JN, Chow LT, Broker TR, Snijders PJ. Transition of human papillomavirus type 16 and 18 transfected human foreskin keratinocytes towards immortality: activation of telomerase and allele losses at 3p, 10p, 11q and/or 18q. *Oncogene* 13:1249–1257, 1996.

Stege GJ, Bosman GJ. The biochemistry of Alzheimer's disease. *Drugs Aging* 14:437–446, 1999.

Stein GH, Drullinger LF, Robetorye RS, Pereira-Smith OM, Smith JR. Senescent cells fail to express cdc2, cycA, and cycB in response to mitogen stimulation. *Proc Natl Acad Sci USA* 88:11012–11016, 1991.

Steinberg D, Parthasarathy S, Carew TE, Khoo JC, Witztum JL. Beyond cholesterol. Modifications of low-density lipoprotein that increase its atherogenicity. *N Engl J Med* 320:915–924, 1989.

Steinberg D, Gotto AM. Preventing coronary artery disease by lowering cholesterol levels. *JAMA* 282:2043–2050, 1999.

Steinert S, Shay JW, Wright WE. Transient expression of human telomerase extends the life span of normal human fibroblasts. *Biochem Biophys Res Commun* 273:1095–1098, 2000.

Steinert S, White DM, Zou Y, Shay JW, Wright WE. Telomere biology and cellular aging in nonhuman primate cells. *Exp Cell Res* 272:146–152, 2002.

Steinsaltz A. *The Essential Talmud*. Harper Colophon Books, New York, 1976.

Stephens P, Cook H, Hilton J, Jones CJ, Haughton MF, Wyllie FS, Skinner JW, Harding KG, Kipling D, Thomas DW. An analysis of replicative senescence in dermal fibroblasts derived from chronic leg wounds predicts that telomerase therapy would fail to reverse their disease-specific cellular and proteolytic phenotype. *Exp Cell Res* 283:22–35, 2003.

Stephenson, J. A role for mitochondria in age-related disorders? *JAMA* 275:1531–1532, 1996.

Stephenson, J. Estrogen as a carcinogen. *JAMA* 285:284, 2001.

Stern L, Allison L, Coppel RL, Dix TI. Discovering patterns in *Plasmodium falciparum* genomic DNA. *Mol Biochem Parasitol* 118:175–186, 2001.

Stern Y, Albert S, Tang MX, Tsai WY. Rate of memory decline in AD is related to education and occupation: cognitive reserve? *Neurology* 53:1942–1947, 1999.

Sternberg SA, Wolfson C, Baumgarten M. Undetected dementia in community-dwelling older people: the Canadian Study of Health and Aging. *J Am Geriatr Soc* 48:1430–1434, 2000.

Stevenson JB, Gottschling DE. Telomeric chromatin modulates replication timing near chromosome ends. *Genes Dev* 13:146–151, 1999.

Stewart N, Bacchetti S. Expression of SV40 large T antigen, but not small t antigen, is required for the induction of chromosomal aberrations in transformed human cells. *Virology* 180:49–57, 1991.

Stewart SA, Ben-Porath I, Carey VJ, O'Connor BF, Hahn WC, Weinberg RA. Erosion of the telomeric single-strand overhang at replicative senescence. *Nat Genet* 33:492–496, 2003.

Stewart SA, Hahn WC, O'Connor BF, Banner EN, Lundberg AS, Modha P, Mizuno H, Brooks MW, Fleming M, Zimonjic DB, Popescu NC, Weinberg RA. Telomerase contributes to tumorigenesis by a telomere length-independent mechanism. *Proc Natl Acad Sci USA* 99:12606–12611, 2002.

Stewart SA, Weinberg RA. Telomerase and human tumorigenesis. *Semin Cancer Biol* 10:399–406, 2000.

Stewart SA, Weinberg RA. Senescence: does it all happen at the ends? *Oncogene* 21:627–630, 2002.

Stoll G, Jander S. The role of microglia and macrophages in the pathophysiology of the CNS. *Prog Neurobiol* 58:233–247, 1999.

Stoll G, Jander S, Schroeter M. Inflammation and glial responses in ischemic brain lesions. *Prog Neurobiol* 56:149–171, 1998.

Stomati M, Rubino S, Spinetti A, Parrini D, Luisi S, Casarosa E, Petraglia F, Genazzani AR. Endocrine, neuroendocrine and behavioral effects of oral dehydroepiandrosterone sulfate supplementation in postmenopausal women. *Gynecol Endocrinol* 13:15–25, 1999.

Stone DJ, Rozovsky I, Morgan TE, Anderson CP, Hajian H, Finch CE. Astrocytes and microglia respond to estrogen with increased apoE mRNA in vivo and in vitro. *Exp Neurol* 143:313–318, 1997.

Stoppler H, Hartmann DP, Sherman L, Schlegel R. The human papillomavirus type 16 E6 and E7 oncoproteins dissociate cellular telomerase activity from the maintenance of telomere length. *J Biol Chem* 272:13332–13337, 1997.

Stoppler H, Stoppler MC, Kisiela M, Holzbach A, Moll I, Houdek P, Moll R. Telomerase activity of Merkel cell carcinomas and Merkel cell carcinoma–derived cell cultures. *Arch Dermatol Res* 293:397–406, 2001.

Strahl-Bolsinger S, Hecht A, Luo K, Grunstein M. SIR2 and SIR4 interactions differ in core and extended telomeric heterochromatin in yeast. *Genes Dev* 11:83–93, 1997.

Straub B, Muller M, Krause H, Goessl C, Schrader M, Heicappell R, Miller K. Molecular staging of pelvic surgical margins after radical prostatectomy: comparison of RT-PCR for prostate-specific antigen and telomerase activity. *Oncol Rep* 9:545–549, 2002.

Straub RH, Cutolo M, Zietz B, Scholmerich J. The process of aging changes the interplay of the immune, endocrine and nervous systems. *Mech Ageing Dev* 122:1591–1611, 2001.

Strauss E. Growing old together. *Science* 292:41–43, 2001.

Street KA, Hall KL, Murphy P, Walter CA. Formamidopyriidine-DNA glycosylate targeted to specific organelles in C2C12 cells. *J Anti-Aging Med* 2:275–285, 1999.

Streit WJ. The role of microglia in regeneration. *Eur Arch Otorhinolaryngol* Suppl:S69–70, 1994.

Streit WJ. Microglial response to brain injury: a brief synopsis. *Toxicol Pathol* 28:28–30, 2000.

Streit WJ. Microglia as neuroprotective, immuno competent cell of the CNS. *Glia* 40:133–139, 2002.

Streit WJ, Sparks DL. Activation of microglia in the brains of humans with heart disease and hypercholesterolemic rabbits. *J Mol Med* 75:130–138, 1997.

Streit WJ, Walter SA, Pennell NA. Reactive microgliosis. *Prog Neurobiol* 57:563–581, 1999.

Strittmatter WJ, Saunders AM, Schmechel D, Pericak-Vance M, Enghild J, Salvesen GS, Roses AD. Apolipoprotein E: high-avidity binding to beta-amyloid and increased frequency of type 4 allele in late-onset familial Alzheimer disease. *Proc Natl Acad Sci USA* 90:1977–1981, 1993.

Strollo F. Hormonal changes in humans during spaceflight. *Adv Space Biol Med* 7:99–129, 1999.

Struhl K. A paradigm for precision. *Science* 293:1054–1055, 2001.

Sturrock RR. Changes in neurologia and myelination in the white matter of aging mice. *J Gerontol* 31:513–522, 1976.

Su IH, Frank R, Gauthier BG, Valderrama E, Simon DB, Lifton RP, Trachtman H. Bartter syndrome and focal segmental glomerulosclerosis: a possible link between two diseases. *Pediatr Nephrol* 14:970–972, 2000.

Suda T, Fujiyama A, Takimoto M, Igarashi M, Kuroiwa T, Waguri N, Kawai H, Mita Y, Aoyagi Y. Interchromosomal telomere length variation. *Biochem Biophys Res Commun* 291:210–214, 2002.

Suda T, Isokawa O, Aoyagi Y, Nomoto M, Tsukada K, Shimizu T, Suzuki Y, Naito A, Igarashi H, Yanagi M, Takahashi T, Asakura H. Quantitation of telomerase activity in hepatocellular carcinoma: a possible aid for a prediction of recurrent diseases in the remnant liver. *Hepatology* 27:402–406, 1998.

Suehara N, Mizumoto K, Tanaka M, Niiyama H, Yokohata K, Tominaga Y, Shimura H, Muta T, Hamasaki N. Telomerase activity in pancreatic juice differentiates ductal carcinoma from adenoma and pancreatitis. *Clin Cancer Res* 3:2479–2483, 1997.

Sugihara S, Mihara K, Marunouchi T, Inoue H, Namba M. Telomere elongation observed in immortalized human fibroblasts by treatment with 60Co gamma rays or 4-nitroquinoline 1-oxide. *Hum Genet* 97:1–6, 1996.

Sugimoto M. Characteristic telomere dynamics of Werner syndrome (WS) cells and telomerase-negative immortalized cells: possible mechanism of telomere elongation in the absence of telomerase. Presented at Telomeres and Telomerase: Implications for Cell Immortality, Cancer, and Age-related Disease. San Francisco, CA, June 1–3, 1998.

Sugita K, Suzuki N, Fujii K, Niimi H. Reduction of unscheduled DNA synthesis and plasminogen activator activity in Hutchinson-Gilford fibroblasts during passaging in vitro: partial correction by interferon-beta. *Mutat Res* 316:133–138, 1995.

Sugiyama S, Takasawa M, Hayakawa M, Ozawa T. Changes in skeletal muscle, heart, and liver mitochondrial electron transport activities in rats and dogs of various ages. *Biochem Mol Biol Int* 30:937–944, 1993.

Suh CI, Shanafelt T, May DJ, Shroyer KR, Bobak JB, Crawford ED, Miller GJ, Markham N, Glode LM. Comparison of telomerase activity and GSTP1 promoter methylation in ejaculate as potential screening tests for prostate cancer. *Mol Cell Probes* 14:211–217, 2000.

Sullivan GW, Sarembock IJ, Linden J. The role of inflammation in vascular diseases. *J Leukoc Biol* 67:591–602, 2000.

Sumida T, Hamakawa H. Telomerase and oral cancer. *Oral Oncol* 37:333–340, 2001.

Sumida T, Hamakawa H, Kayahara H, Zen H, Sogawa K, Tanioka H, Ueda N. Clinical usefulness of telomerase assay for the detection of lymph node metastasis in patients with oral malignancy. *Arch Pathol Lab Med* 124:398–400, 2000.

Sun D. Biotinylated primer for detecting telomerase activity without amplification. In Double JA, Thompson MJ (eds). *Telomeres and Telomerase: Methods and Protocols.* Humana Press, Totowa, NJ, 2002, pp 165–172.

Sunderkotter C, Kalden H, Luger TA. Aging and the skin immune system. *Arch Dermatol* 133:1256–1262, 1997.

Surralles J, Hande MP, Marcos R, Lansdorp PM. Accelerated telomere shortening in the human inactive X chromosome. *Am J Hum Genet* 65:1617–1622, 1999.

Suter H, Tonz O, Scharli A. Geroderma osteodysplastica hereditaria (GOH) in a girl. *Prog Clin Biol Res* 104:327–329, 1982.

Suzuki K, Kashimura H, Ohkawa J, Itabashi M, Watanabe T, Sawahata T, Nakahara A, Muto H, Tanaka N. Expression of human telomerase catalytic subunit gene in cancerous and precancerous gastric conditions. *J Gastroenterol Hepatol* 15:744–751, 2000.

Suzuki K, Oberley TD, Pugh TD, Sempf JM, Weindruch R. Caloric restriction diminishes the age-associated loss of immunoreactive catalase in rat prostate. *Prostate* 33:256–263, 1997.

Suzuki S, Fukushima T, Ami H, Onogi H, Nakamura I, Takenoshita S. New attempt of preoperative differential diagnosis of thyroid neoplasms by telomerase activity measurement. *Oncol Rep* 9:539–544, 2002.

Svendsen CN, Caldwell MA, Ostenfeld T. Human neural stem cells: isolation, expansion and transplantation. *Brain Pathol* 9:499–513, 1999.

Sviderskaya EV, Hill SP, Evans-Whipp TJ, Chin L, Orlow SJ, Easty DJ, Cheong SC, Beach D, DePinho RA, Bennett DC. p16(Ink4a) in melanocyte senescence and differentiation. *J Natl Cancer Inst* 94:446–454, 2002.

Sweet MA, Ntambi JA, Gaumnitz EA, Pugh TD, Weindruch R, Singaram C. Neuropeptide Y- and peptide YY-containing colonic cells increase with ageing in male rats. *Neuropeptides* 30:385–390, 1996.

Syntin P, Chen H, Zirkin BR, Robaire B. Gene expression in brown norway rat Leydig cells: effects of age and of age-related germ cell loss. *Endocrinology* 142:5277–5285, 2001.

Szalai VA, Singer MJ, Thorp HH. Site-specific probing of oxidative reactivity and telomerase function using 7,8-dihydro-8-oxoguanine in telomeric DNA. *J Am Chem Soc* 124:1625–1631, 2002.

Szamosi T, Szollar J, Meggyesi V, Wilhelm O, Bodanszky H, Matyus J. Serum cholesterol and triglyceride levels in progeria as a model of ageing. *Mech Ageing Dev* 28:243–248, 1984.

Szilard L. On the nature of the aging process. *Proc Natl Acad Sci USA* 45:30–45, 1959.

Szutorisz H, Palmqvist R, Roos G, Stenling R, Schorderet DF, Reddel R, Lingner J, Nabholz M. Rearrangements of minisatellites in the human telomerase reverse transcriptase gene are not correlated with its expression in colon carcinomas. *Oncogene* 20:2600–2605, 2001.

Taddei S, Virdis A, Ghiadoni L, Salvetti G, Salvetti A. Endothelial dysfunction in hypertension. *J Nephrol* 13:205–210, 2000.

Taddei S, Virdis A, Mattei P, Ghiadoni L, Fasolo CB, Sudano I, Salvetti A. Hypertension causes premature aging of endothelial function in humans. *Hypertension* 29:736–743, 1997.

Tagawa N, Tamanaka J, Fujinami A, Kobayashi Y, Takano T, Fukata S, Kuma K, Tada H, Amino N. Serum dehydroepiandrosterone, dehydroepiandrosterone sulfate, and pregnenolone sulfate concentrations in patients with hyperthyroidism and hypothyroidism. *Clin Chem* 46:523–528, 2000.

Taggart AK, Teng SC, Zakian VA. Est1p as a cell cycle–regulated activator of telomere-bound telomerase. *Science* 297:1023–1026, 2002.

Tahara E. Molecular mechanism of human stomach carcinogenesis implicated in *Helicobacter pylori* infection. *Exp Toxicol Pathol* 50:375–378, 1998.

Tahara E. Molecular aspects of invasion and metastasis of stomach cancer. *Verh Dtsch Ges Pathol* 84:43–49, 2000.

Tahara H, Kuniyasu H, Yokozaki H, Yasui W, Shay JW, Ide T, Tahara E. Telomerase activity in preneoplastic and neoplastic gastric and colorectal lesions. *Clin Cancer Res* 1:1245–1251, 1995a.

Tahara H, Nakanishi T, Kitamoto M, Nakashio R, Shay JW, Tahara E, Kajiyama G, Ide T. Telomerase activity in human liver tissues: comparison between chronic liver disease and hepatocellular carcinomas. *Cancer Res* 55:2734–2736, 1995b.

Tahara H, Sato E, Noda A, Ide T. Increase in expression level of p21[sdi1/cip1/waf1] with increasing division age in both normal and SV40–transformed human fibroblasts. *Oncogene* 10:835–840, 1995c.

Tahara H, Tokutake Y, Maeda S, Kataoka H, Watanabe T, Satoh M, Matsumoto T, Sugawara M, Ide T, Goto M, Furuichi Y, Sugimoto M. Abnormal telomere dynamics of B-lymphoblastoid cell strains from Werner's syndrome patients transformed by Epstein-Barr virus. *Oncogene* 15:1911–1920, 1997.

Takagi S, Kinouchi Y, Hiwatashi N, Nagashima F, Chida M, Takahashi S, Negoro K, Shimosegawa T, Toyota T. Relationship between microsatellite instability and telomere shortening in colorectal cancer. *Dis Colon Rectum* 43(10 Suppl):S12–17, 2000.

Takahashi M, Kigawa J, Oishi T, Itamochi H, Shimada M, Sato S, Kamazawa S, Akeshima R, Terakawa N. Alteration of telomerase activity in ovarian cancer after chemotherapy. *Gynecol Obstet Invest* 49:204–208, 2000.

Takaishi H, Kitamoto M, Takahashi S, Aikata H, Kawakami Y, Nakanishi T, Nakamura Y, Shimamoto F, Kajiyama G, Ide T. Precancerous hepatic nodules had significant levels of telomerase activity determined by sensitive quantitation using a hybridization protection assay. *Cancer* 88:312–317, 2000.

Takakura M, Kyo S, Kanaya T, Hirano H, Takeda J, Yutsudo M, Inoue M. Cloning of human telomerase catalytic subunit (hTERT) gene promoter and identification of proximal core promoter sequences essential for transcriptional activation in immortalized and cancer cells. *Cancer Res* 59:551–557, 1999.

Takakura M, Kyo S, Kanaya T, Tanaka M, Inoue M. Expression of human telomerase subunits and correlation with telomerase activity in cervical cancer. *Cancer Res* 58:1558–1561, 1998.

Takakura M, Kyo S, Sowa Y, Wang Z, Yatabe N, Maida Y, Tanaka M, Inoue M. Telomerase activation by histone deacetylase inhibitor in normal cells. *Nucleic Acids Res* 29:3006–3011, 2001.

Takashima S. Down syndrome. *Curr Opin Neurol* 10:148–152, 1997.

Takeda T, Hosokawa M, Takeshita S, Irino M, Higuchi K, Matsushita T, Tomita Y, Yashuhira K, Hamamoto H, Shimizu K, Ishii M, Yamamuro T. A new murine model of accelerated senescence. *Mech Aging Dev* 17:183–194, 1981.

Takemoto L, Boyle D. The possible role of alpha-crystallins in human senile cataractogenesis. *Int J Biol Macromol* 22:331–337, 1998.

Takubo K, Izumiyama-Shimomura N, Honma N, Sawabe M, Arai T, Kato M, Oshimura M, Nakamura K. Telomere lengths are characteristic in each human individual. *Exp Gerontol* 37:523–531, 2002.

Takubo K, Nakamura K, Arai T, Nakachi K, Ebuchi M. Telomere length in breast carcinoma of the young and aged [in Japanese]. *Nippon Rinsho* 56:1283–1286, 1998.

Takubo K, Nakamura K, Izumiyama N, Furugori E, Sawabe M, Arai T, Esaki Y, Mafune K, Kammori M, Fujiwara, Kato M, Oshimura M, Sasajima K. Telomere shortening with aging in human liver. *J Gerontol A Biol Sci Med Sci* 55:B533–536, 2000.

Takubo K, Nakamura K, Izumiyama N, Mafune K, Tanaka Y, Miyashita M, Sasajima K, Kato M, Oshimura M. Telomerase activity in esophageal carcinoma. *J Surg Oncol* 66:88–92, 1997.

Takubo K, Nakamura KI, Izumiyama N, Sawabe M, Arai T, Esaki Y, Tanaka Y, Mafune KI, Fujiwara M, Kammori M, Sasajima K. Telomere shortening with aging in human esophageal mucosa. *AGE* 22:95–99, 1999.

Tamura K, Chen YE, Lopez-Ilasaca M, Daviet L, Tamura N, Ishigami T, Akishita M, Takasaki I, Tokita Y, Pratt RE, Horiuchi M, Dzau VJ, Umemura S. Molecular mechanism of fibronectin gene activation by cyclic stretch in vascular smooth muscle cells. *J Biol Chem* 275:34619–34627, 2000.

Tan EM, Rouda S, Hoffren J, Chen YQ, Uitto J, Li K. Extracellular matrix gene expression by human keratinocytes and fibroblasts from donors of varying ages. *Trans Assoc Am Physicians* 106:168–78, 1993.

Tan J, Town T, Paris D, Mori T, Suo Z, Crawford F, Mattson MP, Flavell RA, Mullan M. Microglial activation resulting from CD40-CD40L interaction after -amyloid stimulation. *Science* 286:2352–2355, 1999.

Tan Z. Telomere shortening and the population size-dependency of life span of human cell culture: further implication for two proliferation-restricting telomeres. *Exp Gerontol* 34:831–842, 1999.

Tanaka H, Shimizu M, Horikawa I, Kugoh H, Yokota J, Barrett JC, Oshimura M. Evidence for a putative telomerase repressor gene in the 3p14.2–p21.1 region. *Genes Chromosomes Cancer* 23:123–133, 1998a.

Tanaka J, Fujita H, Matsuda S, Toku K, Sakanaka M, Maeda N. Glucocorticoid- and mineralocorticoid receptors in microglial cells: the two receptors mediate differential effects of corticosteroids. *Glia* 20:23–37, 1997.

Tanaka K, Nakazawa T, Okada Y, Kumahara Y. Roles of nuclear and cytoplasmic environments in the retarded DNA synthesis in Werner syndrome cells. *Exp Cell Res* 127:185–190, 1980.

Tanaka M, Kyo S, Takakura M, Kanaya T, Sagawa T, Yamashita K, Okada Y, Hiyama E, Inoue M. Expression of telomerase activity in human endometrium is localized to epithelial glandular cells and regulated in a menstrual phase-dependent manner correlated with cell proliferation. *Am J Pathol* 153:1985–1991, 1998b.

Tang DG, Tokumoto Y, Apperly JA, Lloyd AC, Raff MC. Lack of replicative senescence in cultured rat oligodendrocyte precursor cells. *Science* 291:868–871, 2001.

Tang M, Jacobs D, Stern Y, Marder K, Schofield P, Gurland B, Andrews H, Mayeux R. Effects of oestrogen during menopause on risk and age at onset of Alzheimer's disease. *Lancet* 348:429–432, 1996a.

Tang MX, Maestre G, Tsai WY, Liu XH, Feng L, Chung WY, Chun M, Schofield P, Stern Y, Tycko B, Mayeux R. Effect of age, ethnicity, and head injury on the association between APOE genotypes and Alzheimer's disease. *Ann NY Acad Sci* 802:6–15, 1996b.

Tang MX, Stern Y, Marder K, Bell K, Gurland B, Lantigua R, Andrews H, Feng L, Tycko B, Mayeux R. The APOE-epsilon4 allele and the risk of Alzheimer disease among African Americans, whites, and Hispanics. *JAMA* 279:751–755, 1998.

Tang SJ, Dumot JA, Wang L, Memmesheimer C, Conwell DL, Zuccaro G, Goormastic M, Ormsby AH, Cowell J. Telomerase activity in pancreatic endocrine tumors. *Am J Gastroenterol* 97:1022–1030, 2002.

Tangkijvanich P, Tresukosol D, Sampatanukul P, Sakdikul S, Voravud N, Mahachai V, Mutirangura A. Telomerase assay for differentiating between malignancy-related and non-malignant ascites. *Clin Cancer Res* 5:2470–2475, 1999.

Tanzi RE. A promising animal model of Alzheimer's disease. *N Engl J Med* 332:1512–1513, 1995.

Tanzi RE, Blacker D. Genetic screening in Alzheimer's disease. *Generations* 24:58–64, 2000.

Tanzi RE, Kovacs DM, Kim TW, Moir RD, Guenette SY, Wasco W. The gene defects responsible for familial Alzheimer's disease. *Neurobiol Dis* 3:159–168, 1996.

Tao LC, Stecker E, Gardner HA. Werner's syndrome and acute myeloid leukemia. *Can Med Assoc J* 105:951–968, 1971.

Tarazona R, Solana R, Ouyang Q, Pawelec G. Basic biology and clinical impact of immunosenescence. *Exp Gerontol* 37:183–189, 2002.

Tardif JC. Insights into oxidative stress and atherosclerosis. *Can J Cardiol* 16(Suppl D):2D–4D, 2000.

Tariot PN, Cummings JL, Katz IR, Mintzer J, Perdomo CA, Schwam EM, Whalen E. A randomized, double-blind, placebo-controlled study of the efficacy and safety of donepezil in patients with Alzheimer's disease in the nursing home setting. *J Am Geriatr Soc* 49:1590–1599, 2001.

Tascilar M, Caspers E, Sturm PD, Goggins M, Hruban RH, Offerhaus GJ. Role of tumor markers and mutations in cells and pancreatic juice in the diagnosis of pancreatic cancer. *Ann Oncol* 10(Suppl 4):107–110, 1999.

Tassin J, Malaise F, Courtois Y. Human lens cells have an in vitro proliferative capacity inversely proportional to the donor age. *Exp Cell Res* 96:1–6, 1979.

Tatar M, Kopelman A, Epstein D, Tu M-P, Yin C-M, Garofalo RS. A mutant *Drosophila* insulin receptor homolog that extends life span and impairs neuroendocrine function. *Science* 292:107–110, 2001.

Tatsumoto N, Hiyama E, Murakami Y, Imamura Y, Shay JW, Matsuura Y, Yokoyama T. High telomerase activity is an independent prognostic indicator of poor outcome in colorectal cancer. *Clin Cancer Res* 6:2696–2701, 2000.

Taylor DH, Ostbye T. The effect of middle- and old-age body mass index on short-term mortality in older people. *J Am Geriatr Soc* 49:1319–1326, 2001.

Taylor DH, Sloan FA. How much do persons with Alzheimer's disease cost Medicare? *J Am Geriatr Soc* 48:639–646, 2000.

Taylor DL, Edwards AD, Mehmet H. Oxidative metabolism, apoptosis and perinatal brain injury. *Brain Pathol* 9:93–117, 1999.

Taylor RS, Ramirez RD, Ogoshi M, Chaffins M, Piatyszek MA, Shay JW. Detection of telomerase activity in malignant and nonmalignant skin conditions. *J Invest Dermatol* 106:759–765, 1996.

Tedgui A, Mallat Z. Anti-inflammatory mechanisms in the vascular wall. *Circ Res* 88:877–887, 2001.

Teillet L, Ribiere P, Gouraud S, Bakala H, Corman B. Cellular signaling, AGE accumulation and gene expression in hepatocytes of lean aging rats fed ad libitum or food-restricted. *Mech Ageing Dev* 123:427–439, 2002.

Teitelbaum SL. Bone resorption by osteoclasts. *Science* 289:1504–1508, 2000.

Teixeira L, Valdez H, McCune JM, Koup RA, Badley AD, Hellerstein MK, Napolitano LA, Douek DC, Mbisa G, Deeks S, Harris JM, Barbour JD, Gross BH, Francis IR, Halvorsen R, Asaad R, Lederman MM. Poor CD4 T cell restoration after suppression of HIV-1 replication may reflect lower thymic function. *AIDS* 15:1749–1756, 2001.

Temple LKF, McLeod RS, Gallinger S, Wright JG. Essays on science and society: defining disease in the genomics era. *Science* 293:807–808, 2001.

Tendian SW, Parker WB. Interaction of deoxyguanosine nucleotide analogs with human telomerase. *Mol Pharmacol* 57:695–699, 2000.

Teng SC, Epstein C, Tsai YL, Cheng HW, Chen HL, Lin JJ. Induction of global stress response in *Saccharomyces cerevisiae* cells lacking telomerase. *Biochem Biophys Res Commun* 291:714–721, 2002.

Teng SC, Kim B, Gabriel A. Retrotransposon reverse transcriptase–mediated repair of chromosomal breaks. *Nature* 383:641–644, 1996.

Teng SC, Zakian VA. Telomere–telomere recombination is an efficient bypass pathway for telomere maintenance in *Saccharomyces cerevisiae*. *Mol Cell Biol* 19:8083–8093, 1999.

Tenover JS. Androgen replacement therapy to reverse and/or prevent age-associated sarcopenia in men. *Baillieres Clin Endocrinol Metab* 12:419–425, 1998.

Teo SH, Jackson SP. Telomerase subunit overexpression suppresses telomere-specific checkpoint activation in the yeast yku80 mutant. *EMBO Rep* 2:197–202, 2001.

Terasaki Y, Okumura H, Ohtake S, Nakao S. Accelerated telomere length shortening in granulocytes. A diagnostic marker for myeloproliferative diseases. *Exp Hematol* 30:1399–1404, 2002.

Terashima M, Takiyama I, Uesugi N, Sasaki N, Takagane A, Hayakawa Y, Abe K, Araya M, Nishizuka S, Shimooki O, Nakaya T, Irinoda T, Yonezawa H, Oyama K, Saito K. Telomerase assay as a possible predictor of the response to anticancer chemotherapy. *Anticancer Res* 20:293–297, 2000.

Terman A, Brunk UT. Lipofuscin: mechanisms of formation and increase with age. *APMIS* 106:265–276, 1998a.

Terman A, Brunk UT. On the degradability and exocytosis of ceroid/lipofuscin in cultured rat cardiac myocytes. *Mech Ageing Dev* 100:145–156, 1998b.

Territo M. The use of autologous transplantation in the treatment of malignant disorders. *J Rheumatol Suppl* 48:36–40, 1997.

Tesmer VM, Ford LP, Holt SE, Frank BC, Yi X, Aisner DL, Ouellette M, Shay JW, Wright WE. Two inactive fragments of the integral RNA cooperate to assemble active telomerase with the human protein catalytic subunit (hTERT) in vitro. *Mol Cell Biol* 19:6207–6216, 1999.

Thakur MK. Estrogen and brain aging. *J Anti-Aging Med* 2:127–132, 1999.

Tham WH, Wyithe JS, Ferrigno PK, Silver PA, Zakian VA. Localization of yeast telomeres to the nuclear periphery is separable from transcriptional repression and telomere stability functions. *Mol Cell* 8:189–199, 2001.

Tham WH, Zakian VA. Transcriptional silencing at *Saccharomyces* telomeres: implications for other organisms. *Oncogene* 21:512–521, 2002.

Thannhauser SJ. Werner's syndrome (progeria of the adult) and Rothmund's syndrome: two types of closely related heredofamilial atrophic dermatoses with juvenile cataracts and endocrine features: a critical study with five new cases. *Ann Intern Med* 23:559–626, 1945.

Theise ND, Nimmakayalu M, Gardner R, Illei PB, Morgan G, Teperman L, Henegariu O, Krause DS. Liver from bone marrow in humans. *Hepatology* 32:11–16, 2000.

Thigpen JT. Limited-stage ovarian carcinoma. *Semin Oncol* 26:29–33, 1999.

Thomas DR. Issues and dilemmas in the prevention and treatment of pressure ulcers: a review. *J Gerontol A Biol Sci Med Sci* 56A:M328–340, 2001.

Thomas E, al-Baker E, Dropcova S, Denyer S, Ostad N, Lloyd A, Kill IR, Faragher RG. Different kinetics of senescence in human fibroblasts and peritoneal mesothelial cells. *Exp Cell Res* 236:355–358, 1997.

Thomas ED. Stem cell transplantation: past, present and future. *Arch Immunol Ther Exp (Warsz)* 45:1–5, 1997.

Thomas M, Yang L, Hornsby PJ. Formation of functional tissue from transplanted adrenocortical cells expressing telomerase reverse transcriptase. *Nat Biotechnol* 18:39–42, 2000a.

Thomas NJ, Morris CM, Scaravilli F, Johansson J, Rossor M, De Lange R, St Clair D, Nicoll J, Blank C, Coulthard A, Bushby K, Ince PG, Burn D, Kalaria RN. Hereditary vascular dementia linked to *notch 3* mutations. CADASIL in British families. *Ann NY Acad Sci* 903:293–298, 2000b.

Thomas T, Thomas G, McLendon C, Sutton T, Mulian M. β-amyloid-mediated vasoactivity and vascular endothelial damage. *Nature* 380:168–171, 1996.

Thomas WE. Brain macrophages: on the role of pericytes and perivascular cells. *Brain Res Brain Res Rev* 31:42–57, 1999.

Thompson JS, Bixler SA, Qian F, Vora K, Scott ML, Cachero TG, Hession C, Schneider P, Sizing ID, Mullen C, Strauch K, Zafari M, Benjamin CD, Tschopp J, Browning JL, Ambrose C. BAFF-R, a newly identified TNF receptor that specifically interacts with BAFF. *Science* 293:2108–2111, 2001.

Thomson JA, Itskovitz-Eldor J, Shapiro SS, Waknitz MA, Swiergiel JJ, Marshall VS, Jones JM. Embryonic stem cell lines derived from human blastocysts. *Science* 282:1145–1147, 1998.

Thorgeirsson SS, Grisham JW. Molecular pathogenesis of human hepatocellular carcinoma. *Nat Genet* 31:339–346, 2002.

Thornley I, Dror Y, Sung L, Wynn RF, Freedman MH. Abnormal telomere shortening in leucocytes of children with Shwachman-Diamond syndrome. *Br J Haematol* 117:189–192, 2002a.

Thornley I, Sutherland R, Wynn R, Nayar R, Sung L, Corpus G, Kiss T, Lipton J, Doyle J, Saunders F, Kamel-Reid S, Freedman M, Messner H. Early hematopoietic reconstitution after clinical stem cell transplantation: evidence for stochastic stem cell behavior and limited acceleration in telomere loss. *Blood* 99:2387–2396, 2002b.

Thornley I, Freedman MH. Telomeres, X-inactivation ratios, and hematopoietic stem cell transplantation in humans: a review. *Stem Cells* 20:198–204, 2002.

Thweatt R, Goldstein S. Werner syndrome and biological ageing: a molecular genetic hypothesis. *Bioessays* 15:421–426, 1993.

Tian XX, Pang JC, Zheng J, Chen J, To SS, Ng HK. Antisense epidermal growth factor receptor RNA transfection in human glioblastoma cells down-regulates telomerase activity and telomere length. *Br J Cancer* 86:1328–1332, 2002.

Tice JA, Ross E, Coxson PG, Rosenberg I, Weinstein MC, Hunink MGM, Goldman PA, Williams L, Goldman L. Cost-effectiveness of vitamin therapy to lower plasma homocysteine levels for the prevention of coronary heart disease. *JAMA* 286:936–943, 2001.

Tilghman SM. The sins of the fathers and mothers: genomic imprinting in mammalian development. *Cell* 96:185–193, 1999.

Tilghman SM. Epigenetics in mammals: genomic imprinting. Presented at Cancer and Molecular Genetics in the Twenty-first Century, Van Andel Research Institute, Grand Rapids, MI, September 5–9, 2000.

Tilvis RS, Kahonen M, Harkonen M. Dehydroepiandrosterone sulfate, diseases and mortality in a general aged population. *Aging (Milano)* 11:30–34, 1999.

Timiras ML. The kidney, the lower urinary tract, the prostate, and body fluids. In Timiras PS (ed). *Physiological Basis of Aging and Geriatrics, 2nd ed.* CRC Press, Boca Raton, FL, 1994a, pp 235–246.

Timiras PS. *Physiological Basis of Aging and Geriatrics, 2nd ed.* CRC Press, Boca Raton, FL, 1994b.

Timiras PS. Steroid-secreting endocrines: adrenal, ovary, testis. In Timiras PS, Quay WB, Vernadakis A (eds). *Hormones and Aging.* CRC Press, Boca Raton, FL, 1995a, pp 25–44.

Timiras PS. Hormones of the thyroid and parathyroid glands. In Timiras PS, Quay WB, Vernadakis A (eds). *Hormones and Aging.* CRC Press, Boca Raton, FL, 1995b, pp 85–106.

Timiras PS, Quay WB, Vernadakis A. *Hormones and Aging.* CRC Press, Boca Raton, FL, 1995.

Tissenbaum HA, Ruvkun G. An insulin-like signaling pathway affects both longevity and reproduction in *Caenorhabditis elegans. Genetics* 148:703–717, 1998.

Tobi M, Chintalapani S, Kithier K, Clapp N. Gastrointestinal tract antigenic profile of cotton-top tamarin, *Saguinus oedipus,* is similar to that of humans with inflammatory bowel disease. *Dig Dis Sci* 45:2290–2297, 2001.

Toklu C, Ozen H, Sahin A, Rastadoskouee M, Erdem E. Factors involved in diagnostic delay of testicular cancer. *Int Urol Nephrol* 31:383–388, 1999.

Tokunaga M, Wakamatsu E, Sato K, Satake S, Aoyama K, Saito K, Sugawara M, Yosizawa Z. Hyaluronuria in a case of progeria (Hutchinson-Gilford syndrome). *J Am Geriatr Soc* 26:296–302, 1978.

Tolar M, Keller JN, Chan S, Mattson MP, Marques MA, Crutcher KA. Truncated apolipoprotein E (ApoE) causes increased intracellular calcium and may mediate ApoE neurotoxicity. *J Neurosci* 19:7100–7110, 1999.

Tollefsbol TO, Andrews LG. Mechanisms for telomerase gene control in aging cells and tumorigenesis. *Med Hypotheses* 56:630–637, 2001.

Tollefsbol TO, Zaun MR, Gracy RW. Increased lability of triosephosphate isomerase in progeria and Werner's syndrome fibroblasts. *Mech Ageing Dev* 20:93–101, 1982.

Tomaska L, Makhov AM, Nosek J, Kucejova B, Griffith JD. Electron microscopic analysis supports a dual role for the mitochondrial telomere-binding protein of *Candida* parapsilosis. *J Mol Biol* 305:61–69, 2001.

Tomaska L, Nosek J, Makhov AM, Pastorakova A, Griffith JD. Extragenomic double-stranded DNA circles in yeast with linear mitochondrial genomes: potential involvement in telomere maintenance. *Nucleic Acids Res* 28:4479–4487, 2000.

Tominaga K, Olgun A, Smith JR, Pereira-Smith OM. Genetics of cellular senescence. *Mech Ageing Dev* 123:927–936, 2002.

Tomita N, Horiuchi M, Tomita S, Gibbons GH, Kim JY, Baran D, Dzau VJ. An oligonucleotide decoy for transcription factor E2F inhibits mesangial cell proliferation in vitro. *Am J Physiol* 275:F278–284, 1998.

Tomoda R, Seto M, Tsumuki H, Iida K, Yamazaki T, Sonoda J, Matsumine A, Uchida A. Telomerase activity and human telomerase reverse transcriptase mRNA expression are correlated with clinical aggressiveness in soft tissue tumors. *Cancer* 95:1127–1133, 2002.

Tong WM, Hande MP, Lansdorp PM, Wang ZQ. DNA strand break-sensing molecule poly(ADP-Ribose) polymerase cooperates with p53 in telomere function, chromosome stability, and tumor suppression. *Mol Cell Biol* 21:4046–4054, 2001.

Toogood AA, Shalet SM. Ageing and growth hormone status. *Baillieres Clin Endocrinol Metab* 12:281–296, 1998.

Toouli CD, Huschtscha LI, Neumann AA, Noble JR, Colgin LM, Hukku B, Reddel RR. Comparison of human mammary epithelial cells immortalized by simian virus 40 T-antigen or by the telomerase catalytic subunit. *Oncogene* 21:128–139, 2002.

Torgerson DJ, Bell-Syer SEM. Hormone replacement therapy and prevention of nonvertebral fractures: a meta-analysis of randomized trials. *JAMA* 285:2891–2897, 2001.

Toussaint O, Remacle J, Dierick JF, Pascal T, Frippiat C, Zdanov S, Magalhaes JP, Royer V, Chainiaux F. From the Hayflick mosaic to the mosaics of ageing. Role of stress-induced premature senescence in human ageing. *Int J Biochem Cell Biol* 34:1415–1429, 2002.

Touyz RM. Oxidative stress and vascular damage in hypertension. *Curr Hypertens Rep* 2:98–105, 2000.

Tran J, Brenner TJ, DiNardo S. Somatic control over the germline stem cell lineage during *Drosophila* spermatogenesis. *Nature* 2000;407:754–757.

Trapp BD, Bo L, Mork S, Chang A. Pathogenesis of tissue injury in MS lesions. *J Neuroimmunol* 98:49–56, 1999.

Travis J. Boning up turning on cells that build bone and turning off ones that destroy it. *Sci News* 157:41–43, 2000.

Treffers WF. Corneal endothelial wound repair in vivo and in vitro. *Ophthalmology* 89:605–613, 1982.

Treon SP, Raje N, Anderson KC. Immunotherapeutic strategies for the treatment of plasma cell malignancies. *Semin Oncol* 27:598–613, 2000.

Tresini M, Mawal-Dewan M, Cristofalo VJ, Sell C. A phosphatidylinositol 3-kinase inhibitor induces a senescent-like growth arrest in human diploid fibroblasts. *Cancer Res* 58:1–4, 1998.

Tresini M, Pignolo RJ, Allen RG, Cristofalo VJ. Effects of donor age on the expression of a marker of replicative senescence (EPC-1) in human dermal fibroblasts. *J Cell Physiol* 179:11–17, 1999.

Treuting PM, Hopkins HC, Ware CA, Rabinovitch PR, Ladiges WC. Generation of genetically altered mouse models for aging studies. *Exp Mol Pathol* 72:49–55, 2002.

Tri TB, Combs DT. Congestive cardiomyopathy in Werner's syndrome. *Lancet* 1:1052–1053, May 13, 1978.

Trinh NH, Hoblyn J, Mohanty S, Yaffe K. Efficacy of cholinesterase inhibitors in the treatment of neuropsychiatric symptoms and functional impairment in Alzheimer disease. *JAMA* 289:210–216, 2003.

Trinkaus-Randall V, Tong M, Thomas P, Cornell-Bell A. Confocal imaging of the alpha 6 and beta 4 integrin subunits in the human cornea with aging. *Invest Ophthalmol Vis Sci* 34:3103–3109, 1993.

Tropepe V, Coles BLK, Chiasson BJ, Jorsford DJ, Elia AJ, McInnes RR, van der Kooy D. Retinal stem cells in the adult mammalian eye. *Science* 287:2032–2036, 2000.

Tryggvason K, Wartiovaara J. Molecular basis of glomerular permselectivity. *Curr Opin Nephrol Hypertens* 10:543–549 , 2001.

Tsai K, Hsu TG, Lu FJ, Hsu CF, Liu TY, Kong CW. Age-related changes in the mitochondrial depolarization induced by oxidative injury in human peripheral blood leukocytes. *Free Radic Res* 35:395–403, 2001.

Tsao SW, Zhang DK, Cheng RY, Wan TS. Telomerase activation in human cancers. *Chin Med J (Engl)* 111:745–750, 1998.

Tseng CJ, Jain S, Hou HC, Liu W, Pao CC, Lin CT, Horng SG, Soong YK, Hsueh S. Applications of the telomerase assay in peritoneal washing fluids. *Gynecol Oncol* 81:420–423, 2001.

Tsien F, Sun B, Hopkins NE, Vedanarayanan V, Figlewicz D, Winokur S, Ehrlich M. Methylation of the FSHD syndrome-linked subtelomeric repeat in normal and FSHD cell cultures and tissues. *Mol Genet Metab* 74:322–331, 2001.

Tsuji A, Ishiko A, Takasaki T, Ikeda N. Estimating age of humans based on telomere shortening. *Forensic Sci Int* 126:197–199, 2002.

Tsujiuchi T, Tsutsumi M, Kido A, Kobitsu K, Takahama M, Majima T, Denda A, Nakae D, Konishi Y. Increased telomerase activity in hyperplastic nodules and hepatocellular carcinomas induced by a choline-deficient L-amino acid–defined diet in rats. *Jpn J Cancer Res* 87:1111–1115, 1996.

Tsujiuchi T, Tsutsumi M, Kido A, Takahama M, Sakitani H, Iki K, Sasaki Y, Denda A, Konishi Y. Induction of telomerase activity during regeneration after partial hepatectomy in the rat. *Cancer Lett* 122:115–120, 1998.

Tsukamoto Y, Taggart AK, Zakian VA. The role of the Mre11-Rad50-Xrs2 complex in telomerase- mediated lengthening of *Saccharomyces cerevisiae* telomeres. *Curr Biol* 11:1328–1335, 2001.

Tsutsui T, Kumakura S, Yamamoto A, Kanai H, Tamura Y, Kato T, Anpo M, Tahara H, Barrett JC. Association of p16(INK4a) and pRb inactivation with immortalization of human cells. *Carcinogenesis* 23:2111–2117, 2002.

Tucker JD, Spruill MD, Ramsey MJ, Director AD, Nath J. Frequency of spontaneous chromosome aberrations in mice: effects of age. *Mutat Res* 425:135–141, 1999.

Tucker V, Jenkins J, Gilmour J, Savoie H, Easterbrook P, Gotch F, Browning MJ. T-cell telomere length maintained in HIV-infected long-term survivors. *HIV Med* 1:116–122, 2000.

Tuft SJ, Gartry DS, Rawe IM, Meek KM. Photorefractive keratectomy: implications of corneal wound healing. *Br J Ophthalmol* 77:243–247, 1993.

Tulina N, Matunis E. Control of stem cell self-renewal in *Drosophila* spermatogenesis by JAK-STAT signaling. *Science* 294:2546–2549, 2002.

Tummala S, Svec F. Correlation between the administered dose of DHEA and serum levels of DHEA and DHEA-S in human volunteers: analysis of published data. *Clin Biochem* 32:355–361, 1999.

Tunstead JR, Hornsby PJ. Relationship of p21WAF1/CIP1/SD11 to cell proliferation in primary cultures of adrenocortical cells. *AGE* 22:39–44, 1999.

Tuntiwechapikul W, Salazar M. Cleavage of telomeric G-quadruplex DNA with perylene-EDTA*Fe(II). *Biochemistry* 40:13652–13658, 2001.

Turkewitz AP, Orias E, Kapler G. Functional genomics: the coming of age for *Tetrahymena thermophila*. *Trends Genet* 18:35–40, 2002.

Turrens JF. Superoxide production by the mitochondrial respiratory chain. In Skulachev V (ed). *Bioscience Report 17*. Plenum Press, New York, 1997, pp 3–8.

Tyler RH, Brar H, Singh M, Latorre A, Graves JL, Mueller LD, Rose MR, Ayala FJ. The effect of superoxide dismutase alleles on aging in *Drosophila*. *Genetica* 91:143–149, 1993.

Tyndall A. Hematopoietic stem cell transplantation in rheumatic diseases other than systemic sclerosis and systemic lupus erythematosus. *J Rheumatol Suppl* 48:94–97, 1997.

Tyner SD, Venkatachalam S, Choi J, Jones S, Ghebranious N, Igelmann H, Lu X, Soron G, Cooper B, Brayton C, Hee Park S, Thompson T, Karsenty G, Bradley A, Donehower LA. p53 mutant mice that display early ageing-associated phenotypes. *Nature* 415:45–53, 2002.

Tzfati Y, Fulton TB, Roy J, Blackburn EH. Template boundary in a yeast telomerase specified by RNA structure. *Science* 288:863–867, 2000.

Tzukerman M, Selig S, Skorecki K. Telomeres and telomerase in human health and disease. *J Pediatr Endocrinol Metab* 15:229–240, 2002.

Uchida W, Matsunaga S, Sugiyama R, Kawano S. Interstitial telomere-like repeats in the *Arabidopsis thaliana* genome. *Genes Genet Syst* 77:63–67, 2002.

Uchino E, Uemura A, Ohba N. Initial stages of posterior vitreous detachment in healthy eyes of older persons evaluated by optical coherence tomography. *Arch Ophthalmol* 119:1475–1479, 2001.

Uchiumi F, Ohta T, Tanuma S. Replication factor C recognizes 5'-phosphate ends of telomeres. *Biochem Biophys Res Commun* 229:310–315, 1996.

Uchiumi F, Watanabe M, Tanuma S. Mammalian proteins that associate with telomeres [in Japanese]. *Nippon Rinsho* 56:1097–1101, 1998.

Uchiumi F, Watanabe M, Tanuma S. Characterization of telomere-binding activity of replication factor C large subunit p140. *Biochem Biophys Res Commun* 258:482–489, 1999.

Ueda M Telomerase in cutaneous carcinogenesis. *J Dermatol Sci* 23:S37–40, 2000.

Uemura H, Kanda F, Ikeda N, Kubota Y. Telomerase activity in prostate cancer [in Japanese]. *Nippon Rinsho* 58:427–429, 2000.

Ueno T, Takahashi H, Oda M, Mizunuma M, Yokoyama A, Goto Y, Mizushina Y, Sakaguchi K, Hayashi H. Inhibition of human telomerase by rubromycins: implication of spiroketal system of the compounds as an active moiety. *Biochemistry* 39:5995–6002, 2000.

Ulaner GA, Giudice LC. Developmental regulation of telomerase activity in human fetal tissues during gestation. *Mol Hum Reprod* 3:769–773, 1997.

Ulaner GA, Hu JF, Vu TH, Giudice LC, Hoffman AR. Telomerase activity in human development is regulated by human telomerase reverse transcriptase (hTERT) transcription and by alternate splicing of hTERT transcripts. *Cancer Res* 58:4168–4172, 1998.

Ullian EM, Sapperstein SK, Christopherson KS, Barres BA. Control of synapse number by glia. *Science* 291:657–661, 2001.

Ulmer SC. Hepatocellular carcinoma. A concise guide to its status and management. *Postgrad Med* 107:117–124, 2000.

Umland EM, Rinaldi C, Parks SM, Boyce EG. The impact of estrogen replacement therapy and raloxifene on osteoporosis, cardiovascular disease, and gynecologic cancers. *Ann Pharmacother* 33:1315–1328, 1999.

Ungar A, Castellani S, Di Serio C, Cantini C, Cristofari C, Vallotti B, La Cava G, Masotti G. Changes in renal autacoids and hemodynamics associated with aging and isolated systolic hypertension. *Prostaglandins Other Lipid Mediat* 62:117–133, 2000.

Untergasser G, Rumpold H, Hermann M, Dirnhofer S, Jilg G, Berger P. Proliferative disorders of the aging human prostate: involvement of protein hormones and their receptors. *Exp Gerontol* 34:275–287, 1999.

Urabe Y, Nouso K, Higashi T, Nakatsukasa H, Hino N, Ashida K, Kinugasa N, Yoshida K, Uematsu S, Tsuji T. Telomere length in human liver diseases. *Liver* 16:293–297, 1996.

Urbanchek MG, Picken EB, Kalliainen LK, Kuzon WM. Specific force deficit in skeletal muscles of old rats is partially explained by the existence of denervated muscle fibers. *J Gerontol A Biol Sci Med Sci* 56:191–197, 2001.

Urquidi V, Tarin D, Goodison S. Telomerase in cancer: clinical applications. *Ann Med* 30:419–430, 1998.

Urquidi V, Tarin D, Goodison S. Role of telomerase in cell senescence and oncogenesis. *Annu Rev Med* 51:65–79, 2000.

Usselmann B, Newbold M, Morris AG, Nwokolo CU. Deficiency of colonic telomerase in ulcerative colitis. *Am J Gastroenterol* 96:1106–1112, 2001.

Valenzuela HF, Effros RB. Loss of telomerase inducibility in antigen-specific memory T cells following multiple encounters with an antigen. *FASEB J* 14:A991, 2000.

Valenzuela HF, Effros RB. Divergent telomerase and CD28 expression patterns in human CD4 and CD8 T cells following repeated encounters with the same antigenic stimulus. *Clin Immunol* 105:117–125, 2002.

Vallejo AN, Nestel AR, Schirmer M, Weyand CM, Goronzy JJ. Aging-related deficiency of CD28 expression in CD4+ T cells is associated with the loss of gene-specific nuclear factor binding activity. *J Biol Chem* 273:8119–8129, 1998.

Valtonen VV. Role of infections in atherosclerosis. *Am Heart J* 138:S431–433, 1999.

Vance ML. The Gordon Wilson Lecture. Growth hormone replacement in adults and other uses. *Trans Am Clin Climatol Assoc* 109:87–96, 1998.

van den Brink GR, de Santa Barbara P, Roberts DJ. Epithelial cell differentiation—a mather [sic] of choice. *Science* 294:2115–2116, 2001.

van der Kooy D, Weiss S. Why stem cells? *Science* 287:1439–1441, 2000.

van Elsas A, Hurwitz AA, Allison JP. Combination immunotherapy of B16 melanoma using anti-cytotoxic T lymphocyte-associated antigen 4 (CTLA-4) and granulocyte/macrophage colony–stimulating factor (GM-CSF)–producing vaccines induces rejection of subcutaneous and metastatic tumors accompanied by autoimmune depigmentation. *J Exp Med* 190:355–366, 1999.

van Geel M, Eichler EE, Beck AF, Shan Z, Haaf T, van Der Maarel SM, Frants RR, de Jong PJ. A cascade of complex subtelomeric duplications during the evolution of the hominoid and Old World monkey genomes. *Am J Hum Genet* 70:269–278, 2002.

van Heek NT, Meeker AK, Kern SE, Yeo CJ, Lillemoe KD, Cameron JL, Offerhaus GJ, Hicks JL, Wilentz RE, Goggins MG, De Marzo AM, Hruban RH, Maitra A. Telomere shortening is nearly universal in pancreatic intraepithelial neoplasia. *Am J Pathol* 161:1541–1547, 2002.

Van Hoften C, Burger H, Peeters PH, Grobbee DE, Van Noord PA, Leufkens HG. Long-term oral contraceptive use increases breast cancer risk in women over 55 years of age: the DOM cohort. *Int J Cancer* 87:591–594, 2000.

van Leeuwen F, Kieft R, Cross M, Borst P. Tandemly repeated DNA is a target for the partial replacement of thymine by beta-D-glucosyl-hydroxymethyluracil in *Trypanosoma brucei*. *Mol Biochem Parasitol* 109:133–145, 2000.

van Leeuwen FW, Hol EM. Molecular misreading of genes in Down syndrome as a model for the Alzheimer type of neurodegeneration. *J Neural Transm Suppl* 57:137–159, 1999.

Van Poppel H, Nilsson S, Algaba F, Bergerheim U, Dal Cin P, Fleming S, Hellsten S, Kirkali Z, Klotz L, Lindblad P, Ljungberg B, Mulders P, Roskams T, Ross RK, Walker C, Wersall P. Precancerous lesions in the kidney. *Scand J Urol Nephrol Suppl* 205:136–165, 2000.

van Staa T-P, Wegman S, de Vries F, Leufkens B, Cooper C. Use of statins and risk of fractures. *JAMA* 285:1850–1855, 2001.

van Steensel B, de Lange T. Control of telomere length by the human telomeric protein TRF1. *Nature* 385:740–743, 1997.

van Steensel B, Smogorzewska A, de Lange T. TRF2 protects human telomeres from end-to-end fusions. *Cell* 92:401–413, 1998.

Van Voorhies WA, Ward S. Genetic and environmental conditions that increase longevity in *Caenorhabditis elegans* decrease metabolic rate. *Proc Natl Acad Sci USA* 96:11399–11403, 1999.

Van Zeeland NL, Wanagat J, Lopez, ME, Aiken JM. Segmental nature of age-associated, skeletal muscle mitochondrial abnormalities necessitates three-dimensional analyses. *J Anti-Aging Med* 2:231–241, 1999.

Vapaatalo H, Mervaala E. Clinically important factors influencing endothelial function. *Med Sci Monit* 7:1075–1085, 2001.

Varley H, Pickett HA, Foxon JL, Reddel RR, Royle NJ. Molecular characterization of inter-telomere and intra-telomere mutations in human ALT cells. *Nat Genet* 30:301–305, 2002.

Vastag B. At polio's end game, strategies differ. *JAMA* 286:2797–2799, 2001a.

Vastag B. Epigenetics is seen as possible key to cloning. *JAMA* 286:1438–1440, 2001b.

Vastag B. Study concludes that moderate PSA levels are unrelated to prostate cancer outcomes. *JAMA* 287:969–970, 2002.

Vaziri H. Critical telomere shortening regulated by the ataxia-telangiectasia gene acts as a DNA damage signal leading to activation of p53 protein and limited life-span of human diploid fibroblasts. A review. *Biochemistry (Mosc)* 62:1306–1310, 1997.

Vaziri H. Extension of life span in normal human cells by telomerase activation: a revolution in cultural senescence. *J Anti-Aging Med* 1:125–130 1998.

Vaziri H, Benchimol S. Reconstruction of telomerase activity in normal cells leads to elongation of telomeres and extended replicative life span. *Cur Biol* 8:279–282, 1998.

Vaziri H, Benchimol S. Alternative pathways for the extension of cellular life span: inactivation of p53/pRb and expression of telomerase. *Oncogene* 18:7676–7680, 1999.

Vaziri H, Dragowska W, Allsopp RC, Thomas TC, Harley CB, Lansdorp PM. Evidence for a mitotic clock in human hematopoetic stem cells: loss of telomeric DNA with age. *Proc Natl Acad Sci USA* 91:9857–9860, 1994.

Vaziri H, Schachter F, Uchida I, Wei L, Zhu X, Effros R, Harley CB. Loss of telomeric DNA during aging of normal and trisomy 21 human lymphocytes. *Am J Hum Genet* 52:661–667, 1993.

Vaziri H, West MD, Allsopp RC, Davison TS, Wu YS, Arrowsmith CH, Poirier GG, Benchimol S. ATM-dependent telomere loss in aging human diploid fibroblasts and DNA damage lead to the post-translational activation of p53 protein involving poly(ADP-ribose) polymerase. *EMBO J* 16:6018–6033, 1997.

Vega-Palas MA, Venditti S, Di Mauro E. Heterochromatin organization of a natural yeast telomere. Changes of nucleosome distribution driven by the absence of Sir3p. *J Biol Chem* 273:9388–9392, 1998.

Vekrellis K, Ye Z, Qiu WQ, Walsh D, Hartley D, Chesneau V, Rosner MR, Selkoe DJ. Neurons regulate extracellular levels of amyloid beta-protein via proteolysis by insulin-degrading enzyme. *J Neurosci* 20:1657–1665, 2000.

Veldhuis JD. Neuroregulatory pathophysiology of impoverished growth hormone (GH) secretion in the aging brain. *J Anti-Aging Med* 1:173–196, 1998.

Veldhuis JD, Iranmanesh A, Mulligan T, Pincus SM. Disruption of the young–adult synchrony between luteinizing hormone release and oscillations in follicle-stimulating hormone, prolactin, and nocturnal penile tumescence (NPT) in healthy older men. *J Clin Endocrinol Metab* 84:3498–3505, 1999.

Veldman T, Horikawa I, Barrett JC, Schlegel R. Transcriptional activation of the telomerase hTERT gene by human papillomavirus type 16 E6 oncoprotein. *J Virol* 75:4467–4472, 2001.

Velicescu M, Dubeau L. p53: a key player in the telomere dynamics. *Cancer Biol Ther* 1:518–519, 2002.

Veltman JA, Schoenmakers EF, Eussen BH, Janssen I, Merkx G, van Cleef B, van Ravenswaaij CM, Brunner HG, Smeets D, van Kessel AG. High-throughput analysis of subtelomeric chromosome rearrangements by use of array-based comparative genomic hybridization. *Am J Hum Genet* 70:1269–1276, 2002.

Venable ME, Obeid LM. Phospholipase D in cellular senescence. *Biochim Biophys Acta* 1439:291–298, 1999.

Venditti S, Di Stefano G, D'Eletto M, Di Mauro E. Genetic remodeling and transcriptional remodeling of subtelomeric heterochromatin are different. *Biochemistry* 41:4901–4910, 2002.

Venditti S, Vega-Palas MA, Di Mauro E. Heterochromatin organization of a natural yeast telomere. Recruitment of Sir3p through interaction with histone H4 N terminus is required for the establishment of repressive structures. *J Biol Chem* 274:1928–1933, 1999a.

Venditti S, Vega-Palas MA, Di Stefano G, Di Mauro E. Imbalance in dosage of the genes for the heterochromatin components Sir3p and histone H4 results in changes in the length and sequence organization of yeast telomeres. *Mol Gen Genet* 262:367–377, 1999b.

Venetsanakos E, Mirza A, Fanton C, Romanov SR, Tlsty T, McMahon M. Induction of tubulogenesis in telomerase-immortalized human microvascular endothelial cells by glioblastoma cells. *Exp Cell Res* 273:21–33, 2002.

Venkatesan RN, Price C. Telomerase expression in chickens: constitutive activity in somatic tissues and down-regulation in culture. *Proc Natl Acad Sci USA* 95:14763–14768, 1998.

Venters HD, Tang Q, Liu Q, VanHoy RW, Dantzer R, Kelley KW. A new mechanism of neurodegeneration: a proinflammatory cytokine inhibits receptor signaling by a survival peptide. *Proc Natl Acad Sci USA* 96:9879–9884, 1999.

Verbeke P, Fonager J, Clark BFC, Rattan SIS. Heat shock response and aging: mechanisms and applications. *Cell Biol Int* 25:845–857, 2001.

Verdery RB, Ingram DK, Roth GS, Lane MA. Caloric restriction increases HDL2 levels in rhesus monkeys (*Macaca mulatta*). *Am J Physiol* 273:E714–719, 1997.

Vermeulen A, Goemaere S, Kaufman JM. Testosterone, body composition and aging. *J Endocrinol Invest* 22:110–116, 1999.

Vertino PM, Issa JP, Pereira-Smith OM, Baylin SB. Stabilization of DNA methyltransferase levels and CpG island hypermethylation precede SV40-induced immortalization of human fibroblasts. *Cell Growth Differ* 5:1395–1402, 1994.

Viard JP, Mocroft A, Chiesi A, Kirk O, Roge B, Panos G, Vetter N, Bruun JN, Johnson M, Lundgren JD, EuroSIDA Study Group. Influence of age on CD4 cell recovery in human immunodeficiency virus–infected patients receiving highly active antiretroviral therapy: evidence from the EuroSIDA study. *J Infect Dis* 183:1290–1294, 2001.

Viel JJ, McManus DQ, Brewer GJ. Age- and concentration-dependent neuroprotection and toxicity by TNF in cortical neurons exposed to β-amyloid. *J Neurosci Res* 64:454–465, 2001.

Vietor M, Winter S, Groscurth P, Naumann U, Weller M. On the significance of telomerase activity in human malignant glioma cells. *Eur J Pharmacol* 407:27–37, 2000.

Vieweg J. The evolving role of dendritic cell therapy in urologic oncology. *Curr Opin Urol* 10:307–312, 2000.

Vijg J. Somatic mutations and aging: a re-evaluation. *Mutat Res* 447:117–135, 2000.

Villa R, Folini M, Lualdi S, Veronese S, Daidone MG, Zaffaroni N. Inhibition of telomerase activity by a cell-penetrating peptide nucleic acid construct in human melanoma cells. *FEBS Lett* 473:241–248, 2000a.

Villa R, Folini M, Perego P, Supino R, Setti E, Daidone MG, Zunino F, Zaffaroni N. Telomerase activity and telomere length in human ovarian cancer and melanoma cell lines: correlation with sensitivity to DNA damaging agents. *Int J Oncol* 16:995–1002, 2000b.

Villa R, Porta CD, Folini M, Daidone MG, Zaffaroni N. Possible regulation of telomerase activity by transcription and alternative splicing of telomerase reverse transcriptase in human melanoma. *J Invest Dermatol* 116:867–873, 2001.

Villanueva JM, Jia X, Yohannes PG, Doetsch PW, Marzilli LG. Cisplatin (cis-Pt(NH(3))(2)Cl(2)) and cis-[Pt(NH(3))(2)(H(2)O)(2)](2+) intrastrand cross-linking reactions at the telomere GGGT DNA sequence embedded in a duplex, a hairpin, and a bulged duplex: use of Mg(2+) and Zn(2+) to convert a hairpin to a bulged duplex. *Inorg Chem* 38:6069–6080, 1999.

Villareal DT, Binder EF, Williams DB, Schechtman KB, Yarasheski KE, Kohrt WM. Bone mineral density response to estrogen replacement in frail elderly women. *JAMA* 286:815–820, 2001.

Villee, DB, Nichols G, Talbot NB. Metabolic studies in two boys with classical progeria. *Pediatrics* 43:207–216, 1969.

Villeponteau B. The heterochromatin loss model of aging. *Exp Gerontol* 32:383–394, 1997.

Virchow RLK. *Die Cellularpathologie in ihrer Begründung auf physiologische und pathologische Gewebelehre.* A. Hirschwald, Berlin, 1858.

Visser M, Deeg DJH, Lips P, Harris TB, Bouter LM. Skeletal muscle mass and muscle strength in relation to lower-extremity performance in older men and women. *J Am Geriatr Soc* 48:381–386, 2000.

Vogel G. In contrast to Dolly, cloning resets telomere clock in cattle. *Science* 288:586–587, 2000.

Vogel H, Lim DS, Karsenty G, Finegold M, Hasty P. Deletion of Ku86 causes early onset of senescence in mice. *Proc Natl Acad Sci USA* 96:10770–10775, 1999.

Vojta PJ, Futreal PA, Annab LA, Kato H, Pereira-Smith OM, Barrett JC. Evidence for two senescence loci on human chromosome 1. *Genes Chromosomes Cancer* 16:55–63, 1996.

Volk MJ, Pugh TD, Kim M, Frith CH, Daynes RA, Ershler WB, Weindruch R. Dietary restriction from middle age attenuates age-associated lymphoma development and interleukin 6 dysregulation in C57BL/6 mice. *Cancer Res* 54:3054–3061, 1994.

Volm M, Mattern J, Koomagi R. Association of telomerase expression with successful heterotransplantation of lung cancer. *Int J Oncol* 16:31–35, 2000.

Volpi E, Mittendorfer B, Rasmussen B, Wolfe R. The response of muscle protein anabolism to combined hyperaminoacidemia and glucose-induced hyperinsulinemia is impaired in the elderly. *J Clin Endocrinol Metab* 85:4481–4490, 2000.

Volpi E, Sheffield-Moore M, Rasmussen BB, Wolfe RR. Basal muscle amino acid kinetics and protein synthesis in healthy young and older men. *JAMA* 286:1206–1212, 2001.

Voltaire. *Candide.* Dover Thrift Editions, Mineola, New York, 1991. Based on the original publication, 1759.

Voltaire. *Philosophical Dictionary.* In Redman, 1977. Based on the original publication, 1764.

von der Leyen HE, Braun-Dullaeus R, Mann MJ, Zhang L, Niebauer J, Dzau VJ. A pressure-mediated nonviral method for efficient arterial gene and oligonucleotide transfer. *Hum Gene Ther* 10:2355–2364, 1999.

von der Leyen HE, Gibbons GH, Morishita R, Lewis NP, Zhang L, Nakajima M, Kaneda Y, Cooke JP, Dzau VJ. Gene therapy inhibiting neointimal vascular lesion: in vivo transfer of endothelial cell nitric oxide synthase gene. *Proc Natl Acad Sci USA* 92:1137–1141, 1995.

von der Leyen HE, Mann MJ, Dzau VJ. Gene inhibition and gene augmentation for the treatment of vascular proliferative disorders. *Semin Interv Cardiol* 1:209–214, 1996.

von Werder K. The somatopause is no indication for growth hormone therapy. *J Endocrinol Invest* 22(5 Suppl):137–141, 1999.

von Zglinicki T. Telomeres: influencing the rate of aging. *Ann NY Acad Sci* 854:318–327, 1998.

von Zglinicki T. Role of oxidative stress in telomere length regulation and replicative senescence. *Ann NY Acad Sci* 908:99–110, 2000.

von Zglinicki T. Oxidative stress shortens telomeres. *Trends Biochem Sci* 27:339–344, 2002.

von Zglinicki T, Pilger R, Sitte N. Accumulation of single-strand breaks is the major cause of telomere shortening in human fibroblasts. *Free Radic Biol Med* 28:64–74, 2000a.

von Zglinicki T, Saretzki G, Docke W, Lotze C. Mild hyperoxia shortens telomeres and inhibits proliferation of fibroblasts: a model for senescence? *Exp Cell Res* 220:186–193, 1995.

von Zglinicki T, Serra V, Lorenz M, Saretzki G, Lenzen-Grossimlighaus R, Gessner R, Risch A, Steinhagen-Thiessen E. Short telomeres in patients with vascular dementia: an indicator of low antioxidative capacity and a possible risk factor? *Lab Invest* 80:1739–1747, 2000b.

Vorchheimer DA, Fuster V. Inflammatory markers in coronary artery disease: let prevention douse the flames. *JAMA* 286: 2154–2156, 2001.

Vulliamy T, Marrone A, Dokal I, Mason PJ. Association between aplastic anaemia and mutations in telomerase RNA. *Lancet* 359:2168–2170, 2002.

Vulliamy T, Marrone A, Goldman F, Dearlove A, Bessler M, Mason PJ, Dokal I. The RNA component of telomerase is mutated in autosomal dominant dyskeratosis congenita. *Nature* 413:432–435, 2001a.

Vulliamy TJ, Knight SW, Mason PJ, Dokal I. Very short telomeres in the peripheral blood of patients with X-linked and autosomal dyskeratosis congenita. *Blood Cells Mol Dis* 27:353–357, 2001b.

Wachsman JT. The beneficial effects of dietary restriction: reduced oxidative damage and enhanced apoptosis. *Mutat Res* 350:25–34, 1996.

Wada E, Hisatomi H, Moritoyo T, Kanamaru T, Hikiji K. Genetic diagnostic test of hepatocellular carcinoma by telomerase catalytic subunit mRNA. *Oncol Rep* 5:1407–1412, 1998.

Wadhwa R, Pereira-Smith OM, Reddel RR, Sugimoto Y, Mitsui Y, Kaul SC. Correlation between complementation group for immortality and the cellular distribution of mortalin. *Exp Cell Res* 216:101–106, 1995.

Wadia JS, Dowdy SF. Protein transduction technology. *Curr Opin Biotechnol* 13:52–56, 2002.

Wagers AJ, Sherwood RI, Christensen JL, Weissman IL. Little evidence for developmental plasticity of adult hematopoietic stem cells. *Science* 297:2256–2259, 2002.

Wagner JD. Rationale for hormone replacement therapy in atherosclerosis prevention. *J Reprod Med* 45(3 Suppl):245–258, 2000.

Wagner JP, Black IB, DiCicco-Bloom E. Stimulation of neonatal and adult brain neurogenesis by subcutaneous injection of basic fibroblast growth factor. *J Neurosci* 19:6006–6016, 1999.

Wagner UG, Koetz K, Weyand CM, Goronzy JJ. Perturbation of the T cell repertoire in rheumatoid arthritis. *Proc Natl Acad Sci USA* 95:14447–14452, 1998.

Wahlin J, Cohn M. Analysis of the RAP1 protein binding to homogeneous telomeric repeats in *Saccharomyces castellii*. *Yeast* 19:241–256, 2002.

Wai-Hong T, WH, Zakian VA. Telomeric tethers. *Nature* 403(6765):34–35, 2000.

Wainwright LJ, Middleton PG, Rees JL. Changes in mean telomere length in basal cell carcinomas of the skin. *Genes Chromosomes Cancer* 12:45–49, 1995.

Wakayama T, Rodriguez I, Perry AC, Yanagimachi R, Mombaerts P. Mice cloned from embryonic stem cells. *Proc Natl Acad Sci USA* 96:14984–14989, 1999.

Wakayama T, Tabar V, Rodriguez I, Perry ACF, Studer L, Mombaerts P. Differentiation of embryonic stem cell lines generated from adult somatic cells by nuclear transfer. *Science* 292:740–742, 2001.

Wakimoto P, Block G. Dietary intake, dietary patterns, and changes with age: an epidemiological perspective. *J Gerontol A Biol Sci Med Sci* 56:65–80, 2001.

Walboomers JM, Meijer CJ, Steenbergen RD, van Duin M, Helmerhorst TJ, Snijders PJ. Human papillomavirus and the development of cervical cancer: concept of carcinogenesis [in Dutch]. *Ned Tijdschr Geneeskd* 144:1671–1674, 2000.

Waldenschmidt TJ, Noelle RJ. Long live the mature B cell—a *BAFF*ling mystery resolved. *Science* 293:2012–2013, 2001.

Walford RL. *The Immunologic Theory of Ageing.* Copenhagen, 1969.

Walford RL. Antibody diversity, histocompatibility systems, disease states, and ageing. *Lancet* 2:1226–1229, 1970.

Wallace D. Science takes cellular approach to exploring aging. Available January 4, 2000 at http://www.cnn.com/2000/ HEALTH/aging/01/03/aging.population.html, 2000. Quoted on p 3 of Morris J, Salvatore S.

Wallace JD, Cuneo RC, Lundberg PA, Rosen T, Jorgensen JO, Longobardi S, Keay N, Sacca L, Christiansen JS, Bengtsson BA, Sonksen PH. Responses of markers of bone and collagen turnover to exercise, growth hormone (GH) administration, and GH withdrawal in trained adult males. *J Clin Endocrinol Metab* 85:124–133, 2000.

Walker DG, Beach TG. Microglial and astrocytic reactions in Alzheimer's disease. In de Vellis J (ed). *Neuroglia in the Aging Brain.* Humana Press, Totowa, NJ, 2002, pp 339–364.

Walker GA, White TM, McColl G, Jenkins NL, Babich S, Candido EPM, Johnson TE, Lithgow GJ. Heat shock protein accumulation is upregulated in a long-lived mutant of *Caenorhabditis elegans. J Gerontol A Biol Sci Med Sci* 56:B281–287, 2001.

Walker RF, Bercu BB. Effectiveness of growth hormone (GH) secretagogues in diagnosing and treating GH secretory deficiency in aging men. *J Anti-Aging Med* 1:219–228, 1998.

Walser M. Creatinine excretion as a measure of protein nutrition in adults of varying age. *JPEN J Parenter Enteral Nutr* 11:73S–78S, 1987.

Wanagat J, Allison DB, Weindruch R. Caloric intake and aging: mechanisms in rodents and a study in nonhuman primates. *Toxicol Sci* 52:35–40, 1999.

Wanagat J, Lopez ME, Aiken JM. Alterations of the mitochondrial genome. In Masoro EJ, Austad SN (eds). *Handbook of the Biology of Aging, 5th ed.* Academic Press, New York, 2001, pp 114–139.

Wanek LJ, Snow MH. Activity-induced fiber regeneration in rat soleus muscle. *Anat Rec* 258:176–185, 2000.

Wang CK, Nelson CF, Brinkman AM, Miller AC, Hoeffler WK. Spontaneous cell sorting of fibroblasts and keratinocytes creates an organotypic human skin equivalent. *J Invest Dermatol* 114:674–680, 2000a.

Wang CS, Goulet F, Lavoie J, Drouin R, Auger F, Champetier S, Germain L, Tetu B. Establishment and characterization of a new cell line derived from a human primary breast carcinoma. *Cancer Genet Cytogenet* 120:58–72, 2000b.

Wang E, Autexier C, Chen E. Apoptosis and aging. In Masoro EJ, Austad SN (eds). *Handbook of the Biology of Aging, 5th ed.* Academic Press, New York, 2001a, pp 246–268.

Wang E, Warner HR (eds). *Growth Control During Cell Aging.* CRC Press, Boca Raton, FL, 1989.

Wang J, Hannon GJ, Beach DH. Risky immortalization by telomerase. *Nature* 405:755–756, 2000c.

Wang, J, Xie L, Allan S, Beach D, Hannon G. Myc activates telomerase. *Genes Dev* 12:1769, 1998a.

Wang L, Evans AE, Ogburn CE, Youssoufian H, Martin GM, Oshima JB. Werner helicase expression in human fetal and adult aortas. *Exp Gerontol* 34:935–941, 1999.

Wang L, Hunt KE, Martin GM, Oshima J. Structure and function of the human Werner syndrome gene promoter: evidence for transcriptional modulation. *Nucleic Acids Res* 26:3480–3485, 1998b.

Wang L, Ogburn CE, Ware CB, Ladiges WC, Youssoufian H, Martin GM, Oshima J. Cellular Werner phenotypes in mice expressing a putative dominant-negative human *WRN* gene. *Genetics* 154:357–362, 2000d.

Wang PS, Solomon DH, Mogun H, Avorn J. HMG-CoA reductase inhibitors and the risk of hip fractures in elderly patients. *JAMA* 283:3211–3216, 2000e.

Wang S, Sun J, Zhang W. Telomerase activity in cervical intraepithelial neoplasia [in Chinese]. *Zhonghua Fu Chan Ke Za Zhi* 36:275–277, 2001b.

Wang SJ, Sakamoto T, Yasuda Si S, Fukasawa I, Ota Y, Hayashi M, Okura T, Zheng JH, Inaba N. The relationship between telomere length and telomerase activity in gynecologic cancers. *Gynecol Oncol* 84:81–84, 2002.

Wang SM, Nishigori C, Yagi T, Takebe H Reduced DNA repair in progeria cells and effects of gamma-ray irradiation on UV-induced unscheduled DNA synthesis in normal and progeria cells. *Mutat Res* 256:59–66, 1991.

Wang SM, Nishigori CK, Zhang JM, Takebe H. Reduced DNA-repair capacity in cells originating from a progeria patient. *Mutat Res* 237:253–257, 1990.

Wang SM, Phillips PD, Sierra F, Cristofalo VJ. Altered expression of the twist gene in young versus senescent human diploid fibroblasts. *Exp Cell Res* 228:138–145, 1996.

Wang SS, Zakian VA. Sequencing of *Saccharomyces* telomeres cloned using T4 DNA polymerase reveals two domains. *Mol Cell Biol* 10:4415–4419, 1990a.

Wang SS, Zakian VA. Telomere–telomere recombination provides an express pathway for telomere acquisition. *Nature* 345:456–458, 1990b.

Wang X, et al. Apolipoprotein E gene polymorphism and its association with human longevity in the Uygur nationality in Xinjiang. *Chinese Med J* 114:817–820, 2001c.

Wang X, Masters JR, Wong YC, Lo AK, Tsao SW. Mechanism of differential sensitivity to cisplatin in nasopharyngeal carcinoma cells. *Anticancer Res* 21:403–408, 2001d.

Wang X, Zhang Z, He M. Location expression of human telomerase reverse transcriptase in lung cancer, benign lesion and normal lung tissue [in Chinese]. *Zhonghua Jie He He Hu Xi Za Zhi* 24:461–464, 2001e.

Wang Z, Kyo S, Takakura M, Tanaka M, Yatabe N, Maida Y, Fujiwara M, Hayakawa J, Ohmichi M, Koike K, Inoue M. Progesterone regulates human telomerase reverse transcriptase gene expression via activation of mitogen-activated protein kinase signaling pathway. *Cancer Res* 60:5376–5381, 2000f.

Wang Z, Ramin SA, Tsai C, Lui P, Herbert PJ, Kyeyune-Nyombi E, Ruckle HC, Beltz RE, Sands JF. Detection of telomerase activity in prostatic fluid specimens. *Urol Oncol* 6:4–9, 2000g.

Wang Z, Ramin SA, Tsai C, Lui P, Ruckle HC, Beltz RE, Sands JF. Telomerase activity in prostate sextant needle cores from radical prostatectomy specimens. *Urol Oncol* 6:57–62, 2001f.

Wang ZQ, Bell-Farrow AD, Sonntag W, Cefalu WT. Effect of age and caloric restriction on insulin receptor binding and glucose transporter levels in aging rats. *Exp Gerontol* 32:671–684, 1997.

Ware TL, Wang H, Blackburn EH. Three telomerases with completely non-telomeric template replacements are catalytically active. *EMBO J* 19:3119–3131, 2000.

Waring GO 3d, Lynn MJ, Nizam A, Kutner MH, Cowden JW, Culbertson W, Laibson PR, McDonald MB, Nelson JD, Obstbaum SA, et al. Results of the Prospective Evaluation of Radial Keratotomy (PERK) Study five years after surgery: the PERK Study Group. *Ophthalmology* 98:1164–1176, 1991.

Warner HR. Aging and regulation of apoptosis. *Curr Top Cell Regul* 35:107–121, 1997.

Warner HR, Campisi J, Cristofalo VJ, Miller RA, Papaconstantinou J, Pereira-Smith O, Smith JR, Wang E. Control of cell proliferation in senescent cells. *J Gerontol A Biol Sci Med Sci* 47:B185–189, 1992.

Warner HR, Hodes RJ. Telomere length, telomerase, and aging: hype, hope, and reality. *Generations* 24:48–53, 2000.

Warner HR, Hodes RJ, Pocinki K. What does cell death have to do with aging? *J Am Geriatr Soc* 45:1140–1146, 1997.

Warner J, Butler R. Alzheimer's disease. *Clin Evidence* 3:419–425, 2000.

Warnholtz A, Mollnau H, Oelze M, Wendt M, Munzel T. Antioxidants and endothelial dysfunction in hyperlipidemia. *Curr Hypertens Rep* 3:53–60, 2001.

Wasserman SA, DiNardo S. Staying a boy forever. *Science* 294:2495–2496, 2002.

Watabe-Rudolph M, Rudolph KL, Averbeck T, Buhr T, Lenarz T, Stover T. Telomerase activity, telomere length, and apoptosis: a comparison between acquired cholesteatoma and squamous cell carcinoma. *Otol Neurotol* 23:793–798, 2002.

Watanabe H, Pan ZQ, Schreiber-Agus N, DePinho RA, Hurwitz J, Xiong Y. Suppression of cell transformation by the cyclin-dependent kinase inhibitor p57KIP2 requires binding to proliferating cell nuclear antigen. *Proc Natl Acad Sci USA* 95:1392–1397, 1998.

Watanabe N. Telomerase, cell immortality and cancer [in Japanese]. *Hokkaido Igaku Zasshi* 76:127–132, 2001.

Watanabe Y, Lee SW, Detmar M, Ajioka I, Dvorak HF. Vascular permeability factor/vascular endothelial growth factor (VPF/VEGF) delays and induces escape from senescence in human dermal microvascular endothelial cells. *Oncogene* 14:2025–2032, 1997.

Waters DD, Alderman EL, Hsia J, Howard BV, Cobb FR, Rogers WJ, Ouyang P, Thompson P, Tardif JC, Higginson L, Bittner V, Steffes M, Gordon DJ, Proschan M, Younes N, Verter JI. Effects of hormone replacement therapy and antioxidant vitamin supplements on coronary atherosclerosis in postmenopausal women. *JAMA* 288:2432–2440, 2002.

Watson JD. *The Double Helix*. Mentor, New York, 1968.

Watson JD. Origin of concatameric T7 DNA. *Nature: New Biology* 239:197–201, 1972.

Watt FM, Hogan BLM. Out of Eden: stem cells and their niches. *Science* 287:1427–1430, 2000.

Weaver DT. Telomeres: moonlighting by DNA repair proteins. *Curr Biol* 8:R492–494, 1998.

Weber KT, Sun Y. Remodeling of the cardiac interstium in ischemic cardiomyopathy. In Hosenpud JD, Greenberg BH (eds). *Congestive Heart Failure*. Lippincott Williams & Wilkins, Philadelphia, 2000, pp 117–136.

Webley K, Bond JA, Jones CJ, Blaydes JP, Craig A, Hupp T, Wynford-Thomas D. Posttranslational modifications of p53 in replicative senescence overlapping but distinct from those induced by DNA damage. *Mol Cell Biol* 20:2803–2808, 2000.

Webster S, Bradt B, Rogers J, Cooper N. Aggregation state-dependent activation of the classical complement pathway by the amyloid beta peptide. *J Neurochem* 69:388–398, 1997.

Webster S, Rogers J. Relative efficacies of amyloid beta peptide (A beta) binding proteins in A beta aggregation. *J Neurosci Res* 46:58–66, 1996.

Wei MC, Zong W-X, Cheng E H-Y, Lindsten T, Panoutsakopoulou V, Ross AJ, Roth KA, MacGregor GR, Thompson CB, Korsmeyer SJ. Proapoptotic BAX and BAK: a requisite gateway to mitochondrial dysfunction and death. *Science* 292:727–730, 2001a.

Wei W, Hemmer RM, Sedivy JM. Role of p14(ARF) in replicative and induced senescence of human fibroblasts. *Mol Cell Biol* 21:6748–6757, 2001b.

Weinberg RA. Telomeres. Bumps on the road to immortality. *Nature* 396:23–24, 1998.

Weindruch R. Effect of caloric restriction on age-associated cancers. *Exp Gerontol* 27:575–581, 1992.

Weindruch R. Interventions based on the possibility that oxidative stress contributes to sarcopenia. *J Gerontol A Biol Sci Med Sci* 50(Spec No):157–161, 1995.

Weindruch R. The retardation of aging by caloric restriction: studies in rodents and primates. *Toxicol Pathol* 24:742–745, 1996.

Weindruch R, Albanes D, Kritchevsky D. The role of calories and caloric restriction in carcinogenesis. *Hematol Oncol Clin North Am* 5:79–89, 1991.

Weindruch R, Keenan KP, Carney JM, Fernandes G, Feuers RJ, Floyd RA, Halter JB, Ramsey JJ, Richardson A, Roth GS, Spindler SR. Caloric restriction mimetics: metabolic interventions. *J Gerontol A Biol Sci Med Sci* 56A:B20–33, 2001.

Weindruch R, Lane MA, Ingram DK, Ershler WB, Roth GS. Dietary restriction in rhesus monkeys: lymphopenia and reduced mitogen-induced proliferation in peripheral blood mononuclear cells. *Aging (Milano)* 9:304–308, 1997.

Weindruch R, Walford RL. *The Retardation of Aging and Disease by Dietary Restriction*. CC Thomas, Springfield, IL, 1988.

Weinrich SL, Pruzan R, Ma L, Ouellette M, Tesmer VM, Holt SE, Bodnar AG, Lichtsteiner S, Kim NW, Trager JB, Taylor RD, Carlos R, Andrews WH, Wright WE, Shay JW, Harley CB, Morin GB. Reconstitution of human telomerase with the template RNA component hTR and the catalytic protein subunit hTRT. *Nat Genet* 17:498–502, 1997.

Weinstein BS, Ciszek D. The reserve-capacity hypothesis: evolutionary origins and modern implications of the trade-off between tumor-suppression and tissue-repair. *Exp Gerontol* 37:615–627, 2002.

Weirach-Schwaiger H, Weirich HG, Gruber B, Schweiger M, Hirsch-Kauffmann M. Correlation between senescence and DNA repair in cells from young and old individuals and in premature aging syndromes. *Mutat Res* 316:37–48, 1994.

Weismann A. *Uber Leben und Tod*. Jena, 1884.

Weissman IL. Translating stem and progenitor cell biology to the clinic: barriers and opportunities. *Science* 287:1442–1446, 2000.

Welle S. Growth hormone and insulin-like growth factor-I as anabolic agents. *Curr Opin Clin Nutr Metab Care* 1:257–262, 1998.

Wellinger RJ, Ethier K, Labrecque P, Zakian VA. Evidence for a new step in telomere maintenance. *Cell* 85:423–433, 1996.

Wellinger RJ, Wolf AJ, Zakian VA. Use of non-denaturing Southern hybridization and two dimensional agarose gels to detect putative intermediates in telomere replication in *Saccharomyces cerevisiae*. *Chromosoma* 102(1 Suppl):S150–156, 1992.

Wellinger RJ, Wolf AJ, Zakian VA. Origin activation and formation of single-strand TG1-3 tails occur sequentially in late S phase on a yeast linear plasmid. *Mol Cell Biol* 13:4057–4065, 1993a.

Wellinger RJ, Wolf AJ, Zakian VA. *Saccharomyces* telomeres acquire single-strand TG1-3 tails late in S phase. *Cell* 72:51–60, 1993b.

Wellinger RJ, Wolf AJ, Zakian VA. Structural and temporal analysis of telomere replication in yeast. *Cold Spring Harb Symp Quant Biol* 58:725–732, 1993c.

Wen J, Cong YS, Bacchetti S. Reconstitution of wild-type or mutant telomerase activity in telomerase-negative immortal human cells. *Hum Mol Genet* 7:1137–1141, 1998.

Weng N. Interplay between telomere length and telomerase in human leukocyte differentiation and aging. *J Leukoc Biol* 70:861–867, 2001.

Weng NP. Regulation of telomerase expression in human lymphocytes. *Springer Semin Immunopathol* 24:23–33, 2002.

Weng NP, Granger L, Hodes RJ. Telomere lengthening and telomerase activation during human B cell differentiation. *Proc Natl Acad Sci USA* 94:10827–10832, 1997a.

Weng NP, Hathcock KS, Hodes RJ. Regulation of telomere length and telomerase in T and B cells: a mechanism for maintaining replicative potential. *Immunity* 9:151–157, 1998.

Weng NP, Hodes RJ. The role of telomerase expression and telomere length maintenance in human and mouse. *J Clin Immunol* 20:257–267, 2000.

Weng NP, Levine BL, June CH, Hodes RJ. Human naive and memory T lymphocytes differ in telomeric length and replicative potential. *Proc Natl Acad Sci USA* 92:11091–11094, 1995.

Weng NP, Levine BL, June CH, Hodes RJ. Regulated expression of telomerase activity in human T lymphocyte development and activation. *J Exp Med* 183:2471–2479, 1996.

Weng N, Levine BL, June CH, Hodes RJ. Regulation of telomerase RNA template expression in human T lymphocyte development and activation. *J Immunol* 158:3215–3220, 1997b.

Weng NP, Palmer LD, Levine BL, Lane HC, June CH, Hodes RJ. Tales of tails: regulation of telomere length and telomerase activity during lymphocyte development, differentiation, activation, and aging. *Immunol Rev* 160:43–54, 1997c.

Wenz C, Enenkel B, Amacker M, Kelleher C, Damm K, Lingner J. Human telomerase contains two cooperating telomerase RNA molecules. *EMBO J* 20:3526–3534, 2001.

Werner CWO. Ueber Kataract in Verbindung mit Sclerodermie. Schmidt and Karnig, Kiel, Germany, 1904.

Werninghaus K, Meydani M, Bhawan J, Margolis R, Blumberg JB, Gilchrest BA. Evaluation of the photoprotective effect of oral vitamin E supplementation. *Arch Dermatol* 130:1257–1261, 1994.

West CD, Brown H, Simons EL, Carter DB, Kumagai LF, Englert E Jr. Adrencortical function and cortisol metabolism in old age. *J Clin Endocrinol Metab* 21:1197, 1961.

West MD. The cellular and molecular biology of skin aging. *Arch Dermatol* 130:87–95, 1994.

West MD, Pereira-Smith OM, Smith JR. Replicative senescence of human skin fibroblasts correlates with a loss of regulation and overexpression of collagenase activity. *Exp Cell Res* 184:138–147, 1989.

West MD, Shay JW, Wright WE, Linskens MH. Altered expression of plasminogen and plasminogen activator inhibitor during cellular senescence. *Exp Gerontol* 31:175–193, 1996.

Westendorp RG, Kirkwood TB. Human longevity at the cost of reproductive success. *Nature* 396:743–746, 1998.

Westerman KA, Leboulch P. Reversible immortalization of mammalian cells mediated by retroviral transfer and site-specific recombination. *Proc Natl Acad Sci USA* 93:8971–8976, 1996.

Westerterp KR, Meijer EP. Physical activity and parameters of aging: a physiological perspective. *J Gerontol A Biol Sci Med Sci* 56:B7–12, 2001.

Weyand CM, Brandes JC, Schmidt D, Fulbright JW, Goronzy JJ. Functional properties of CD4+CD28– T cells in the aging immune system. *Mech Ageing Dev* 102:131–147, 1998.

Whikehart DR, Register SJ, Chang Q, Montgomery B. Relationship of telomeres and p53 in aging bovine corneal endothelial cell cultures. *Invest Ophthalmol Vis Sci* 41:1070–1075, 2000.

White L, Petrovitch H, Ross GW, Masaki KH, Abbott RD, Teng EL, Rodriguez BL, Blanchette PL, Havlik RJ, Wergowske G, Chiu D, Foley DJ, Murdaugh C, Curb JD. Prevalence of dementia in older Japanese American men in Hawaii. *JAMA* 276:955–960, 1996.

Wick G, Jansen-Durr P, Berger P, Blasko I, Grubeck-Loebenstein B. Diseases of aging. *Vaccine* 18:1567–1583, 2000.

Wick M, Zubov D, Hagen G. Genomic organization and promoter characterization of the gene encoding the human telomerase reverse transcriptase (hTERT). *Gene* 232:97–106, 1999.

Widrick JJ, Maddalozzo GF, Lewis D, Valentine BA, Garner DP, Stelzer JE, Shoepe TC, Snow CM. Mophological and functional characteristics of skeletal muscle fibers from hormone-replaced and nonreplaced postmenopausal women. *J Gerontol A Biol Sci Med Sci* 58:3–10, 2003.

Wiemann SU, Satyanarayana A, Tsahuridu M, Tillmann HL, Zender L, Klempnauer J, Flemming P, Franco S, Blasco MA, Manns MP, Rudolph KL. Hepatocyte telomere shortening and senescence are general markers of human liver cirrhosis. *FASEB J* 16:935–942, 2002.

Wierzba-Bobrowicz T, Lewandowska E, Schmidt-Sidor B, Gwiazda E. The comparison of microglia maturation in CNS of normal human fetuses and fetuses with Down's syndrome. *Folia Neuropathol* 37:227–234, 1999.

Wiesel E. *Legends of Our Time*. Avon Books, New York, 1968.

Wilde, O. *The Picture of Dorian Gray*. 1890.

Wildy KS, Wasko MC. Current concepts regarding pharmacologic treatment of rheumatoid and osteoarthritis. *Hand Clin* 17:321–338, xi, 2001.

Wiley EA, Zakian VA. Extra telomeres, but not internal tracts of telomeric DNA, reduce transcriptional repression at *Saccharomyces* telomeres. *Genetics* 139:67–79, 1995.

Williams B. A potential role for angiotensin II–induced vascular endothelial growth factor expression in the pathogenesis of diabetic nephropathy? *Miner Electrolyte Metab* 24:400–405, 1998.

Williams JR. The effects of dehydroepiandrosterone on carcinogenesis, obesity, the immune system, and aging. *Lipids* 35:325–331, 2000.

Williams K, Dooley N, Ulvestad E, Becher B, Antel JP. IL-10 production by adult human derived microglial cells. *Neurochem Int* 29:55–64, 1996.

Williams O. *Immortal Poems of the English Language*. Washington Square Press, New York, 1952.

Wilmoth JR, Deegan LJ, Lundstrom H, Horiuchi S. Increase of maximum life span in Sweden, 1861–1999. *Science* 289:2366–2368, 2000.

Wilmut I, Clark J, Harley CB. Laying hold on eternal life? *Nat Biotechnol* 18:599–600, 2000.

Wilson CA, Ramos L, Villasenor MR, Anders KH, Press MF, Clarke K, Karlan B, Chen JJ, Scully R, Livingston D, Zuch RH, Kanter MH, Cohen S, Calzone FJ, Slamon DJ. Localization of human BRCA1 and its loss in high-grade, non-inherited breast carcinomas. *Nat Genet* 21:236–240, 1999.

Wilson PWF. Homocysteine and coronary heart disease: how great is the hazard? *JAMA* 288:2042–2043, 2002.

Wilson RS, Mendes de Leon CF, Barnes LL, Schneider JA, Bienias JL, Evans DA, Bennett DA. Participation in cognitively stimulating activities and risk of incident Alzheimer disease. *JAMA* 287:742–748, 2002.

Wilt T, Brawer M: Prostate cancer: non-metastatic. *Clin Evidence* 3:410–417, 2000.

Wingo PA, Ries LAG, Rosenberg HM, Miller DS, Edwards BK. Cancer incidence and mortality, 1973–1995. *Cancer* 82:1197–1207, 1998.

Winkler BS, Boulton ME, Gottsch JD, Sternberg P. Oxidative damage and age-related macular degeneration. *Mol Vis* 5:32, 1999.

Winkles JA, O'Connor ML, Friesel R. Altered regulation of platelet-derived growth factor A-chain and c-*fos* gene expression in senescent progeria fibroblasts. *J Cell Physiol* 144:313–325, 1990.

Wirak DO, Bayney R, Kundel CA, Lee A, Scangos GA, Trapp BD, Unterbeck AJ. Regulatory region of human amyloid precursor protein (APP) gene promotes neuron-specific gene expression in the CNS of transgenic mice. *EMBO J* 10:289–296, 1991.

Wise PM. Nathan Shock Memorial Lecture 1991. Changing neuroendocrine function during aging: impact on diurnal and pulsatile rhythms. *Exp Gerontol* 29:13–19, 1994.

Wise PM. Neuroendocrine involvement in the aging: evidence from studies of reproductive aging and caloric restriction. *Neurobiol Aging* 16:853; discussion 855–856, 1995.

Wise PM. Neuroendocrine modulation of the "menopause": insights into the aging brain. *Am J Physiol* 277:E965–970, 1999.

Wise PM, Kashon ML, Krajnak KM, Rosewell KL, Cai A, Scarbrough K, Harney JP, McShane T, Lloyd JM, Weiland NG. Aging of the female reproductive system: a window into brain aging. *Recent Prog Horm Res* 52:279–303; discussion 303–305, 1997.

Wise PM, Krajnak KM, Kashon ML. Menopause: the aging of multiple pacemakers. *Science* 273:67–70, 1996.

Wise PM, Scarbrough K, Lloyd J, Cai A, Harney J, Chiu S, Hinkle D, McShane T. Neuroendocrine concomitants of reproductive aging. *Exp Gerontol* 29:275–283, 1994.

Wise PM, Smith MJ, Dubal DB, Wilson ME, Krajnak KM, Rosewell KL. Neuroendocrine influences and repercussions of the menopause. *Endocr Rev* 20:243–248, 1999.

Wiseman BS, Werb Z. Stromal effects on mammary development and breast cancer. *Science* 296:1046–1049, 2002.

Wisman GB, De Jong S, Meersma GJ, Helder MN, Hollema H, De Vries EG, Keith WN, Van Der Zee AG. Telomerase in (pre)neoplastic cervical disease. *Hum Pathol* 31:1304–1312, 2000.

Wisman GB, Hollema H, de Jong S, ter Schegget J, Tjong-A-Hung SP, Ruiters MH, Krans M, de Vries EG, van der Zee AG. Telomerase activity as a biomarker for (pre)neoplastic cervical disease in scrapings and frozen sections from patients with abnormal cervical smear. *J Clin Oncol* 16:2238–2245, 1998.

Wisman GB, Knol AJ, Helder MN, Krans M, de Vries EG, Hollema H, de Jong S, van Der Zee AG. Telomerase in relation to clinicopathologic prognostic factors and survival in cervical cancer. *Int J Cancer* 91:658–664, 2001.

Wistrom C, Villeponteau B. Cloning and expression of SAG: a novel marker of cellular senescence. *Exp Cell Res* 199:355–362, 1992.

Wistrom D, Feng J, Villeponteau B. Proliferative capacity of human fibroblasts when cultured in serum from young or old cows. *J Gerontol A Biol Sci Med Sci* 44:B160–163, 1989.

Wisuthsarewong W, Viravan S. Hutchinson-Gilford progeria syndrome. *J Med Assoc Thai* 82:96–102, 1999.

Wittgenstein L. *Philosophical Investigations, 3rd ed.* Anscombe GEM (trans). MacMillan Company, New York, 1958.

Wittman CW, Wszolek MF, Shulman JM, Salvaterra PM, Lewis J, Hutton M, Feany MB. Taupathy in *Drosophila*: neurodegeneration without neurofibrillary tangles. *Science* 293:711–714, 2001.

Wojtyk RI, Goldstein S. Fidelity of protein synthesis does not decline during aging of cultured human fibroblasts. *J Cell Physiol* 103:299–303, 1980.

Wolf NS, Pendergrass WR. The relationships of animal age and caloric intake to cellular replication in vivo and in vitro: a review. *J Gerontol A Biol Sci Med Sci* 54:B502–517, 1999.

Wolf NS, Li Y, Pendergrass W, Schmeider C, Turturro A. Normal mouse and rat strains as models for age-related cataract and the effect of caloric restriction on its development. *Exp Eye Res* 70:683–692, 2000.

Wolf NS, Penn PE, Jiang D, Fei RG, Pendergrass WR. Caloric restriction: conservation of in vivo cellular replicative capacity accompanies life-span extension in mice. *Exp Cell Res* 217:317–323, 1995.

Wolfe J. Growth hormone: a physiological fountain of youth? *J Anti-Aging Med* 1:9–26, 1998.

Wolff DJ, Clifton K, Karr C, Charles J. Pilot assessment of the subtelomeric regions of children with autism: detection of a 2q deletion. *Genet Med* 4:10–14, 2002.

Wolkow CA, Kimura KD, Lee M-S, Ruvkun G. Regulation of *C. elegans* life span by insulin-like signaling in the nervous system. *Science* 290:147–150, 2000.

Wollheim FA. Serum markers of articular cartilage damage and repair. *Rheum Dis Clin North Am* 25:417–432, 1999.

Wollheim FA. Approaches to rheumatoid arthritis in 2000. *Curr Opin Rheumatol* 13:193–201, 2001.

Wollina U, Reuter A, Schaarschmidt H, Muller E, Maak B, Schmidt U. Hutchinson-Gilford syndrome [in German]. *Hautarzt* 43:453–457, 1992.

Wolozin B, Kellman W, Ruosseau P, Celesia GG, Siegel G. Decreased prevalence of Alzheimer disease associated with 3-hydroxy-3-methyglutaryl coenzyme A reductase inhibitors. *Arch Neurol* 57:1439–1443, 2000.

Wolthers KC, Bea G, Wisman A, Otto SA, de Roda Husman AM, Schaft N, de Wolf F, Goudsmit J, Coutinho RA, van der Zee AG, Meyaard L, Miedema F. T cell telomere length in HIV-1 infection: no evidence for increased CD4+ T cell turnover. *Science* 274:1543–1547, 1996.

Wolthers KC, Miedema F. Telomeres and HIV-1 infection: in search of exhaustion. *Trends Microbiol* 6:144–147, 1998.

Wolthers KC, Schuitemaker H, Miedema F. Rapid CD4+ T-cell turnover in HIV-1 infection: a paradigm revisited. *Immunol Today* 19:44–48, 1998.

Wong JM, Kusdra L, Collins K. Subnuclear shuttling of human telomerase induced by transformation and DNA damage. *Nat Cell Biol* 4:731–736, 2002.

Wong KK, Chang S, Weiler SR, Ganesan S, Chaudhuri J, Zhu C, Artandi SE, Rudolph KL, Gottlieb GJ, Chin L, Alt FW, DePinho RA. Telomere dysfunction impairs DNA repair and enhances sensitivity to ionizing radiation. *Nat Genet* 26:85–88, 2000.

Wood LD, Halvorsen TL, Dhar S, Baur JA, Pandita RK, Wright WE, Hande MP, Calaf G, Hei TK, Levine F, Shay JW, Wang JJ, Pandita TK. Characterization of ataxia telangiectasia fibroblasts with extended life span through telomerase expression. *Oncogene* 20:278–288, 2001a.

Wood RD, Mitchell M, Sgouros J, Lindahl T. Human DNA repair genes. *Science* 291: 1284–1289, 2001b.

Woodbury D, Schwarz EJ, Prockop DJ, Black IB. Adult rat and human bone marrow stromal cells differentiate into neurons. *J Neurosci Res* 61:364–370, 2000.

World Health Organization. Assessment of Fracture Risk and its Application to Screening for Postmenopausal Osteoporosis. WHO Technical Report Series 843. World Health Organization, Geneva, 1994.

Worzala K, Hiller R, Sperduto RD, Mutalik K, Murabito JM, Moskowitz M, D'Agostino RB, Wilson PW. Postmenopausal estrogen use, type of menopause, and lens opacities: the Framingham studies. *Arch Intern Med* 161:1448–1454, 2001.

Wright JH, Gottschling DE, Zakian VA. *Saccharomyces* telomeres assume a non-nucleosomal chromatin structure. *Genes Dev* 6:197–210, 1992.

Wright JH, Zakian VA. Protein–DNA interactions in soluble telosomes from *Saccharomyces cerevisiae*. *Nucleic Acids Res* 23:1454–1460, 1995.

Wright TC Jr, Cox JT, Massad LS, Twiggs LB, Wilkinson EJ; ASCCP-Sponsored Consensus Conference. 2001 Consensus Guidelines for the management of women with cervical cytological abnormalities. *JAMA* 287:2120–2129, 2002.

Wright WE, Brasiskyte D, Piatyszek MA, Shay JW. Experimental elongation of telomeres extends the life span of immortal × normal cell hybrids. *EMBO J* 15:1734–1741, 1996a.

Wright WE, Hayflick L. Nuclear control of cellular aging demonstrated by hybridization of anucleate and whole cultured normal human fibroblasts. *Exp Cell Res* 96:113–121, 1975.

Wright WE, Pereira-Smith OM, Shay JW. Reversible cellular senescence: implications for immortalization of normal human diploid fibroblasts. *Mol Cell Biol* 9:3088–3092, 1989.

Wright WE, Piatyszek MA, Rainey WE, Byrd W, Shay JW. Telomerase activity in human germline and embryonic tissues and cells. *Dev Genet* 18:173–179, 1996b.

Wright WE, Shay JW. Telomere positional effects and the regulation of cellular senescence. *Trends Genet* 8:193–197, 1992a.

Wright WE, Shay JW. The two-stage mechanism controlling cellular senescence and immortalization. *Exp Gerontol* 27:383–389, 1992b.

Wright WE and Shay JW. Mechanisms of escaping senescence in human diploid cells. In Holbrook JJ, Martin GR, Lockshin RA (eds). *Modern Cell Biology Series, Cellular Aging and Cell Death.* John Wiley & Sons, New York, 1996, pp 153–167.

Wright WE, Shay JW. Telomere dynamics in cancer progression and prevention: fundamental differences in human and mouse telomere biology. *Nat Med* 6:849–851, 2000.

Wright WE, Shay JW. Historical claims and current interpretations of replicative aging. *Nat Biotechnol* 20:682–688, 2002.

Wright WE, Shay JW, Piatyszek MA. Modifications of a telomeric repeat amplification protocol (TRAP) result in increased reliability, linearity and sensitivity. *Nucleic Acids Res* 23:3794–3795, 1995.

Wright WE, Tesmer VM, Huffman KE, Levene SD, Shay JW. Normal human chromosomes have long G-rich telomeric overhangs at one end. *Genes Dev* 11:2801–2809, 1997.

Wright WE, Tesmer VM, Liao ML, Shay JW. Normal human telomeres are not late replicating. *Exp Cell Res* 251:492–499, 1999.

Wright WW, Fiore C, Zirkin BR. The effect of aging on the seminiferous epithelium of the Brown Norway rat. *J Androl* 14:110–117, 1993.

Writing Group for the Women's Health Initiative Investigators. Risks and benefits of estrogen plus progestin in healthy postmenopausal women. Principal results from the Women's Health Initiative randomized controlled trial. *JAMA* 288:321–333, 2002.

Wu A, Ichihashi M, Ueda M. Correlation of the expression of human telomerase subunits with telomerase activity in normal skin and skin tumors. *Cancer* 86:2038–2044, 1999a.

Wu K, Lund M, Bang K, Thestrup-Pedersen K. Telomerase activity and telomere length in lymphocytes from patients with cutaneous T-cell lymphoma. *Cancer* 86:1056–1063, 1999b.

Wu KD, Hansen ER. Shortened telomere length is demonstrated in T-cell subsets together with a pronounced increased telomerase activity in CD4 positive T cells from blood of patients with mycosis fungoides and parapsoriasis. *Exp Dermatol* 10:329–336, 2001.

Wu KJ, Grandori C, Amacker M, Simon-Vermot N, Polack A, Lingner J, Dalla-Favera R. Direct activation of TERT transcription by c-MYC. *Nat Genet* 21:220–224, 1999c.

Wu WJ, Liu LT, Huang CN, Huang CH, Chang LL. The clinical implications of telomerase activity in upper tract urothelial cancer and washings. *BJU Int* 86:213–219, 2000a.

Wu XX, Kakehi Y, Takahashi T, Habuchi T, Ogawa O. Telomerase activity in urine after transurethral resection of superficial bladder cancer and early recurrence. *Int J Urol* 7:210–217, 2000b.

Wyllie FS, Jones CJ, Skinner JW, Haughton MF, Wallis C, Wynford-Thomas D, Faragher RG, Kipling D. Telomerase prevents the accelerated cell ageing of Werner syndrome fibroblasts. *Nat Genet* 24:16–17, 2000.

Wymenga LF, Wisman GB, Veenstra R, Ruiters MH, Mensink HJ. Telomerase activity in needle biopsies from prostate cancer and benign prostates. *Eur J Clin Invest* 30:330–335, 2000.

Wynford-Thomas D. Cellular senescence and cancer. *J Pathol* 187:100–111, 1999.

Wynford-Thomas D. Replicative senescence: mechanisms and implications for human cancer. *Pathol Biol (Paris)* 48:301–307, 2000.

Wynford-Thomas D, Kipling D. Cancer and the knockout mouse. *Nature* 389:551–552, 1997.

Wynn RF, Cross MA, Hatton C, Will AM, Lashford LS, Dexter TM, Testa NG. Accelerated telomere shortening in young recipients of allogenic bone-marrow transplants. *Lancet* 351:178–181, 1998.

Wyrick JJ, Holstege FC, Jennings EG, Causton HC, Shore D, Grunstein M, Lander ES, Young RA. Chromosomal landscape of nucleosome-dependent gene expression and silencing in yeast. *Nature* 402:418–421, 1999.

Xia MQ, Berezovska O, Kim TW, Xia WM, Liao A, Tanzi RE, Selkoe D, Hyman BT. Lack of specific association of presenilin 1 (PS-1) protein with plaques and tangles in Alzheimer's disease. *J Neurol Sci* 158:15–23, 1998.

Xia SJ, Shammas MA, Shmookler Reis RJ. Reduced telomere length in ataxia-telangiectasia fibroblasts. *Mutat Res* 364:1–11, 1996.

Xiang H, Wang J, Mao Y, Liu M, Reddy VN, Li DW. Human telomerase accelerates growth of lens epithelial cells through regulation of the genes mediating RB/E2F pathway. *Oncogene* 21:3784–3791, 2002.

Xinarianos G, Scott FM, Liloglou T, Prime W, Turnbull L, Walshaw M, Field JK. Evaluation of telomerase activity in bronchial lavage as a potential diagnostic marker for malignant lung disease. *Lung Cancer* 28:37–42, 2000.

Xu D, Neville R, Finkel T. Homocysteine accelerates endothelial cell senescence. *FEBS Lett* 470:20–24, 2000a.

Xu D, Popov N, Hou M, Wang Q, Bjorkholm M, Gruber A, Menkel AR, Henriksson M. Switch from Myc/Max to Mad1/Max binding and decrease in histone acetylation at the telomerase reverse transcriptase promoter during differentiation of HL60 cells. *Proc Natl Acad Sci USA* 98:3826–3831, 2001a.

Xu D, Zheng C, Bergenbrant S, Holm G, Bjorkholm M, Yi Q, Gruber A. Telomerase activity in plasma cell dyscrasias. *Br J Cancer* 84:621–625, 2001b.

Xu L, Pirollo KF, Tang WH, Rait A, Chang EH. Transferrin-liposome-mediated systemic *p53* gene therapy in combination with radiation results in regression of human head and neck cancer xenografts. *Hum Gene Ther* 10:2941–2952, 1999.

Xu W, Gong L, Haddad MM, Bischof O, Campisi J, Yeh ET, Medrano EE. Regulation of microphthalmia-associated transcription factor MITF protein levels by association with the ubiquitin-conjugating enzyme hUBC9. *Exp Cell Res* 255:135–143, 2000b.

Xu X, Sonntag WE. Growth hormone–induced nuclear translocation of Stat-3 decreases with age: modulation by caloric restriction. *Am J Physiol* 271(5 Pt 1):E903–E909, 1996a.

Xu X, Sonntag WE. Moderate caloric restriction prevents the age-related decline in growth hormone receptor signal transduction. *J Gerontol A Biol Sci Med Sci* 51:B167–174, 1996b.

Yaar M. Molecular mechanisms of skin aging. *Adv Dermatol* 10:63–75; discussion 76, 1995.

Yaar M, Arora J, Garmyn M, Gilani A, Gilchrest BA. Influence of aging and malignant transformation on keratinocyte gene expression. *Recent Results Cancer Res* 128:205–214, 1993.

Yaar M, Gilchrest BA. Cellular and molecular mechanisms of cutaneous aging. *J Dermatol Surg Oncol* 16:915–922, 1990.

Yaar M, Gilchrest BA. Human melanocytes as a model system for studies of Alzheimer disease. *Arch Dermatol* 133:1287–1291, 1997.

Yaar M, Gilchrest BA. Aging versus photoaging: postulated mechanisms and effectors. *J Investig Dermatol Symp Proc* 3:47–51, 1998.

Yaar M, Gilchrest BA. Skin aging: postulated mechanisms and consequent changes in structure and function. *Clin Geriatr Med* 17:617–630, 2001.

Yaar M, Zhai S, Pilch PF, Doyle SM, Eisenhauer PB, Fine RE, Gilchrest BA. Binding of beta-amyloid to the p75 neurotrophin receptor induces apoptosis. A possible mechanism for Alzheimer's disease. *J Clin Invest* 100:2333–2340, 1997.

Yablonka-Reuveni Z, Seger R, Rivera AJ. Fibroblast growth factor promotes recruitment of skeletal muscle satellite cells in young and old rats. *J Histochem Cytochem* 47:23–42, 1999.

Yahata N, Ohyashiki K, Ohyashiki JH, Iwama H, Hayashi S, Ando K, Hirano T, Tsuchida T, Kato H, Shay JW, Toyama K. Telomerase activity in lung cancer cells obtained from bronchial washings. *J Natl Cancer Inst* 90:684–690, 1998.

Yajima T, Yagihashi A, Kameshima H, Furuya D, Kobayashi D, Hirata K, Watanabe N. Establishment of quantitative reverse transcription–polymerase chain reaction assays for human telomerase–associated genes. *Clin Chim Acta* 290:117–127, 2000.

Yajima T, Yagihashi A, Kameshima H, Kobayashi D, Hirata K, Watanabe N. Telomerase reverse transcriptase and telomeric-repeat binding factor protein 1 as regulators of telomerase activity in pancreatic cancer cells. *Br J Cancer* 85:752–757, 2001.

Yamada K, Yajima T, Yagihashi A, Kobayashi D, Koyanagi Y, Asanuma K, Yamada M, Moriai R, Kameshima H, Watanabe N. Role of human telomerase reverse transcriptase and telomeric-repeat binding factor proteins 1 and 2 in human hematopoietic cells. *Jpn J Cancer Res* 91:1278–1284, 2000.

Yamada O, Motoji T, Mizoguchi H. Up-regulation of telomerase activity in human lymphocytes. *Biochim Biophys Acta* 1314:260–266, 1996.

Yamaguchi Y, Nozawa K, Savoysky E, Hayakawa N, Nimura Y, Yoshida S. Change in telomerase activity of rat organs during growth and aging. *Exp Cell Res* 242:120–127, 1998.

Yamanishi Y, Hiyama K, Ishioka S, Maeda H, Yamanaka T, Kurose Y, Yamakido M. Telomerase activity in the synovial tissues of chronic inflammatory and non-inflammatory rheumatic diseases. *Int J Mol Med* 4:513–517, 1999.

Yamanishi Y, Hiyama K, Maeda H, Ishioka S, Murakami T, Hiyama E, Kurose Y, Shay JW, Yamakido M. Telomerase activity in rheumatoid synovium correlates with the mononuclear cell infiltration level and disease aggressiveness of rheumatoid arthritis. *J Rheumatol* 25:214–220, 1998.

Yamashita J, Itoh H, Hirashima M, Ogawa M, Nishikawa Satomi, Yurugi T, Naito M, Nakao K, Nishikawa S. Flk1-positive cells derived from embryonic stem cells serve as vascular progenitors. *Nature* 408:92–96, 2000.

Yan LJ, Sohal RS. Mitochondrial adenine nucleotide translocase is modified oxidatively during aging. *Proc Natl Acad Sci USA* 95:12896–12901, 1998.

Yan P, Benhattar J, Coindre JM, Guillou L. Telomerase activity and hTERT mRNA expression can be heterogeneous and does not correlate with telomere length in soft tissue sarcomas. *Int J Cancer* 98:851–856, 2002.

Yan Y, Ouellette MM, Shay JW, Wright WE. Age-dependent alterations of c-fos and growth regulation in human fibroblasts expressing the HPV16 E6 protein. *Mol Biol Cell* 7:975–983, 1996.

Yan Y, Shay JW, Wright WE, Mumby MC. Inhibition of protein phosphatase activity induces p53–dependent apoptosis in the absence of p53 transactivation. *J Biol Chem* 272:15220–15226, 1997.

Yanagihara T. Vascular dementia [in Japanese]. *Rinsho Shinkeigaku* 39:1197–1199, 1999.

Yang CT, You L, Yeh CC, Chang JW, Zhang F, McCormick F, Jablons DM. Adenovirus-mediated p14(ARF) gene transfer in human mesothelioma cells. *J Natl Cancer Inst* 92:636–641, 2000.

Yang H, Kyo S, Takatura M, Sun L. Autocrine transforming growth factor beta suppresses telomerase activity and transcription of human telomerase reverse transcriptase in human cancer cells. *Cell Growth Differ* 12:119–127, 2001a.

Yang J, Chang E, Cherry AM, Bangs CD, Oei Y, Bodnar A, Bronstein A, Chiu CP, Herron GS. Human endothelial cell life extension by telomerase expression. *J Biol Chem* 274:26141–26148, 1999a.

Yang J, Nagavarapu U, Relloma K, Sjaastad MD, Moss WC, Passaniti A, Herron GS. Telomerized human microvasculature is functional in vivo. *Nat Biotechnol* 19:219–224, 2001b.

Yang L, Suwa T, Wright WE, Shay JW, Hornsby PJ. Telomere shortening and decline in replicative potential as a function of donor age in human adrenocortical cells. *Mech Ageing Dev* 122:1685–1694, 2001c.

Yang P, Becker D. Telomerase activity and expression of apoptosis and anti-apoptosis regulators in the progression pathway of human melanoma. *Int J Oncol* 17:913–919, 2000.

Yang Q, Bermingham NA, Finegold MJ, Zoghbi HY. Requirement of Math1 for secretory cell lineage commitment in the mouse intestine. *Science* 294:2155–2158, 2001d.

Yang SM, Fang DC, Yang JL, Liang GP, Lu R, Luo YH, Liu WW. Effect of antisense human telomerase RNA on malignant phenotypes of gastric carcinoma. *J Gastroenterol Hepatol* 17:1144–1152, 2002a.

Yang X, Tahin Q, Hu YF, Russo IH, Balsara BR, Mihaila D, Slater C, Barrett JC, Russo J. Functional roles of chromosomes 11 and 17 in the transformation of human breast epithelial cells in vitro. *Int J Oncol* 15:629–638, 1999b.

Yang Y, Chen Y, Zhang C, Huang H, Weissman SM. Nucleolar localization of hTERT protein is associated with telomerase function. *Exp Cell Res* 277:201–209, 2002b.

Yang Y, Wilson DL. Characterization of a life-extending mutation in *age-2*, a new aging gene in *Caenorhabditis elegans*. *J Gerontol A Biol Sci Med Sci* 54:B137–142, 1999.

Yao H, Wu B, Wu Q. Study and detection of telomerase activity in oral squamous cell carcinomas and precancerous lesions [in Chinese]. *Zhonghua Kou Qiang Yi Xue Za Zhi* 34:328–330, 1999.

Yashima K, Ashfaq R, Nowak J, Von Gruenigen V, Milchgrub S, Rathi A, Albores-Saavedra J, Shay JW, Gazdar AF. Telomerase activity and expression of its RNA component in cervical lesions. *Cancer* 82:1319–1327, 1998a.

Yashima K, Litzky LA, Kaiser L, Rogers T, Lam S, Wistuba II, Milchgrub S, Srivastava S, Piatyszek MA, Shay JW, Gazdar AF. Telomerase expression in respiratory epithelium during the multistage pathogenesis of lung carcinomas. *Cancer Res* 57:2373–2377, 1997a.

Yashima K, Maitra A, Rogers BB, Timmons CF, Rathi A, Pinar H, Wright WE, Shay JW, Gazdar AF. Expression of the RNA component of telomerase during human development and differentiation. *Cell Growth Differ* 9:805–813, 1998b.

Yashima K, Maitra A, Timmons CF, Rogers BB, Pinar H, Shay JW, Gazdar AF. Expression of the RNA component of telomerase in Wilms tumor and nephrogenic rest recapitulates renal embryogenesis. *Hum Pathol* 29:536–542, 1998c.

Yashima K, Milchgrub S, Gollahon LS, Maitra A, Saboorian MH, Shay JW, Gazdar AF. Telomerase enzyme activity and RNA expression during the multistage pathogenesis of breast carcinoma. *Clin Cancer Res* 4:229–234, 1998d.

Yashima K, Piatyszek MA, Saboorian HM, Virmani AK, Brown D, Shay JW, Gazdar AF. Telomerase activity and in situ telomerase RNA expression in malignant and non-malignant lymph nodes. *J Clin Pathol* 50:110–117, 1997b.

Yashin AI, De Benedictis G, Vaupel JW, Tan Q, Andreev KF, Iachine IA, Bonafe M, Velensin S, De Luca M, Carotenuto L, Franseschi C. Genes and longevity: lessons from studies of centenarians. *J Gerontol A Biol Sci Med Sci* 55:B319–B328, 2000.

Yasui W, Yokozaki H, Fujimoto J, Naka K, Kuniyasu H, Tahara E. Genetic and epigenetic alterations in multistep carcinogenesis of the stomach. *J Gastroenterol* 35:111–115, 2000.

Yasumoto S, Kunimura C, Kikuchi K, Tahara H, Ohji H, Yamamoto H, Ide T, Utakoji T. Telomerase activity in normal human epithelial cells. *Oncogene* 13:433–439, 1996.

Yaswen P, Stampfer MR. Epigenetic changes accompanying human mammary epithelial cell immortalization. *J Mammary Gland Biol Neoplasia* 6:223–234, 2001.

Yatabe N, Kyo S, Kondo S, Kanaya T, Wang Z, Maida Y, Takakura M, Nakamura M, Tanaka M, Inoue M. 2–5A antisense therapy directed against human telomerase RNA inhibits telomerase activity and induces apoptosis without telomere impairment in cervical cancer cells. *Cancer Gene Ther* 9:624–630, 2002.

Yates JR, Moore AT. Genetic susceptibility to age related macular degeneration. *J Med Genet* 37:83–87, 2000.

Yazawa M, Okuda M, Setoguchi A, Iwabuchi S, Nishimura R, Sasaki N, Masuda K, Ohno K, Tsujimoto H. Telomere length and telomerase activity in canine mammary gland tumors. *Am J Vet Res* 62:1539–1543, 2001.

Yazawa M, Okuda M, Setoguchi A, Nishimura R, Sasaki N, Hasegawa A, Watari T, Tsujimoto H. Measurement of telomerase activity in dog tumors. *J Vet Med Sci* 61:1125–1129, 1999.

Yaziji H, Gown AM. Immunohistochemical analysis of gynecologic tumors. *Int J Gynecol Pathol* 20:64–78, 2001.

Ye L, Miki T, Nakura J, Oshima J, Kamino K, Rakugi H, Ikegami H, Higaki J, Edland SD, Martin GM, Ogihara T. Association of a polymorphic variant of the Werner helicase gene with myocardial infarction in a Japanese population. *Am J Med Genet* 68:494–498, 1997.

Yeager TR, Neumann AA, Englezou A, Huschtscha LI, Noble JR, Reddel RR. Telomerase-negative immortalized human cells contain a novel type of promyelocytic leukemia (PML) body. *Cancer Res* 59:4175–4179, 1999.

Yeats WB. *The Collected Poems of W. B. Yeats, 2nd ed.* The MacMillan Company, New York, 1963.

Yegorov YE. Around telomerase. *Mol Biol (Mosc)* 33:333–339, 1999.

Yegorov YE, Akimov SS, Akhmalisheva AK, Semenova IV, Smirnova YB, Kraevsky AA, Zelenin AV. Blockade of telomerase function in various cells. *Anticancer Drug Des* 14:305–316, 1999.

Yegorov YE, Akimov SS, Hass R, Zelenin AV, Prudovsky IA. Endogenous β-galactosidase activity in continuously nonproliferating cells. *Exp Cell Res* 243:207–211, 1998.

Yegorov YE, Chernov DN, Akimov SS, Akhmalisheva AK, Smirnova YB, Shinkarev DB, Semenova IV, Yegorova IN, Zelenin AV. Blockade of telomerase function by nucleoside analogs. *Biochemistry (Moscow)* 62:1296–1305, 1997.

Yen TC, Su JH, King KL, Wei YH. Ageing-associated 5-kb deletion in human liver mitochondrial DNA. *Biochem Biophys Res Commun* 178:124–131, 1991.

Yermakova AV, Rollins J, Callahan LM, Rogers J, O'Banion MK. Cyclooxygenase-1 in human Alzheimer and control brain: quantitative analysis of expression by microglia and CA3 hippocampal neurons. *J Neuropathol Exp Neurol* 58:1135–1146, 1999.

Yi SY, Joeng KS, Kweon JU, Cho JW, Chung IK, Lee J. A single-stranded telomere binding protein in the nematode *Caenorhabditis elegans*. *FEBS Lett* 505:301–306, 2001.

Yi X, Tesmer VM, Savre-Train I, Shay JW, Wright WE. Both transcriptional and posttranscriptional mechanisms regulate human telomerase template RNA levels. *Mol Cell Biol* 19:3989–3997, 1999.

Yi X, White DM, Aisner DL, Baur JA, Wright WE, Shay JW. An alternate splicing variant of the human telomerase catalytic subunit inhibits telomerase activity. *Neoplasia* 2:433–440, 2000.

Yin D. Biochemical basis of lipofuscin, ceroid, and age pigment-like fluorophores. *Free Radic Biol Med* 21:871–888, 1996.

Yokoyama Y, Takahashi Y, Shinohara A, Wan X, Takahashi S, Niwa K, Tamaya T. The 5'-end of hTERT mRNA is a good target for hammerhead ribozyme to suppress telomerase activity. *Biochem Biophys Res Commun* 273:316–321, 2000.

Yokozaki H, Yasui W, Tahara E. Genetic and epigenetic changes in stomach cancer. *Int Rev Cytol* 204:49–95, 2001.

Yoo SH, Adamis AP. Retinal manifestations of aging. *Int Ophthalmol Clin* 38:95–101, 1998.

Yoshikawa TT. Epidemiology of aging and infectious disease. In Yoshikawa TT, Norman DC (eds). *Infectious Disease in the Aging*. Totowa, NJ, 2001, pp 3–6.

Yoshikawa TT, Norman DC. *Infectious Disease in the Aging*. Humana Press, Totowa, NJ, 2001.

Yoshimi N, Ino N, Suzui M, Hara A, Nakatani K, Sato S, Mori H. Telomerase activity of normal tissues and neoplasms in rat colon carcinogenesis induced by methylazoxymethanol acetate and its difference from that of human colonic tissues. *Mol Carcinog* 16:1–5, 1996.

You YO, Lee G, Min BM. Retinoic acid extends the in vitro life span of normal human oral keratinocytes by decreasing p16(INK4A) expression and maintaining telomerase activity. *Biochem Biophys Res Commun* 268:268–274, 2000.

Young EA. DHEA: mood, memory, and aging. *Biol Psychiatry* 45:1531–1532, 1999.

Young JB. Aging and the sympathoadrenal system. In Masoro EJ, Austad SN (eds). *Handbook of the Biology of Aging, 5th ed.* Academic Press, New York, 2001, pp 269–296.

Youngman LD, Park JY, Ames BN. Protein oxidation associated with aging is reduced by dietary restriction of protein or calories. *Proc Natl Acad Sci USA* 89:9112–9116, 1992.

Younus J, Gilchrest BA. Modulation of mRNA levels during human keratinocyte differentiation. *J Cell Physiol* 152:232–239, 1992.

Yu BP. *Free Radicals in Aging*. CRC Press, Boca Raton, FL, 1993.

Yu BP. Approaches to anti-aging intervention: the promises and the uncertainties. *Mech Ageing Dev* 111:73–87, 1999.

Yu CC, Lo SC, Wang TC. Telomerase is regulated by protein kinase C-ζ in human nasopharyngeal cancer cells. *Biochem J* 355:459–464, 2001.

Yu CE, Oshima J, Fu YH, Wijsman EM, Hisama F, Alisch R, Matthews S, Nakura J, Miki T, Ouais S, Martin GM, Mulligan J, Schellenberg GD. Positional cloning of the Werner's syndrome gene. *Science* 272:258–262, 1996.

Yu CE, Oshima J, Wijsman EM, Nakura J, Miki T, Piussan C, Matthews S, Fu YH, Mulligan J, Martin GM, Schellenberg GD. Mutations in the consensus helicase domains of the Werner syndrome gene. Werner's Syndrome Collaborative Group. *Am J Hum Genet* 60:330–341, 1997.

Yu GL, Blackburn EH. Developmentally programmed healing of chromosomes by telomerase in *Tetrahymena*. *Cell* 67:823–832, 1991.

Yu GL, Bradley JD, Attardi LD, Blackburn EH. In vivo alteration of telomere sequences and senescence caused by mutated *Tetrahymena* telomerase RNAs. *Nature* 344:126–132, 1990.

Yu JL, Rak JW, Coomber BL, Hicklin DJ, Kerbel RS. Effect of p53 status on tumor response to antiangiogenic therapy. *Science* 295:1526–1528, 2002.

Yuan HT, Kaneko T, Matsuo M. Relevance of oxidative stress to the limited replicative capacity of cultured human diploid cells: the limit of cumulative population doublings increases under low concentrations of oxygen and decreases in response to aminotriazole. *Mech Ageing Dev* 81:159–168, 1995.

Yudoh K, Matsuno H, Nakazawa F, Katayama R, Kimura T. Reconstituting telomerase activity using the telomerase catalytic subunit prevents the telomere shorting and replicative senescence in human osteoblasts. *J Bone Miner Res* 16:1453–1464, 2001.

Yudoh K, Matsuno H, Osada R, Nakazawa F, Katayama R, Kimura T. Decreased cellular activity and replicative capacity of osteoblastic cells isolated from the periarticular bone of rheumatoid arthritis patients compared with osteoarthritis patients. *Arthritis Rheum* 43:2178–2188, 2000.

Yui J, Chiu CP, Lansdorp PM. Telomerase activity in candidate stem cells from fetal liver and adult bone marrow. *Blood* 91:3255–3262, 1998.

Zack DJ, Dean M, Molday RS, Nathans J, Redmond TM, Stone EM, Swaroop A, Valle D Weber BH. What can we learn about age-related macular degeneration from other retinal diseases? *Mol Vis* 5:30, 1999.

Zaffaroni N, Lualdi S, Villa R, Bellarosa D, Cermele C, Felicetti P, Rossi C, Orlandi L, Daidone MG. Inhibition of telomerase activity by a distamycin derivative: effects on cell proliferation and induction of apoptosis in human cancer cells. *Eur J Cancer* 38:1792–1801, 2002.

Zakian VA. Structure and function of telomeres. *Annu Rev Genet* 23:579–604, 1989.

Zakian VA. Telomeres: beginning to understand the end. *Science* 270:1601–1607, 1995.

Zakian VA. Structure, function, and replication of *Saccharomyces cerevisiae* telomeres. *Annu Rev Genet* 30:141–172, 1996.

Zakian VA. Life and cancer without telomerase. *Cell* 91:1–3, 1997.

Zalla JA. Werner's syndrome. *Cutis* 25:275–278, 1980.

Zaman Z, Heid C, Ptashne M. Telomere looping permits repression "at a distance" in yeast. *Curr Biol* 12:930–933, 2002.

Zandi PP, Carlson MC, Plassman BL, Welsh-Bohmer KA, Mayer LS, Steffens DC, Breitner JC; Cache County Memory Study Investigators. Hormone replacement therapy and incidence of Alzheimer disease in older women: the Cache County Study. *JAMA* 288:2123–2129, 2002.

Zebrower ME, Kieras FJ, Brown WT. Analysis by high-performance liquid chromatography of hyaluronic acid and chondroitin sulfates. *Anal Biochem* 157:93–99, 1986a.

Zebrower ME, Kieras FJ, Brown WT. Urinary hyaluronic acid elevation in Huthinson-Gilford progeria syndrome. *Mech Ageing Dev* 35:39–46, 1986b.

Zeitzer JM, Daniels JE, Duffy JF, Klerman EB, Shanahan TL, Dijk DJ, Czeisler CA. Do plasma melatonin concentrations decline with age? *Am J Med* 107:432–436, 1999.

Zeng G, Millis AJT. Differential regulation of collagenase and stromelysin mRNA in late passage cultures of human fibroblasts. *Exp Cell Res* 222:150–156, 1996.

Zenilman JM. Chlamydia and cervical cancer: a real association? *JAMA* 285:81–83, 2001.

Zentgraf U, Hinderhofer K, Kolb D. Specific association of a small protein with the telomeric DNA–protein complex during the onset of leaf senescence in *Arabidopsis thaliana*. *Plant Mol Biol* 42:429–438, 2000.

Zhang A, Zheng C, Lindvall C, Hou M, Ekedahl J, Lewensohn R, Yan Z, Yang X, Henriksson M, Blennow E, Nordenskjold M, Zetterberg A, Bjorkholm M, Gruber A, Xu D. Frequent amplification of the telomerase reverse transcriptase gene in human tumors. *Cancer Res* 60:6230–6235, 2000.

Zhang DK, Ngan HY, Cheng RY, Cheung AN, Liu SS, Tsao SW. Clinical significance of telomerase activation and telomeric restriction fragment (TRF) in cervical cancer. *Eur J Cancer* 35:154–160, 1999a.

Zhang F, Deng Z, Jia Z, Wei Y, Fan J, Wu H. Telomere length and DCC gene mRNA expression of human large intestine cancers [in Chinese]. *Zhonghua Yi Xue Yi Chuan Xue Za Zhi* 18:187–190, 2001a.

Zhang F, Jia Z, Deng Z, Wei Y, Zheng R, Yu L. In vitro modulation of telomerase activity, telomere length and cell cycle in MKN45 cells by verbascoside. *Planta Med* 68:115–118, 2002a.

Zhang P, Liegeois NJ, Wong C, Finegold M, Hou H, Thompson JC, Silverman A, Harper JW, DePinho RA, Elledge SJ. Altered cell differentiation and proliferation in mice lacking p57KIP2 indicates a role in Beckwith-Wiedemann syndrome. *Nature* 387:151–158, 1997.

Zhang R, Brennan M-L, Fu X, Aviles RJ, Pearce GL, Penn MS, Topol EJ, Sprecher DL, Hazen SL. Association between myeloperoxidase levels and risk of coronary artery disease. *JAMA* 286:2136–2142, 2001b.

Zhang R, Wang X, Guo L, Xie H. Growth inhibition of BEL-7404 human hepatoma cells by expression of mutant telomerase reverse transcriptase. *Int J Cancer* 97:173–179, 2002b.

Zhang RG, Guo LX, Wang XW, Xie H. Telomerase inhibition and telomere loss in BEL-7404 human hepatoma cells treated with doxorubicin. *World J Gastroenterol* 8:827–831, 2002c.

Zhang RG, Zhang RP, Wang XW, Xie H. Effects of cisplatin on telomerase activity and telomere length in BEL-7404 human hepatoma cells. *Cell Res* 12:55–62, 2002d.

Zhang S, Dong M, Teng X, Chen T. Quantitative assay of telomerase activity in head and neck squamous cell carcinoma and other tissues. *Arch Otolaryngol Head Neck Surg* 127:581–585, 2001c.

Zhang SZ, Huang PC, Xu Y, Chen J, Cai KR. Effects of telomerase sense and antisense oligodeoxynucleotides on growth and differentiation of nasopharyngeal carcinoma cells [in Chinese]. *Ai Zheng* 21:493–497, 2002e.

Zhang W, Funk WD, Wright WE, Shay JW, Deisseroth AB. Novel DNA binding of p53 mutants and their role in transcriptional activation. *Oncogene* 8:2555–2559, 1993a.

Zhang W, Guo XY, Hu GY, Liu WB, Shay JW, Deisseroth AB. A temperature-sensitive mutant of human p53. *EMBO J* 13:2535–2544, 1994.

Zhang W, Piatyszek MA, Kobayashi T, Estey E, Andreeff M, Deisseroth AB, Wright WE, Shay JW. Telomerase activity in human acute myelogenous leukemia: inhibition of telomerase activity by differentiation-inducing agents. *Clin Cancer Res* 2:799–803, 1996.

Zhang W, Shay JW, Deisseroth A. Inactive p53 mutants may enhance the transcriptional activity of wild-type p53. *Cancer Res* 53:4772–4775, 1993b.

Zhang WW, Klotz L. Telomerase activity in needle biopsies from prostate cancer and benign prostates: the influence of sampling bias. *Eur J Clin Invest* 30:275–276, 2000.

Zhang X, Mar V, Zhou W, Harrington L, Robinson MO. Telomere shortening and apoptosis in telomerase-inhibited human tumor cells. *Genes Dev* 13:2388–2399, 1999b.

Zhao JQ, Glasspool RM, Hoare SF, Bilsland A, Szatmari I I, Keith WN. Activation of telomerase RNA gene promoter activity by NF-Y, Sp1, and the retinoblastoma protein and repression by Sp3. *Neoplasia* 2:531–539, 2000a.

Zhao P, Li X, Yang Z, Wang D. Telomerase activity in radiation-induced chronic human skin ulcers. *J Environ Pathol Toxicol Oncol* 18:17–19, 1999.

Zhao X, Wan D, Jiang H. Analysis on loss of heterozygosity of chromosome 17p13.3 in hepatocellular carcinoma and construction of genomic contig in the deleted region [in Chinese]. *Zhonghua Zhong Liu Za Zhi* 22:377–380, 2000b.

Zheng PS, Iwasaka T, Yamasaki F, Ouchida M, Yokoyama M, Nakao Y, Fukuda K, Matsuyama T, Sugimori H. Telomerase activity in gynecologic tumors. *Gynecol Oncol* 64:171–175, 1997a.

Zheng PS, Iwasaka T, Yokoyama M, Nakao Y, Pater A, Sugimori H. Telomerase activation in in vitro and in vivo cervical carcinogenesis. *Gynecol Oncol* 66:222–226, 1997b.

Zhou J, Allred DC, Avis I, Martinez A, Vos MD, Smith L, Treston AM, Mulshine JL. Differential expression of the early lung cancer detection marker, heterogeneous nuclear ribonucleoprotein-A2/B1 (hnRNP-A2/B1) in normal breast and neoplastic breast cancer. *Breast Cancer Res Treat* 66:217–224, 2001.

Zhou JQ, Monson EK, Teng SC, Schulz VP, Zakian VA. Pif1p helicase, a catalytic inhibitor of telomerase in yeast. *Science* 289:771–774, 2000.

Zhou XZ, Lu KP. The Pin2/TRF1–interacting protein PinX1 is a potent telomerase inhibitor. *Cell* 107:347–359, 2001.

Zhu H, Fu W, Mattson MP. The catalytic subunit of telomerase protects neurons against amyloid β-peptide–induced apoptosis. *J Neurochem* 75:117–124, 2000a.

Zhu H, Guo Q, Mattson MP. Dietary restriction protects hippocampal neurons against the death-promoting action of a presenilin-1 mutation. *Brain Res* 842:224–229, 1999a.

Zhu J, Wang H, Bishop JM, Blackburn EH. Telomerase extends the life span of virus-transformed human cells without net telomere lengthening. *Proc Natl Acad Sci USA* 96:3723–3728, 1999b.

Zhu L, Hathcock KS, Hande P, Lansdorp PM, Seldin MF, Hodes RJ. Telomere length regulation in mice is linked to a novel chromosome locus. *Proc Natl Acad Sci USA* 95:8648–8653, 1998.

Zhu L, Smith S, de Lange T, Seldin MF. Chromosomal mapping of the tankyrase gene in human and mouse. *Genomics* 57:320–321, 1999c.

Zhu X, Raina AK, Boux H, Simmons ZL, Takeda A, Smith MA. Activation of oncogenic pathways in degenerating neurons in Alzheimer disease. *Int J Dev Neurosci* 18:433–437, 2000b.

Zhu X, Rottkamp CA, Boux H, Takeda A, Perry G, Smith MA. Activation of p38 kinase links tau phosphorylation, oxidative stress, and cell cycle–related events in Alzheimer disease. *J Neuropathol Exp Neurol* 59:880–888, 2000c.

Zhu X, Rottkamp CA, Raina AK, Brewer GJ, Ghanbari HA, Boux H, Smith MA. Neuronal CDK7 in hippocampus is related to aging and Alzheimer disease. *Neurobiol Aging* 21:807–813, 2000d.

Zietman AL, Thakral H, Wilson L, Schellhammer P. Conservative management of prostate cancer in the prostate specific antigen era: the incidence and time course of subsequent therapy. *J Urol* 166:1702–1706, 2001.

Zijlmans JM, Martens UM, Poon SS, Raap AK, Tanke HJ, Ward RK, Lansdorp PM. Telomeres in the mouse have large inter-chromosomal variations in the number of T2AG3 repeats. *Proc Natl Acad Sci USA* 94:7423–7428, 1997.

Zimonjic D, Brooks MW, Popescu N, Weinberg RA, Hahn WC. Derivation of human tumor cells in vitro without widespread genomic instability. *Cancer Res* 61:8838–8844, 2001.

Zink MC, Suryanarayana K, Mankowski JL, Shen A, Piatak M Jr, Spelman JP, Carter DL, Adams RJ, Lifson JD, Clements JE. High viral load in the cerebrospinal fluid and brain correlates with severity of simian immunodeficiency virus encephalitis. *J Virol* 73:10480–10488, 1999a.

Zink WE, Zheng J, Persidsky Y, Poluektova L, Gendelman HE. The neuropathogenesis of HIV-1 infection. *FEMS Immunol Med Microbiol* 26:233–241, 1999b.

Zipursky A. Telomerase, immortality, and cancer. *Pediatr Res* 47:174, 2000.

Zirkin BR, Chen H. Regulation of Leydig cell steroidogenic function during aging. *Biol Reprod* 63:977–981, 2000.

Zochbauer-Muller S, Minna JD. The biology of lung cancer including potential clinical applications. *Chest Surg Clin North Am* 10:691–708, 2000.

Zou Y, Yi X, Wright WE, Shay JW. Human telomerase can immortalize Indian muntjac cells. *Exp Cell Res* 281:63–76, 2002.

Zs-Nagy I. The membrane hypothesis of aging: its relevance to recent progress in genetic research. *J Mol Med* 75:703–714, 1997.

Zubenko GS, Henderson R, Stiffler JS, Stabler S, Rosen J, Kaplan BB. Association of the APOE epsilon 4 allele with clinical subtypes of late life depression. *Biol Psychiatry* 40:1008–1016, 1996.

Zucchini A, Bonfiglioli G, Masigna Ricciardi MG. Hutchinson-Gilford progeria. A rare case of neonatal occurrence [in Italian]. *Pediatr Med Chir* 8:583–585, 1986.

Index

Abacavir, 116
Accelerator, 77
ACE (angiotensin converting enzyme), 173
Acetylcholine, 166, 225
Acetylcholinesterase, 240
ABCR gene, 273
Accelerated aging, 7, 134
Acquired immune deficiency syndrome (AIDS),
    83, 204–205, 237
Acridines, 117
Acrogeria, 129, 130
Acrometageria, 129
ACTH (adrenocorticotropic hormone), 164, 209
Actin, 253, 255
Actinic keratosis, 83
Activity-dependent neurotropic factor (ADNF),
    236
Acute lymphoid leukemia (ALL), 85
Acute myelogeneous leukemia (AML), 84, 85,
    109
Acute phase reactants, 237
Ad libitum diet, 8, 11, 70
Adalimumab, 190
Adenocarcinoma, 85, 87, 96, 99
Adenosylmethionine, 270
Adenovirus, 76, 113, 176, 270, 282, 285
ADH (antidiuretic hormone), 209, 214, 217
Adhesion, 142, 145, 154, 156, 168, 170–172,
    177

Adhesion molecules, 147, 155, 170–172, 177,
    194, 196, 236, 269, 279
Adipocytes, 261, 264
Adjuvant chemotherapy, 76, 119–120
Adrenal axis, 209, 219
Adrenal gland, 165, 209, 215, 219
Adrenocortical cells, 164, 219–220, 285
Adrenocorticotropic hormone (ACTH), 164,
    209
Adriamycin, 117
African sleeping sickness, 123, 124
age-1, 9, 10
Age since fertilization, 46–47
Age since-last-division, 46
Aggregates, 230
Aggregation, 115, 185, 276
Aging biomarkers, 9, 96, 275, 28
Aging cascade, 66–74, 125–126, 163, 165–168,
    186, 190, 214, 229, 230, 232, 234,
    236, 242, 280
Aging disease, 3, 4, 7, 70, 126, 128, 290
Age-related disease, 3, 4, 9, 15, 31, 55–57, 61,
    70–74, 120, 123, 125–128, 146–149,
    160, 161, 181, 183, 190, 207, 209,
    215, 217, 220, 223, 224, 233, 234,
    236, 238, 239, 277, 281, 283, 285,
    288–290
Age resetting, 7, 13, 41, 55, 59–61, 70, 128,
    155–157, 177, 207, 218, 284–288

Age reversal, 4, 41, 43, 57, 67, 69, 128, 132, 133, 137, 157, 159, 164, 175, 189, 219, 223, 240, 269–270, 284, 290

Aglet, 17

AIDS, 83, 204–205, 237

AIDS dementia, 237

Airway abnormalities, 135

Albumin, 246

Alcoholic hepatitis, 264–265

Aldosterone, 209, 215

Alkaline phosphatase, 184–185, 188

ALL (acute lymphoid leukemia), 85

Allogenic cells, 202

Alopecia, 150, 151, 160

Alpha crystallins, 276

Alpha fetal protein, 101

Alpha-hydroxy acid, 158

Alternate lengthening of telomeres (ALT), 31, 80–81, 111, 131, 159

Altitude, 36, 192

Alzheimers dementia (or disease), 63, 64, 130, 182, 216, 227–244, 255, 273, 284

Ames dwarf mice, 222

Amifostine, 112

AML (acute myelogenous leukemia), 84, 85, 109

Amniotic fluid cells, 53

Amyloid, 235–237, 239

Amyloid precursor, 230–232, 234, 239, 243, 244

Anaerobic metabolism, 69

Anabolism, 145, 254

Anagen, 150, 151, 160

Anaphase, 17

Anaplastic astrocytoma, 105, 106

Anaplastic oligodendroglioma, 106

Androgens, 90, 91, 215, 216, 217

Anemia, 53, 69, 121, 202, 203, 245, 248, 264, 285

Aneuploidy, 78, 81, 88, 100, 105, 138, 170, 285

Aneurysm, 135, 163, 165

Angina, 14, 126, 165, 255

Angiogenesis 35, 75, 76, 102, 110, 136

Angiography, 101, 166

Angiomyolipoma, 99

Angioplasty, 127, 175

Angiotensin, 168, 169, 171, 173, 176, 178, 209, 245

Angiotensin converting enzyme (ACE), 173

Anoxia, 69

Antagonistic pleiotropy, 77

Anterior chamber, 271, 274, 275

Anthraquinones, 117

Anthrax, 126

Antibiotics, 6, 62, 114, 116, 128, 174, 242

Antidiuretic hormone (ADH), 209, 214, 217

Antigens, 90, 112, 117, 118, 135, 142, 184, 191, 192, 195, 196, 197, 198, 200

Antigenic determinants, 38

Antiinflammatory drugs, 189, 229, 241, 242. *See specific drugs*

Antioxidant production, 11

Antioxidant supplementation, 158, 164, 175, 243, 270, 274

Antisense oligonucleotides, 113, 114, 115, 167, 176

Antisense telomeric RNA, 114, 115

AP1 transcription factor, 72, 73

Apheresis, 190

Aplastic anemia, 121, 202, 203

Apolipoprotein, 166, 229, 239

Apoptosis, 9, 19, 20, 21, 26, 35, 53, 55, 56, 57, 64, 69, 75, 76, 79, 94, 110, 113, 114, 115, 116, 117, 119, 168, 169, 172, 175, 178, 195, 206, 207, 230, 232, 235, 238, 239, 242, 243, 263, 265, 267, 269, 274, 280

APP (amyloid precursor protein), 230–232, 234, 239, 243, 244

Appendicular muscle, 265

Appendix, 263

Arabidopsis, 61

Ara-C, 115

Arachidonic acid, 237

Arginine vasopressin secreting cells, 218

Arsenic, 114

Arterial endothelium, 46, 57, 59, 138, 163, 170, 173

Arthritis, 14, 128, 179–181, 183–190, 194, 233, 255, 284. *See specific arthritides*

Arthropods, 123

Articular tissue, 185–186, 189

Artificial chromosome, 14

Ascorbate (ascorbic acid), 48, 246

Aspirin (acetyl salicylic acid), 174, 191, 241

Asthenia, 62

Astigmatism, 275

Astrocytes, 225, 227, 232–237

Astrocytoma, 105–106

Ataxia telangiectasia (ATM), 43, 44, 129

Ateleiosis, 138

Atherogenesis, 14, 45, 63, 127, 167–178, 233

Atheroma, 127, 170, 175–176

Atherosclerosis, 9, 56–58, 61, 69–72, 125–127, 130, 134–135, 138, 140, 157, 161–178, 213, 215, 222–223, 228–229, 235–236, 240, 258, 265, 275–277

Atherosclerosis in progeria, 130, 134–135, 138

ATM (ataxia telangiectasia), 43, 44, 129

ATM kinase, 21. *See* Tel1p and Mec1p

ATP, 42, 54, 58, 68, 253, 273

ATPase, 231

Atrial cells, 176
Atrial fibrillation, 163
Atrium, 161
Atypical nevi, 82
Autism, 51
Autocrine hormones, 74, 112, 200
Autoimmune disease, 186, 192, 193, 195, 214, 249
Autoreactivity, 193, 195
Autosomal genes, 130, 133, 150, 238
Axons, 141, 142, 225, 226, 272
5-azacytidine, 116
Azidothymidine, 116
Azothioprine, 190

B lymphocytes, 25, 192, 198, 200–201, 205–206
Babesia, 123
Bacteria, 6, 13, 62, 71, 122, 263, 284
Balantidium, 123
Baldness, 135, 150, 151, 160
Basal cell carcinoma, 82, 83
Basal cells, 30, 82, 83, 141, 149, 150
Basal forebrain, 239
Basal keratinocytes, 46, 82
Basal metabolism, 12, 136
Base pairs, 29, 31, 39, 47, 48, 49, 51, 267, 268
Basement membrane, 136, 165, 229, 246–247, 248, 249, 277
Basic fibroblast growth factor (bFGF), 154, 236
Basilar skin cells, 81, 145, 151
Bax, 94, 117, 168
Bcl-2, 85, 94, 104, 109, 239, 265, 287
Beckwith-Wiedemann syndrome, 60, 138
Benign proliferative lesions, 83, 93
Beta amyloid (β amyloid), 229–233, 235–237, 243
Beta amyloid precursor (β amyloid precursor), 230–232, 234, 239, 243, 244
Beta cells, 284
Beta-D-glucosyl-hydroxymethyluracil, 21
Beta galactosidase (β-gal), 20, 42, 55, 116, 153, 156, 170, 184, 186, 277, 279
Bicalutamide, 91
Bilharziasis, 98, 123
Biliary tract tumors, 102, 103
Binswanger's disease 228
Biological age, 64
Biological immortality, 67
Biomarkers, 9, 96, 167, 275, 283
Biopsy, 41, 80, 87, 88, 89, 91, 92, 94, 97, 102, 103, 104, 138, 268
Bipolar cells, 278
Birds, 34
Bisphosphonates, 180, 187, 188

Bladder cancer, 78, 97–98, 114, 118, 123, 136
Blastocyst, 54
Blindness, 124, 273, 274, 275, 276
Blood–brain barrier, 165, 229
Blood pressure, 125. *See* Hypertension
Bloom's syndrome, 129, 130, 285
Body mass, 11, 88, 247
Body temperature, 12, 143
Body weight, 141, 261
Bone density, 182, 187, 221
Bone marrow, 35, 45, 79, 83, 84, 109, 121, 149, 176, 179, 188, 189, 191–193, 195, 196, 197, 199, 200, 202–203, 207, 227, 245, 262, 284
Bone turnover, 180, 223
Borrelia, 13
Botulinum toxin (Botox), 158
Bowen's disease, 83
Brakes, 57
Breast cancer, 76, 84, 87–90, 109, 112, 113, 114, 116
Breast epithelial cells, 32, 114, 115
Breast lobular epithelium, 30
Bromodeoxyuridine, 116
Bronchial washings, 87
Burkitt's lymphoma, 33
Bulge area, 151
Bullae, 144, 154, 156
Burn rate, 48
Burns, 140, 154
Butyrylcholinesterase, 240

CAAT box, 132, 286
Cachexia, 62
Cadmium, 112
Caenorhabditis elegans (nematode), 8–12, 20, 66, 70, 213
Calcification, 166
Calcitonin, 187, 210
Calcitriol (vitamin D), 154, 184–185, 187, 210, 245, 248
Calcium (Ca^{2+}), 132, 179, 180, 187, 209, 210, 231, 234, 245, 276
Caloric restriction (CR), 7–13, 44, 51, 70, 158, 188, 195, 206, 210, 215, 223, 233, 238, 250, 254, 259, 281
Cancer. *See specific cancers*
Cancer therapy, 110–121, 290
Capillaries, 143, 144, 147, 163, 165, 168, 177, 183, 208, 215, 229, 236, 255, 256, 258, 276
Capillary endothelium, 162, 163, 166, 168, 177, 255, 258
Carbon tetrachloride, 270
Carbovir, 116

Carcinogenesis, 28, 34, 75–79, 84, 101, 102, 104, 110–111, 120, 160, 213

Carcinoma, 29, 32, 76, 79, 82–83, 85–89, 92, 96, 98–104, 107–109, 112–115, 118, 120

Cardiac failure, 163, 165, 172

Cardiac hypertrophy, 163–164

Cardiomyopathy, 130

Cardiovascular aging, 131, 162–173, 178, 228, 253

Cardiovascular cell senescence, 168–173

Cardiovascular interventions, 173–178

Carnitine, 58

Cartilage, 181, 183

Caspase, 114, 117, 242

Catabolism, 62, 145, 231, 237, 254, 278

Catagen, 151, 160

Catalase, 66, 69, 133

Cataract, 130, 135, 274, 276, 279, 280, 281–282

Cathepsin, 279

Cats, 48, 272, 279

Causation, 4, 27, 57–58, 113, 126, 169, 173, 185, 219, 223, 232, 234, 236

CD4, 186, 194, 198, 204–205

CD8, 196, 198, 204–205

CD28, 194, 196, 197, 199, 201, 205, 206

CD34, 192, 199, 202, 206

CD38, 199, 202, 206

CD40, 201

cdc2, 73, 145

Cdc13p, 19

Cdk (cyclin-dependent kinase), 26, 28, 53, 76, 154, 175

Cecum, 263, 268

Celecoxib, 242

Cell cycle, 14, 17, 18, 20, 21, 25, 26, 31, 33, 38–39, 40, 41, 4, 44, 51, 53, 55, 63, 72, 73, 75–76, 77, 90, 107, 110, 120, 138, 141, 152, 156, 159, 167, 175, 176, 178, 199, 200, 233, 287

Cell cycle braking, 26, 33, 53, 75, 76, 77

Cell cycle checkpoints, 19, 20, 21, 53, 75–76, 79, 94

Cell cycle deceleration, 38, 39, 41, 43

Cell cycle defects, 44, 76, 113

Cell differentiation, 13, 24, 25, 31, 33, 37, 45, 54, 60, 64, 73, 79, 83, 84, 87, 91, 99, 101, 106, 107, 109, 112, 115, 141, 145, 149, 154, 159, 160, 171, 176, 177, 178, 185, 188, 192, 197, 198, 199, 200, 201, 202, 215, 256, 257, 260, 270, 277, 278, 281, 284, 285

Cell donor, 27, 59, 60, 87, 104, 145–146, 150, 152, 154, 155, 170, 188, 194, 199, 201, 202, 219, 234, 243, 257, 259, 278, 284

Cell morphology, 20, 33, 38, 39, 40, 115, 138, 166, 184, 226, 236, 283

Cell quiescence, 38, 199

Cell rescue, 25, 41, 53, 55, 160, 203, 285, 288

Cell senescence, defining, 25, 26, 38–45, 47, 49, 53

Cell signaling, 10, 19, 20, 27, 53, 187, 196, 200, 241, 245, 256, 269, 280, 286

Cell take, 285

Cellulitis, 62, 126

Central nervous system (CNS), 10, 104–107, 165, 215, 224–244, 261, 272, 284

Central nervous system cancers, 104–107

Centromere, 22, 106

Ceramide, 55

Cerebrospinal fluid (CSF), 104

Cerebrovascular accident (stroke), 14, 57, 134, 135, 140, 164, 165, 173, 223, 227, 228

Cervical cancer, 32, 92–95, 97

Cervical lipodysplasia, 129

Cestodes, 123

c-fos, 72, 73, 79, 132, 137, 145, 201, 218

Chaga's disease, 123

Chaperones, 30, 91, 276, 287

Checkpoint, 19, 20, 21, 53, 75–76, 79, 94

Checkpoint arrest, 18, 26, 76, 115

Checkpoint kinase, 26, 76, 154, 175, 233

Chemotactic factors, 171

CHF. *See* Congestive heart failure

Chicken cells, 24, 40

Chickens, 24, 34, 40

Chinese hamsters, 22

Chlamydia, 167, 242

Cholangiocellular carcinoma, 100

Cholesterol, 4, 56–58, 62, 71–72, 125–127, 135, 166–170, 173, 210, 262, 265, 273, 276

Cholinergic neurons, 230, 239

Chondrocytes, 128, 138, 139, 181, 183–186, 189–190, 285

Chondroitin, 189

Chorion, 53

Choroid, 271, 274, 277, 280

Chromatids, 17, 22, 131

Chromatin, 21, 22, 40, 44, 46, 49, 50–52, 57, 80, 90, 139, 286

Chromatin extrusions, 139

Chromatin, telomeric, 22, 44, 46, 50–52, 80

Chromophores, 117

Chromosome 1, 25, 32, 82, 106

Chromosome 2, 22

Chromosome 3, 8, 29, 32, 79, 98, 287

Chromosome 4, 25, 32

Chromosome 5, 30, 32, 286

Chromosome 6, 32, 51, 81, 94
Chromosome 7, 25, 98
Chromosome 8, 131
Chromosome 10, 106, 287
Chromosome 14, 106
Chromosome 17, 32, 98
Chromosome 22, 106
Chromosome healing. *See* Chromosome repair
Chromosome integrity, 17, 19, 23
Chromosome repair, 13, 14, 18, 21, 30, 42–45,
        48, 53, 54, 58, 63, 70, 75–77, 111,
        131, 137, 138, 206
Chromosome stability, 17, 20, 21, 40, 44, 49,
        76, 78, 110, 116, 120, 121, 172, 202,
        288
Chromosome structure, 11, 13, 17–19, 21, 22,
        28, 34, 50, 51, 115, 117, 131
Chromosome x, 81, 98, 138
Chromosome y, 98
Chronic lymphocytic leukemia (CLL), 84–85
Chronic myelogenous leukemia (CML), 109,
        203
Chronological age, 46
Ciliary muscles, 271, 272, 276
Ciliary margin cells, 278
Ciliates, 20, 21
CIP1, 25
Circadian cycles, 218
Cirrhosis, 81, 101, 128, 264, 265, 267–270
Circular chromosomes, 58
Circulation half life, 192
Cisplatin, 91, 115, 116
c-jun, 72
Claudication, 165
Clinical staging, 78, 81, 82, 87–89, 92–93, 96–
        99, 100–102, 104
Clk. *See* Clock gene
CLL (chronic lymphocytic leukemia), 84, 85
Clock, 24, 27, 48, 57, 59, 70, 210, 217, 218,
        219
Clock gene, 10
Clone viability, 59–60
Clones, 52, 59–60, 201, 220
Clotting, 191, 262
CML. *See* Chronic myelogenous leukemia
c-Myc, 31–33, 79, 80, 88, 90, 91, 94, 106, 107,
        109, 112, 113, 117, 137, 286, 287
CNS. *See* Central nervous system
Cockayne's syndrome, 129
Coenzyme Q, 8
Cognitive dysfunction, 239
Collagen, 55, 136, 137, 139, 141–143, 145–
        148, 155, 156, 158, 162, 166, 184,
        185, 188, 221, 229, 246, 250, 269,
        270, 272, 278–280
Collagen cross linking, 185, 276

Collagenase, 55, 116, 146, 155
Colon, 78, 212, 222, 263, 265, 268
Colon cancer, 78, 95, 103, 104, 112, 188, 222,
        263, 265
Colony stimulating factor (CSF), 113, 180, 193,
        211
Colorectal cancer, 88, 100–101, 104, 111
Complement, 25, 194, 237, 242
Complementation groups, 25
Compliance, 166, 169
Cones, 272
Congestive heart failure (CHF), 163, 245, 255
Connective tissue, 107, 137, 141, 155, 163, 229,
        266
Constitutive expression, 31, 32, 34, 73, 94, 95,
        146, 152, 155, 195, 204, 230, 241,
        279, 281, 286
Constitutive senescence, 61
Copper, 112, 233
Copy switching, 111
Core promoter, 31, 112, 286, 287
Cornea, 141, 271, 274, 275, 277, 278, 280, 282,
        284, 285
Corneal endothelial cells, 38, 275, 277
Corneal equivalent, 282
Coronary arteries, 63, 69, 71, 74, 126–128,
        161–166, 168, 170–172, 174, 253,
        264
Coronary stenosis, 62, 167, 171, 175, 176
Corticosteroids, 7, 210, 212, 234, 242, 243,
        252
Cortisol, 182, 210, 220
Cosmetic issues, 90, 140, 157–159, 283
Costs of longevity, 12
Cow (bovine), 5, 220, 277
COX (cyclooxygenase), 189, 241, 242
COX-1 inhibitors, 241, 242
COX-2 inhibitors, 183, 189, 241, 242
Coxsackie virus, 167, 178
cpG island, 31, 286
CPT-11, 115
c-reactive protein, 167
Creatinine, 245–248
CRH (corticotropin releasing hormone), 209
Crisis, 26, 40, 49, 80, 116, 118, 119
Critically short telomeres, 18, 33, 39, 61, 69,
        200, 285
Criticism, 3, 11, 61–63, 91, 113, 126, 234, 283
Crohn's disease, 268
Cross linking, 185, 276
Crypt cells, 54, 81, 263, 267
Crypts of Lieberkühn, 263, 267
CSF. *See* Cerebrospinal fluid
CSF. *See* Colony stimulating factor
CTF, 73
Cutaneous lymphoma, 83

Cyanocobalamin, 175, 264
Cyclic dependent kinases, 26, 28, 53, 76, 154, 175
Cyclins, 28, 53, 72, 76, 154
Cyclooxygenase. *See* COX
Cyclophosphamide, 115, 190
Cytochrome c oxidase, 69, 234
Cytokines, 54, 55, 74, 121, 141, 146, 149, 152, 170, 171, 178, 193, 194, 195, 197, 199, 200, 206, 211, 225, 227, 236, 27, 242, 250, 264, 268, 269, 270, 279
Cytomegalovirus, 167
Cyclophosphamide, 115, 190
Cyclosporin, 190
Cytoplasts, 25

D1Z2, 82
Daf, 9, 10
Dapsone, 241
Dauer phase, 9, 10, 12
Daughter cells, 26, 54, 64, 192, 199, 257
Dead man switch, 76
Decubitus ulcers, 140, 157, 158
Dehydroepiandrosterone (DHEA), 210, 215, 217, 221, 222, 223, 250, 259
Dementia. *See specific types*
Demethylating agents, 116, 287
Dendrimers, 285
De novo chromosomes, 14
Dentate gyrus, 243
Deoxyglucose, 9
Dermal cancer. *See* Skin cancer
Dermal epidermal junction (epidermal dermal junction), 142, 144, 154, 156
Dermal papilla, 151
Dermatitis, 5, 83, 150
Dermis, 141–144, 147, 150, 155, 194
Descemet's membrane, 275
DHEA. *See* Dehydroepiandrosterone
Diabetes, 56, 71, 73, 102, 125, 127, 130, 135, 157, 165, 167, 169, 173, 174, 210, 216, 217, 220, 221, 222, 224, 230, 247, 249, 250, 258, 270, 273, 275, 276, 277, 284, 285
Diabetic skin ulcers, 285
Dialysis, 245, 250
Diastolic pressure, 162, 169
Dietary restriction. *See* Caloric restriction
Dietary supplements, 7, 88, 136, 158, 164, 187, 206, 211, 213, 215, 221, 223, 239, 240, 243, 259, 274, 276, 281
Differentiation, 11, 24–25, 31, 33, 37, 45, 54, 60, 64, 73, 79, 84, 87, 91, 99, 101, 105–107, 109, 112, 115, 141, 145, 146, 149, 154, 159–160, 171, 176–

178, 185, 188, 192, 197–202, 215, 256–257, 260, 270, 277–278, 281, 284–285
Dihydrofolate reductase, 72
Disease-modifying antirheumatic drugs (DMARDs), 189
Disposable soma, 77
Distamycin, 116
Diverticulitis, 263, 268
Diverticulosis, 268
DKC (dyskeratosis congenita), 149–150, 285
DMP, 72
DMSO, 62
DNA circles, 11, 13. *See* Extrachromosomal ribosomal circles
DNA damage, 18, 20, 33, 35, 40, 43, 53, 57–59, 69, 75–76, 94, 110, 131, 255, 267
DNA mismatch, 111, 120, 138
DNA-PKCs (DNA-dependent protein kinase catalytic subunits), 21, 287
DNA primer, 18, 22, 28
DNA repair, 13, 14, 18, 21, 30, 42–45, 48, 53, 54, 58, 63, 70, 75–77, 111, 131, 137, 138, 206
DNA synthesis, 25, 29, 33, 131, 137, 178, 200
Dogs, 80
Donepezil, 241
Dopamine, 209, 224, 225
Double-edged sword, 77
Double-strand break repair, 21, 43, 116
Doublings. *See* Population doublings
Down's syndrome (Trisomy 21), 12, 13, 129, 203, 231, 237
Doxorubicin, 109, 117
DP, 72–73
Drosophila melanogaster (fruit fly), 7, 8, 10, 11, 13, 22, 28, 70
Duchenne muscular dystrophy, 257, 260. *See also* Muscular dystrophy
Ductal carcinoma, 103
Dukes classification, 104
Duodenum, 212, 262, 263
Duplex DNA, 18, 19, 20, 51
Dyskeratosis congenita (DKC), 149–150, 285
Dyskerin, 150
Dysplasia, 93, 99, 102, 129, 195

E-box, 286
E2F, 32, 40, 72–73, 145, 154, 175, 176
EBV (Epstein Barr virus), 99, 118, 121
E-Cbs, 21
Echinococcus, 123
Ectothelium, 24
Edema, 245, 274
Edmonson-Steiner staging, 101

EGF, 137, 141, 154. *See also* Epidermal growth factor
Eicosanoids, 237, 264
Elastin, 55, 136, 137, 142, 143, 146–148, 155–156, 162
Elastase, 55, 155
Electrolytes, 209, 210, 225, 245, 248, 249, 272
Embryonic stem cells, 24, 27, 35, 59–60, 174, 176, 284
End organ pathology, 163, 165, 166, 168, 258
End replication problem, 23
Endocarditis, 194
Endocrine aging, 211–223
Endocrinological catastrophe, 59
Endogenous hTERT, 29
Endometrial cancer, 95, 188
Endothelial cells, 25, 38, 45, 46, 55, 59, 62, 63, 64, 69, 71, 74, 128, 138, 139, 155, 161–173, 175–178. 235, 236, 246, 247, 249, 251, 257, 258, 262, 263, 265, 275, 277, 280
Endothelin, 169
Energy metabolism, 8–10, 13, 41, 152, 209
eNOS (endothelial nitric oxide synthase), 170, 177
Entomoeba, 123
Entropy, 6
Ependymoma, 107
Epidemiology, 8, 9, 130, 133, 167, 182, 188, 221, 230, 241
Epidermal dermal junction, 142, 144, 154, 156
Epidermal growth factor (EGF), 105, 112, 137, 141, 145, 151, 154
Epidermis, 30, 45, 48, 63, 73, 82–83, 141–145, 147, 149, 150, 153–156, 223
Epigallocatechin gallate, 116
Epigenetic effects, 12, 59–60, 77, 126, 138, 139
Epigenetic mosaicism, 138
Epinephrine, 209, 211
Epstein Barr virus (EBV), 99, 118, 121
Eptastigmine, 241
Equilibrium, 44
ERCs (extrachromosomal ribosomal circles), 13
Erosive dermatitis, 35
Error catastrophe theory, 26, 43, 137
Erythropoietin, 74, 192, 209
Esophageal cancer, 99
Esophagus, 99, 261, 263, 267
Estradiol, 88, 91, 188, 239, 240, 287
Estriol, 188
Estrogen, 7, 31, 74, 87–88, 95, 166, 170, 172, 173, 174, 179, 180, 182, 184, 187, 188, 206, 209, 211, 212, 213, 215, 216, 218, 219, 221, 223, 231, 239, 240, 242, 259, 260, 262, 273, 281, 287
Etanercept, 190
Ethics, Foreword, 4, 8, 206, 207, 284, 290
Etoposide, 115
Euchromatin, 49
Eugenics, 8
Eukaryotes, 6, 23, 49, 50, 51, 66–68
Evolutionary costs, 10, 12, 77
Evolutionary pressure, 14, 22, 78
Ex vivo telomerization, 284
Excision damage, 137, 138
Exercise, 70, 71, 72, 125, 158, 166, 167, 173, 174, 180, 187, 198, 216, 221, 252, 254–256, 258–259
Exogenous hTERT, 29, 32, 78, 111
Exons, 31
Explosives, 48
Extracellular matrix, 49, 55, 63–64, 110, 142, 145–146, 155, 156, 159, 166, 180, 257, 262, 269, 280
Extrachromosomal ribosomal circles (ERCs), 11, 13
Extending cellular lifespan, 27, 30, 40, 111, 120, 121, 151, 154, 171, 188, 189, 257
Extending lifespan, 4–5, 8–13, 16, 36, 66, 188, 222, 288, 290
Extracellular defenses, 75, 112
Exudates, 274
Eye aging, 273–282
Eye structure, 271–273

FADD (Fas associated protein with death domain), 117
Failure to thrive, 134
Falciparum malaria, 49, 123
Familial Alzheimer's dementia, 231
Fanconi's anemia, 53, 285
Fas, 117, 168
Fas associated protein with death domain. *See* FADD
Fascia, 141, 142
Fatty acids, 261, 262, 270
Fatty streaks, 166
F-box protein, 30
FDA (Food and Drug Administration), 289
Fecal blood, 103
Fecundity, 12
Fenestrations, 246
Fertility, 10, 35, 61
Fertilization, 7, 36, 37, 46–48, 52, 59–61, 63, 69, 138, 139
Fetal development, 35, 37, 53, 60

Fiber packing, 276
Fibroblasts, 13, 25, 27–28, 34, 39–40, 42–43, 46, 53, 55, 56, 63, 72–73, 78–79, 82, 96, 114, 115–117, 119–120, 128, 131–133, 137–139, 141–142, 144–146, 149, 151–156, 158–160, 162, 171, 173, 176–178, 179–180, 183, 186, 190, 219, 236, 257–258, 265, 269, 271, 277–279, 281, 286–287
Fibrocystic disease, 89
Fibromodulin, 139
Fibronectin, 116, 136, 155, 279
Fibrous layer, 162
Fidelity of protein synthesis, 43, 137
Filtration slits, 246
Finches, 34
Fine vessel disease, 163
Flanking regions, 286
Flow cytometry, 81
Flukes, 123
Foam cells, 126, 166, 167, 170, 233
Folate, 175
Follicle stimulating hormone (FSH), 209
Follicles, 54, 110, 143, 151, 152, 160, 216, 219
Follicular adenomas, 108
Food and Drug Administration (FDA), 289
Fork replication, 79
Fountain of youth, 11
Fovea, 272
Fractures, 144, 179, 181–182, 187, 217, 255, 258
Free nerve endings, 142–143, 271
Free radical accumulation, 6, 14, 216, 283
Free radical damage, 6, 13, 15, 42, 59, 62, 66–67, 69, 90, 164, 168, 229, 233–234, 237
Free radical metabolism, 8, 12, 13, 69, 70
Free radical production, 6, 11, 42–43, 48, 58, 68, 70, 75, 142, 234, 239
Free radical repair, 42–43
Free radical scavenging, 42–43, 210
Free radical sequestration, 42–43, 55, 63, 69, 75
Free radical theory, 6, 26, 56–58, 66
French-American-British subtype, 85, 109
Fried eggs, 39
Fruit fly (*Drosophila melanogaster*) 7, 8, 10, 11, 13, 22, 28, 70
FSH (follicle stimulating hormone), 209
Fuch's endothelial dystrophy, 277
Functional mismatch, 165, 180, 288
Fungal disease, 123, 124
Furosemide, 248
Fused cells, 25, 111
Fuses, 48

G0 phase, 38, 141
G1 phase, 26, 38, 72, 73, 76
G-quartet, 19, 21, 117
Galantamine, 241
Gamma rays, 138
Gamma-glutamyl transpeptidase (gamma-GT), 152
Ganglion cells, 274, 278, 280
Ganglioneuroma, 105, 106
Gas, 57, 77
Gastric cancer (gastric carcinoma), 99–100, 104
Gastrointestinal cancer, 99–104
Gene copy number, 29
Gene gun, 285
Generations, 35, 47, 61, 19
Genes. *See specific gene*
General model, 45, 56–59
Genetic alteration, 8, 13, 70, 105, 207
Genetic catastrophe, 76, 77
Genetic errors, 75, 135
Genetic instability, 33, 35, 40, 44, 54, 56, 75, 78, 80, 84, 106, 109, 111, 120–121, 130, 132, 149–150, 156, 202, 268, 287
Genistein, 78, 115
Genital cancer, 90–97
Genomic stability, 17, 20, 21, 40, 44, 49, 76, 78, 110, 116, 120, 121, 172, 202, 288
Germ cells, 6–7, 10, 23–27, 35–37, 53–54, 55–56, 59, 64, 66, 67, 80, 119, 202, 215, 219, 289. *See* Ova and Sperm
Germ line, 6–7, 24, 35, 55, 59, 66, 67, 119, 202
Germinal centers, 110, 201, 205
Germinative cells, 141, 143, 279
Gerontogenes, 185
GFAP, 236, 242. *See* Glial fibrillary acidic protein
GFR (glomerular filtration rate), 247
Giardia lamblia, 123
Ginkgo biloba, 241
Glaucoma, 274–275, 280–281
Glia. *See specific types of glia*
Glial fibrillary acidic protein (GFAP), 236, 242
Glioblastoma, 33, 104, 112, 113
Glioblastoma multiforme, 105, 106
Glomerular filtration rate (GFR), 247
Glomerulonephritis, 249
Glomerulosclerosis, 249
Glomeruli, 99, 219, 245–250
Glucagon, 209
Glucocorticoids, 209, 210, 215, 219, 222, 239, 242
Gluconeogenesis, 270
Glucosamine, 189
Glucose, 9, 10, 11, 70, 71, 152, 208, 209, 210, 216, 231, 245, 252, 261
Glucose metabolism, 11, 70, 209, 210
Glucose mimetics, 9

Glucose-6-phosphate dehydrogenase (G6PDH), 152
Glutamate, 231, 233, 235
Glutathione peroxidase, 133
Glutathione reductase (GSSG-RD), 152
Glutathione-S-transferase (GSH-S-T), 152
Glycation, 11, 169, 232, 275
Glycolysis, 10, 252, 254
Glycoprotein, 137, 172, 192, 209, 246
Glycosylation, 137
GnRH (gonadotropin-inhibiting hormone), 209
Gold compounds, 190
Golgi-Mazzoni receptors, 143
Gonadal axis, 209
Granular leukocytes, 192
Granule cells, 243
Granulocyte-macrophage colony-stimulating factor, 113
Granulocytes, 83, 85, 194, 202, 203
Granulosa cells, 219
GREBP, 73
GRH (growth hormone releasing hormone), 209
Growth arrest, 17, 21, 72, 76, 115, 287
Growth hormone (GH), 7, 70, 136, 209, 211, 212, 213, 214–215, 217, 218, 221–222, 252, 255, 259
GSH peroxidase (GPx), 69

H1, 51
H2, 51
H3, 51
H4, 51
HAART (highly active anti-retroviral therapy), 204
HAECs (human aortic endothelial cells), 177
Hair, 54, 130, 151, 160
Hair follicles, 54, 81, 143, 151, 152, 155
Hairpin, 28
Hammerhead ribozyme, 113
Hamsters, 22, 34, 35, 60
Hardening of the arteries, 166
Hashimoto's thyroiditis, 108
Hayflick limit, 24, 26
HDL (high density lipoprotein), 135, 168
Head and neck tumors, 76, 107–108
Healing, 9, 14, 35, 61, 130, 133, 135, 140, 142, 147, 154, 157, 158, 159, 180, 226, 278, 281
Heart disease. See Atherosclerosis
Heat loss, 157, 158
Heat shock protein (HSP), 12, 30, 91, 198, 287
Heavy chain protein, 254
HeLa cells, 32, 33, 94, 115, 116
Helicase, 13, 43, 51, 79, 80 , 130–133, 260
Helicobacter pylori, 99, 167, 267

Hemagglutinating viruses, 176
Hemangioblastoma, 98
Hematocrit, 202, 245
Hematopoesis, 61, 84, 139, 191–192
Hematopoetic stem cells, 24, 35, 83, 139, 150, 192, 195–197, 199–200, 202, 227
Hemidesmosomes, 156, 279
Hemodialysis, 245, 250
Hemorrhagic stroke, 228
Heparin, 243
Hepatic cancer, 100–102, 264, 265
Hepatic cirrhosis, 81, 128, 267, 269, 270
Hepatic regeneration, 31, 81, 269
Hepatitis, 81, 100, 101, 184, 264–265, 269
Hepatocyte, 10, 25, 38, 56, 68, 132, 257, 262, 264, 265, 268–270
Hepatoma, 114, 115
Hepato-renal failure, 262
HER2/neu, 88
Herbimycin A, 32
Hereditary non-polyposis colorectal cancer, 103
Herpes papilloma virus (HPV), 79, 86, 93, 94, 95
Herpesvirus, 167, 176
hEST2, 29. See hTERT
Heterochromatin, 22, 49– 52, 57
Hippocampus, 219, 226, 242
Histones, 46, 51, 58
Histone deacetylase inhibitors, 112
HIV (human immunodeficiency virus; see also AIDS), 123, 202, 204, 205, 207, 232, 260, 284
HIV reverse transcriptase, 28
HLA, 135, 170, 202
HLH proteins, 33
HMG-CoA reductase inhibitors, 187, 241. See Statins
hnRNPs (heterogenous nuclear ribonucleoproteins), 19
Hodgkin's disease, 110
Homeostasis, 19, 52, 55, 56, 67, 145, 158, 186, 209, 217, 231, 236, 245, 246, 261, 272
Homocysteine, 166, 168, 169
Holoenzyme, 30, 78
Hormesis, 12
Hominids, 5, 24
Homo sapiens (human), 24
Hormonal intervention, 7, 211, 259
Hormones. See specific hormone
Horse (equine) telomeres, 14
Hourglasses, 48
HPV (human papilloma virus), 79, 93, 94, 95, 282
H-ras oncogene, 48, 78

HSP (heat shock protein), 12, 30, 91, 198, 287
hTERT, 14, 21–24, 27–33, 40–41, 43, 54, 72,
    78–79, 81–83, 85–86, 88–89, 91–103,
    105–108, 112–115, 117–121, 131,
    150–152, 154–157, 159–160, 170–
    171, 177–178, 188–189, 194, 198,
    200, 205–207, 219–220, 223, 251,
    260, 270, 281, 284–288. *See also*
    Telomerase
hTERT expression, 29–32, 78–79, 86, 88, 91–
    92, 94–102, 105, 107, 113, 115, 118,
    120, 156, 170, 188, 205, 284–288
hTERT induction, 31, 112, 116, 120, 159, 178,
    200–201, 260, 282, 285–286, 290
hTERT knockout, 31, 34–35, 37, 47, 52, 61, 63,
    205, 268, 269, 287
hTERT levels, 30, 31, 82, 88, 95
hTERT mutants, 114
hTERT recruitment, 30, 78
hTERT sequence, 10, 14, 17–18, 22–23, 28–30,
    114–115, 118, 124
hTERT splicing transcripts, 54
hTERT transcription, 32, 33, 94, 112, 118, 287
hTERT transport, 30, 78
HTLV (human T cell leukemia virus), 85
hTR, 14, 21, 23, 28, 29, 30, 33, 78, 81, 82, 85,
    88–89, 93, 95–102, 107, 113–115,
    118, 150, 200, 287. *See* Telomerase
hTR expression, 29, 30, 78, 82, 85, 88–89, 95–
    102, 107, 113–115, 118, 150
hTR gene, 29, 287
hTR half-life, 29, 98
hTR mutant, 28
hTR non-template bases, 28
hTR transcription rate, 29, 118
Humpty-Dumpty phenomenon, 240, 288
Huperzine, 241
Hurthle cell adenoma, 108
Hutchinson-Gilford syndrome (progeria), 12,
    13, 53, 61, 129–130, 133–139, 167,
    195, 199, 278, 285
HUVEC cells, 285
Hyaluronan, 279
Hyaluronic acid, 132, 136
Hyaluronidase, 136
Hydrogen peroxide, 40, 58, 69, 164
Hydroxycholoquine, 189
Hyperacusis, 135
Hyperlipidemia, 71, 169, 217
Hyperoxia, 7, 40, 69
Hyperplasia, 81, 88, 93, 101, 175, 256, 257,
    265, 267
Hypertension, 14, 56, 71, 126, 127, 135, 164,
    165, 166, 167, 168–170, 173, 174,
    222, 248, 249, 250, 264, 273, 277
Hypertrophy, 91, 163, 164, 176, 236, 256, 257

Hypokalemia, 248
Hyponatremia, 248
Hypoperfusion, 166
Hypothalamus, 59, 145, 209, 210, 211, 214,
    218–219
Hypoxia, 40, 62, 69, 76, 79, 172, 248, 279
Hysterectomy, 239

Ibuprofen, 128, 241, 248
ICAM (intercellular adhesion molecules), 171,
    177
Id, 33
IDE (insulin degrading enzyme), 233
IGF-1, 211, 215, 221
IgM antibodies, 193
IL (interleukin), 112, 146, 178, 195, 198, 200,
    201
Ileum, 263
Imatinib, 84
Immigrant cells, 141
Immune aging, 120, 192–207
Immune response, 35, 183, 184, 186, 194, 201,
    205, 241, 242
Immune senescence, 120, 192–207
Immune surveillance, 75, 78, 112, 144, 196, 288
Immunity, 117, 144, 192, 193, 194, 289
Immunization, 6, 70, 127, 174, 196, 205, 270
Immunocompromise, 123, 159
Immunosuppression, 205
Imprinting, 60
Incontinence, 14
Indigenous antigens, 192
Indigenous cells, 141, 142, 144, 155, 166, 171,
    184, 190
Indomethacin, 241
Infarction, 4, 57, 61–64, 74, 127, 131, 140,
    161–173, 178, 226, 253, 258, 274
Infection, 7, 14, 31, 62, 71, 92, 93, 94, 98, 100,
    120, 122, 123, 124, 139, 140, 151,
    157, 158, 161, 167, 174, 178, 183,
    191, 192, 193, 194, 196, 198, 203,
    204, 205, 213, 216, 228, 230, 237,
    242, 245, 248, 250, 253, 255, 265,
    267, 275, 286, 289
Infectious senescence, 56
Infliximab, 190
INK4a, 35
Insects, 13, 57
Insulin, 10, 11, 70, 74, 102, 138, 208, 209, 210,
    212, 216–217, 220, 221, 223, 233,
    270, 284
Insulin-like receptor, 10
Insulin-like growth factor 136, 152, 185, 211,
    215, 229, 242, 257, 259, 279
Insulin signaling, 10

Insulin receptor, 10
Insulin degrading enzyme (IDE), 233
Insulinoma, 103
Integrins, 177, 180, 236, 269, 279
Intercellular adhesion molecules, 171, 177. *See* ICAM
Interdigitations, 142, 144, 156
Interferon, 33, 84, 154
Interleukin (IL), 112, 146, 178, 195, 198, 200, 201
Intestinal angina, 165
Intimal cells, 170, 175, 178
Intracellular defenses, 53, 76
Intrinsic aging, 53, 76
Intrinsic factor, 167, 264
Introns, 58, 79, 285
Iodine, 210
Ionic fountains, 52
Iris, 271, 272, 274, 275, 277
Ischemia, 69, 163, 165, 167, 223, 231, 235, 238, 239, 252, 253, 265, 268, 274, 275, 276, 280, 288
Ischemic bowel, 265, 268
Islet of Langerhans, 73, 210
Isoflavones, 79, 115, 187
Isomerase, 113, 132, 137
Isospora, 123
Ito cells, 262

Jejunum, 263
Junk cells, 56

Kaposi's sarcoma, 83
Keratin, 141, 142
Keratinocyte growth factor, 141, 145
Keratinocytes, 32, 33, 46, 48, 71, 82, 120, 141–146, 149–156, 15–160, 274, 278
Klinefelter's syndrome, 129
Kluyveromyces lactis, 19
Knockouts, 31, 34, 35, 37, 47, 52, 61, 63, 205, 268, 269, 287
KRAB, 214, 287
K-ras mutation, 102
Krause end bulbs, 143
Ku, 21
Kwashiorkor, 264

L5, 73
L7, 73
La, 21
Lactate, 136, 235, 252, 261
Lactic acid, 136, 235, 252, 261. *See also* Lactate
Lamin-A, 139

Langerhans cells, 73, 142, 144, 154, 210
Large vessel disease, 163, 165
Laser, 281
Lead (Pb), 114, 115, 238
Leflunomide, 190
Leiomyoma, 93
Leishmania, 124
Lens, 135, 271, 272, 274,-279, 281
Leprosy, 241
Leukemia, 81, 84–85, 109, 113, 176, 202–204
Leukocyte, 24, 25, 40, 73, 83–86, 102, 104, 109, 139, 150, 171–173, 192–195, 197–199, 202–204, 206
Leydig cells, 215, 216, 219
LH (luteinizing hormone), 209, 219
LHRH (luteinizing hormone releasing hormone), 209
Li-Fraumeni syndrome, 76, 114, 115
Lifespan determination, 10–11
Limited model, 45–56
Linear chromosomes, 14, 16, 17, 22, 23, 58, 122, 123
Linkage, 36, 46, 49, 50, 52–53, 59–61, 75, 139, 183, 235
Lipids, 9, 69, 71, 74, 126, 166–170, 174, 215, 225
Lipid membrane, 9, 42, 44–45, 67, 229
Lipid membrane turnover, 9, 44, 45
Lipid oxidation, 9, 68, 236
Lipid peroxidation, 45, 57, 69, 169, 231, 232, 234, 243, 264
Lipid turnover, 45, 152
Lipofuscin, 126, 136, 164, 215, 225, 233, 278, 280
Lipoma, 62
Liposarcoma, 107
Liposomes, 176, 285
Liver cancer, 100–102. *See also* Hepatic cancer
Liver disease, 81, 128, 264–265, 267, 269, 270
Loa, 123
Longevity, 12, 21, 6, 67, 69
Longevity genes, 6
Loop diuretics, 248
Low density lipoprotein, 168
Lumbar puncture, 104
Lung cancer, 76, 85–87, 106, 109
Lupus, 284. *See also* Systemic lupus erythematosus
Luteinizing hormone, 209, 219. *See* LH
Lymph nodes, 89, 91, 95, 104, 108
Lymphoblastoid cells, 138
Lymphocytes, 13, 25, 30, 35, 38, 54, 59, 82, 101, 110, 117–119, 131, 137, 138, 155, 166, 180, 186, 192, 194, 196–199, 201, 203–207, 237, 284, 285
Lymphokines, 54, 119, 199, 211
Lymphoproliferative cancer, 149
Lysosomes, 68, 274

M1 (mortality stage 1), 26, 49
M2 (mortality stage 2), 26
Macrophage, 116, 144, 166–167, 180–181, 195, 232, 265
Macrophage colony stimulating factor (M-CSF), 113, 193
Macula, 272–276
Macular degeneration, 272–276, 278–282
Mad1, 32, 112
Magic bullet, 76, 80, 119
Magnesium, 245
Maillard reactions, 276
Malaria, 123–124, 126, 190
Malignancy, 14, 30, 32, 34–35, 53, 61–63, 75–121, 130, 135, 140, 142, 149, 150, 178, 194–195, 200, 204, 207, 213, 215, 222, 264–265, 269, 281, 284
Malignant transformation, 26, 35, 53, 77, 78, 85, 90, 104, 106, 107, 110, 120, 142, 144, 171, 176, 177, 201, 202, 207, 220, 270, 281
Mammary gland. See Breast
Marrow transplantation, 121, 195, 202–203, 207, 284
Matrix, 49, 55, 59, 6, 64, 110, 16, 142, 145–149, 154–155, 159, 162, 166, 179–183, 185, 186, 246, 257, 262, 269, 275, 280
Maximum lifespan, 5–6, 12, 70, 14, 289–290
MCF7 breast cancer cells, 116
M-CSF. See Macrophage colony stimulating factor
MDS, 84. See Myelodysplastic syndrome
Mean lifespan, 5, 6, 63, 70
Mec1p, 21
Medulloblastoma, 104
MEFs (mouse embryonic fibroblasts), 34
Meiotic spindle, 20
Meissner's corpuscles, 143
Melanin, 142, 143, 158
Melanocytes, 82, 141–142, 144, 154, 155, 158, 231
Melanocytic nevi, 82
Melanoma, 35, 82–83, 113, 118, 124
Melatonin, 7, 70, 210, 211, 212, 215, 221, 241
Memory, 64, 222, 225, 239–242
Memory cells, 184, 194, 196, 198, 200, 201
Meningioma, 105, 106
Meningitis, 194
Menopause, 88, 95, 96, 173, 182, 187, 212, 215–219, 222, 239, 259, 273
Mental retardation, 51
Mercaptopurine, 116
Merkel's cells, 143
Merkel's tumor, 82
Mesangial cells, 247
Mesenchyma, 141

Mesenteric adenopathy, 268
Mesothelioma, 33
Mesothelium, 24
Metabolic rate, 10, 11, 14, 48, 63, 136, 208
Metabolic regulators, 10
Metageria, 129, 130
Metalloproteinases, 137, 155, 159
Metastases, 81, 82, 95, 100, 104, 108, 110
Metastatic melanoma, 82
Methotrexate, 190
Methylation, 26, 32, 33, 57, 60, 138
Metrifonate, 241
MeWo cells, 116
Microarrays, 156, 270
Microbes, 24, 158, 289
Microglia, 45, 63, 64, 170, 204, 225, 227, 232–239, 241–244
Microinfarct dementia, 227, 228, 235
Microtubules, 20
Microvessel disease, 172
Mineralization, 179
Mismatch. See Functional mismatch
Mismatch repair, 111, 120, 138
Mitochondria, 6, 13, 14, 42, 57, 58, 67–69, 126, 229, 253, 254
Mitochondrial ATP, 58, 68
Mitochondrial damage, 11, 13, 42, 55, 58, 59, 67–69, 136, 145, 163, 165, 233, 234, 243, 255
Mitochondrial degradation, 67–69
Mitochondrial energy expenditure, 11, 14
Mitochondrial genes, 14, 58, 67–69, 195, 234, 255
Mitochondrial membranes, 42, 45, 55, 67–68
Mitochondrial proliferation, 17, 67–69
Mitochondrial protein synthesis, 58, 67
Mitochondrial ROS, 42, 54, 58, 66, 75
Mitochondrial tagging, 67–68
Mitochondrial turnover, 58, 67–69
Mitochondrial volume, 58, 67, 216, 262
Mitogens, 26, 28, 72, 79, 137, 145, 154, 200, 206
Mitosis, 25, 49
Mitotic spindles, 20
Molecular turnover, 44–45
Monoclonal antibodies, 117, 121, 152
Monoclonal gammopathy of undetermined significance (MGUS), 85
Monocytes, 83, 166, 170–172, 177, 180, 186, 192, 199, 227, 232, 235
Morbidity, 58, 63, 88, 106, 122, 140, 163, 165, 174, 182, 183, 194, 196, 210, 213, 221, 227, 237, 242, 255, 258, 259
MORF-4 (Mortality factor 4), 25, 234
Mortalin, 25, 116
Mortality, 7–10, 12, 25, 26, 61–63, 88, 90, 92, 98, 103, 106, 123, 126, 140, 157, 161, 163, 165, 172, 174, 175, 182, 191,

194, 214, 221, 227, 242, 253, 255,
    258, 259, 283, 289
Mortality factor 4 (MORF-4), 25, 234
Mortality stages (M1, M2), 26, 49
Morula, 53
Mosaic disease, 130, 138, 139, 153
Motor neuron, 224, 226, 252
Mouse, 7, 22, 30–31, 34, 40, 47, 60, 61, 63, 66,
    70, 73, 131, 155, 159, 256, 278. *See*
    Mus musculus and spretus
M phase, 115
MRE11, 19
MRX complex, 19
mSin3, 33
mtDNA, 58, 59, 67, 69, 234. *See* Mitochondria
mTERT, 19, , 30, 34, 35, 40, 79, 205, 235, 256
Multiple myeloma, 85, 118
Multiple sclerosis, 233, 237
Mus musculus, 22, 47, 63. *See also* Mouse
Mus spretus, 22, 47, 63. *See also* Mouse
Muscle, 4, 45, 68, 143, 158, 161, 162, 165–166,
    168–172, 176, 178, 179, 182, 183,
    208, 210, 221, 224, 229, 248, 252–
    260, 261, 263, 265, 266, 271, 272,
    275, 276, 284, 288
Muscle aging, 253–260
Muscle cell senescence, 256–258
Muscle interventions, 258–260
Muscular dystrophy, 257, 260, 281
Myb, 20
Myc/Max, 286
Myelocytes, 192, 198
Myelodysplastic syndrome (MDS), 78, 84, 85, 202
Myeloperoxidase, 167
Myoblasts, 175, 256–257, 260
Myocardial infarction, 4, 57, 61–64, 74, 127,
    131, 140, 161–168, 172, 178, 258
Myocyte, 25, 38, 46, 48, 56, 61, 63–64, 68–69,
    139, 163–164, 172, 174, 175–176,
    178, 252, 254–259, 284
Myofibrils, 253
Myosin, 253–255, 258
Myotonic dystrophy, 129
Myxedema, 210, 227
MZF-2 (myeloid-specific zinc finger protein 2),
    112, 287
MZ-5-156, 33, 113

NADH, 69, 264
Naegleria, 123
Nagana, 123
Naive T cells, 184, 186, 194, 197, 198, 205
Naproxen, 241
Nasopharyngeal carcinomas, 108, 114, 116
Natural killer (NK) cells, 194

Necrosis, 74, 135, 166, 222, 230, 264, 265, 268
Needle biopsy, 89, 102
Nematode, 8, 123. *See Caenorhabditis elegans*
Neovascularization, 274, 280
Nephrin, 246
Nephrons, 246, 249
Nephrotic syndrome, 249
Neprilysin, 237
Nerve growth factor (NGF), 211, 239
Neural precursor cells, 226, 234
Neural tube, 61, 139
Neuroblastoma, 80, 105–106, 108–109
Neurodegeneration, 230, 234
Neurofibrillary tangle (NFT), 126, 230–232,
    237, 241
Neuromuscular innervation, 252, 255, 258
Neurons, 25, 38, 45, 46, 48, 56, 63, 64, 69, 104,
    139, 141, 208, 210, 214, 219, 224–
    244, 252, 255, 258, 272, 274, 277,
    278, 288
Neurotoxins, 236
NF-kappa B, 73, 236
NFT (neurofibrillary tangle), 126, 230–232,
    237, 241
Nijmegen breakage syndrome (NMS), 21, 44
Nitric oxide (NO), 169–170, 176, 236, 237,
    242
Nitric oxide synthase, 170, 176–177
NGF (nerve growth factor), 211, 239
NK cells (natural killer cells), 194
NO (nitric oxide), 169–170, 176, 236, 237, 242
Nondividing cells, 63, 256, 287
Norepinephrine, 209, 216
Non-Hodgkin's lymphoma, 110
Nonmetastatic cutaneous squamous cell
    carcinoma, 82
Non-small cell lung cancer, 86, 109
NSAIDs (nonsteroidal antiinflammatory drugs),
    189, 242
Nuclear clumps, 16
Nuclear envelope, 139
Nuclear membrane, 52, 118, 286
Nuclear ring structures, 81
Nucleolus, 13, 14, 131
Nucleotides, 18, 29
Nucleus, 16, 30, 52, 58, 59, 67, 69, 75, 78, 79,
    95, 115, 118, 139, 218, 286
Nutrients, 6, 8, 183, 192, 252, 263, 271
Nutrition, 141, 182, 206, 214, 215, 227, 228,
    230, 248, 255, 264, 266

Obesity, 7, 102, 166, 183, 221, 273
OctBP, 73
Ocular stromal keratinocytes, 38, 277
Oligodendrocytes, 64, 225–227, 284

Oligodendrogliomas (oligodendroglial tumors), 78, 104–106
Oligonucleotides, 27, 113, 114–115, 175–176
Oligonucleotide antisense, 114–115, 167, 175
Oligonucleotide length, 115
Oligonucleotide normal sense, 115
Oocyte, 53, 218–219
Oncogene, 32, 33, 48, 76, 78–80, 90, 93–95, 108, 110, 111, 113, 137, 239, 287
Oncogene activation, 48, 80
Oncotherapeutic agents, 62, 114, 115, 118
Oncotherapy, 102, 112, 120, 213
Oocytes, 53, 218, 219
Opacification, 281
OPG (osteoprotegerin), 180
Optic nerve, 272, 275
Opticin, 139
Optimal diet, 9, 158
Oral tumors, 108
Orchestra, 49, 53, 55, 180, 218
Organismal aging, 13, 56–59, 122, 264
Organogenesis, 35
Organotypic human skin equivalent, 156
Orthopedic system, 175–190
Orthopedic system aging, 181–187
Orthopedic system interventions, 187–190
Osteoarthritis, 128, 179, 181, 183, 185–186, 189–190, 233
Osteoblasts, 43, 179–181, 183–185, 187–190, 233, 247, 285
Osteoblastic tumors, 107
Osteocalcin, 184, 185
Osteoclastogenesis, 180
Osteoclasts, 139, 179–181, 183–184, 187–188, 223, 247
Osteolysis, 135
Osteopenia, 135, 182, 185–187, 222
Osteoporosis, 130, 135, 158, 179–185, 187–190, 213, 216, 217, 222, 254, 255, 258, 285
Osteoprotegerin (OPG), 180
Osteosarcoma, 118
Ova, 24, 209, 218
Ovarian cancer, 91, 96–97, 103, 114, 115, 119
Ovarian failure, 218–219
Ovary, 92, 211, 212, 218, 219
Overhang, 18–19, 132
Oxidative damage, 9, 11, 12, 19, 21, 36, 40, 48, 54, 62, 67, 68, 255, 274, 276, 281
Oxidative phosphorylation, 136
Oxidative tagging, 69
Oxygen, 8, 12, 42, 58, 66, 69, 161, 164, 165, 171, 183, 189, 191, 192, 231, 241, 242, 252, 253, 255, 267, 275, 279
Oxygen consumption, 12, 255, 264

p1, 73
p14, 72
p15, 153
p16, 26, 28, 40, 76, 153, 154, 159, 160, 287
p19, 76
p21, 25, 28, 53, 76, 116, 153, 154, 199, 287
p23, 30
p27, 40, 154
p53, 18, 20, 25, 26, 32, 33, 53, 76–77, 85, 86, 94, 96, 103, 110, 113, 120, 153, 267, 277, 287
p73, 76
p80, 21
p95, 21
p107, 72
Pacific salmon, 59
Pacinian corpuscles, 143
Paget's disease, 187
Pancreatic cancer, 102–103, 109, 210
Pancreatic islet cells, 220, 285
Pancreatitis, 102–103
Papanicolaou smear, 87, 92–94
Papillary carcinoma, 108
Paracrine hormones, 74, 269
Paragonimus westermani, 123
Parapsoriasis, 83
Parasitic disease, 122–124
Parathyroid gland, 210, 220
Parathyroid hormone, 179, 182, 185, 187, 209
Parathyroid tumors, 108
Parenchyma, 86, 246, 262
Parkinson's disease, 32, 76, 79, 80, 117, 120, 153, 224, 227–229, 238, 243
PARP (poly [ADP-ribose] polymerase), 21, 76
Pathological fractures, 181
PCR, 80 89, 91, 93, 98, 104, 106, 114
PDGF (platelet-derived growth factor), 137
Pedicularis striata 116
Penclomedine, 113
Penguins, 34
Penicillamine, 190
Peptide nucleic acids (PNAs), 114–115
Perhydroxyl formation, 68
Periarticular osteopenia, 185–186
Peripheral vascular disease, 135, 162–166, 224
Peritelomeric region, 51, 132, 133
Peritoneal fluid, 96, 97, 102
Perivascular microglia, 227, 236
Pernicious anemia, 264
PET scan (positron emission tomography), 229
Petrels, 34
Perylene diimides, 117
Phagocytosis, 67, 68, 194, 225, 236, 262, 272, 275
Pharmacokinetics, 118
Pheochromocytoma, 69, 243

Platelet-derived growth factor (PDGF), 137
Philadelphia (Ph) chromosome, 203
Philadelphia (Ph) translocation, 84
Phospholipids, 164
Phosphorothioate oligomers, 115
Phosphorothioate oligonucleotide (PTO), 114
Phosphorylation, 33, 95, 136, 137, 154, 194
Photoaging, 7, 145, 147, 157–158, 278
Photon interference, 276
Physical activity, 11, 102, 183, 248. *See also* Exercise
Physostigmine, 241
Pick's disease, 227
PIH (prolactin inhibiting hormone), 209
Pin2, 20. *See also* TRF1
Pineal gland, 210
Pinworms, 123
PinX1, 20
Pituitary, 59, 208–210, 212, 214, 216, 218, 219
Placenta, 53, 210
Plants, 4, 17, 19, 20, 21, 61
Plaque, 71, 149, 166, 170, 171, 230, 232, 233, 237, 241
Plasma cell dyscrasia, 85, 118
Plasmids, 31, 176, 286
Plasminogen activator, 63, 146
Plasmodium falciparum, 49
Platelets, 171, 174, 191, 192
Platinum, 114, 115
Platyhelminthes, 122
Pleuripotent cells, 196, 200
Ploidy, 105, 120
PNAs, 114–115. *See* Peptide nucleic acids
Pneumocystis, 123
Pneumonia, 123, 128, 194, 204
Podocytes, 246–247, 249, 251
Poison ivy dermatitis, 83
Pol, 286. *See also* Polymerase
Poliomyelitis (polio), 284
Polyclonal cancers, 75
Polycomb-group proteins, 2
Polycythemia vera, 85
Polyenylphosphatidylcholine, 270
Polymerase, 21, 29, 138, 286
Polyps, 103–104, 222
Polyvalent antigens, 118
Population doublings (Pds), 27, 38–39, 41–42, 46–47, 60, 113, 119, 132, 137, 156–157, 188, 197, 200, 279, 285
Porphyrins, 116, 117, 119
Portal veins, 262
Post-mitotic cells, 67–69, 197
Postponing aging, 9, 70, 131
Post-replicative cells, 64
Post-reproductive, 77
Post-transcriptional mechanisms, 30, 98

Post-translational modifications, 276
Pot1, 20
Potassium, 132, 245
Precursor cells, 54, 82, 117, 118, 180, 188, 192, 226, 232, 234, 285
Pregnenolone, 210
PRELP, 139
Presbyopia, 274–276, 280
Presenilins, 230–231
PRH (prolactin releasing hormone), 209
Primary melanoma, 82
Primate, 8, 9, 14, 4, 47, 51, 182, 204, 227, 230, 279
Primate telomeres, 14, 34, 47, 51
Procollagen, 185, 188
Procreative energy, 16
Progeria, 7, 12, 129–139, 167
Progeric atherosclerosis, 130, 134–135, 138, 167
Progeroid syndromes, 129, 132, 136
Progesterone, 88, 95, 188, 210, 259
Progestin, 174
Prolactin (PRL), 209
Promoter, 31–33, 72, 79, 95, 112–113, 116–118, 121, 132, 146, 213, 220, 251, 286–287
Promyelocytic leukemia, 81
Prophase, 52
Prostacyclin, 169
Prostaglandins, 242, 280
Prostanoids, 169
Prostate cancer (or tumors), 76, 90–92, 98, 109, 114, 118, 119, 213
Prostate specific antigen (PSA), 90, 91
Protease, 137, 171, 237, 244, 269
Proteins, 12, 141, 142, 167, 171, 177, 181, 185, 209, 220. *See specific proteins*
    apolipoprotein, 166, 229, 239
    cell cycle, 21, 25, 33, 41, 72, 73, 233
    CNS, 230–234, 236–237, 239, 242–244
    context, 57
    defective, 69, 146, 186
    degradation, 44–45, 146–147, 155, 156, 163
    DNA damage, 53, 69, 76
    equilibrium, 44
    fidelity, 43, 137
    filtration, 246, 249–250
    heat shock (HSPs), 12, 198
    histone, 46, 51, 58
    intake, 262, 264
    loss, 140
    mitochondrial, 58, 67
    muscle, 253–255, 258
    ocular, 271, 275–276, 280–281
    oxidation, 9
    pools, 44–45, 145–146, 148
    progeric, 132, 136, 137

Proteins (*continued*)
    receptors, 269
    repair, 18
    senescent, 27, 54, 73, 94, 132, 145, 154
    silencing, 50–51, 131
    structure 17
    synthesis, 12, 42–45, 58, 70, 73, 118, 137,
        145, 186, 219, 221, 254, 286
    telomere, 17, 19–21, 23, 26, 28–33, 43, 51–
        52, 58, 80–81, 84, 95–98, 102, 104,
        117, 287
    tumor markers, 101, 107, 117
    turnover, 9, 44–45, 57, 69, 145–146, 148,
        155, 186, 254, 261
    zinc finger, 112, 287
Proteinuria, 249, 250
Proteolysis, 30, 31, 73, 79, 155, 200
Proteosomes, 45, 231, 237
Protooncogenes, 32, 137
Proton pumps, 68
PSA (prostate-specific antigen), 90, 91
Psoralen, 26
Psoriasis, 149
PTO (phosphorothioate oligonucleotide), 114
Ptolemy, 47
Puberty, 72
Puerperal fever, 126
Pulmonary cancer, 76, 85–87, 106, 109. *See
        also* Lung cancer
Purpuromycin, 116
Pyridoxine, 175

QM, 72
Quadruplex compounds, 117, 119
Quadruplex telomeric DNA, 117, 131
Quantal processes, 39, 147

Racemization, 276
Rad50p, 19, 80
Rad52p, 80
Radiation
Radiation damage, 43, 149, 203, 267
Radiation resistance, 22, 76
Radiation therapy, 108, 116, 119, 121, 263
Radiosensitivity, 44
Raf, 40
Raloxifene, 187
RANKL (receptor for activating nuclear factor
        Kappa B ligand), 180
Rap (repressor/activator protein), 51, 52
Ras, 40
Rat, 64, 73, 78, 91, 164, 172, 216, 219, 226,
        250, 256, 257
Rate of aging, 6, 8, 196, 290

Rb (retinoblastoma), 26, 33, 73, 77, 85, 94, 287
Reactive oxygen species (ROS), 8, 42, 54, 58,
        66, 157, 171, 231, 267, 275
Reactive senescence, 56, 62, 157, 164, 278
Receptor for activating nuclear factor Kappa B
        ligand (RANKL), 180
Recombination, 6, 11, 49, 51, 111, 112
Reconstitution
    hematopoetic system, 197, 202
    immune, 121, 202, 207
    muscle tissue, 259
    skin, 156, 158, 159, 283, 284
    telomerase activity, 30
    tissue, 288
recQ, 131
Regeneration, 178
    bone, 189
    cells, 30
    hepatic, 31, 81, 264, 268, 269
    intestinal, 267
    muscle, 255, 256, 257, 259
    neural, 226
Regulators
    cell division, 46, 141, 152, 156, 175, 180,
        209, 263
    DNA repair, 53, 76, 138
    endocrine, 59, 209, 217, 218, 219
    energy production, 70
    growth, 46, 72, 73, 88, 109
    metabolic, 10
    peritelomeric genes, 51
    stem cell, 25
    telomerase activity, 30, 31, 54, 82, 91, 93–95,
        98, 112–113, 116, 172, 200–205, 286–
        287
    telomerase expression, 26, 29, 30–33, 51, 73,
        79, 85, 93–96, 98, 112–113, 118, 131,
        133, 172, 197, 198, 200–205, 256,
        286–287
    telomere length, 26, 34, 50, 52, 84, 288
    transcriptional, 10, 25
Regulatory obstacles, 124, 206, 288–289
Rejection, 203, 269, 270, 282
Remodeling, 20, 40, 137, 147, 155, 180, 183,
        236, 268, 285
Renal and urinary tract cancers, 97–99
Renal cell carcinoma, 32, 98–99, 112, 118
Renal cortical cells, 250
Renal failure, 245, 249, 250, 262
Renal osteodystrophy, 248
Renal transplantation, 250
Renin, 209, 245, 248
Replication factors, 21, 55
Replicative limit, 24–25, 27, 77, 139, 270, 281,
        286, 287
Replicometers, 48

Reporter genes, 49
Repressor, 31, 32, 33, 51, 72, 79, 94
Reproduction, 5, 12, 77, 88, 188, 209, 210, 218, 239
Rescue, 25, 41, 53, 55, 160, 203, 285, 288
Resetting aging, 7, 60–61, 68
Resetting gene expression, 36, 37, 49, 59–61, 68,
    128, 131, 139, 156, 157, 177, 218, 284
Resetting linkage, 60–61, 139
Resetting mitochondria, 68
Resetting senescence, 41, 70, 131, 155, 156,
    177, 207, 218
Resetting telomere length, 13, 55, 155, 199,
    284, 285
Restenosis, 167, 171, 175, 176
Rete pegs, 158
Rete ridges, 154
Reticulocyte count, 202
Retina, 107, 271, 272–282
Retinal cells, 121, 272–282
Retinal detachment
Retinal disease, 210, 224, 273–282
Retinal pigmented epithelial cells (RPEs), 27, 42,
    73, 120, 153, 177, 272, 274, 278–281
Retinitis pigmentosa, 273
Retinoblastoma protein (Rb), 26, 33, 73, 77, 85,
    94, 287
Retinoic acid, 113, 151, 158, 283
Retinol, 158, 182, 272, 280
Retroelements, 28
Retrograde response, 67
Retroposons, 28
Retrotransposition, 111
Retrotransposons, 28
Retrovirus, 31, 115, 131, 156, 157, 159, 177,
    204, 270, 286
Retroviral transformation, 157, 270
Retroviral vectors, 159
Reverse transcriptase, 23, 28, 29
Reverse transcriptase inhibitors, 116
Rhesus macaques (Rhesus monkeys), 9, 11, 243
Rheumatoid arthritis, 180–181, 183–186, 189–
    190, 284
Ribozyme, 113, 119
Rif, 52
Ring chromosomes, 58, 106, 122, 151
Risedronate, 187
Rivastigmine, 241
River blindness, 124
RNA polymerase, 29, 286
RNA template, 23, 28, 114
Robertsonian translocations, 150
Rods, 272, 273, 278
Rofecoxib, 24, 242
Rolling circle mechanism, 80
Rothmund's syndrome, 129
Roundworms, 123

Rubromycin, 116
Ruffini endings, 143
Rust, 59

s3, 73
s6, 73
s10, 73
S phase, 22
Saccharomyces cerevisiae, 6, 8, 11, 19, 21, 49,
    50, 116
Saccharomyces pombe, 20
Salmon, 59
Sarcoma, 78, 83, 107
Sarcopenia, 128, 130, 217, 224, 248, 253–260,
    265, 266, 275, 276
Satellite cells, 64, 68, 79, 172, 256–259, 233
Saturated fats, 135
Schistosoma mansoni, 123
Schistosoma haematobium, 98, 123
Schistosoma japonicum, 12
Schwannoma, 107
Sclera, 271–272
Scleroderma, 149, 284
Sclerosis, 9, 149, 233, 237, 276
Sebaceous glands, 141
Seborrhoeic warts, 83
Sebum, 223
Secondary follicles, 110
Secondary pathology, 77, 168, 258, 264, 277
Secondary vascular aging, 235
Secretase, 244
Segmental progeria, 12, 130, 135, 138
Seip's syndrome, 129
Selective breeding, 8–9, 11, 70
Selectins, 236
Selegiline, 241
Selenium, 115
Seminal vesicle, 91
Sendai virus, 176, 285
SENs, 152–153
Senescence
    accelerated, 8, 13, 56, 121, 132–133, 138–
        139, 144, 154, 169, 186, 202–204,
        237–238, 265, 268, 270, 278
    definition, 25, 26, 38–45, 47, 49, 53
sepsis, 62, 140, 194
Septic arthritis, 194
SERMs (selective estrogen receptor
        modulators), 187, 188
Serotonin, 212, 224
Sertoli cells, 215, 219
Serum lipids, 9
Severe combined immune deficiency (SCID),
        177, 220
Sexual steroids, 188, 210, 215, 216, 217

SGS1 helicase, 79, 131
Shear stress, 142, 144, 163, 165, 168, 169, 177
Shwachman-Diamond syndrome, 195
Signal transduction, 110, 194, 200, 269
Silencing, 7, 11, 49–52, 75, 79, 112, 131, 139, 287
Simian immune virus, 204, 232
Sinclair swine cutaneous melanoma, 82
Single strand breaks, 19, 48
Sinusoids, 262
Sir (silent information regulatory) proteins, 11, 51, 52, 131, 283
Sister chromatid, 22, 131
Skin, 140–160
Skin aging, 143–160
Skin cancer, 82–83, 150
Skin reconstitution, 156
SLE (systemic lupus erythematosus), 284
Sleeping sickness, 123, 124
Slime molds, 18
Slit diaphragm, 246
Smooth muscle, 162, 166, 168–171, 176, 178, 229, 259, 266
Sodium butyrate, 112
Solid tumors, 75, 78, 79, 83, 90, 109, 204
Soluble factors, 45
Somatic cells, 6, 7 24–27, 29–31, 33–37, 38, 42, 45, 47, 53–55, 60, 64, 66–67, 70, 73, 81, 119, 122, 150, 178, 196–197, 199, 269, 284, 289
Somatostatin, 11, 209, 212
Sp1, 31, 79, 286
spe-26, 10
Sperm, 24, 61, 139, 209, 215, 219
Spermatogenesis, 61, 19
Spinal stenosis, 165
Spleen, 192
Splenic atrophy, 205
Splice variants, 22, 79, 106
Spontaneous immortality, 34, 114, 115
Squamous cells, 82, 141, 145
Squamous cell carcinomas, 76, 79, 82, 87, 107
Starvation, 8, 9, 44
Statins, 11, 175, 187, 241
Staurosporine, 115
Stellate cells, 262, 265, 269–270
Stem cells, 24–26, 30, 45, 54, 64, 73, 81, 119, 187
  bone, 187
  embryonic, 24, 176, 284
  gastrointestinal, 54, 81, 263, 267–268
  hair follicle, 54, 81, 151
  hematopoetic, 24, 54, 81, 83, 121, 192, 195–197, 199–200, 202, 205–207
    erythrocyte, 68
    leukocyte, 24, 25, 83, 84, 119, 139, 150, 284
  hepatic, 54, 81
  muscle, 64, 256
  myocardial, 64, 172, 176
  neural, 64, 226, 234, 243, 284–285
  ocular, 278, 281
  skin, 30, 54, 81, 145, 151, 154
  therapeutic, 284–285
  transit cells, 25
Stem mitochondria, 65
Stenosis, 62
Steroids, 7, 91, 132, 146, 188, 190, 209, 210, 212, 215, 216, 217, 219, 234, 242, 243, 252, 275. *See also specific hormones*
Stochastic process, 26, 39, 67, 107, 147, 230
Storm petrels, 34
Stratified columnar cells, 141
Strawman arguments, 62
Stress, 7, 71, 144, 165, 167, 173, 202, 248, 266
  hypothermic, 140
  immune, 197, 248, 263, 265
  oxidative, 12, 64, 156, 164, 168, 206, 259, 274, 275
  physiologic, 128, 180, 202, 234, 242, 248, 249, 255, 267
  shear, 142, 144, 156, 162, 163, 165, 168–170, 177
Stroke, 57, 164, 173, 223, 228
Stroma, 38, 89, 95, 97, 99, 180, 188, 219, 277, 278, 282
Stromolysin, 155
Subendothelial cells, 59, 63, 74, 166, 168, 170, 171
Substantia nigra, 224, 238
Subtelomere, 30, 49, 50, 51, 80, 82, 124
"Successful" aging, 284
Sudoriparous glands, 141
Sulfasalazine, 190
Sun screens, 158
Superoxide, 58, 63, 66, 69, 133, 169, 216
Superoxide dismutase (SOD), 58, 63, 66, 133
Supertwisted DNA, 13
Suprachiasmatic nucleus, 218
Surgical menopause, 239
Survival curves, 5
SV40, 26, 27, 33, 99, 138, 188, 220, 282, 285
Swallows, 34
Sympathetic system, 147, 209
Synapses, 225, 226, 231, 232, 233, 236, 239
Syncytial cells, 253, 257
Synergistic activators, 286
Synovial antigens, 184
Synuclein, 238
Syrian hamsters, 34
Systemic lupus erythematosus (SLE), 284
Systolic pressure, 162, 169, 252

T cell receptor (TCR), 184, 199
T cell receptor rearrangement excision circles (TREC), 186

Tabula rasa, 60
Tacrine, 240, 241
Tamarin, 34
Taenia, 123
Tamoxifen, 91, 95, 113
Tandem repeats, 29, 58
Tangles, 126, 230, 231, 232, 237, 241
Tankyrase, 21, 79
T antigen, 26, 33, 99, 118, 142, 188, 220, 282, 285
Tapetum, 272
Tapeworms, 123
TATA, 31, 132, 286
Tau protein, 230
Taz1p, 20
TCR (T cell receptor), 199
Teeth, 135
Tel1, 21
Telogen, 151
Telomerase. *See also* telomere terminal
        transferase, hTERT, and hTR
    activity, 21, 29–35, 40, 53–54, 61, 78–119,
        124, 150, 154, 158–159, 172, 186,
        197, 199–202, 204–205, 219, 227,
        234, 256, 268–270, 277–279, 287, 290
    baseline activity, 34, 83, 99
    catalytic component, 22–23, 28–31
    components, 19, 23, 28–31
    dimeric, 23, 28
    expression, 20, 25, 32, 34–36, 54, 62, 77–
        121, 131, 133, 149, 151, 159, 160,
        171–172, 178, 188, 198–206, 250,
        267, 268, 279
    holoenzyme, 30, 78
    induction, 31, 112, 116, 120, 159, 178, 200–
        201, 260, 282, 285, 290
    inhibition, 30, 32, 4, 80, 95, 111–121, 122–
        124, 169
    knockout, 31, 34–5, 37, 47, 52, 61, 63, 205,
        268, 269, 287
    non-template regions, 28–29
    null, 19, 34–35
    promoter, 31–33, 72, 79, 95, 112–113, 116–
        118, 121, 220, 251, 286–287
    proteolysis, 30–31, 73, 79, 155, 200
    repression, 29, 31–34, 40, 52, 72–73, 79, 81,
        94, 112–113, 200–201, 286–287
    template, 19, 23, 28–29, 114–115
    transduction, 110, 287
    transfection, 27, 29, 31, 37, 41, 114, 117,
        119–120, 138, 155, 159, 177–178,
        188, 189, 206–207, 219–220, 223,
        243, 257, 260, 270, 281, 282, 285
    transcription, 22, 29–33, 52, 54, 72–73, 94,
        112, 116, 118, 200, 286–287
Telomeres
    absolute length, 35–36, 49, 52
    associated DNA, 19, 50
    associated proteins, 19, 29, 30, 51, 81, 95,
        102, 117
    attrition, 121, 124, 170, 172
    binding proteins, 19, 20, 52, 58, 81
    buffer, 35
    capping, 17, 18, 21, 30, 40, 119
    complex, 17, 19, 50
    critical length (short), 84, 111
    deletion, 17, 40
    d-loop, 18–20
    DNA, 17, 28, 39, 52, 81, 88, 90, 117
    Drosophila, 11, 13, 22, 28
    duplex, 18–20, 51
    erosion, 23, 46–49, 54, 66, 118, 151, 169,
        186, 197, 199, 201, 204, 269
    G-quartet, 19, 21, 117
    heterochromatin, 22, 49–52, 57
    hypervariable, 47
    lagging strand, 22
    leading strand, 22
    -like sequences, 10
    linear chromosomes, 14
    loss, 17–20, 23, 36, 40, 41, 47–49, 54, 56,
        60–61, 64–65, 78, 82, 85, 116, 121,
        132, 172, 195–198, 200–203, 205,
        219–220, 257, 267, 269
    maintenance, 13, 17, 20–23, 29, 35, 43–44,
        47, 53, 60, 69, 77, 80, 84, 88, 108,
        110–116, 121, 124, 131, 133, 139,
        149–150, 159, 200–201, 203–204,
        268, 288
    mean length, 39, 63, 83, 198, 204, 269, 279
    non-canonical mechanisms, 13
    overhang, 18–19, 40, 132
    position effect, 49–50
    relative length, 5–36, 47, 48, 60
    resetting, 13
    since fertilization, 36
    proteins, 17, 19–21, 23, 26, 28–33, 43, 51–
        52, 58, 80–81, 84, 95–98, 102, 104,
        117, 287
    repair, 18, 30, 48
    restriction fragments (TRFs), 90, 99, 202,
        204, 279
    structure, 13, 16, 17–19, 21–22, 28, 34, 115,
        117, 131
    tether, 17
    t-loop, 18–19, 26
Telomeric bouquets, 52
Telomeric heterochromatin, 22, 44, 46, 49–52,
        57, 80
Telomeric probes, 51
Telomeric repeat amplification protocol
        (TRAP), 81, 82, 84, 87, 89, 91, 97–98,
        103, 106, 114, 117

Telomerization, 37, 41, 53, 69, 71, 128, 188, 243, 259, 281, 282, 284, 285
TeloRZ, 113. *See* Hammerhead ribozyme
Temperature, 12, 143, 214, 255
TEPs (telomere associated proteins), 28, 30, 77, 86, 95, 100, 102, 113, 115
Terminal differentiation, 31, 73, 141, 199, 277
Testes, 68, 150, 210, 212, 215, 219
Testicular cancer, 90–91
Testosterone, 91, 136, 160, 182, 209, 211, 212, 215, 217, 221, 252, 259
Tetanus, 126–128, 174–175
Tetrahymena, 14, 17, 21, 28, 58
TFIID, 73
TGF (transforming growth factor), 137, 146, 152, 185, 236, 242
Thalassemia, 202
Thapsigargin, 115
6–thioguanine, 116
Thorny-headed worms, 123
Thrombocytes, 191
Thrombosis, 161, 167, 170, 174, 175, 228, 276
Thymidine kinase, 118, 137
Thymocytes, 198
Thymoma, 118
Thyroid neoplasia (thyroid tumors), 108
Thyroid stimulating hormone (TSH), 209, 210
Thyroxine (T4), 210
Time bombs, 48
TIN2, 21
Tissue-type plasminogen activator (t-PA), 146
Tithynos, 4–5
TMPyP4, 116, 119
TNF (tumor necrosis factor), 145, 146, 170, 177, 186, 190, 195, 206, 236, 265
Tobacco, 14, 71, 102, 127, 135, 157, 166–169, 174, 230, 273
Tocopherols, 58, 158, 167, 243
Topoisomerase, 113, 185
Toxins, 7, 71, 118, 151, 158, 168, 169, 230, 236–239, 245, 263, 265
Toxoplasma, 123
tPA (tissue-type plasminogen activator), 146
Trabeculae, 181, 184
Transcription
    fidelity, 43, 137
    forkhead family, 10
    regulation, 10, 25, 29–33, 52, 54, 69, 72–73, 91, 94, 112, 116, 118, 200, 286–287
    silencing, 7, 11, 49–52, 75, 79, 112, 131, 139, 287
    switching, 31, 287
Transfection, 27, 29, 31, 37, 41, 114, 117, 119–120, 138, 155, 159, 177–178, 188, 189, 206–207, 219–220, 223, 243, 257, 260, 270, 281, 282, 285

Transforming growth factor (TGF), 137, 146, 152, 185, 236, 242
Transgenics, 29, 78, 118, 198, 244
Transit cells, 25
Translocation, 4, 51, 79, 84, 95, 137, 150
Transplantation, 100, 121, 127, 174, 175, 178, 189, 195, 202–203, 207, 220, 223, 250, 270, 282, 284, 485
TRAP telomeric repeat amplification protocol), 81, 82, 84, 87, 89, 91, 97–98, 103, 106, 114, 117
Trauma, 7, 62, 71, 128, 142, 151, 157, 158, 160, 183, 186, 226, 232, 238, 253, 275
TREC (T cell receptor rearrangement excision circles), 186
Trematodes, 122–123
Tretinoin, 158
TRFs (telomere restriction fragments), 90, 99, 202, 204, 279
TRH (thyroid releasing hormone), 209
Trichinella, 123
Trichomonas vaginalis, 123
Triiodothyronine (T), 210
Trisomy 21 (Down's syndrome), 12, 13, 129, 203, 231, 237
Trophic factors, 64, 74, 154, 170, 173, 208, 211, 236, 242, 243, 247, 280
Trophoblasts, 53
Tropoelastin, 136, 137
Trypanosomes, 18, 123, 124
Trypsin, 17
TSH (thyroid stimulating hormone), 209, 210
Tuberculosis, 86, 194
Tubules, 99, 215, 245–246, 249, 251
Tumor necrosis factor (TNF), 145, 146, 170, 177, 186, 190, 195, 206, 236, 265
Tumor suppressor, 33, 35, 75, 79, 80, 94, 160, 287
Turner's syndrome, 129
Turnover
    cell, 71–74, 78, 83, 128, 144, 154, 197, 202–203, 268–269, 277
    equations, 44
    lipid, 45, 152
    membranes, 9, 44, 45
    mitochondria, 9, 44–45, 57, 69, 145–146, 148, 155, 186, 254, 261
    protein, 9, 44–45, 57, 69, 145–146, 148, 155, 186, 254, 261
Tyrosine kinase, 10, 171

U937 cells, 113, 116
Ubiquination, 45
Ubiquitin, 238

Ulcers, 140, 149, 158, 267, 285
Ultraviolet (UV), 7, 43, 48, 58, 61–63, 137, 142, 144, 146, 151, 154, 157, 158, 159, 278, 279, 281
Univalent antigens, 118
Unscheduled DNA synthesis, 137
Urea, 245, 246
Urinary hyaluronic acid, 136
Urokinase-type plasminogen activator (u-PA), 146
Urothelial, 97
Uterus, 92, 259
Uvea, 82, 272, 274

v-Myc-estrogen receptor protein, 1, 287
Vaccine, 118, 194, 244
Vascular dementia, 228, 231, 235
Vascular endothelial growth factor (VEGF), 247
Vascular insufficiency, 136, 147, 151, 235
Vascular regulation, 143, 147
Vasculitic stroke, 228
Vasculopathy, 276
Vasoactive intestinal polypeptide secreting cells, 218
Veins, 133, 135, 161, 170, 174, 175, 213, 245, 258, 261, 262, 275, 278
Venous stasis, 285
Ventricle, 161, 162, 228
Verbascoside, 116
Verteporfin, 281
Viral hepatitis, 81, 100, 101, 264, 265
Vitagenes, 36
Vitamin D, 184, 185, 187. *See* Calcitriol
Vitamins, 154, 158, 175, 184, 210, 245, 248, 272, 274
Vivax malaria, 123
Von Hippel-Lindau suppressor gene, 98

WAF1, 25, 76, 287
Waldenstrom's macroglobulinemia, 118
Warts, 83
Watchmaker's masterpiece, 48
Water clefts, 276
Wear-and-tear, 46, 53, 55, 59, 67, 160, 183, 290
Weight lifting, 255
Werner syndrome, 12, 13, 53, 79, 129–133, 136, 138, 260, 278
Wernicke-Korsakoff syndrome, 227, 264
Whales, 276
Whipworms, 123
Wiedemann-Rautenstrauch syndrome, 129
Wilms' tumor, 3
WHO (World Health Organization), 105
Wound healing 9, 14, 35, 61, 130, 133, 135, 140, 142, 147, 154, 157, 158, 159, 180, 226, 278, 281
Wrinkles, 142, 157–158
WRN, 131–132
WT1, 33
Wuchereria, 123

Xrs2p, 19

Yeast. *See Saccharomyces cerevisiae or other species*
    budding, 20
    fission, 20

ZFQR, 287
Zinc, 274
Zinc fingers, 112, 287
Zygote, 60, 61, 231